Medical Epigenetics

Medical Epigenetics

Edited by Augustus Drew

AMERICAN
MEDICAL PUBLISHERS
www.americanmedicalpublishers.com

American Medical Publishers,
41 Flatbush Avenue,
1st Floor, New York,
NY 11217, USA

Visit us on the World Wide Web at:
www.americanmedicalpublishers.com

ISBN: 978-1-63927-255-6

Cataloging-in-Publication Data

Medical epigenetics / edited by Augustus Drew.
p. cm.
Includes bibliographical references and index.
ISBN 978-1-63927-255-6
1. Epigenetics. 2. Medical genetics. 3. Genetics. I. Drew, Augustus.
RB155 .M43 2022
616.042--dc23

Table of Contents

Preface

Epigenetics is the study that deals with the heritable phenotype changes which do not involve changes in DNA sequence. Epigenetics usually shows changes that affect the activity of gene and expression but are also used to describe any heritable phenotypic change. Epigenetics in medicine consists of the use of drugs and epigenome influencing techniques in order to treat medical conditions. Epigenetic mechanisms have three categories - DNA methylation, histone modifications and regulatory RNA. It influences many diseases like cancer, diabetes, mental illness and heart diseases. In such situation, medical epigenetics helps in influencing these pathways. This book brings forth some of the most innovative concepts and elucidates the unexplored aspects of epigenetics. The various advancements in epigenetics in medicine are glanced at and their applications as well as ramifications are looked at in detail. This book, with its detailed analyses and data, will prove immensely beneficial to professionals and students involved in this area at various levels.

All of the data presented henceforth, was collaborated in the wake of recent advancements in the field. The aim of this book is to present the diversified developments from across the globe in a comprehensible manner. The opinions expressed in each chapter belong solely to the contributing authors. Their interpretations of the topics are the integral part of this book, which I have carefully compiled for a better understanding of the readers.

At the end, I would like to thank all those who dedicated their time and efforts for the successful completion of this book. I also wish to convey my gratitude towards my friends and family who supported me at every step.

Editor

1

Regional differences in mitochondrial DNA methylation in human post-mortem brain tissue

Matthew Devall[1], Rebecca G. Smith[1], Aaron Jeffries[1,2], Eilis Hannon[1], Matthew N. Davies[3], Leonard Schalkwyk[4], Jonathan Mill[1,2], Michael Weedon[1] and Katie Lunnon[1*]

Abstract

Background: DNA methylation is an important epigenetic mechanism involved in gene regulation, with alterations in DNA methylation in the nuclear genome being linked to numerous complex diseases. Mitochondrial DNA methylation is a phenomenon that is receiving ever-increasing interest, particularly in diseases characterized by mitochondrial dysfunction; however, most studies have been limited to the investigation of specific target regions. Analyses spanning the entire mitochondrial genome have been limited, potentially due to the amount of input DNA required. Further, mitochondrial genetic studies have been previously confounded by nuclear-mitochondrial pseudogenes. Methylated DNA Immunoprecipitation Sequencing is a technique widely used to profile DNA methylation across the nuclear genome; however, reads mapped to mitochondrial DNA are often discarded. Here, we have developed an approach to control for nuclear-mitochondrial pseudogenes within Methylated DNA Immunoprecipitation Sequencing data. We highlight the utility of this approach in identifying differences in mitochondrial DNA methylation across regions of the human brain and pre-mortem blood.

Results: We were able to correlate mitochondrial DNA methylation patterns between the cortex, cerebellum and blood. We identified 74 nominally significant differentially methylated regions ($p < 0.05$) in the mitochondrial genome, between anatomically separate cortical regions and the cerebellum in matched samples ($N = 3$ matched donors). Further analysis identified eight significant differentially methylated regions between the total cortex and cerebellum after correcting for multiple testing. Using unsupervised hierarchical clustering analysis of the mitochondrial DNA methylome, we were able to identify tissue-specific patterns of mitochondrial DNA methylation between blood, cerebellum and cortex.

Conclusions: Our study represents a comprehensive analysis of the mitochondrial methylome using pre-existing Methylated DNA Immunoprecipitation Sequencing data to identify brain region-specific patterns of mitochondrial DNA methylation.

Keywords: 5-mC, 5-Methylcytosine, Blood, Brain, DNA methylation, Epigenetics, MeDIP-seq, Mitochondria, *NUMTs*

Introduction

Mitochondria are unique organelles in that they have their own circular genome, approximately 16.6 kb in size [1]. Mitochondrial DNA (mtDNA) consists of 37 genes, 22 encoding for transfer RNAs (tRNAs), two for ribosomal RNAs (rRNAs) and 13 encoding for proteins important in the electron transport chain. Each of these 13 proteins are directly involved in the regulation of cellular respiration, generating the majority of ATP required for the process. However, mitochondria have an array of other important cellular roles such as calcium homeostasis [2] and neural stem cell differentiation [3]. As such, abnormal mitochondrial function, dynamics and trafficking have been associated with a number of brain disorders including Alzheimer's disease [4, 5], schizophrenia [6], bipolar disorder [7] and major depressive disorder [8].

* Correspondence: k.lunnon@exeter.ac.uk
[1]University of Exeter Medical School, RILD, University of Exeter, Barrack Road, Devon, UK
Full list of author information is available at the end of the article

Epigenetic processes mediate the reversible regulation of gene expression, occurring independently of DNA sequence variation, acting principally through chemical modifications to DNA and nucleosomal histone proteins and orchestrate a diverse range of important physiological functions. DNA methylation is the best characterized and most stable epigenetic modification modulating the transcription of mammalian genomes and, because it can be robustly assessed using existing genomic DNA resources, is the focus of most human epidemiological epigenetic research to date [9]. The most widely used method for epigenome-wide analysis of DNA methylation is the Illumina 450K methylation array, and a number of studies have recently shown differential DNA methylation of the nuclear genome (ncDNA), between different tissue types [10–12] and also in a range of complex diseases, from brain disorders such as Alzheimer's disease [13–15] and schizophrenia [16, 17], to systemic diseases such as type 2 diabetes [18] and Crohn's disease [19]. However, with no representation of the mitochondrial genome on this platform, as well as a lack of analysis on other genome-wide platforms, the role of mtDNA methylation has been largely neglected [20, 21].

Since the identification of 5-methylcytosine (5-mC) in mitochondria, research into mtDNA methylation as an independent and potentially relevant mark has received more regular attention [22, 23]. However, most research is either focussed on low resolution, global DNA methylation, or candidate gene DNA methylation changes using techniques such as bisulfite pyrosequencing [20]. These recent publications have indicated that differences in mtDNA methylation are present in a variety of different phenotypes [24–29] and may have potential utility as a biomarker [30]. In addition, a recent study has explored the use of Methylated DNA Immunoprecipitation Sequencing (MeDIP-seq) to investigate changes in mtDNA methylation across 39 cell lines and tissues from publicly available data [31]. At present, genome-wide sequencing technologies have not yet been used to interrogate alterations in the mtDNA methylome across tissues in the same individuals.

A high proportion of current, publicly available, genome-wide DNA methylation data has been generated through the use of MeDIP-seq, a method designed to interrogate genome-wide changes in methylation at high throughput and low cost [32]. However, given the presence of nuclear-mitochondrial pseudogenes (*NUMTs*), regions of the nuclear genome that share a high sequence homology with their mitochondrial paralogue [33, 34], mitochondrial reads are often discarded from further analysis. The development of bioinformatic pipelines to investigate regions of differential mtDNA methylation from whole genome data would provide a novel way in which to interrogate the mtDNA methylome in publicly available data. Here, we control for the presence of *NUMTs* in a previously published MeDIP-seq dataset, to investigate differential DNA methylation across the mitochondrial genome in human post-mortem brain samples.

Results

MtDNA methylation patterns are correlated between the cortex, cerebellum and blood

To date, no study has investigated differences in mtDNA methylation across different matched regions of human brain and blood samples. Our sample (Table 1) consisted of MeDIP-seq data from three individuals, free of any neuropathology and neuropsychiatric disease, for five different regions of the cortex (Brodmann areas (BA) 8, 9 and 10, superior temporal gyrus (STG) and entorhinal cortex (ECX)), the cerebellum (CER) and pre-mortem blood [35]. Given that MeDIP-seq data has been generated from standardly extracted total genomic DNA and thus contains a mixture of ncDNA and mtDNA [36], we initially controlled for regions of high sequence homology between the two genomes within our data by realigning mtDNA reads to a series of custom reference genomes using an in-house pipeline (see the Methods section) to specifically analyze mtDNA methylation (Fig. 1). Briefly, after an initial alignment to the GRCH37 reference genome using BWA, uniquely mapped reads were extracted and aligned to a custom GRCH37 reference genome not containing the mitochondrial sequence. Reads that did not map to this custom genome were found to share less homology with the nuclear genome and were taken forward and realigned once more to the full reference genome. Initially, we were interested to investigate whether changes in mtDNA across the mitochondrial genome were highly correlated between different tissue types. Using principal component analysis (PCA), we found that mtDNA methylation patterns are highly correlated between different cortical regions ($r > 0.99$, $p < 2.2E-16$), with a slightly weaker correlation between the cerebellum and cortex ($r > 0.97$, $p < 2.2E-16$) (Fig. 2). Due to the small number of blood samples available, deriving a significance level for the correlations between the cerebellum and blood could not be made.

Table 1 Demographic information

Individual	Age at death (years)	Age at bloods sampled (years)	Post-mortem delay (hours)	Gender
1	82	79	43	Female
2	92	N/A	17	Female
3	78	78	10	Male

MeDIP-seq data was available from post-mortem brain samples obtained from three individuals free of any neuropathology and neuropsychiatric disease. Data was available for five different regions of the cortex (Brodmann areas (BA) 8, 9 and 10, superior temporal gyrus (STG), entorhinal cortex (ECX), the cerebellum (CER) and pre-mortem blood (BLD). MeDIP-seq data was available for all individuals from cortical and cerebellar samples; however, blood MeDIP-seq data was not available for individual 2. Data is freely available to download from http://epigenetics.iop.kcl.ac.uk/brain

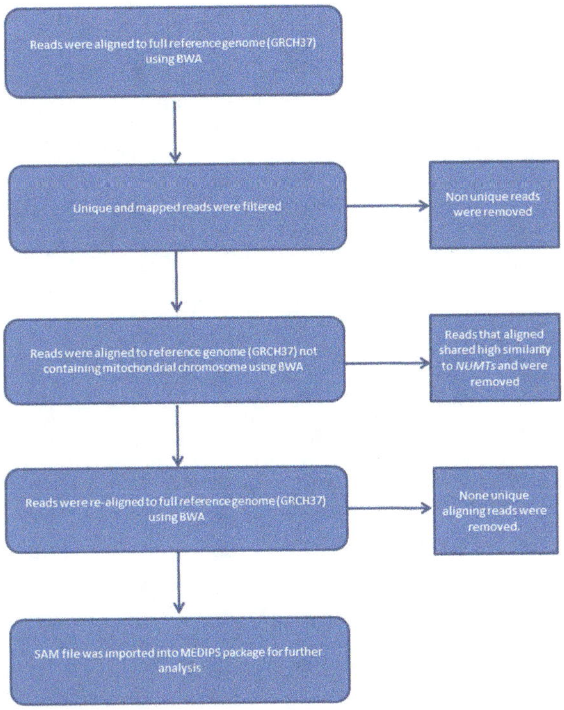

Fig. 1 Overview of the analysis pipeline

Instead, in an attempt to explore the similarity between matched blood and cerebellum samples, the direction of differential methylation with respect to the cortex was used. Here, we found that 93.1% of the windows analyzed in the cerebellum and blood had the same direction of methylation difference with respect to the cortex, further suggesting a strong correlation between the two tissue types.

Differentially methylated regions of the mitochondrial genome can be identified between anatomically distinct cortical regions and the cerebellum

Having identified correlated mtDNA methylation patterns across different brain regions, we were interested to investigate whether we could identify differentially methylated regions (DMRs) in the mitochondrial genome between different regions of the cortex and cerebellum. To identify such tissue-specific DMRs within the mitochondrial genome, paired t tests were performed across matched cortical and cerebellum samples at 100 bp windows across the mitochondrial genome (see the Methods section). In total, we identified 74 nominally significant DMRs ($p < 0.05$) between the five individual cortical regions and the cerebellum (Table 2; Fig. 3). Of these DMRs, seven (Table 2, bold face) were found to be present across all prefrontal cortex areas (BA8, BA9, BA10). Furthermore, the direction of methylation

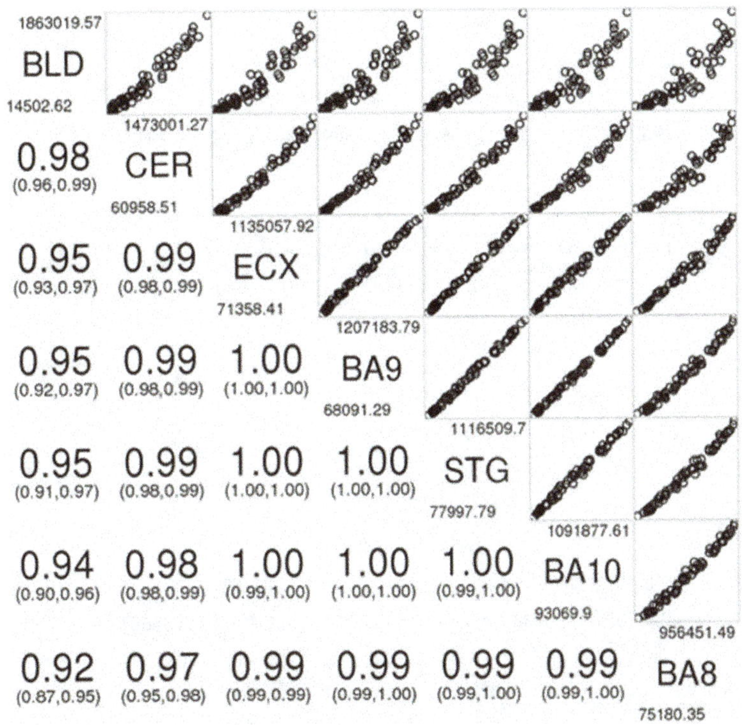

Fig. 2 MtDNA methylation patterns are correlated between the cortex, cerebellum and blood. Samples were ordered based upon the similarity of their principal components, RPKM values, with r calculated for the correlations between each tissue. *BLD* blood, *BA8* Brodmann area 8, *BA9* Brodmann area 9, *BA10* Brodmann area 10, *CER* cerebellum, *CTX* cortex, *ECX* entorhinal cortex, *STG* superior temporal gyrus

Table 2 List of DMRs identified between five anatomically discreet cortical regions and cerebellum

Start (bp)	Stop (bp)	Gene(s)	BA8		BA9		BA10		EC		STG	
			p value	Δ RPKM	*p* value	Δ RPKM	*p* value	Δ RPKM	*p* value	Δ RPKM	*p* value	Δ RPKM
1	100	D-Loop	-	-	-	-	-	-	-	-	-	-
101	200	D-Loop	-	-	-	-	-	-	-	-	-	-
201	300	D-Loop	-	-	-	-	-	-	-	-	-	-
301	400	D-Loop	-	-	-	-	-	-	-	-	-	-
401	500	D-Loop	-	-	-	-	-	-	-	-	-	-
501	600	MT-TF	-	-	-	-	-	-	-	-	-	-
601	700	MT-TF/MT-RNR1	-	-	-	-	-	-	-	-	-	-
701	800	MT-RNR1	-	-	-	-	-	-	3.21E−02	79156	-	-
801	900	MT-RNR1	4.31E−02	94246	2.93E−02	−43592	-	-	-	-	1.79E−02	95257
901	1000	MT-RNR1	ND	ND	ND	ND	ND	ND	ND	ND	ND	ND
1001	1100	MT-RNR1	ND	ND	ND	ND	ND	ND	ND	ND	ND	ND
1101	1200	MT-RNR1	ND	ND	ND	ND	ND	ND	ND	ND	ND	ND
1201	1300	MT-RNR1	ND	ND	ND	ND	ND	ND	ND	ND	ND	ND
1301	1400	MT-RNR1	ND	ND	ND	ND	ND	ND	ND	ND	ND	ND
1401	1500	MT-RNR1	ND	ND	ND	ND	ND	ND	ND	ND	ND	ND
1501	1600	MT-RNR1	ND	ND	ND	ND	ND	ND	ND	ND	ND	ND
1601	1700	MT-RNR1/MT-TV/MT-RNR2	ND	ND	ND	ND	ND	ND	ND	ND	ND	ND
1701	1800	MT-RNR2	ND	ND	ND	ND	ND	ND	ND	ND	ND	ND
1801	1900	MT-RNR2	ND	ND	ND	ND	ND	ND	ND	ND	ND	ND
1901	2000	MT-RNR2	ND	ND	ND	ND	ND	ND	ND	ND	ND	ND
2001	2100	MT-RNR2	ND	ND	ND	ND	ND	ND	ND	ND	ND	ND
2101	2200	MT-RNR2	ND	ND	ND	ND	ND	ND	ND	ND	ND	ND
2201	2300	MT-RNR2	ND	ND	ND	ND	ND	ND	ND	ND	ND	ND
2301	**2400**	**MT-RNR2**	**2.54E−02**	**−97351**	**3.20E−02**	**−29509**	**4.31E−02**	**−82048**	-	-	-	-
2401	2500	MT-RNR2	8.90E−03	70950	-	-	-	-	-	-	-	-
2501	2600	MT-RNR2	3.30E−03	51937	-	-	-	-	-	-	-	-
2601	2700	MT-RNR2	ND	ND	ND	ND	ND	ND	ND	ND	ND	ND
2701	2800	MT-RNR2	ND	ND	ND	ND	ND	ND	ND	ND	ND	ND
2801	2900	MT-RNR2	-	-	-	-	-	-	-	-	-	-
2901	3000	MT-RNR2	-	-	-	-	-	-	-	-	-	-
3001	3100	MT-RNR2	-	-	-	-	-	-	-	-	-	-
3101	3200	MT-RNR2	ND	ND	ND	ND	ND	ND	ND	ND	ND	ND
3201	3300	MT-RNR2/MT-TL	-	-	-	-	-	-	2.09E−02	242424	-	-
3301	3400	MT-TL1/MT-ND1	-	-	-	-	-	-	-	-	-	-
3401	3500	MT-ND1	-	-	1.54E−02	864685	-	-	-	-	-	-
3501	3600	MT-ND1	4.41E−02	1180914	-	-	1.72E−02	226066	-	-	-	-
3601	**3700**	**MT-ND1**	**4.73E−02**	**1250436**	**4.52E−02**	**1228936**	**3.73E−02**	**1183681**	-	-	-	-
3701	3800	MT-ND1	-	-	-	-	2.16E−02	20818	-	-	-	-
3801	3900	MT-ND1	-	-	-	-	-	-	-	-	-	-
3901	4000	MT-ND1	-	-	-	-	-	-	-	-	-	-
4001	4100	MT-ND1	2.41E−02	−39498	1.55E−02	−38704	-	-	4.68E−02	−49753	1.56E−02	243767
4101	4200	MT-ND1	ND	ND	ND	ND	ND	ND	ND	ND	ND	ND

Table 2 List of DMRs identified between five anatomically discreet cortical regions and cerebellum *(Continued)*

4201	4300	MT-ND1/MT-TI	ND	ND	ND	ND	ND	ND	ND	ND	ND	ND
4301	4400	MT-TI/MT-TQ	ND	ND	ND	ND	ND	ND	ND	ND	ND	ND
4401	4500	MT-TM/MT-ND2	ND	ND	ND	ND	ND	ND	ND	ND	ND	ND
4501	4600	MT-ND2	ND	ND	ND	ND	ND	ND	ND	ND	ND	ND
4601	4700	MT-ND2	ND	ND	ND	ND	ND	ND	ND	ND	ND	ND
4701	4800	MT-ND2	ND	ND	ND	ND	ND	ND	ND	ND	ND	ND
4801	4900	MT-ND2	ND	ND	ND	ND	ND	ND	ND	ND	ND	ND
4901	5000	MT-ND2	ND	ND	ND	ND	ND	ND	ND	ND	ND	ND
5001	5100	MT-ND2	ND	ND	ND	ND	ND	ND	ND	ND	ND	ND
5101	5200	MT-ND2	ND	ND	ND	ND	ND	ND	ND	ND	ND	ND
5201	5300	MT-ND2	ND	ND	ND	ND	ND	ND	ND	ND	ND	ND
5301	5400	MT-ND2	ND	ND	ND	ND	ND	ND	ND	ND	ND	ND
5401	5500	MT-ND2	ND	ND	ND	ND	ND	ND	ND	ND	ND	ND
5501	5600	MT-ND2/MT-TW/MT-TA	ND	ND	ND	ND	ND	ND	ND	ND	ND	ND
5601	5700	MT-TA/MT-TN	ND	ND	ND	ND	ND	ND	ND	ND	ND	ND
5701	5800	MT-TN/MT-TC	ND	ND	ND	ND	ND	ND	ND	ND	ND	ND
5801	5900	MT-TC/MT-TY	ND	ND	ND	ND	ND	ND	ND	ND	ND	ND
5901	6000	MT-CO1	ND	ND	ND	ND	ND	ND	ND	ND	ND	ND
6001	6100	MT-CO1	ND	ND	ND	ND	ND	ND	ND	ND	ND	ND
6101	6200	MT-CO1	ND	ND	ND	ND	ND	ND	ND	ND	ND	ND
6201	6300	MT-CO1	ND	ND	ND	ND	ND	ND	ND	ND	ND	ND
6301	6400	MT-CO1	ND	ND	ND	ND	ND	ND	ND	ND	ND	ND
6401	6500	MT-CO1	ND	ND	ND	ND	ND	ND	ND	ND	ND	ND
6501	6600	MT-CO1	ND	ND	ND	ND	ND	ND	ND	ND	ND	ND
6601	6700	MT-CO1	ND	ND	ND	ND	ND	ND	ND	ND	ND	ND
6701	6800	MT-CO1	ND	ND	ND	ND	ND	ND	ND	ND	ND	ND
6801	6900	MT-CO1	ND	ND	ND	ND	ND	ND	ND	ND	ND	ND
6901	7000	MT-CO1	ND	ND	ND	ND	ND	ND	ND	ND	ND	ND
7001	7100	MT-CO1	ND	ND	ND	ND	ND	ND	ND	ND	ND	ND
7101	7200	MT-CO1	ND	ND	ND	ND	ND	ND	ND	ND	ND	ND
7201	7300	MT-CO1	ND	ND	ND	ND	ND	ND	ND	ND	ND	ND
7301	7400	MT-CO1	ND	ND	ND	ND	ND	ND	ND	ND	ND	ND
7401	7500	MT-CO1/MT-TS1	ND	ND	ND	ND	ND	ND	ND	ND	ND	ND
7501	7600	MT-TS1/MT-TD/MT-CO2	ND	ND	ND	ND	ND	ND	ND	ND	ND	ND
7601	7700	MT-CO2	ND	ND	ND	ND	ND	ND	ND	ND	ND	ND
7701	7800	MT-CO2	ND	ND	ND	ND	ND	ND	ND	ND	ND	ND
7801	7900	MT-CO2	ND	ND	ND	ND	ND	ND	ND	ND	ND	ND
7901	8000	MT-CO2	ND	ND	ND	ND	ND	ND	ND	ND	ND	ND
8001	8100	MT-CO2	ND	ND	ND	ND	ND	ND	ND	ND	ND	ND
8101	8200	MT-CO2	ND	ND	ND	ND	ND	ND	ND	ND	ND	ND
8201	8300	MT-CO2/MT-TK	ND	ND	ND	ND	ND	ND	ND	ND	ND	ND
8301	8400	MT-TK/MT-ATP8	ND	ND	ND	ND	ND	ND	ND	ND	ND	ND
8401	8500	MT-ATP8	ND	ND	ND	ND	ND	ND	ND	ND	ND	ND

Table 2 List of DMRs identified between five anatomically discreet cortical regions and cerebellum *(Continued)*

8501	8600	MT-ATP8/MT-ATP6	ND	ND	ND	ND	ND	ND	ND	ND	ND	ND
8601	8700	MT-ATP6	ND	ND	ND	ND	ND	ND	ND	ND	ND	ND
8701	8800	MT-ATP6	ND	ND	ND	ND	ND	ND	ND	ND	ND	ND
8801	8900	MT-ATP6	ND	ND	ND	ND	ND	ND	ND	ND	ND	ND
8901	9000	MT-ATP6	ND	ND	ND	ND	ND	ND	ND	ND	ND	ND
9001	9100	MT-ATP6	ND	ND	ND	ND	ND	ND	ND	ND	ND	ND
9101	9200	MT-ATP6	ND	ND	ND	ND	ND	ND	ND	ND	ND	ND
9201	9300	MT-ATP6/MT-CO3	ND	ND	ND	ND	ND	ND	ND	ND	ND	ND
9301	9400	MT-CO3	ND	ND	ND	ND	ND	ND	ND	ND	ND	ND
9401	9500	MT-CO3	ND	ND	ND	ND	ND	ND	ND	ND	ND	ND
9501	9600	MT-CO3	ND	ND	ND	ND	ND	ND	ND	ND	ND	ND
9601	9700	MT-CO3	ND	ND	ND	ND	ND	ND	ND	ND	ND	ND
9701	9800	MT-CO3	ND	ND	ND	ND	ND	ND	ND	ND	ND	ND
9801	9900	MT-CO3	-	-	-	-	-	-	-	-	-	-
9901	10000	MT-CO3/MT-TG	-	-	-	-	-	-	-	-	-	-
10001	10100	MT-TG/MT-ND3	-	-	-	-	-	-	-	-	-	-
10101	10200	MT-ND3	-	-	-	-	-	-	-	-	-	-
10201	10300	MT-ND3	4.68E−02	−662126	-	-	-	-	3.14E−02	−591067	7.30E−03	−57012
10301	**10400**	**MT-ND3/MT-TR/MT-ND4L**	**3.61E−02**	**−132719**	**3.61E−02**	**−135759**	**4.02E−02**	**−115364**	1.40E−02	−73063	3.36E−02	−105106
10401	10500	MT-ND4L	-	-	4.68E−02	−71246	-	-	-	-	-	-
10501	10600	MT-ND4L	-	-	-	-	-	-	-	-	-	-
10601	10700	MT-ND4L	ND	ND	ND	ND	ND	ND	ND	ND	ND	ND
10701	10800	MT-ND4L/MT-ND4	ND	ND	ND	ND	ND	ND	ND	ND	ND	ND
10801	10900	MT-ND4	ND	ND	ND	ND	ND	ND	ND	ND	ND	ND
10901	11000	MT-ND4	ND	ND	ND	ND	ND	ND	ND	ND	ND	ND
11001	11100	MT-ND4	ND	ND	ND	ND	ND	ND	ND	ND	ND	ND
11101	11200	MT-ND4	ND	ND	ND	ND	ND	ND	ND	ND	ND	ND
11201	11300	MT-ND4	-	-	1.94E−02	−68903	1.84E−02	−79625	4.71E−02	58742	-	-
11301	11400	MT-ND4	-	-	4.78E−02	−139847	-	-	-	-	-	-
11401	11500	MT-ND4	ND	ND	ND	ND	ND	ND	ND	ND	ND	ND
11501	11600	MT-ND4	ND	ND	ND	ND	ND	ND	ND	ND	ND	ND
11601	11700	MT-ND4	ND	ND	ND	ND	ND	ND	ND	ND	ND	ND
11701	11800	MT-ND4	ND	ND	ND	ND	ND	ND	ND	ND	ND	ND
11801	11900	MT-ND4	ND	ND	ND	ND	ND	ND	ND	ND	ND	ND
11901	12000	MT-ND4	ND	ND	ND	ND	ND	ND	ND	ND	ND	ND
12001	12100	MT-ND4	ND	ND	ND	ND	ND	ND	ND	ND	ND	ND
12101	12200	MT-ND4/MT-TH	ND	ND	ND	ND	ND	ND	ND	ND	ND	ND
12201	12300	MT-TS2/MT-TL2	ND	ND	ND	ND	ND	ND	ND	ND	ND	ND
12301	12400	MT-TL2/MT-ND5	4.71E−02	1787	-	−197592	-	-	-	-	-	-
12401	12500	MT-ND5	-	-	-	-	-	-	-	-	-	-
12501	12600	MT-ND5	-	-	-	-	-	-	-	-	-	-
12601	12700	MT-ND5	-	-	-	-	-	-	-	-	-	-
12701	12800	MT-ND5	2.05E−02	−5702	-	-	4.58E−02	−388706	-	-	4.36E−02	−394978
12801	12900	MT-ND5	2.26E−02	−89668	-	-	-	-	-	-	-	-

Table 2 List of DMRs identified between five anatomically discreet cortical regions and cerebellum *(Continued)*

12901	13000	MT-ND5	-	-	3.10E−02	−130016	-	-	-	-	-	-
13001	13100	MT-ND5	ND	ND	ND	ND	ND	ND	ND	ND	ND	ND
13101	13200	MT-ND5	ND	ND	ND	ND	ND	ND	ND	ND	ND	ND
13201	13300	MT-ND5	ND	ND	ND	ND	ND	ND	ND	ND	ND	ND
13301	13400	MT-ND5	1.48E−02	−175917	-	-	9.80E−03	−144949	3.40E−02	−133604		
13401	13500	MT-ND5	3.64E−02	−104010	-	-	3.40E−02	−81264	-	-	-	-
13501	13600	MT-ND5	-	-	-	-	-	-	-	-	-	-
13601	13700	MT-ND5	-	-	-	-	-	-	-	-	-	-
13701	13800	MT-ND5	1.31E−02	−422610	-	-	1.20E−03	3714	-	-	-	-
13801	13900	MT-ND5	-	-	3.72E−02	708761	2.59E−02	123249	-	-	-	-
13901	14000	MT-ND5	-	-	-	-	2.17E−02	−75118	-	-	-	-
14001	14100	MT-ND5	-	-	-	-	-	-	-	-	-	-
14101	14200	MT-ND5/MT-ND6	-	-	-	-	-	-	-	-	4.18E−02	−534766
14201	14300	MT-ND6	-	-	-	-	-	-	-	-	-	-
14301	14400	MT-ND6	-	-	-	-	-	-	-	-	-	-
14401	14500	MT-ND6	-	-	-	-	-	-	-	-	-	-
14501	14600	MT-ND6	-	-	-	-	-	-	-	-	4.86E−02	−82767
14601	14700	MT-ND6/MT-TE	-	-	-	-	-	-	-	-	-	-
14701	14800	MT-TE/MT-CYB	-	-	-	-	-	-	-	-	-	-
14801	14900	MT-CYB	ND	ND	ND	ND	ND	ND	ND	ND	ND	ND
14901	15000	MT-CYB	ND	ND	ND	ND	ND	ND	ND	ND	ND	ND
15001	15100	MT-CYB	ND	ND	ND	ND	ND	ND	ND	ND	ND	ND
15101	15200	MT-CYB	-	-	-	-	-	-	-	-	-	-
15201	15300	MT-CYB	-	-	-	-	-	-	1.20E−02	254183	-	-
15301	15400	MT-CYB	-	-	-	-	-	-	-	-	-	-
15401	15500	MT-CYB	4.38E−02	10628	-	-	2.10E−02	−554527	-	-	3.28E−02	−554225
15501	15600	MT-CYB	3.73E−02	−671707	-	-	1.23E−02	−685630	3.82E−02	9301	3.51E−02	−695515
15601	15700	MT-CYB	-	-	-	-	4.33E−02	−746270	-	-	-	-
15701	15800	MT-CYB	-	-	-	-	-	-	-	-	-	-
15801	15900	MT-CYB/MT-TT	-	-	-	-	-	-	-	-	-	-
15901	16000	MT-TT/MT-TP	-	-	-	-	-	-	-	-	-	-
16001	16100	MT-TP	-	-	-	-	-	-	-	-	-	-
16101	16200	D-Loop	-	-	3.40E−03	3014	-	-	-	-	-	-
16201	**16300**	**D-Loop**	**4.64E−02**	**380407**	**2.50E−02**	**1117943**	**3.68E−02**	**296890**	-	-	-	-
16301	**16400**	**D-Loop**	**3.65E−02**	**−941720**	**1.38E−02**	**−112453**	**2.73E−02**	**−177146**	-	-	-	-
16401	**16500**	**D-Loop**	**4.29E−02**	**444051**	**2.20E−02**	**1151402**	**1.68E−02**	**313156**	-	-	-	-
16501	**16600**	**D-Loop**	**3.71E−02**	**784572**	**2.10E−02**	**764994**	**2.46E−02**	**836662**	-	-	-	-

Shown is the location of the DMR within the mitochondrial genome (ChrM) (based on GENCODE), the gene(s) residing within the 100 bp window, and p value from paired t tests between each of the five cortical regions: Brodmann areas 8, 9 and 10 (BA8, BA9, BA10), entorhinal cortex (ECX) and superior temporal gyrus (STG) compared to the cerebellum (CER). Results are displayed in order of genomic position. RPKM and corresponding p values are shown for windows if $p < 0.05$. Key: - denotes data not significant ($p > 0.05$); ND denotes not determined as the window was not included in analysis due to removal in *NUMT* pipeline. Results shown in bold represent those found to be present across all prefrontal cortex areas (BA8, BA9, BA10)

difference was maintained in all Brodmann area regions, with three conserved regions of hypomethylation and four conserved regions of hypermethylation, with respect to the cerebellum. Furthermore, four of the seven conserved regions were adjacent to each other within the mitochondrial displacement loop (D-Loop) (16201–16600 bp), a region associated with gene transcription and DNA replication.

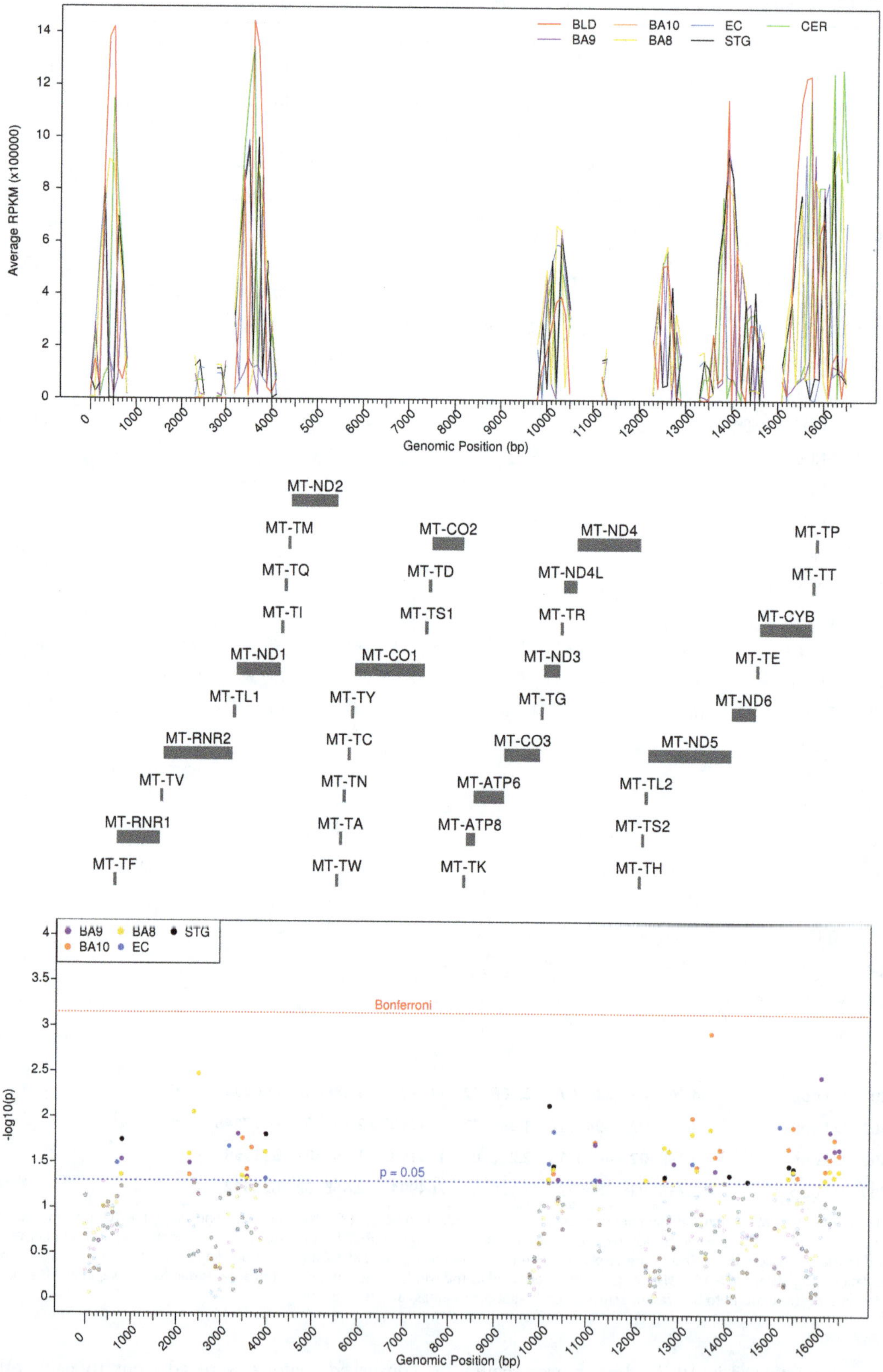

Fig. 3 (See legend on next page.)

(See figure on previous page.)
Fig. 3 DNA methylation differences are seen in the mitochondrial genome between brain regions and blood. Average raw RPKM values across the mitochondrial genome for each individual cortical brain region alongside matched blood and cerebellum samples are shown in the *top panel*, with gene positions downloaded from GENCODE shown in the *middle panel*. For each 100 bp window, paired *t* tests were performed to compare each cortical brain region and the cerebellum, with -log10 (*p*) shown in the *bottom panel*. *BLD* blood, *BA8* Brodmann area 8, *BA9* Brodmann area 9, *BA10* Brodmann area 10, *CER* cerebellum, *CTX* cortex, *ECX* entorhinal cortex, *RPKM* reads per kilobase of transcript per million mapped reads, *STG* superior temporal gyrus. *Red dashed line* denotes the Bonferroni significance, whilst *blue dashed line* denotes $p < 0.05$ in the *lower panel*

A number of differentially methylated regions in mtDNA can be observed between the cortex and cerebellum

We were also interested to see whether total cortical tissue was significantly different to matched cerebellum samples. Given the paired nature of the different anatomical regions of the cortex, we used a multilevel mixed effects model to compare total cortex to cerebellum (see the Methods section). This analysis revealed 48 nominally significant ($p < 0.05$) windows (Table 3; Fig. 4), of which eight passed the Bonferroni correction (Table 3, bold face). Interestingly, three of these eight were adjacent to each other, lying between 10301 and 10600 bp and covering MT-ND3/MT-ND4L and MT-TR. We also saw a Bonferroni significant difference in DNA methylation in the D-Loop, where we earlier noted DNA methylation changes across all three Brodmann area regions.

MtDNA methylation patterns can distinguish between tissue types

Although we have shown that mtDNA methylation patterns are highly similar between distinct anatomical regions of the human brain and blood, we were also interested to identify whether mtDNA methylation patterns could distinguish between these tissue types. Through unsupervised hierarchical clustering, we showed that average mtDNA methylation patterns can segregate these tissues (Fig. 5a). Importantly, ncDNA methylation profiles in the same samples have also been previously shown to separate the cortex, cerebellum and blood [35]. Interestingly, when we performed unsupervised hierarchical clustering on the individual samples, we found that, in most cases, intra-individual differences across tissue types are greater than inter-individual differences within each tissue type, as the cortex, cerebellum and blood samples clustered with their own tissue type, respectively (Fig. 5b).

Discussion

The availability of publicly available epigenomic data provides a great resource for mitochondrial epigenetics, a field that is relatively nascent and has yet to be thoroughly investigated in a range of complex diseases. Here, we present evidence that mtDNA methylation patterns across mtDNA are brain region specific. However, data such as that presented here is confounded by a lack of isolation of mtDNA prior to antibody enrichment and sequencing. As such, the potential of including *NUMTs* in datasets derived from data generated using total genomic DNA could lead to misleading results. Here, we controlled for regions of high sequence homology between the nuclear and mitochondrial genomes. However, this approach is likely over-conservative and does lead to the generation of a somewhat truncated consensus sequence. PCA of the mitochondrial epigenome after corrections for nuclear homology was able to separate individuals belonging to the three main tissue types, the blood, cortex and cerebellum based on mtDNA methylation variation among tissue types. This tissue specificity is further highlighted by the identification of eight DMRs that pass the Bonferroni correction for multiple testing between total cortex and cerebellum. MtDNA methylation has been shown to be cell line dependent in the past. [31] Although overall DNA methylation levels were low in all tissues, it is worth noting that the study was performed on non bisulfite-treated DNA. As such, the low percentage of mtDNA methylation is not a pitfall due to a lack of a total bisulfite treatment efficiency. One limitation of the current study is the unavailability of publicly available MeDIP-seq datasets of matched cortical and cerebellum tissue from other cohorts for validation purposes. Future work would aim to replicate our findings in additional study cohorts and also to investigate the relationship between mitochondrial DNA methylation and gene expression.

Despite a number of nominally significant windows being identified between each individual cortical region and the cerebellum, these did not pass the Bonferroni correction, although it is likely this method is too stringent. Nevertheless, the conservation of seven nominally significant windows across each Brodmann area is interesting to note. Four of these windows lie adjacent to each other and correspond to the mitochondrial D-Loop, a region containing the only two mitochondrial promoters which is typically associated with gene transcription and DNA replication. However, one limitation of this study is owed to the use of antibody-based enrichment, resulting in the analysis being limited to a window-based approach. Despite this, studies of the nuclear genome have shown high correlation between window-based approaches and, more sensitive, single-site assays such as the Illumina 450K beadarray [32]. However, given the small size of the mitochondrial genome and that

Table 3 List of DMRs identified between total cortex and cerebellum

Start (bp)	Stop (bp)	Gene(s)	*p* value
1	100	D-Loop	-
101	200	D-Loop	-
201	300	D-Loop	-
301	400	D-Loop	-
401	500	D-Loop	7.99E−03
501	600	MT-TF	4.49E−03
601	700	MT-TF/MT-RNR1	1.16E−02
701	800	MT-RNR1	3.22E−03
801	**900**	**MT-RNR1**	**1.91E−04**
901	1000	MT-RNR1	ND
1001	1100	MT-RNR1	ND
1101	1200	MT-RNR1	ND
1201	1300	MT-RNR1	ND
1301	1400	MT-RNR1	ND
1401	1500	MT-RNR1	ND
1501	1600	MT-RNR1	ND
1601	1700	MT-RNR1/MT-TV/MT-RNR2	ND
1701	1800	MT-RNR2	ND
1801	1900	MT-RNR2	ND
1901	2000	MT-RNR2	ND
2001	2100	MT-RNR2	ND
2101	2200	MT-RNR2	ND
2201	2300	MT-RNR2	ND
2301	2400	MT-RNR2	8.10E−03
2401	2500	MT-RNR2	7.50E−03
2501	2600	MT-RNR2	5.14E−03
2601	2700	MT-RNR2	ND
2701	2800	MT-RNR2	ND
2801	2900	MT-RNR2	-
2901	3000	MT-RNR2	-
3001	3100	MT-RNR2	-
3101	3200	MT-RNR2	-
3201	3300	MT-RNR2/MT-TL	1.51E−03
3301	3400	MT-TL1/MT-ND1	-
3401	3500	MT-ND1	1.37E−02
3501	3600	MT-ND1	4.27E−03
3601	3700	MT-ND1	5.56E−03
3701	3800	MT-ND1	8.21E−03
3801	3900	MT-ND1	-
3901	4000	MT-ND1	-
4001	**4100**	**MT-ND1**	**3.07E−06**
4101	4200	MT-ND1	-
4201	4300	MT-ND1/MT-TI	ND

Table 3 List of DMRs identified between total cortex and cerebellum *(Continued)*

4301	4400	MT-TI/MT-TQ	ND
4401	4500	MT-TM/MT-ND2	ND
4501	4600	MT-ND2	ND
4601	4700	MT-ND2	ND
4701	4800	MT-ND2	ND
4801	4900	MT-ND2	ND
4901	5000	MT-ND2	ND
5001	5100	MT-ND2	ND
5101	5200	MT-ND2	ND
5201	5300	MT-ND2	ND
5301	5400	MT-ND2	ND
5401	5500	MT-ND2	ND
5501	5600	MT-ND2/MT-TW/MT-TA	ND
5601	5700	MT-TA/MT-TN	ND
5701	5800	MT-TN/MT-TC	ND
5801	5900	MT-TC/MT-TY	ND
5901	6000	MT-CO1	ND
6001	6100	MT-CO1	ND
6101	6200	MT-CO1	ND
6201	6300	MT-CO1	ND
6301	6400	MT-CO1	ND
6401	6500	MT-CO1	ND
6501	6600	MT-CO1	ND
6601	6700	MT-CO1	ND
6701	6800	MT-CO1	ND
6801	6900	MT-CO1	ND
6901	7000	MT-CO1	ND
7001	7100	MT-CO1	ND
7101	7200	MT-CO1	ND
7201	7300	MT-CO1	ND
7301	7400	MT-CO1	ND
7401	7500	MT-CO1/MT-TS1	ND
7501	7600	MT-TS1/MT-TD/MT-CO2	ND
7601	7700	MT-CO2	ND
7701	7800	MT-CO2	ND
7801	7900	MT-CO2	ND
7901	8000	MT-CO2	ND
8001	8100	MT-CO2	ND
8101	8200	MT-CO2	ND
8201	8300	MT-CO2/MT-TK	ND
8301	8400	MT-TK/MT-ATP8	ND
8401	8500	MT-ATP8	ND
8501	8600	MT-ATP8/MT-ATP6	ND
8601	8700	MT-ATP6	ND

Table 3 List of DMRs identified between total cortex and cerebellum *(Continued)*

8701	8800	MT-ATP6	ND
8801	8900	MT-ATP6	ND
8901	9000	MT-ATP6	ND
9001	9100	MT-ATP6	ND
9101	9200	MT-ATP6	ND
9201	9300	MT-ATP6/MT-CO3	ND
9301	9400	MT-CO3	ND
9401	9500	MT-CO3	ND
9501	9600	MT-CO3	ND
9601	9700	MT-CO3	ND
9701	9800	MT-CO3	ND
9801	9900	MT-CO3	-
9901	10000	MT-CO3/MT-TG	-
10001	10100	MT-TG/MT-ND3	1.81E−02
10101	10200	MT-ND3	1.39E−02
10201	**10300**	**MT-ND3**	**3.53E−04**
10301	**10400**	**MT-ND3/MT-TR/MT-ND4L**	**1.19E−05**
10401	**10500**	**MT-ND4L**	**2.61E−04**
10501	10600	MT-ND4L	9.05E−04
10601	10700	MT-ND4L	ND
10701	10800	MT-ND4L/MT-ND4	ND
10801	10900	MT-ND4	ND
10901	11000	MT-ND4	ND
11001	11100	MT-ND4	ND
11101	11200	MT-ND4	ND
11201	**11300**	**MT-ND4**	**8.86E−05**
11301	11400	MT-ND4	1.65E−03
11401	11500	MT-ND4	ND
11501	11600	MT-ND4	ND
11601	11700	MT-ND4	ND
11701	11800	MT-ND4	ND
11801	11900	MT-ND4	ND
11901	12000	MT-ND4	ND
12001	12100	MT-ND4	ND
12101	12200	MT-ND4/MT-TH	ND
12201	12300	MT-TS2/MT-TL2	ND
12301	12400	MT-TL2/MT-ND5	-
12401	12500	MT-ND5	-
12501	12600	MT-ND5	-
12601	12700	MT-ND5	-
12701	12800	MT-ND5	1.81E−03
12801	12900	MT-ND5	1.05E−02
12901	13000	MT-ND5	8.23E−03
13001	13100	MT-ND5	ND

Table 3 List of DMRs identified between total cortex and cerebellum *(Continued)*

13101	13200	MT-ND5	ND
13201	13300	MT-ND5	ND
13301	13400	MT-ND5	1.44E−03
13401	13500	MT-ND5	9.13E−04
13501	13600	MT-ND5	1.61E−02
13601	13700	MT-ND5	3.89E−02
13701	**13800**	**MT-ND5**	**2.77E−04**
13801	13900	MT-ND5	2.80E−03
13901	14000	MT-ND5	1.88E−02
14001	14100	MT-ND5	9.31E−03
14101	14200	MT-ND5/MT-ND6	-
14201	14300	MT-ND6	-
14301	14400	MT-ND6	1.04E−02
14401	14500	MT-ND6	1.99E−02
14501	14600	MT-ND6	2.26E−02
14601	14700	MT-ND6/MT-TE	3.82E−03
14701	14800	MT-TE/MT-CYB	1.92E−02
14801	14900	MT-CYB	ND
14901	15000	MT-CYB	ND
15001	15100	MT-CYB	ND
15101	15200	MT-CYB	3.30E−02
15201	15300	MT-CYB	-
15301	15400	MT-CYB	-
15401	15500	MT-CYB	8.52E−04
15501	15600	MT-CYB	7.43E−04
15601	15700	MT-CYB	1.16E−02
15701	15800	MT-CYB	2.24E−02
15801	15900	MT-CYB/MT-TT	-
15901	16000	MT-TT/MT-TP	-
16001	16100	MT-TP	-
16101	16200	D-Loop	2.23E−03
16201	**16300**	**D-Loop**	**5.02E−04**
16301	16400	D-Loop	1.84E−03
16401	16500	D-Loop	1.12E−03
16501	16600	D-Loop	2.20E−03

Shown is the location of the DMR within ChrM (based on GENCODE), the gene(s) residing within the 100 bp window, and p value from a multilevel mixed effects model. Results are displayed in order of genomic position. RPKM and corresponding p values are shown for windows if $p < 0.05$. Key: - denotes data not significant ($p > 0.05$); ND denotes not determined as the window was not included in analysis due to removal in *NUMT* pipeline; bold denotes windows that reached our Bonferroni significant threshold of $p < 7.04E{-}04$

23 of the 37 genes present in the genome are below 100 bp in size, this window-based approach may not be the most appropriate for future studies designed to specifically assess mtDNA methylation as it can result

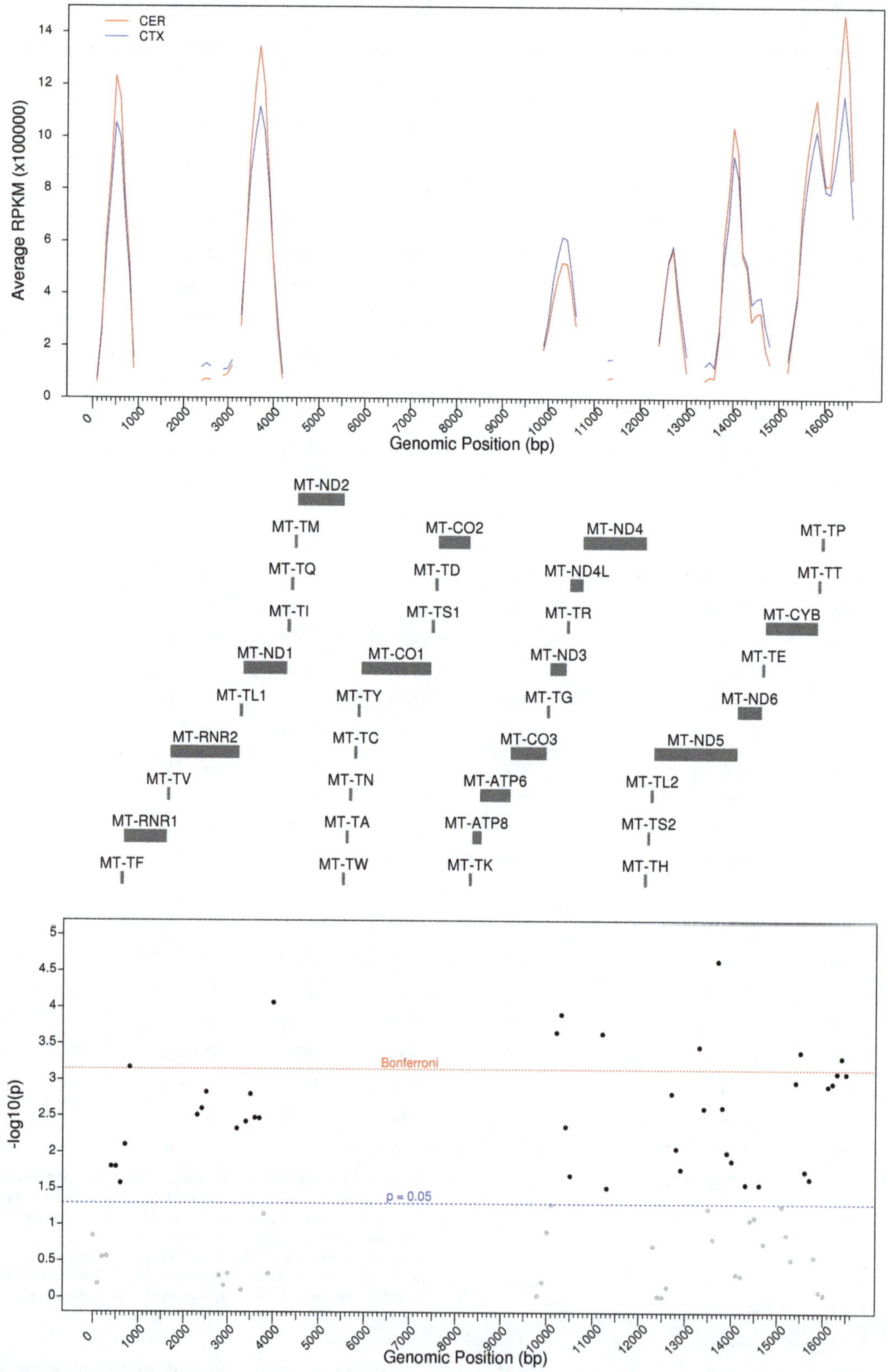

Fig. 4 (See legend on next page.)

(See figure on previous page.)
Fig. 4 DNA methylation differences are seen in the mitochondrial genome between the cerebellum and cortex. RPKM values in the total cortex and cerebellum across the mitochondrial genome are shown in the *top panel*, with gene positions downloaded from GENCODE shown in the *middle panel*. For each 100 bp window, paired *t* tests were performed to compare the cortex to the cerebellum, with -log10 (*p*) shown in the *bottom panel*. *BLD* blood, *BA8* Brodmann area 8, *BA9* Brodmann area 9, *BA10* Brodmann area 10, *CER* cerebellum, *CTX* cortex, *ECX* entorhinal cortex, *RPKM* reads per kilobase of transcript per million mapped reads, *STG* superior temporal gyrus. *Red dashed line* denotes the Bonferroni significance, whilst *blue dashed line* denotes $p < 0.05$ in the *lower panel*

in a window intersecting two genes in the polycistronic transcript.

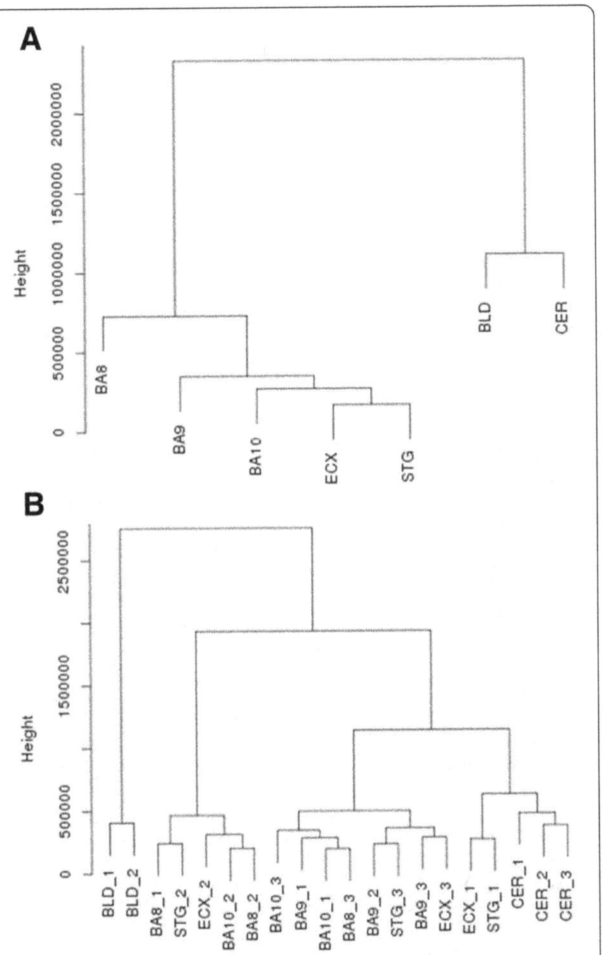

Fig. 5 MtDNA methylation patterns can distinguish between tissue types. **a** Average RPKM values for each cortical brain region, cerebellum and blood samples were clustered based upon the Euclidean distance, identifying two major clusters; the cortex and blood-cerebellum. **b** When clustering RPKM values in the individual samples from the cortex, cerebellum and blood, we observed that individual cortex samples clustered together, whilst cerebellum and blood samples formed separate clusters. This highlights that tissue-specific differences between the cortex, cerebellum and blood are greater than intra-individual variability within a tissue. *BLD* blood, *BA8* Brodmann area 8, *BA9* Brodmann area 9, *BA10* Brodmann area 10, *CER* cerebellum, *CTX* cortex, *ECX* entorhinal cortex, *RPKM* reads per kilobase of transcript per million mapped reads, *STG* superior temporal gyrus

Conclusions

This method provides a conservative approach to determine mtDNA methylation across the genome for data previously generated using next-generation sequencing approaches such as MeDIP-seq. Its conservative nature reduces the risk of the inclusion of *NUMTs* in the final analysis of whole genome data but may also lead to the inclusion of false negatives as well as potential gaps in the reference sequence. As such, it is best suited to analyzing previously generated whole genome data and is not a replacement for the isolation of mitochondrial DNA [36] prior to targeted methylation studies, which would be the optimal approach for investigating mitochondrial epigenomics. However, our method has allowed the identification of novel brain-region-specific DMRs in a previously generated publicly available dataset. Furthermore, the identification of brain region-specific mtDNA methylation patterns across the mitochondrial epigenome suggests the importance of a focussed, tissue-specific study design when investigating mtDNA methylation. As previously discussed, one caveat when utilizing MeDIP-seq data is the segregation of data into neighbouring windows, meaning that determining the exact corresponding gene of a DMR is difficult and, as such, future studies should aim to sequence the mitochondrial DNA methylome at single-base resolution to address this.

Methods

Data collection

We utilized publicly available MeDIP-seq data from Davies et al. [35]. In brief, this data was generated using 5 μg fragmented gDNA, which, following end repair <A> base addition and adaptor ligation, was immunoprecipitated using an anti-5-mC antibody (Diagenode, Liège, Belgium). MeDIP DNA was purified and then amplified using adaptor-mediated PCR, with DNA fragments between 220 and 320 bp subjected to highly parallel 50 bp paired-end sequencing on the Illumina Hi-Seq platform. The paired-end, raw fasta files were provided by the authors and quality checked using FastQC. Sample information is provided in Table 1.

Quality control and *NUMT* exclusion

Fasta files were subjected to adaptor and Phred score ($q < 20$) trimming. In an attempt to remove any potential contamination of possible *NUMTs*, multiple alignments to the reference genome were undertaken. Paired fasta files were aligned to GRCH37 using BWA. Unique and mapped reads aligning to the mitochondria were then re-mapped to a custom GRCH37 reference without the mitochondrial chromosome. Reads not mapping to the custom reference were then taken forward and realigned to the full GRCH37 reference to eliminate the possibility of homologous regions mapping falsely to the mitochondrial genome (Fig. 1). All alignments were carried out using BWA mem and default settings. Reads per kilobase of transcript per million mapped reads (RPKM) values for each sample were calculated using the MEDIPS package [37]. Methylation was averaged across 100 bp non-overlapping windows (default parameter setting in MEDIPS), and only windows with read counts >10 were considered for analysis. Due to the non-normal distribution of all cohorts, RPKM values were $\log^2$ transformed before statistical analysis.

Statistical analyses

All analyses were performed in the *R* statistical environment version 3.2.1 [38]. For all analyses, a nominally significant threshold of $p < 0.05$ and a Bonferroni significant threshold of $p < 7.04E{-}04$ were used. Given the matched sample nature of this cohort, two-tailed, paired *t* tests were performed at each window along the mitochondrial genome to identify DMRs between the individual cortical regions and cerebellum. To compare the total cortex to cerebellum, we performed a multilevel mixed effects model in the Lme4 package in *R* [39], using the brain region as the random effect and individual as the fixed effect. To assess the similarity of the brain regions, we used the *R* function "hclust" to cluster average RPKM values for the brain regions using the Euclidean distance. We used the *R* function "corrgram" within the corrgram package [40] to order samples based upon the similarity of their principal components.

Abbreviations

5-mC: 5-methylcytosine; BA: Brodmann area; DMR: Differentially methylated region; MeDIP-seq: Methylated DNA Immunoprecipitation Sequencing; mtDNA: Mitochondrial DNA; ncDNA: Nuclear DNA; *NUMTs*: Nuclear-mitochondrial DNA; PCA: Principal component analysis; rRNA: Ribosomal ribonucleic acid; tRNA: Transfer ribonucleic acid

Acknowledgements

Not applicable.

Funding

This work was funded by an Alzheimer's Society project grant to KL (grant number AS-PG-14-038), an Alzheimer's Research UK pilot grant to KL (grant number ARUK-PPG2013A-5) and an Alzheimer's Association New Investigator Research Grant to KL (grant number NIRG-14-320878).

Authors' contributions

MD, MW, RS, AJ and EH undertook the data analysis and bioinformatics. MD and MW developed the pipeline for the analysis. MND and JM provided the data for the analysis. KL conceived and supervised the project. MD and KL drafted the manuscript. All authors read and approved the final submission.

Competing interests

The authors declare that they have no competing interests.

Author details

[1]University of Exeter Medical School, RILD, University of Exeter, Barrack Road, Devon, UK. [2]Institute of Psychiatry, Psychology and Neuroscience, King's College London, De Crespigny Park, London, UK. [3]Department of Twin Research & Genetic Epidemiology, King's College London, Lambeth Palace Road, London, UK. [4]School of Biological Sciences, University of Essex, Essex, UK.

References

1. Anderson S, Bankier AT, Barrell BG, de Bruijn MH, Coulson AR, Drouin J, Eperon IC, Nierlich DP, Roe BA, Sanger F, et al. Sequence and organization of the human mitochondrial genome. Nature. 1981;290:457–65.
2. Murgia M, Rizzuto R. Molecular diversity and pleiotropic role of the mitochondrial calcium uniporter. Cell Calcium. 2015;58:11–7.
3. Wang W, Esbensen Y, Kunke D, Suganthan R, Rachek L, Bjoras M, Eide L. Mitochondrial DNA damage level determines neural stem cell differentiation fate. J Neurosci. 2011;31:9746–51.
4. Lunnon K, Ibrahim Z, Proitsi P, Lourdusamy A, Newhouse S, Sattlecker M, Furney S, Saleem M, Soininen H, Kloszewska I, et al. Mitochondrial dysfunction and immune activation are detectable in early Alzheimer's disease blood. J Alzheimers Dis. 2012;30:685–710.
5. Lunnon K, Keohane A, Pidsley R, Newhouse S, Riddoch-Contreras J, Thubron EB, Devall M, Soininen H, Kloszewska I, Mecocci P, et al. Mitochondrial genes are altered in blood early in Alzheimer's disease. Neurobiol Aging. 2017;53:36–47.
6. Prabakaran S, Swatton JE, Ryan MM, Huffaker SJ, Huang JT, Griffin JL, Wayland M, Freeman T, Dudbridge F, Lilley KS, et al. Mitochondrial dysfunction in schizophrenia: evidence for compromised brain metabolism and oxidative stress. Mol Psychiatry. 2004;9:684–97. 643.
7. Clay HB, Sillivan S, Konradi C. Mitochondrial dysfunction and pathology in bipolar disorder and schizophrenia. Int J Dev Neurosci. 2011;29:311–24.
8. Chang CC, Jou SH, Lin TT, Lai TJ, Liu CS. Mitochondria DNA change and oxidative damage in clinically stable patients with major depressive disorder. PLoS One. 2015;10:e0125855.
9. Lunnon K, Mill J. Epigenetic studies in Alzheimer's disease: current findings, caveats, and considerations for future studies. Am J Med Genet B Neuropsychiatr Genet. 2013;162B:789–99.
10. Lunnon K, Hannon E, Smith RG, Dempster E, Wong C, Burrage J, Troakes C, Al-Sarraj S, Kepa A, Schalkwyk L, Mill J. Variation in 5-hydroxymethylcytosine across human cortex and cerebellum. Genome Biol. 2016;17:27.
11. Lowe R, Slodkowicz G, Goldman N, Rakyan VK. The human blood DNA methylome displays a highly distinctive profile compared with other somatic tissues. Epigenetics. 2015;10:274–81.
12. Lokk K, Modhukur V, Rajashekar B, Martens K, Magi R, Kolde R, Koltsina M, Nilsson TK, Vilo J, Salumets A, Tonisson N. DNA methylome profiling of human tissues identifies global and tissue-specific methylation patterns. Genome Biol. 2014;15:r54.
13. Lunnon K, Smith R, Hannon EJ, De Jager PL, Srivastava G, Volta M, Troakes C, Al-Sarraj S, Burrage J, Macdonald R, et al. Methylomic profiling implicates cortical deregulation of ANK1 in Alzheimer's disease. Nat Neurosci. 2014;17:1164–70.
14. De Jager PL, Srivastava G, Lunnon K, Burgess J, Schalkwyk LC, Yu L, Eaton ML, Keenan BT, Ernst J, McCabe C, et al. Alzheimer's disease: early alterations in brain DNA methylation at ANK1, BIN1, RHBDF2 and other loci. Nat Neurosci. 2014;17:1156–63.

15. Smith AR, Smith RG, Condliffe D, Hannon E, Schalkwyk L, Mill J, Lunnon K. Increased DNA methylation near TREM2 is consistently seen in the superior temporal gyrus in Alzheimer's disease brain. Neurobiol Aging. 2016;47:35–40.
16. Pidsley R, Viana J, Hannon E, Spiers HH, Troakes C, Al-Saraj S, Mechawar N, Turecki G, Schalkwyk LC, Bray NJ, Mill J. Methylomic profiling of human brain tissue supports a neurodevelopmental origin for schizophrenia. Genome Biol. 2014;15:483.
17. Hannon E, Spiers H, Viana J, Pidsley R, Burrage J, Murphy TM, Troakes C, Turecki G, O'Donovan MC, Schalkwyk LC, et al. Methylation QTLs in the developing brain and their enrichment in schizophrenia risk loci. Nat Neurosci. 2016;19:48–+.
18. Florath I, Butterbach K, Heiss J, Bewerunge-Hudler M, Zhang Y, Schottker B, Brenner H. Type 2 diabetes and leucocyte DNA methylation: an epigenome-wide association study in over 1,500 older adults. Diabetologia. 2016;59:130–8.
19. Adams AT, Kennedy NA, Hansen R, Ventham NT, O'Leary KR, Drummond HE, Noble CL, El-Omar E, Russell RK, Wilson DC, et al. Two-stage genome-wide methylation profiling in childhood-onset Crohn's Disease implicates epigenetic alterations at the VMP1/MIR21 and HLA loci. Inflamm Bowel Dis. 2014;20:1784–93.
20. Devall M, Mill J, Lunnon K. The mitochondrial epigenome: a role in Alzheimer's disease? Epigenomics. 2014;6:665–75.
21. Devall M, Roubroeks J, Mill J, Weedon M, Lunnon K. Epigenetic regulation of mitochondrial function in neurodegenerative disease: New insights from advances in genomic technologies. Neurosci Lett. 2016;625:47–55.
22. Shock LS, Thakkar PV, Peterson EJ, Moran RG, Taylor SM. DNA methyltransferase 1, cytosine methylation, and cytosine hydroxymethylation in mammalian mitochondria. Proc Natl Acad Sci U S A. 2011;108:3630–5.
23. Chestnut BA, Chang Q, Price A, Lesuisse C, Wong M, Martin LJ. Epigenetic regulation of motor neuron cell death through DNA methylation. J Neurosci. 2011;31:16619–36.
24. Feng S, Xiong L, Ji Z, Cheng W, Yang H. Correlation between increased ND2 expression and demethylated displacement loop of mtDNA in colorectal cancer. Mol Med Rep. 2012;6:125–30.
25. Pirola CJ, Gianotti TF, Burgueno AL, Rey-Funes M, Loidl CF, Mallardi P, Martino JS, Castano GO, Sookoian S. Epigenetic modification of liver mitochondrial DNA is associated with histological severity of nonalcoholic fatty liver disease. Gut. 2013;62:1356–63.
26. Infantino V, Castegna A, Iacobazzi F, Spera I, Scala I, Andria G, Iacobazzi V. Impairment of methyl cycle affects mitochondrial methyl availability and glutathione level in Down's syndrome. Mol Genet Metab. 2011;102:378–82.
27. Wong M, Gertz B, Chestnut BA, Martin LJ. Mitochondrial DNMT3A and DNA methylation in skeletal muscle and CNS of transgenic mouse models of ALS. Front Cell Neurosci. 2013;7:279.
28. Wen SL, Zhang F, Feng S. Decreased copy number of mitochondrial DNA: a potential diagnostic criterion for gastric cancer. Oncol Lett. 2013;6:1098–102.
29. Blanch M, Mosquera JL, Ansoleaga B, Ferrer I, Barrachina M. Altered mitochondrial DNA methylation pattern in Alzheimer disease-related pathology and in Parkinson disease. Am J Pathol. 2016;186:385–97.
30. Iacobazzi V, Castegna A, Infantino V, Andria G. Mitochondrial DNA methylation as a next-generation biomarker and diagnostic tool. Mol Genet Metab. 2013;110:25–34.
31. Ghosh S, Sengupta S, Scaria V. Comparative analysis of human mitochondrial methylomes shows distinct patterns of epigenetic regulation in mitochondria. Mitochondrion. 2014;18:58–62.
32. Clark C, Palta P, Joyce CJ, Scott C, Grundberg E, Deloukas P, Palotie A, Coffey AJ. A comparison of the whole genome approach of MeDIP-seq to the targeted approach of the Infinium HumanMethylation450 BeadChip® for methylome profiling. PLoS One. 2012;7:e50233.
33. Thangaraj K, Joshi MB, Reddy AG, Rasalkar AA, Singh L. Sperm mitochondrial mutations as a cause of low sperm motility. J Androl. 2003;24:388–92.
34. Yao YG, Kong QP, Salas A, Bandelt HJ. Pseudomitochondrial genome haunts disease studies. J Med Genet. 2008;45:769–72.
35. Davies MN, Volta M, Pidsley R, Lunnon K, Dixit A, Lovestone S, Coarfa C, Harris RA, Milosavljevic A, Troakes C, et al. Functional annotation of the human brain methylome identifies tissue-specific epigenetic variation across brain and blood. Genome Biol. 2012;13:R43.
36. Devall M, Burrage J, Caswell R, Johnson M, Troakes C, Al-Sarraj S, Jeffries AR, Mill J, Lunnon K. A comparison of mitochondrial DNA isolation methods in frozen post-mortem human brain tissue-applications for studies of mitochondrial genetics in brain disorders. Biotechniques. 2015;59:241–6.
37. Lienhard MGC, Morkel M, Herwig R, Chavez L. MEDIPS: genome-wide differential coverage analysis of sequencing data derived from DNA enrichment experiments. Bioinformatics. 2014;30:284–6.
38. R Development Core Team. R: a language and environment for statistical computing. Vienna: R Foundation for Statistical Computing; 2012. p. 2012.
39. Vazquez AI, Bates DM, Rosa GJ, Gianola D, Weigel KA. Technical note: an R package for fitting generalized linear mixed models in animal breeding. J Anim Sci. 2010;88:497–504.
40. Wright K. Package corrgram. R package version 1.9. 2016. Available from. https://cran.r-project.org/web/packages/corrgram/index.html. Accessed 30 Sept 2016.

2

Epigenetic modifications in *KDM* lysine demethylases associate with survival of early-stage NSCLC

Yongyue Wei[1,2,3†], Junya Liang[1,2†], Ruyang Zhang[1,2,3†], Yichen Guo[3], Sipeng Shen[1,2,3], Li Su[2], Xihong Lin[4], Sebastian Moran[5], Åslaug Helland[6], Maria M. Bjaanæs[6], Anna Karlsson[7], Maria Planck[7], Manel Esteller[5], Thomas Fleischer[6], Johan Staaf[7], Yang Zhao[1,2,3], Feng Chen[1,2,3*] and David C. Christiani[2,3,8*]

Abstract

Background: *KDM* lysine demethylase family members are related to lung cancer clinical outcomes and are potential biomarkers for chemotherapeutics. However, little is known about epigenetic alterations in *KDM* genes and their roles in lung cancer survival.

Methods: Tumor tissue samples of 1230 early-stage non-small cell lung cancer (NSCLC) patients were collected from the five independent cohorts. The 393 methylation sites in *KDM* genes were extracted from epigenome-wide datasets and analyzed by weighted random forest (Ranger) in discovery phase and validation dataset, respectively. The variable importance scores (VIS) for the sites in top 5% of both discovery and validation sets were carried forward for Cox regression to further evaluate the association with patient's overall survival. TCGA transcriptomic data were used to evaluate the correlation with the corresponding DNA methylation.

Results: DNA methylation at sites cg11637544 in *KDM2A* and cg26662347 in *KDM1A* were in the top 5% of VIS in both discovery phase and validation for squamous cell carcinomas (SCC), which were also significantly associated with SCC survival ($HR_{cg11637544} = 1.32$, 95%CI, 1.16–1.50, $P = 1.1 \times 10^{-4}$; $HR_{cg26662347} = 1.88$, 95%CI, 1.37–2.60, $P = 3.7 \times 10^{-3}$), and correlated with corresponding gene expression (cg11637544 for *KDM2A*, $P = 1.3 \times 10^{-10}$; cg26662347 for *KDM1A* $P = 1.5 \times 10^{-5}$). In addition, by using flexible criteria for Ranger analysis followed by survival classification tree analysis, we identified four clusters for adenocarcinomas and five clusters for squamous cell carcinomas which showed a considerable difference of clinical outcomes with statistical significance.

Conclusions: These findings highlight the association between somatic DNA methylation in *KDM* genes and early-stage NSCLC patient survival, which may reveal potential epigenetic therapeutic targets.

Keywords: *KDM*, Lysine demethylase, DNA methylation, Lung cancer, Survival

Background

Lung cancer, a highly invasive, rapidly metastasizing cancer, accounting for more than one million deaths each year, has been the leading cause of cancer deaths worldwide for decades [1]. Rapidly developing radiological techniques and strengthened consciousness of health screening result in an increased numbers of lung cancer patients diagnosed at early stage. Early-stage lung cancer patients are expected to have a better prognosis compared with those at late stage [2]. However, significant heterogeneity has been observed for clinical outcomes among the early-stage patients, which may have molecular mechanisms not well understood yet [3]. Epigenetic alterations—particularly methylation in target organ tissues—is a potential causation of this phenomenon [4].

Of particular interest, methylation changes at histone demethylase *KDM* gene family are broadly involved in

* Correspondence: fengchen@njmu.edu.cn; dchris@hsph.harvard.edu
†Equal contributors
1Department of Biostatistics, School of Public Health, Nanjing Medical University, Nanjing 211166, China
2China International Cooperation Center (CICC) for Environment and Human Health, Nanjing Medical University, Nanjing 211166, China
Full list of author information is available at the end of the article

cancer development [5, 6]. Because methylation is reversible, it provides a source of potential biomarkers and therapeutic targets in cancer [7, 8]. Most recent publications show a great potential of epigenetic modifiable agencies in cancer therapy [9, 10]. HumanN6-methyllysine residue demethylation is catalyzed by two distinct subfamilies of demethylases—the flavin-dependent *KDM1* subfamily and the JmjC-domain containing *KDM2-8* subfamily, which regulate the chromatin state at specific loci, and impact gene expression, DNA repair, DNA replication, and genome stability [6]. Emerging evidence connects *KDMs* to cancers, including lung cancer [11–17]. DNA methylation is an important gene regulator that provides epigenetic therapeutic targets in cancer. However, to date, no studies have examined the role of DNA methylation in *KDM* demethylase genes and its relationship to clinical outcomes of lung cancer patients.

Therefore, we performed a large-scale association analysis between somatic DNA methylation in *KDM* gene family members and overall survival of non-small cell lung cancer (NSCLC) patients. The study was performed in a discovery set combining four independent Caucasian populations, followed by an independent replication in the data from The Cancer Genome Atlas (TCGA).

Table 1 Demographic and clinic pathological descriptions for study populations

Variables	Discovery set					Validation set
	Harvard (*N* = 151)	Spain (*N* = 226)	Norway (*N* = 133)	Sweden (*N* = 103)	All (*N* = 613)	TCGA (*N* = 617)
Age (years), mean ± SD	67.67 ± 9.92	65.67 ± 10.58	65.52 ± 9.34	67.54 ± 9.99	66.44 ± 10.08	66.51 ± 9.47
Gender, *n* (%)						*
Female	67 (44.37)	105 (46.46)	71 (53.38)	54 (52.43)	297 (48.45)	255 (41.33)
Male	84 (55.63)	121 (53.54)	62 (46.62)	49 (47.57)	316 (51.55)	362 (58.67)
Smoking status, *n* (%)						*
Never	18 (11.92)	30 (13.57)	17 (12.78)	18 (17.48)	83 (13.65)	55 (9.18)
Former	81 (53.64)	120 (54.30)	74 (55.64)	54 (52.43)	329 (54.11)	376 (62.77)
Current	52 (34.44)	71 (32.13)	42 (31.58)	31 (30.10)	196 (32.24)	168 (28.05)
Unknown	0	5	0	0	5	18
TNM stage, *n* (%)						*
I	104 (68.87)	183 (80.97)	93 (69.92)	95 (92.23)	475 (77.49)	393 (63.70)
II	47 (31.13)	43 (19.03)	40 (30.08)	8 (7.77)	138 (22.51)	224 (36.30)
Histology, *n* (%)						*
Adenocarcinoma (AC)	96 (63.58)	183 (80.97)	133 (100.00)	80 (77.67)	492 (80.26)	332 (53.81)
Squamous cell carcinoma (SCC)	55 (36.42)	43 (19.03)	0 (0.00)	23 (22.33)	121 (19.74)	285 (46.19)
Chemotherapy, *n* (%)						*
No	142 (94.04)	177 (90.77)	102 (76.69)	67 (90.54)	488 (88.25)	194 (76.98)
Yes	9 (5.96)	18 (9.23)	31 (23.31)	7 (9.46)	65 (11.75)	58 (23.02)
Unknown	0	31	0	29	60	365
Radiotherapy, *n* (%)						
No	132 (87.42)	184 (94.36)	132 (99.25)	74 (100.00)	522 (94.39)	239 (94.84)
Yes	19 (12.58)	11 (5.64)	1 (0.75)	0 (0.00)	31 (5.61)	13 (5.16)
Unknown	0	31	0	29	60	365
Adjuvant therapy, *n* (%)						*
No	127 (84.11)	168 (86.15)	101 (75.94)	67 (90.54)	463 (83.73)	187 (74.21)
Yes	24 (15.89)	27 (13.85)	32 (24.06)	7 (9.46)	90 (16.27)	65 (25.79)
Unknown	0	31	0	29	60	365
Survival year, month						
Median (95%CI)	6.66 (5.41–7.87)	7.12 (5.06–9.63)	7.36 (6.77–7.95)*	7.39 (4.98–9.12)	7.39 (6.50–8.23)	4.54 (3.68–5.41)
Dead, *n* (%)	122 (80.79)	101 (44.69)	42 (31.58)	58 (31.58)	323 (52.69)	142 (23.01)

*Statistically significant difference ($P \leq 0.05$) was observed between combined discovery set and validation set (TCGA)

Methods

Lung cancer study populations

Harvard

The Harvard Lung Cancer Study cohort was described previously [18]. Briefly, all cases were recruited at Massachusetts General Hospital (MGH) since 1992 and were newly diagnosed, histologically confirmed primary NSCLC. Snap-frozen tumor samples were collected from NSCLC patients during curative surgery with complete resection. There were151 early-stage (TNM stage I, II) cases selected for this study which had complete survival information. Tumor DNA was extracted from 5-μm-thick histopathologic sections. Each specimen was evaluated by an MGH pathologist for amount (tumor cellularity > 70%) and quality of tumor cells and histologically classified using WHO criteria.

Spain

Study population was reported previously [19]. In brief, tumors were collected by surgical resection from patients who provided consent and under approval by the institutional review boards. The median clinical follow-up was 7.2 years.

Norway

As described previously [20], participants were patients with operable lung cancer tumors who were seen at Oslo University Hospital-Riks hospitalet, Norway, from 2006 to 2011. Only early-stage (stage I, II) patients were selected for the current study.

Sweden

Tumor tissue specimens were collected from patient's early-stage lung cancer who underwent operation at the Skane University Hospital, Lund, Sweden [21].

TCGA

We used The Cancer Genome Atlas (TCGA) resources for validation, including 332 early-stage lung adenocarcinomas (AC) and 285 early-stage squamous cell carcinomas (SCC) which had survival information and common covariates. Level-1 HumanMethylation450 DNA methylation data (image data) of each patient were downloaded on October 01, 2015.

Quality control process for DNA methylation data

DNA methylation was assessed using Illumina Infinium HumanMethylation450 BeadChips (Illumina Inc., San Diego, CA, USA). Raw image data were imported into Genome Studio Methylation ModuleV1.8 (Illumina Inc.) to calculate methylation signals and to perform normalization, background subtraction, and quality control. Unqualified probes were excluded, if they fit the following quality control (QC) criteria: (i) failed detection ($P > 0.05$) in ≥ 5% samples, (ii) coefficient of variance (CV) < 5%, (iii) methylated or unmethylated in all samples, (iv) common single nucleotide polymorphisms located in probe sequence or in 10-bp flanking regions, (v) or cross-reactive probes [22]. Samples with > 5% undetectable probes were excluded. Methylation signals were further processed for quantile normalization, type I and II correction, and batch effects adjustment using *ComBat* correction [23, 24]. Those QC and normalization processes were performed at each site separately using the same R code with identical settings. In addition, the site information was included as one of the covariates in the following models to control for potential site heterogeneity. Details of QC processes are described in Additional file 1: Figure S1.

Gene expression data

In the TCGA cohort, all 332 AC and 285 SCC early-stage patients had complete mRNA sequencing data. TCGA mRNA sequencing data processing and quality control was done by the TCGA workgroup. Raw counts were normalized using RNA Sequencing by Expectation Maximization (RSEM). Level-3 (gene level) gene quantification data were downloaded from TCGA data portal and were further checked for quality. Expression of *KDM* genes was extracted and $\log_2$ transformed before analysis.

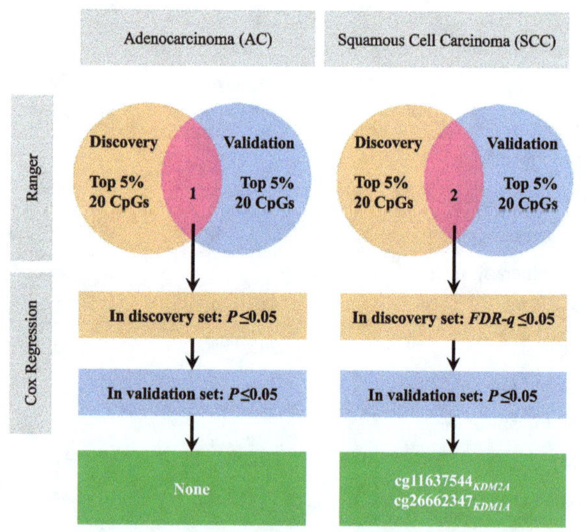

Fig. 1 Analysis work flow. Adenocarcinoma and squamous cell carcinoma samples from Harvard, Spain, Norway, and Sweden cohorts were used for the discovery phase of analysis. Data from The Cancer Genome Atlas (TCGA) were used for validation. Ranger is a weighted version of random forest for controlling for the covariates including age, gender, smoking status, and histological stage. Variable importance score (VIS) was estimated for each CpG site and was ranked in descending order. CpG sites ranked in top 5% in both discovery and validation sets were selected for further evaluation by Cox regression. Multiple testing correction by false discovery rate (FDR) method was used if necessary

Statistical analysis

Continuous variables were summarized as mean ± standard deviation (SD); categorical variables were described as *n* (%). Ranger, a weighted version of random forest for controlling for the potential confounders, was employed in discovery and validation set, respectively, to evaluate the importance of each individual methylation CpG site [25, 26]. A weight of 100% was given to each covariate to ensure a 100% chance to be selected into each tree. Variable importance score (VIS) for each methylation site was estimated and ranked in a descending order. CpG sites that were in top 5% in both discovery and validation set were identified as candidates and carried forward for traditional Cox regression.

The candidate methylation probes were further evaluated by Cox regression with adjustment for covariates including age, gender, smoking status, and stage. Results were described as hazard ratio (*HR*) and 95% confidence interval (95%CI) per 1% increment of methylation. Multiple testing corrections were performed using false discovery rate method (FDR; measured by FDR-*q* value) among results from discovery set. The sites with FDR-$q \leq 0.05$ in discovery set were, in turn, validated in TCGA samples, with a statistical significance level of 0.05. Further, correlations between the DNA methylation of the validated sites and corresponding gene expression level was evaluated by linear regression using TCGA data. Only TCGA samples had both epigenome and transcriptome data, so the methylation-expression analysis was only performed in TCGA cohort.

In addition, flexible criteria were hired for further exploration: (1) CpG sites that were in top 10% in both discovery and validation set were identified as candidates, (2) candidates with FDR-$q \leq 0.1$ in discovery set, and (3) *P* value ≤ 0.05 in validate set. Classification and regression tree (CART) was used to identify clusters with heterogeneous survival outcome. Kaplan-Meier method was used to illustrate the survival curves of different clusters.

All analyses were performed in R Version 3.2.4 (The R Foundation).

Results

We analyzed 393 DNA methylation probes (Additional file 2: Table S1) in 17 *KDM* gene family members located on autosomal chromosomes (Additional file 3: Table S2). Analysis was performed on 1230 tumor DNA samples from early-stage NSCLC patients recruited from five lung cancer study cohorts. Demographics and clinical characteristics are

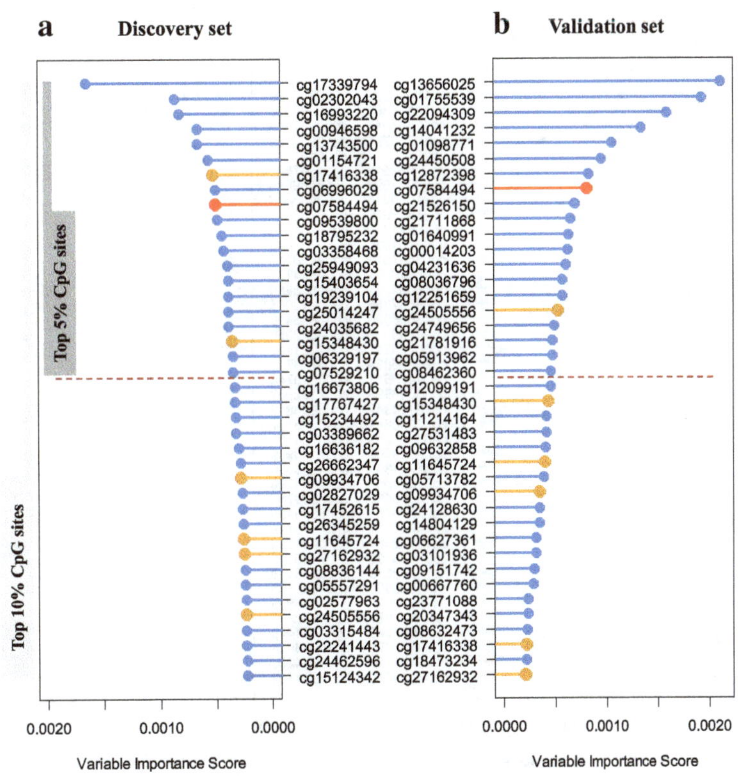

Fig. 2 Ranger in discovery (**a**) or validation (**b**) in adenocarcinomas. Weighted random forest (Ranger, where confounders like age, gender, smoking status, and stage are adjusted with given 100% weight) was employed in discovery phase (**a**) and validation set (**b**) to evaluate the importance of variables. Ranger provides VIS (variable importance score) for each methylation sites. Variables that were in top 5% (red lollipop) or top 10% (yellow lollipop, a flexible criterion) in both discovery phase (**a**) and validation (**b**) would be carried forward

described in Table 1. Figure 1 shows a flow chart for overall analysis. Samples from the Harvard, Spain, Norway, and Sweden studies were combined together for discovery.

Among AC samples, only one common CpG site, cg07584494 in *KDM4B*, was identified of which the importance ranked in the top 5% both in discovery and validation sets (Fig. 2). This CpG was further evaluated by Cox regression, meanwhile, did not reach the stringent criteria of *P* value ≤ 0.05 in both discovery and validation sets.

For SCC samples, the two common probes, cg11637544 within the first exon of *KDM2A* and cg26662347 at TSS200 region of *KDM1A*, were ranked in the top 5% in both discovery and validation sets (Fig. 3). These two CpG sites were further evaluated by Cox regression in discovery set and showed a significant association with SCC patients' survival [$cg11637544_{KDM2A}$, hazard ratio (*HR*) per 1% methylation increment = 1.38, 95% confidence interval (95%CI) 1.15–1.66, $P = 0.0006$, FDR-q = 0.0011; $cg26662347_{KDM1A}$, *HR* = 2.12, 95%CI 1.26–3.57, $P = 0.0045$, FDR-q = 0.0090]. Both CpG sites were replicated with statistical significance in validation set from TCGA ($HR_{cg11637544} = 1.26$, 95%CI 1.05–1.52, $P = 0.0136$; $HR_{cg26662347} = 1.75$, 95%CI 1.16–2.64, $P = 0.007$). Meta-analysis combining the evidences from the discovery and validation sets further showed a stronger association between worse SCC patient's survival and hypermethylation at $cg11637544_{KDM2A}$ ($HR = 1.32$, 95%CI, 1.16–1.50, $P = 1.1 \times 10^{-4}$; Fig. 4a) and at $cg26662347_{KDM1A}$ ($HR = 1.88$, 95%CI, 1.37–2.60, $P = 3.7 \times 10^{-3}$; Fig. 4b). Furthermore, altered DNA methylation at sites $cg11637544_{KDM2A}$ ($r = 0.37$, $P = 1.3 \times 10^{-10}$) (Fig. 4c) and $cg26662347_{KDM1A}$ ($r = 0.25$, $P = 1.5 \times 10^{-5}$) (Fig. 4d) were positively correlated with the corresponding gene expression.

In addition to the stringent criteria, we also comprehensively explored the data using Ranger with relatively flexible criteria, followed by survival classification tree analysis which can consider both linear and non-linear patterns, and both individual and interaction effects of CpG sites simultaneously (Additional file 4: Figure S2). CpG sites of which the variable importance score ranked in the top 10% in both discovery and validation set were selected, including seven CpG sites for AC samples (Fig. 2) and five for SCC samples (Fig. 3). Among AC cases, seven CpG sites as well as covariates were used to build a survival classification tree using the merged data of discovery and validation sets (Fig. 5a). Four clusters were identified with significantly different survival curves (Fig. 5b) and outcome (Fig. 5c). Among these seven CpG sites, none showed a

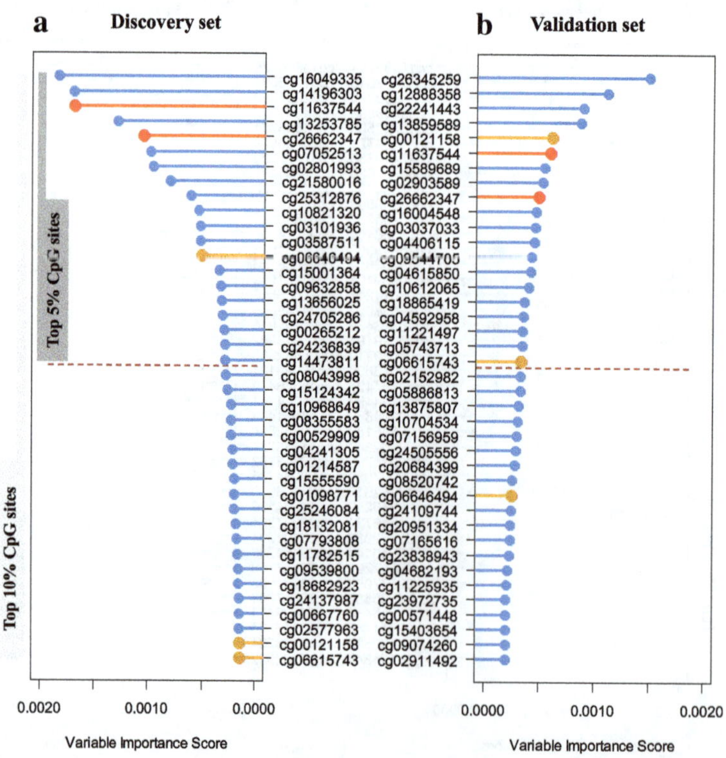

Fig. 3 Ranger in discovery (**a**) or validation (**b**) in squamous cell carcinomas. Weighted random forest (Ranger, where confounders like age, gender, smoking status, and stage are adjusted with given 100% weight) was employed in discovery phase (**a**) and validation set (**b**) to evaluate the importance of variables. Ranger provides VIS (variable importance score) for each methylation sites. Variables that were in top 5% (red lollipop) or top 10% (yellow lollipop, a flexible criterion) in both discovery phase (**a**) and validation (**b**) would be carried forward

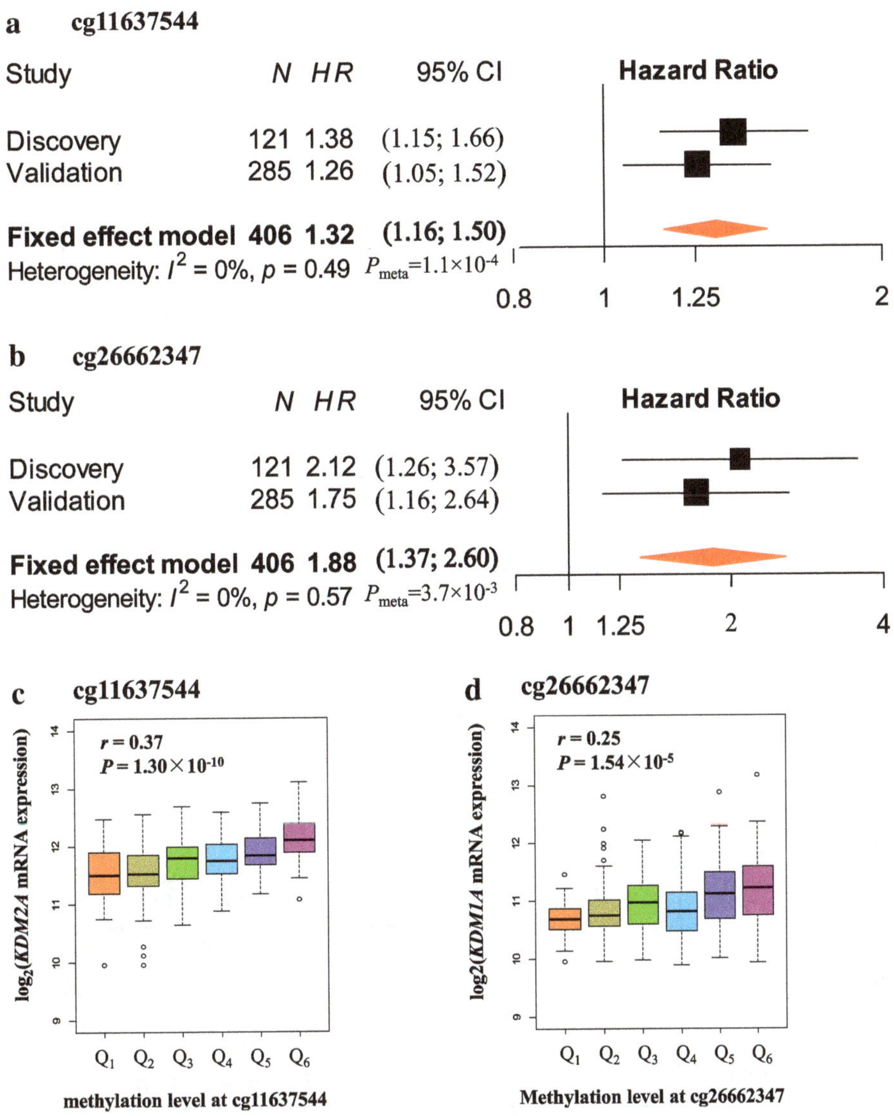

Fig. 4 Association between DNA methylation at sites cg11637544 in *KDM2A* and cg26662347 in *KDM1A* with overall survival of squamous cell carcinomas and correlation between these two sites and their corresponding gene expression. Fixed-effects meta-analysis was used to combine the results from discovery and validation sets for squamous cell carcinomas (SCC) (**a** cg11637544$_{KDM2A}$; **b** cg26662347$_{KDM1A}$). I^2 and corresponding *P* value were used to evaluate heterogeneity across studies. DNA methylation level was categorized to six quantiles, and box plot for gene expression was drawn for each quantile. Pearson correlation was used to estimate the correlation coefficient (*r*) and the *P* value; gene expression was log2 transformed before analysis (**c** cg11637544$_{KDM2A}$; **d** cg26662347$_{KDM1A}$)

correlation with corresponding gene's expression. Similarly, among SCC cases, five CpG sites, three of which were newly identified, and covariates were used to build the classification tree (Fig. 6a), which identified five clusters and statistically distinguished patient's survival (Fig. 6b, c). Among the three newly identified CpG sites for SCC samples (Additional file 4: Figure S2), two of which were correlated with their corresponding gene expression with statistical significance ($r_{cg00121158} = 0.24$, $P_{cg00121158} = 4.38 \times 10^{-5}$; $r_{cg06615743} = -0.17$, $P_{cg06615743} = 0.004$; Additional file 5: Figure S3A-B).

Discussion

Several non-hypothesis-based epigenome-wide studies have analyzed lung cancer prognosis [19–21] and have identified several potential epigenetic biomarkers to help better understand the etiology of NSCLC. To the best of our knowledge, this is the first population-based study integrating five independent cohorts that suggested the relationship between tumor DNA methylation alterations at the *KDM* gene family members and NSCLC overall survival. The results expand our current understanding of the *KDM* gene family in lung cancer etiology.

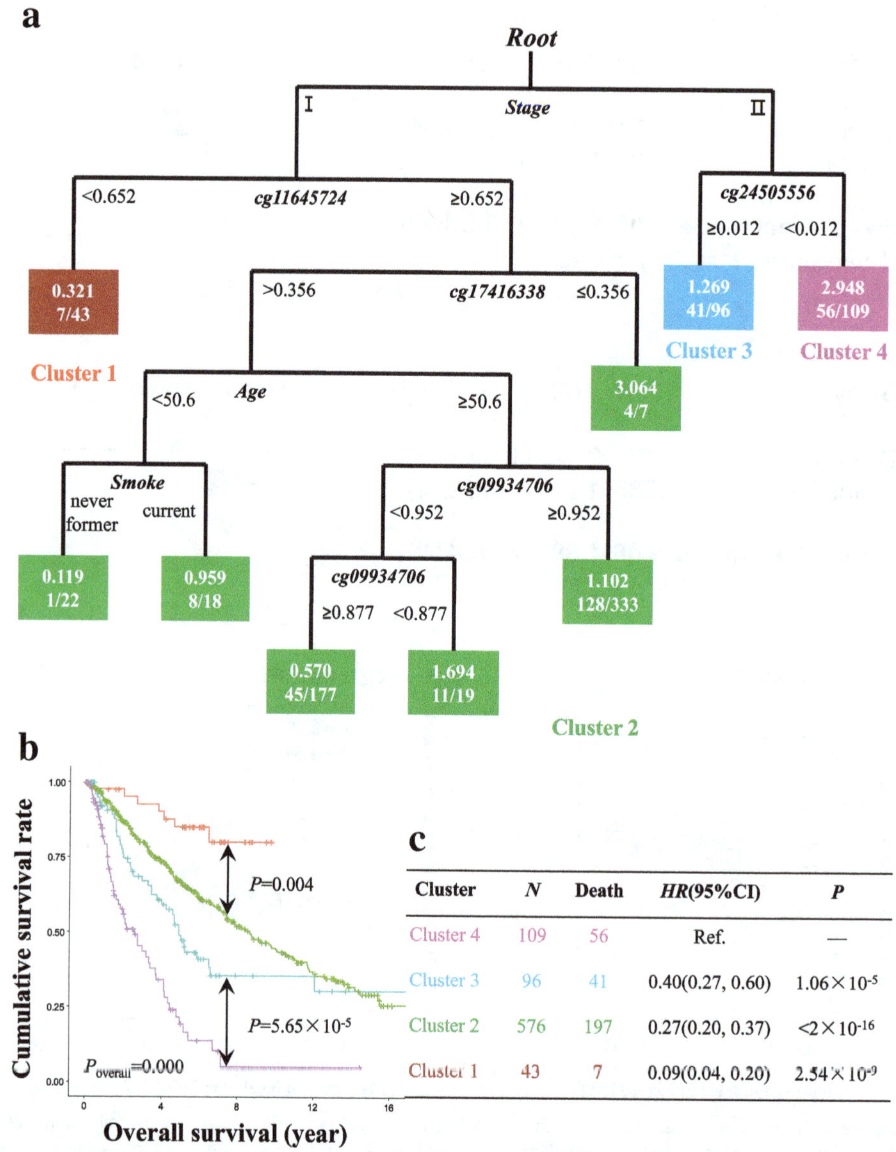

c

Cluster	N	Death	HR(95%CI)	P
Cluster 4	109	56	Ref.	—
Cluster 3	96	41	0.40(0.27, 0.60)	1.06×10^{-5}
Cluster 2	576	197	0.27(0.20, 0.37)	$<2\times10^{-16}$
Cluster 1	43	7	0.09(0.04, 0.20)	2.54×10^{-9}

Fig. 5 Survival classification tree for adenocarcinomas. Survival classification tree was built with seven CpG sites as well as covariates using the merged data of discovery and validation sets among adenocarcinoma cases (**a**), which identified five clusters with significantly different survival curves (**b**). Cox regression was used to compare the outcomes among clusters (cluster 4 as reference) and represented by hazard ratio (*HR*), 95% confidence interval (95%CI), and the *P* value (**c**)

DNA methylation surrounding the transcriptional start site (TSS) has been investigated extensively [27]; generally, hyper-methylation blocks transcription initiation and reduces gene expression [27, 28]. However, DNA methylation at cg11637544 in the first exon of *KDM2A* and at cg26662347 in the 200-kb TSS region of *KDM1A* elevates corresponding expression in tumor tissues. The function of gene body methylation remains unclear. However, functional elements could be in the gene body and could modulate expression through enhancers, transcription factor binding sites, and repetitive elements [29]. Gene body DNA methylation may maintain nucleosome stabilization in transcribed regions and increase transcriptional efficiency either by elongation or by splicing, which, in turn, leads to altered outcomes [30]. Although promoter-associated hyper-methylation mostly downregulates gene expression, a small part of methylation surrounding TSS region upregulates expression [31]. This phenomenon may be mediated by affecting the binding activity of upstream transcription factors [32], which warrants further well-designed functional studies.

As previously reported, overexpression of *KDM1A* and *KDM2A* in NSCLC cells increases cell

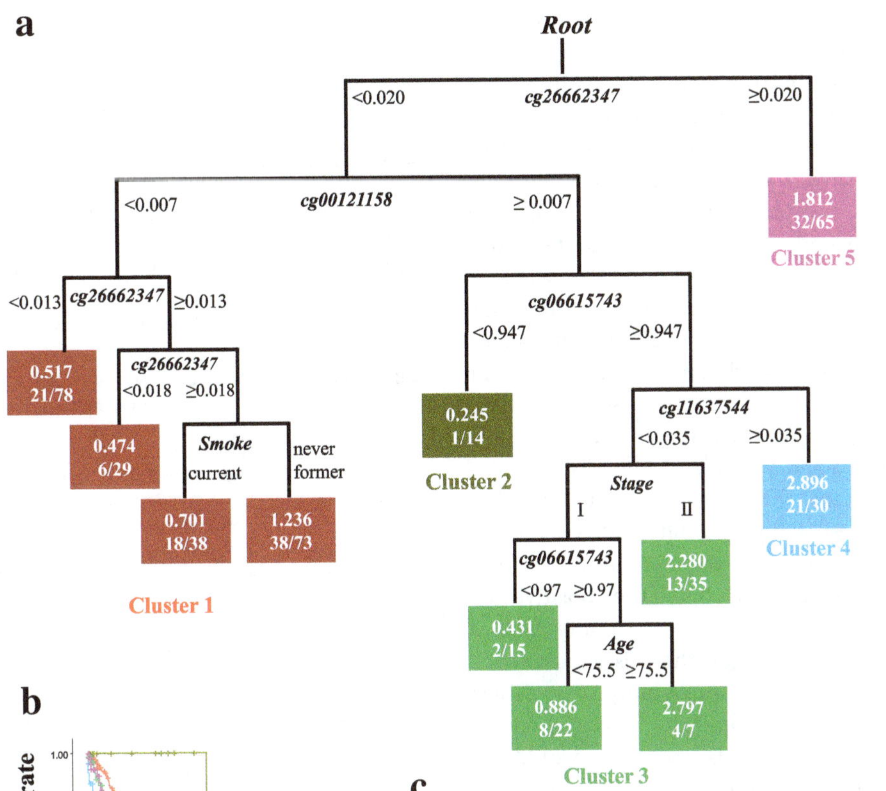

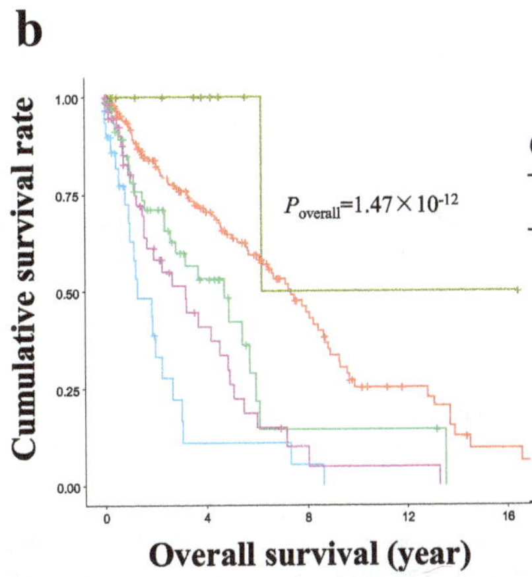

c

Cluster	*N*	Death	*HR*(95%CI)	*P*
Cluster 4	30	21	Ref.	—
Cluster 5	65	32	0.57(0.33, 0.99)	0.047
Cluster 3	79	27	0.39(0.22, 0.70)	0.001
Cluster 1	218	83	0.21(0.13, 0.34)	5.58×10^{-10}
Cluster 2	14	1	0.04(0.01, 0.30)	0.002

Fig. 6 Survival classification tree for squamous cell carcinomas. Survival classification tree was built with five CpG sites as well as covariates using the merged data of discovery and validation sets among adenocarcinoma cases (**a**), which identified four clusters with significantly different survival curves (**b**). Cox regression was used to compare the outcomes among clusters (cluster 4 as reference) and represented by hazard ratio (*HR*), 95% confidence interval (95%CI), and the *P* value (**c**)

proliferation and invasiveness and promotes cancer metastasis [12, 13]. Here, we provided further evidence that those associations appear to be generalizable to patient population. However, functional studies are needed to evaluate the mechanisms that underlie the associations between methylation alterations and survival and the mediating pathway affecting gene transcription. Nevertheless, no promising individual CpG site was identified for adenocarcinoma patients following the stringent criteria, which may due to underlying epigenetic heterogeneity between adenocarcinomas and squamous cell carcinomas [33, 34].

In addition, a comprehensive survival classification tree analysis were also performed to further explore the data by including more potentially associated CpG sites, which identified clusters with significantly different clinical outcome for both adenocarcinomas and squamous cell carcinomas. More *KDM* genes, including *KDM4B*, *KDM2B*, and *KDM4A* for adenocarcinomas and *KDM2B*, *KDM4C*, and *KDM4B* for squamous cell carcinomas, appear to be associated with patients' survival. So far, *KDM2B* has been involved in mechanisms, independently or interactively with microRNAs, for cancers of the blood [35], pancreas [36], breast [37], or stomach [38]. However, the direct impact of *KDM2B* DNA methylation on SCC survival is not well understood and therefore is an area that needs further exploration. *KDM4* histone demethylases is emerging as key regulatory modifiers to histone trimethylated residues that have an important role in cancer development and as a potential therapeutic targets [39]. *KDM4A* is related to mTOR inhibitor sensitivity in SCC patients and impacts copy gains of drug-resistant regions in the genome [17, 40]. *KDM4B* encodes a DNA damage response protein that confers a survival advantage following γ-irradiation [41]. *KDM4C* inhibition by curcuminoids is an adjuvant therapy that can benefit colon cancer patients [42]. However, methylation signals in *KDM4* family members are not individually associated with NSCLC survival, which indicates that there may have interactions of *KDM4* and the other elements.

A major strength of this study is that we used weighted random forest (Ranger) to filter DNA methylation signals. Random forest (RF) is powerful in handling high-dimensional genetic data, but false positive or spurious association may occur if confounding factors are not corrected [43]. In Ranger, there is a parameter from 0 to 1 that represents the probability of variables selected for splitting the tree [26]. If the weight of covariate is given a value of 1, this covariate would be involved in each tree with 100% chance, and thus be controlled. In addition, survival classification tree, a nonparametric and decision-tree-based data mining approach, was used which can improve statistical power and indicate potential interactions between the CpG sites in this study [44, 45]. However, further studies need to be done to validate authenticity and how they interact, which is another area that needs further exploration.

We acknowledge some limitations in our study. First, the positive association between methylation and corresponding gene expression lacks biological evidence. The association should be interpreted with caution, and thus warrants further functional experiments. Second, the censored rate of TCGA cohort is relatively high. Early-stage NSCLC patients could be followed longer to obtain more precise estimates in future. In addition, clinical therapy information after surgery is under informative and not included in this study. Finally, our study did not include other races rather than Caucasian. The findings of this study should be interpreted with caution among other populations. Further studies are needed to investigate their possible differences among multiple ethnicities.

Conclusions

In conclusion, this study highlights the role of somatic epigenetic alterations of *KDM* gene family members on NSCLC overall survival. The findings indicate potential dynamic and reversible therapeutic targets for lung cancer patients and may suggest a high-risk early-stage NSCLC population for adjuvant therapies.

Additional files

Additional file 1: Figure S1. Quality control processes for DNA methylation chip data. Quality control measures and exclusion criteria as applied to Harvard, Spain, Norway, Sweden, and The Cancer Genome Atlas (TCGA) sample cohorts.

Additional file 2: Table S1. Annotation of CpG sites in KDM gene family.

Additional file 3: Table S2. Distributions of CpG sites in KDM genes.

Additional file 4: Figure S2. Analysis work flow. Adenocarcinoma and squamous cell carcinoma samples from Harvard, Spain, Norway, and Sweden cohorts were used for the discovery phase of analysis. Data from The Cancer Genome Atlas (TCGA) were used for Validation. Ranger is a weighted version of random forest for controlling for the covariates including age, gender, smoking status, and histological stage. Variable importance score (VIS) was estimated for each CpG site and was ranked in descending order. CpG sites ranked in top 10% in both discovery and validation sets were selected for further evaluation by Cox regression. Multiple testing correction by false discovery rate (FDR) method was used if necessary.

Additional file 5: Figure S3. DNA methylation probes identified by flexible criterion in squamous cell carcinoma and their correlation with corresponding gene expression. Three more sites were identified in SCC samples under flexible criterion: cg06646494 in *KDM2B*, cg00121158 in *KDM4C*, and cg06615743 in *KDM4B*. The cg00121158 (A) and cg06615743 (B) showed a statistical correlation with the corresponding gene expression. DNA methylation level was categorized to six quantiles and box plot for gene expression was drawn for each quantile. Pearson correlation was used to estimate the correlation coefficient (r) and the *P* value, Gene expression was log2 transformed before analysis.

Abbreviations

95%CI: 95% confidence interval; AC: Lung adenocarcinomas; CART: Classification and regression tree; CV: Coefficient of variance; FDR: False discovery rate; *HR*: Hazard ratio; MGH: Massachusetts General Hospital; NSCLC: Non-small cell lung cancer; QC: Quality control; RF: Random forest; RSEM: RNA Sequencing by Expectation Maximization; SCC: Squamous cell carcinomas; SD: Standard deviation; TCGA: The Cancer Genome Atlas; TSS: Transcriptional start site; VIS: Variable importance scores

Acknowledgements

The authors thank TCGA for contributing the clinical, DNA methylation, and RNA sequencing data as well as all of the study subjects who participated in Harvard LCS and external replication studies.

Funding

This study was supported by the National Natural Science Foundation of China (81530088 and 81473070 to F.C., 81402764 to Y.W., 81402763 to R.Z., and 81373102 to Y.Z.), the National Institute of Health (CA092824 and CA209414 to D.C.C.), State's Key Project of Research and Development Program (2016YFE0204900 to F.C.), Natural Science Foundation of the Jiangsu Higher Education Institutions of China (14KJA310002 to F.C.) and A Project Funded by the Priority Academic Program Development of Jiangsu Higher Education Institutions (PAPD). Y.W. and R.Z. were partially supported by the Outstanding Young Teachers Training Program of Nanjing Medical University. The sponsors had no role in the design of the study, collection and analysis of data, or preparation of the manuscript.

Authors' contributions

YW, JL, RZ, FC, and DCC contributed to the conception and design. DCC, LS, ME, AH, and JS contributed to the collection of samples and assembly of data. YW, JL, RZ, YG, SS, ZW, MT, YZ, FC, XL, SMS, TF, MMB, AK, and MP contributed to the data management and data analysis and interpretation. All coauthors contributed to the manuscript writing, review, and revision. DCC contributed to the financial support and study supervision. All coauthors contributed to the final approval of manuscript.

Competing interests

The authors declare that they have no competing interests.

Author details

[1]Department of Biostatistics, School of Public Health, Nanjing Medical University, Nanjing 211166, China. [2]China International Cooperation Center (CICC) for Environment and Human Health, Nanjing Medical University, Nanjing 211166, China. [3]Department of Environmental Health, Harvard T.H. Chan School of Public Health, Harvard University, Boston, MA 02115, USA. [4]Department of Biostatistics, Harvard T.H. Chan School of Public Health, Harvard University, Boston, MA 02115, USA. [5]Cancer Epigenetics and Biology Program (PEBC), Bellvitge Biomedical Research Institute (IDIBELL), 08908 L'Hospitalet, Barcelona, Catalonia, Spain. [6]Department of Genetics, Institute for Cancer Research, Oslo University Hospital, Oslo, Norway. [7]Division of Oncology and Pathology, Department of Clinical Sciences Lund, Lund University, Medicon Village, SE 22381 Lund, Sweden. [8]Pulmonary and Critical Care Unit, Massachusetts General Hospital, Department of Medicine, Harvard Medical School, Boston, MA 02114, USA.

References

1. Siegel R, Ma J, Zou Z, Jemal A. Cancer statistics, 2014. CA Cancer J Clin. 2014;64(1):9–29. https://doi.org/10.3322/caac.21208:1542-4863.
2. Rami-Porta R, Asamura H, Travis WD, Rusch VW. Lung cancer—major changes in the American Joint Committee on Cancer eighth edition cancer staging manual. CA Cancer J Clin. 2017;67:138–55.
3. Tang S, Pan Y, Wang Y, Hu L, Cao S, Chu M, Dai J, Shu Y, Xu L, Chen J, et al. Genome-wide association study of survival in early-stage non-small cell lung cancer. Ann Surg Oncol. 2015;22:630–5.
4. Heyn H, Esteller M. DNA methylation profiling in the clinic: applications and challenges. Nat Rev Genet. 2012;13:679–92.
5. Bannister AJ, Kouzarides T. Regulation of chromatin by histone modifications. Cell Res. 2011;21:381–95.
6. Thinnes CC, England KS, Kawamura A, Chowdhury R, Schofield CJ, Hopkinson RJ. Targeting histone lysine demethylases—progress, challenges, and the future. Biochim Biophys Acta. 1839;2014:1416–32.
7. Hojfeldt JW, Agger K, Helin K. Histone lysine demethylases as targets for anticancer therapy. Nat Rev Drug Discov. 2013;12:917–30.
8. Black JC, Whetstine JR. Tipping the lysine methylation balance in disease. Biopolymers. 2013;99:127–35.
9. Topper MJ, Vaz M, Chiappinelli KB, DeStefano Shields CE, Niknafs N, Yen RC, Wenzel A, Hicks J, Ballew M, Stone M, et al. Epigenetic therapy ties MYC depletion to reversing immune evasion and treating lung cancer. Cell. 2017; 171:1284–300. e1221
10. Kalin JH, Wu M, Gomez AV, Song Y, Das J, Hayward D, Adejola N, Wu M, Panova I, Chung HJ, et al. Targeting the CoREST complex with dual histone deacetylase and demethylase inhibitors. Nat Commun. 2018;9:53.
11. Maes T, Mascaro C, Ortega A, Lunardi S, Ciceri F, Somervaille TC, Buesa C. KDM1 histone lysine demethylases as targets for treatments of oncological and neurodegenerative disease. Epigenomics. 2015;7:609–26.
12. Kong L, Zhang P, Li W, Yang Y, Tian Y, Wang X, Chen S, Yang Y, Huang T, Zhao T, et al. KDM1A promotes tumor cell invasion by silencing TIMP3 in non-small cell lung cancer cells. Oncotarget. 2016;7:16.
13. Wagner KW, Alam H, Dhar SS, Giri U, Li N, Wei Y, Giri D, Cascone T, Kim JH, Ye Y, et al. KDM2A promotes lung tumorigenesis by epigenetically enhancing ERK1/2 signaling. J Clin Invest. 2013;123:5231–46.
14. Dhar SS, Alam H, Li N, Wagner KW, Chung J, Ahn YW, Lee MG. Transcriptional repression of histone deacetylase 3 by the histone demethylase KDM2A is coupled to tumorigenicity of lung cancer cells. J Biol Chem. 2014;289:7483–96.
15. Black JC, Van Rechem C, Whetstine JR. Histone lysine methylation dynamics: establishment, regulation, and biological impact. Mol Cell. 2012;48:491–507.
16. Van Rechem C, Black JC, Greninger P, Zhao Y, Donado C, Burrowes PD, Ladd B, Christiani DC, Benes CH, Whetstine JR. A coding single nucleotide polymorphism in lysine demethylase KDM4A associates with increased sensitivity to mTOR inhibitors. Cancer Discov. 2015;5:10.
17. Van Rechem C, Black JC, Boukhali M, Aryee MJ, Graslund S, Haas W, Benes CH, Whetstine JR. Lysine demethylase KDM4A associates with translation machinery and regulates protein synthesis. Cancer Discov. 2015;5(3):255-63.
18. Asomaning K, Miller DP, Liu G, Wain JC, Lynch TJ, Su L, Christiani DC. Second hand smoke, age of exposure and lung cancer risk. Lung Cancer. 2008;61:13–20.
19. Sandoval J, Mendez-Gonzalez J, Nadal E, Chen G, Carmona FJ, Sayols S, Moran S, Heyn H, Vizoso M, Gomez A, et al. A prognostic DNA methylation signature for stage I non-small-cell lung cancer. J Clin Oncol. 2013;31:4140–7.
20. Bjaanaes MM, Fleischer T, Halvorsen AR, Daunay A, Busato F, Solberg S, Jorgensen L, Kure E, Edvardsen H, Borresen-Dale AL, et al. Genome-wide DNA methylation analyses in lung adenocarcinomas: association with EGFR, KRAS and TP53 mutation status, gene expression and prognosis. Mol Oncol. 2016;10:330–43.
21. Karlsson A, Jonsson M, Lauss M, Brunnstrom H, Jonsson P, Borg A, Jonsson G, Ringner M, Planck M, Staaf J. Genome-wide DNA methylation analysis of lung carcinoma reveals one neuroendocrine and four adenocarcinoma epitypes associated with patient outcome. Clin Cancer Res. 2014;20:6127–40.
22. Chen YA, Lemire M, Choufani S, Butcher DT, Grafodatskaya D, Zanke BW, Gallinger S, Hudson TJ, Weksberg R. Discovery of cross-reactive probes and polymorphic CpGs in the Illumina Infinium HumanMethylation450 microarray. Epigenetics. 2013;8:203–9.
23. Marabita F, Almgren M, Lindholm ME, Ruhrmann S, Fagerstrom-Billai F, Jagodic M, Sundberg CJ, Ekstrom TJ, Teschendorff AE, Tegner J, Gomez-Cabrero D. An evaluation of analysis pipelines for DNA methylation profiling using the Illumina HumanMethylation450 BeadChip platform. Epigenetics. 2013;8:333–46.
24. Johnson WE, Li C, Rabinovic A. Adjusting batch effects in microarray expression data using empirical Bayes methods. Biostatistics. 2007;8:118–27.
25. Breiman L. Random forests. Mach Learn. 2001;45:5–32.
26. Wright MN, Ziegler A. Ranger: a fast implementation of random forests for high dimensional data in C++ and R. J Stat Softw. 2017;077:1–17.
27. Baylin SB, Jones PA. A decade of exploring the cancer epigenome—biological and translational implications. Nat Rev Cancer. 2011;11:726–34.
28. Brenet F, Moh M, Funk P, Feierstein E, Viale AJ, Socci ND, Scandura JM. DNA methylation of the first exon is tightly linked to transcriptional silencing. PLoS One. 2011;6:e14524.
29. Lomelin D, Jorgenson E, Risch N. Human genetic variation recognizes functional elements in noncoding sequence. Genome Res. 2010;20:311–9.
30. Yang X, Han H, De Carvalho DD, Lay FD, Jones PA, Liang G. Gene body methylation can alter gene expression and is a therapeutic target in cancer. Cancer Cell. 2014;26:577–90.
31. Wagner JR, Busche S, Ge B, Kwan T, Pastinen T, Blanchette M. The relationship between DNA methylation, genetic and expression inter-individual variation in untransformed human fibroblasts. Genome Biol. 2014;15:R37.
32. Maurano MT, Wang H, John S, Shafer A, Canfield T, Lee K, Stamatoyannopoulos JA. Role of DNA methylation in modulating transcription factor occupancy. Cell Rep. 2015;12:1184–95.
33. Cancer Genome Atlas Research N. Comprehensive genomic characterization of squamous cell lung cancers. Nature. 2012;489:519–25.
34. Devarakonda S, Morgensztern D, Govindan R. Genomic alterations in lung adenocarcinoma. Lancet Oncol. 2015;16:e342–51.
35. He J, Nguyen AT, Zhang Y. KDM2b/JHDM1b, an H3K36me2-specific demethylase, is required for initiation and maintenance of acute myeloid leukemia. Blood. 2011;117:3869–80.
36. Tzatsos A, Paskaleva P, Ferrari F, Deshpande V, Stoykova S, Contino G, Wong KK, Lan F, Trojer P, Park PJ, Bardeesy N. KDM2B promotes pancreatic cancer via Polycomb-dependent and -independent transcriptional programs. J Clin Invest. 2013;123:727–39.

37. Kottakis F, Foltopoulou P, Sanidas I, Keller P, Wronski A, Dake BT, Ezell SA, Shen Z, Naber SP, Hinds PW, et al. NDY1/KDM2B functions as a master regulator of polycomb complexes and controls self-renewal of breast cancer stem cells. Cancer Res. 2014;74:3935–46.
38. Hong X, Xu Y, Qiu X, Zhu Y, Feng X, Ding Z, Zhang S, Zhong L, Zhuang Y, Su C, et al. MiR-448 promotes glycolytic metabolism of gastric cancer by downregulating KDM2B. Oncotarget. 2016;7:22092–102.
39. Berry WL, Janknecht R. KDM4/JMJD2 histone demethylases: epigenetic regulators in cancer cells. Cancer Res. 2013;73:2936–42.
40. Black JC, Manning AL, Van Rechem C, Kim J, Ladd B, Cho J, Pineda CM, Murphy N, Daniels DL, Montagna C, et al. KDM4A lysine demethylase induces site-specific copy gain and rereplication of regions amplified in tumors. Cell. 2013;154:541–55.
41. Young LC, McDonald DW, Hendzel MJ. Kdm4b histone demethylase is a DNA damage response protein and confers a survival advantage following gamma-irradiation. J Biol Chem. 2013;288:21376–88.
42. Kim TD, Fuchs JR, Schwartz E, Abdelhamid D, Etter J, Berry WL, Li C, Ihnat MA, Li PK, Janknecht R. Pro-growth role of the JMJD2C histone demethylase in HCT-116 colon cancer cells and identification of curcuminoids as JMJD2 inhibitors. Am J Transl Res. 2014;6:236–47.
43. Zhao Y, Chen F, Zhai R, Lin X, Wang Z, Su L, Christiani DC. Correction for population stratification in random forest analysis. Int J Epidemiol. 2012;41:1798–806.
44. Wu X, Gu J, Grossman HB, Amos CI, Etzel C, Huang M, Zhang Q, Millikan RE, Lerner S, Dinney CP. Bladder cancer predisposition: a multigenic approach to DNA-repair and cell-cycle–control genes. Am J Hum Genet. 2006;78:464.
45. Chen M, Kamat AM, Huang M, Grossman HB, Dinney CP, Lerner SP, Wu X, Gu J. High-order interactions among genetic polymorphisms in nucleotide excision repair pathway genes and smoking in modulating bladder cancer risk. Carcinogenesis. 2007;28:2160–5.

Aberrant expression and DNA methylation of lipid metabolism genes in PCOS: a new insight into its pathogenesis

Jie-Xue Pan[1,2,4], Ya-Jing Tan[1], Fang-Fang Wang[2], Ning-Ning Hou[2], Yu-Qian Xiang[1], Jun-Yu Zhang[1], Ye Liu[1], Fan Qu[2], Qing Meng[2], Jian Xu[2], Jian-Zhong Sheng[2,3] and He-Feng Huang[1,2*]

Abstract

Background: Polycystic ovary syndrome (PCOS), whose etiology remains uncertain, is a highly heterogenous and genetically complex endocrine disorder. The aim of this study was to identify differentially expressed genes (DEGs) in granulosa cells (GCs) from PCOS patients and make epigenetic insights into the pathogenesis of PCOS.

Results: Included in this study were 110 women with PCOS and 119 women with normal ovulatory cycles undergoing in vitro fertilization acting as the control group. RNA-seq identified 92 DEGs unique to PCOS GCs in comparison with the control group. Bioinformatic analysis indicated that synthesis of lipids and steroids was activated in PCOS GCs. 5-Methylcytosine analysis demonstrated that there was an approximate 25% reduction in global DNA methylation of GCs in PCOS women (4.44 ± 0.65%) compared with the controls (6.07 ± 0.72%; $P < 0.05$). Using MassArray EpiTYPER quantitative DNA methylation analysis, we also found hypomethylation of several gene promoters related to lipid and steroid synthesis, which might result in the aberrant expression of these genes.

Conclusions: Our results suggest that hypomethylated genes related to the synthesis of lipid and steroid may dysregulate expression of these genes and promote synthesis of steroid hormones including androgen, which could partially explain mechanisms of hyperandrogenism in PCOS.

Keywords: Polycystic ovary syndrome, RNA-seq, Methylation, Hyperandrogenism, Synthesis of lipid and steroid

Background

Polycystic ovary syndrome (PCOS), characterized by chronic anovulation and hyperandrogenism, is one of the most prevalent endocrine disorders in women of reproductive age [1]. It is also thought to be the leading cause of anovulatory infertility [1]. There is no single etiologic factor that fully accounts for the pathogenesis of PCOS, and several lines of evidence demonstrate that PCOS is a complex and multifactorial disorder with a high degree of heritability [2]. The high degree of familial aggregation of PCOS suggests that genetic factor plays an important role in its etiology [3, 4]. Recent genetic studies have been performed without adding significant new knowledge to the field [5, 6].

There is evidence indicating that epigenetic alterations, including aberrant DNA methylation might contribute to the development of PCOS [7]. DNA methylation is a highly tissue-specific phenomenon that varies with time on the basis of environmental fluctuations [8]. It is involved in the stability of gene expression during organismal development [9, 10]. Specific genes such as *LHR* [11], *EPHX1* [12], and *CYP19A1* [13] have been demonstrated to be associated with PCOS with aberrant DNA methylation in distinct tissues. In a recent genome-wide study, Wang et al. reported that DNA methylation and gene expression differences exist between PCOS and non-PCOS ovaries [14]. Our previous work has also indicated that epigenetic alterations of several important transcription factors are involved in the follicular development in granulosa cells (GCs) that contribute to PCOS [7].

* Correspondence: huanghefg@hotmail.com
[1]The International Peace Maternity and Child Health Hospital, School of Medicine, Shanghai Jiao Tong University, Shanghai 200030, China
[2]The Key Laboratory of Reproductive Genetics, Ministry of Education (Zhejiang University), Hangzhou, Zhejiang 310006, China
Full list of author information is available at the end of the article

Ovarian androgen excess is the most typical pathological manifestation of PCOS [1, 15]. The mechanisms underlying androgen excess and abnormal follicular development in PCOS remain to be elucidated. In this study, we identified differentially expressed genes (DEGs) with global transcriptome sequencing and highlighted the abnormal biological pathways among these DEGs in the GCs of PCOS women. We compared global DNA methylation of GCs between control and PCOS groups. Furthermore, DNA methylation levels of selected genes were evaluated with MassArray EpiTYPER. The correlations between gene expression and differential methylation of CpG sites were also analyzed. The altered expression level of genes related to lipid metabolism and steroid synthesis combined with the disarranged DNA methylation in GCs of PCOS women suggest that abnormal lipid metabolism and steroid synthesis and epigenetic dysregulation play important roles in the pathogenesis of PCOS.

Results

Patient demographic data and clinical features

The clinical characteristics of PCOS women and controls are shown in Table 1. Enrolled cases and controls were of comparable age and fasting glucose levels. Significant differences between the two groups ($P < 0.05$) were found in menstrual cycle length, body mass index (BMI), antral follicle count (AFC), fasting insulin, HOMA-IR (homeostasis model assessment of insulin resistance), ratio of serum luteinizing hormone (LH)/follicle-stimulating hormone (FSH), serum TT (total testosterone) levels on the third day of spontaneous menstrual cycle, and concentration of TT, sex hormone-binding globulin (SHBG), FAI (free androgen index), and insulin in the follicular fluids (FFs). All these values mentioned above were greater for PCOS group than those in controls except for SHBG, which is lower in PCOS women.

Identification of DEGs in GCs between PCOS patients and controls

To determine DEGs, GCs from three non-obese PCOS and three comparable control women were studied. Clinical characteristics of each participant are presented in Additional file 1: Table S3. According to the inspected RNA-seq data, all the quality control parameters were within the acceptable ranges. A total of 23,675 annotated Ensembl genes were detected and included in subsequent analysis (Additional file 2: Dataset S1), of which 12,814 genes were upregulated and 10,861 genes were downregulated in GCs of PCOS women (Fig. 1a). After

Table 1 Demographic data and clinic characteristics of the IVF patients who participated in the study

Items	Control ($n = 119$)	PCOS ($n = 110$)	P value
Age	29.85 ± 0.37	29.11 ± 0.35	0.149
Body mass index	21.74 ± 0.29	22.79 ± 0.36	0.024
Cycle length (days)	29.00 ± 0.22	67.73 ± 6.40	< 0.001
Duration of infertility	4.24 ± 0.30	3.91 ± 0.26	0.416
Fasting glucose (mmol/L)	4.65 ± 0.04	4.75 ± 0.05	0.068
Fasting insulin (pmol/L)*	70.29 ± 2.99	100.19 ± 5.35	< 0.001
HOMA-IR*	2.00 ± 0.09	2.96 ± 0.16	< 0.001
Day 3 LH/FSH	0.72 ± 0.04	1.48 ± 0.09	< 0.001
Day 3 TT (nmol/L)	0.78 ± 0.03	3.02 ± 0.14	< 0.001
Day 3 DHEA-S (μmol/L)	6.61 ± 0.24	7.62 ± 0.33	0.013
Day 3 E_2 (pmol/L)	130.69 ± 4.63	148.47 ± 7.96	0.055
AFC	9.92 ± 0.30	20.45 ± 0.39	< 0.001
Androstenedione (ng/ml) in FF#	6.62 ± 1.06	7.25 ± 1.28	0.345
TT (ng/ml) in FF#	4.87 ± 0.49	9.25 ± 1.21	0.022
SHBG (nmol/L) in FF#	57.70 ± 3.01	53.06 ± 3.14	0.042
FAI in FF#	31.63 ± 4.34	69.28 ± 13.81	0.024
Insulin (mU/L) in FF#	37.51 ± 3.13	48.45 ± 3.50	0.024
Retrieved oocyte number	12.58 ± 0.64	17.63 ± 0.89	< 0.001

Values are presented as mean ± SE. P value was determined by Student's t tests

HOMA-IR homeostasis model assessment of insulin resistance, *Day 3* the third day of spontaneous menstrual cycle, *LH* luteinizing hormone, *FSH* follicle stimulating hormone, *TT* total testosterone, *DHEA-S* dehydroepiandrosterone-sulfate, E_2 estradiol, *AFC* antral follicle count, *FF* follicular fluid, *SHBG* sex hormone binding globulin, *FAI* free androgen index

*$n = 53$ in control and $n = 50$ in PCOS

#$n = 50$ in control and $n = 71$ in PCOS

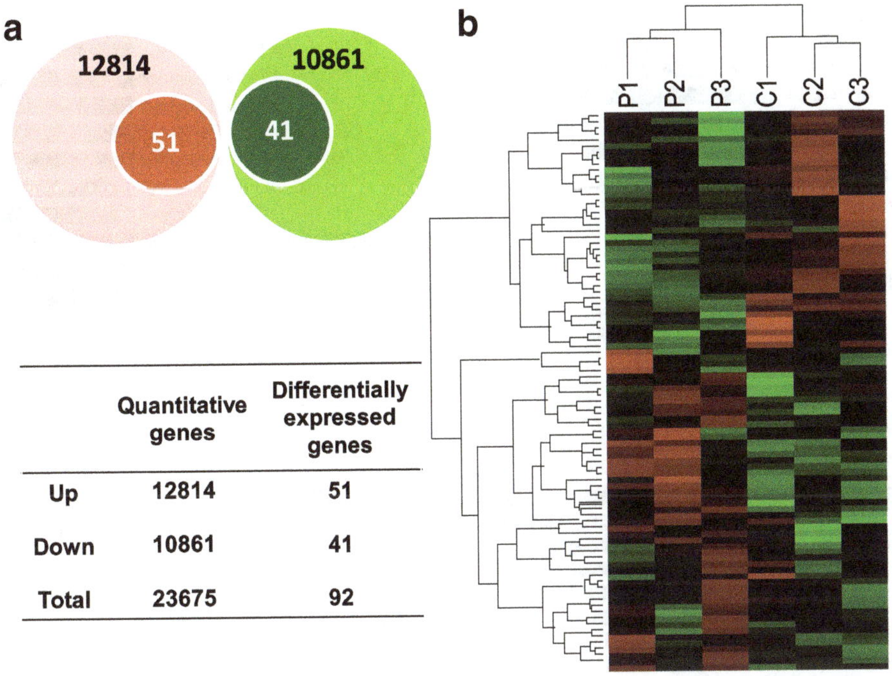

	Quantitative genes	Differentially expressed genes
Up	12814	51
Down	10861	41
Total	23675	92

Fig. 1 Differentially expressed genes in GCs between PCOS and control women. **a** Venn diagram showing the number of differentially expressed genes in GCs between the PCOS and control group. Red indicates upregulated genes, and green denotes downregulated genes. **b** Hierarchal clustering presentation of differentially expressed genes identified in GCs. Each row represents a single gene, and each column represents an experimental sample. Increasing green intensities denote genes that decrease in expression, and increasing red intensities denote gene that increases in expression in PCOS samples compared with control samples

applying statistical analysis ($P < 0.05$), a fold change (FC) criterion (fold change in gene expression levels between pathological and control GCs) > 1.5, and the false discovery rate (FDR) < 0.05, 92 genes were significantly differentially expressed in GCs of PCOS compared with controls, including 51 upregulated genes and 41 downregulated genes (Additional file 3: Dataset S2). Hierarchical clustering was performed on the dataset of DEGs (Fig. 1b). The results showed a striking separation between the two groups into two major opposite branches, indicating that the genes expressed in GCs of PCOS women were significantly different from those of controls.

Bioinformatic analysis of DEGs

To better understand the potential function of the 92 DEGs, Ingenuity Pathway Analysis (IPA) was used to further analyze the expression data in the context of known biological responses as well as other higher order response pathways to assign functional information and biological relevance to these DEGs. These results are presented as negative logarithm of the significance level, which is a statistical score measuring the likelihood of the genes in a given network being found together through Fisher's exact test. Based on the expression data of 92 DEGs, functional analysis showed that these DEGs were enriched in the category of diseases and disorder, molecular and cellular functions, and physiological system development and function (Fig. 2a–c). Within the category of diseases and disorders, the inflammatory response, reproductive system disease, and endocrine system disorders were included on the top ten related dysfunctions. Within the category of molecular and cell functions, cell death and survival, cell-to-cell signaling and interaction, cellular movement, and lipid metabolism were listed in the top related functions. Within the category of development and functions, the endocrine system development and function was also involved. The further downstream effect analysis of DEGs between the PCOS and control groups predicated that the synthesis of lipid was activated (z score = 2.014) in the PCOS group (Fig. 2d). The other lipid metabolism biological processes, such as steroidogenesis of hormone (z score = 1.253), the quantity of steroid (z score = 1.411), synthesis of steroid (z score = 1.253), and synthesis of terpenoid (z score = 1.253) might also be activated in the PCOS group (Fig. 2d). These alterations were in accordance with the hyperandrogenism of PCOS.

Validation of DEGs related to lipid and steroid metabolism with qPCR

To confirm the RNA-seq results, 12 upregulated genes and three downregulated genes related to lipid

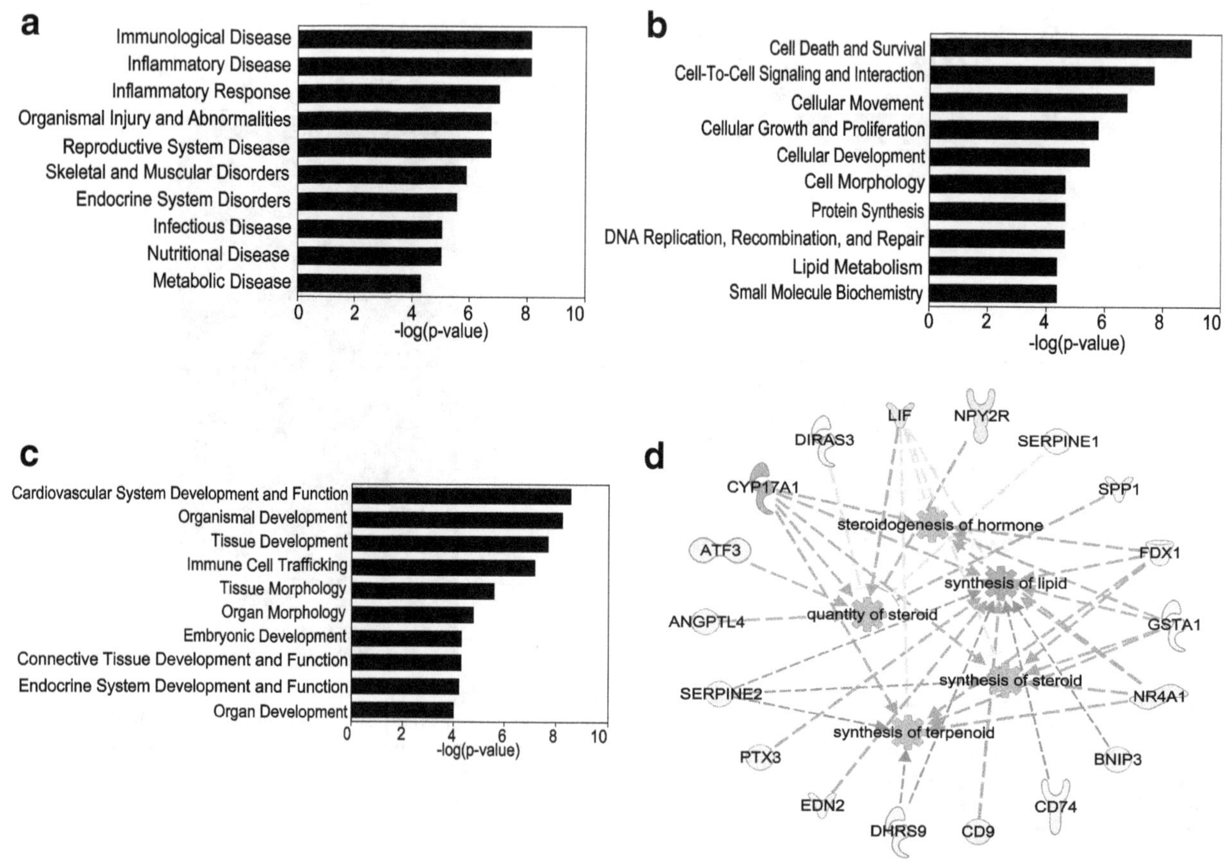

Fig. 2 Bioinformatic analysis of the RNA-seq results. Ingenuity Pathway Analysis was used, which analyzes the expression data in the context of known biological response and regulatory networks as well as other higher order response pathways, to assign functional information and biological relevance. **a**–**c** Functional analysis of 92 DEGs. The top 10 influenced biofunctions are grouped by disease and disorder (**a**), molecular and cell functions (**b**), and physiological system development and functions (**c**). Results are shown as the negative logarithm of significance, which is a statistical score and a measure of the likelihood of the genes in a given network being found together as a result of chance, as determined by Fisher's exact test. Downstream effects analysis of DEGs predicts activated lipid metabolism in GCs from PCOS women (**d**)

and steroid metabolism were identified with qPCR (Fig. 3). GCs from 93 control and 79 PCOS women were enrolled in this part of the study. The results of qPCR showed that the expression of related genes were in accordance with the RNA-seq analysis results.

Global DNA methylation of GCs from PCOS women and controls

To compare the global DNA methylation level of the GCs between PCOS and controls, we assessed the levels of 5-mC in the genomic DNA of GCs by ELISA with antibody specific to 5-mC. As shown in Fig. 4, the global DNA methylation levels were $6.07 \pm 0.72\%$ and $4.44 \pm 0.65\%$ in the GCs from control and PCOS groups, respectively. We observed a significant reduction of approximately 25% in the level of 5-mC in GCs from PCOS women compared with controls ($P < 0.05$).

MassArray EpiTYPER quantitative DNA methylation analysis of target genes

We analyzed DNA methylation of 15 DEGs related to lipid metabolism and synthesis of steroid hormones, including *GSTA1, CD74, ANGPTL4, CD9, NR4A1, EDN2, PTX3, LIF, SLC12A8, PEX3, CYP17A1, SERPINE1, DIRAS3, BNIP3*, and *SPP1*. With the UCSC Genome Browser (http://www.genome.ucsc.edu/) and online primer designer—Epidesigner (http://www.epidesigner.com), we found that *GSTA1* and *CD74* possessed no obvious CpG islands or intensive CpG clusters in their promoter regions. We then investigated the methylation level of each CpG site or cluster in the promoters of the other 13 DEGs verified by qPCR (*ANGPTL4, CD9, NR4A1, EDN2, PTX3, LIF, SLC12A8, PEX3, CYP17A1, SERPINE1, DIRAS3, BNIP3, SPP1*) in 16 GC DNA samples (8 PCOS women and 8 controls, the first cohort). We found no significant differences in the methylation levels of CpG sites or clusters of *ANGPTL4, CYP17A1, PEX3, DIRAS3, PTX3*, and *SLC12A8* and amplicon for

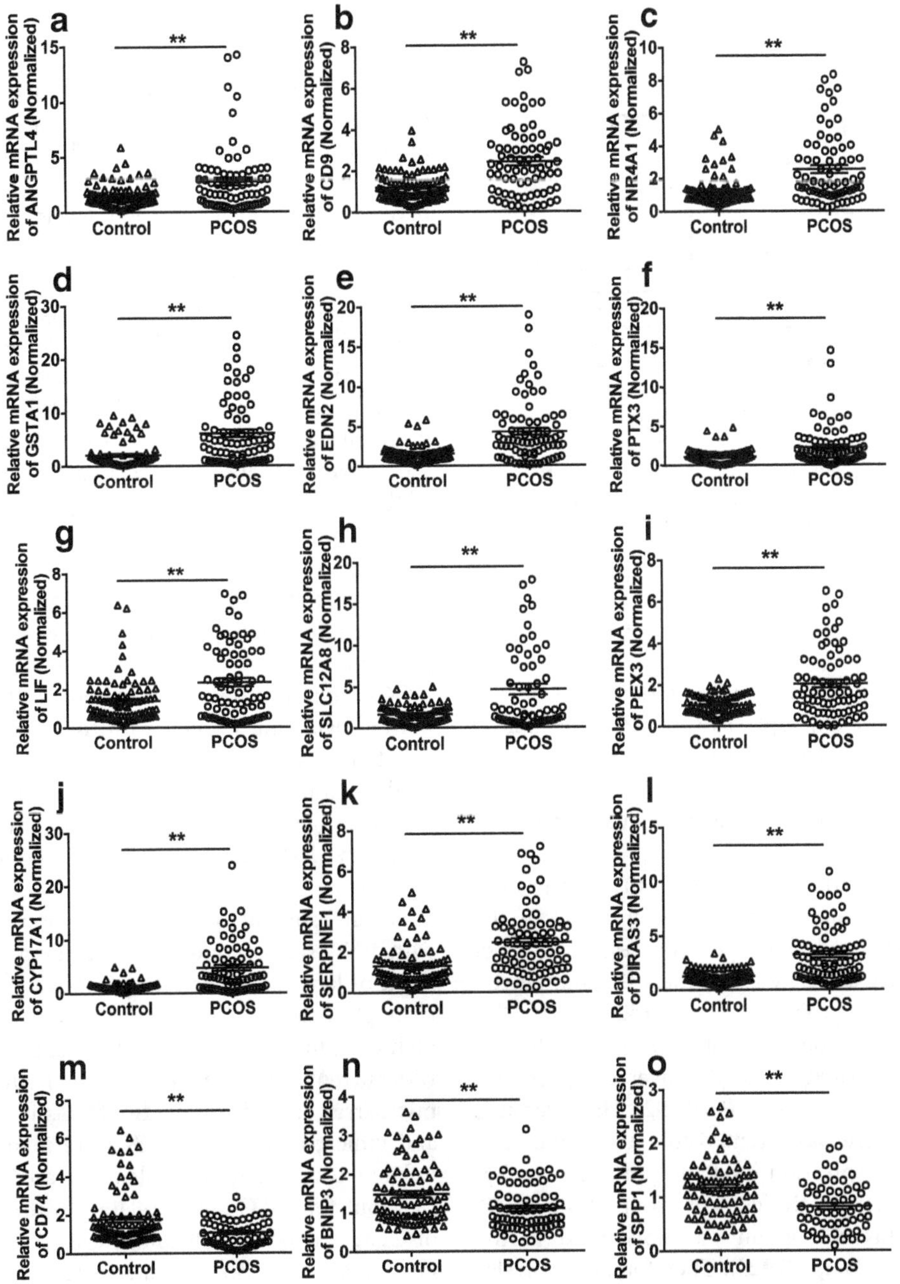

Fig. 3 Verification of 15 differentially expressed genes related to lipid metabolism and steroid synthesis identified by RNA-seq. The mRNA expression levels for 15 DEGs in GCs of control ($n = 93$) and PCOS women ($n = 79$). **a–l** are upregulated and **m–o** are downregulated in transcription analysis and qPCR. Data are presented as mean ± SE. P value is determined by independent samples t test. *, **, $P < 0.05$ and $P < 0.01$, compared with the corresponding controls, respectively

SPP1 (primer 1) in the GCs between PCOS and control women (Additional file 4: Figure S1a–h). Although two CpG sites in the promoter of *SERPINE1* were hypomethylated, it is probably meaningless for such a low methylation level of these sites (Additional file 4: Figure S1i). Significant differences were found in the methylation levels of some CpG sites or clusters in the promoter regions of *CD9*, *BNIP3*, *EDN2*, *NR4A1*, *LIF*, and *SPP1* (primer 2) between PCOS and control women. To confirm these differences, we further validated the significance of the results in a second cohort consisting of 30 controls and 39 PCOS women. We found that a cluster of CpG sites in the promoter regions of *CD9*, *NR4A1*, *EDN2*, and *BNIP3* were hypomethylated (Fig. 5a–c, e) and that a single CpG site (CpG_8, -780) in the promoter region of LIF was also hypomethylated (Fig. 5d).

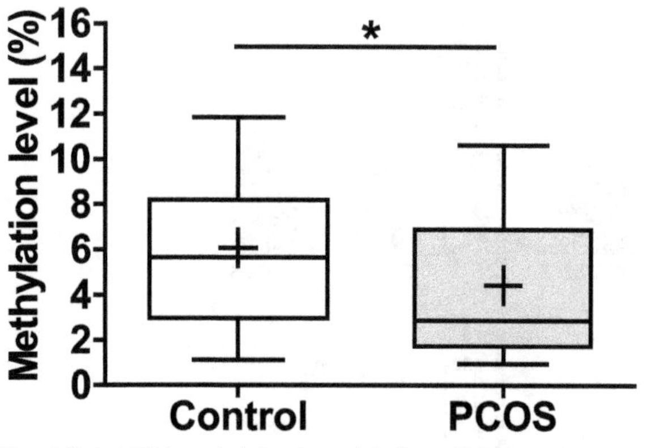

Fig. 4 Global DNA methylation box plots. For each group, the bottom and top bars indicate the 10th and 90th percentiles, respectively. The bottom and top of each box indicate the 25th and 75th percentiles, the line through the middle of each box represents the median, and the mean value for each group is noted by (+) in each box. Thirty GC genomic DNA from controls and 39 GC genomic DNA from PCOS women were analyzed. *P* value is determined by Mann-Whitney *U* test. *, $P < 0.05$, compared with the controls

However, we did not find significant difference in the methylation level of any CpG site of *SPP1* (primer 2) between PCOS and control women (Fig. 5f).

The influence of promoter methylation status on gene expression

We analyzed the relationship between the methylation levels of CpG sites and gene expression levels of the differentially methylated genes. The expression level of *CD9* was negatively correlated with the average methylation level of *CD9* promoter ($R = -0.420$, $P = 0.023$) (Fig. 5a). The expression level of *BNIP3* was also, to some extent, correlated with the average promoter methylation status ($R = -0.186$, $P = 0.292$). However, it is noteworthy that there was a remarkably negative correlation between the expression level and promoter methylation level of *BNIP3* in the control group ($R = -0.740$, $P = 0.001$), but this correlation was not found in the PCOS group ($R = 0.23$, $P = 0.923$). Therefore, the correlations of these two groups are fully independent of each other. We did not observe significant correlation between the expression level and promoter methylation level of *EDN2*. The expression of *LIF* was negatively correlated with the promoter methylation level ($R = -0.565$, $P = 0.001$) (Fig. 5d). There is a mildly negative correlation between the expression level and promoter methylation level of *NR4A1* ($R = -0.355$, $P = 0.054$).

Discussion

In the present study, we identified 92 DEGs in GCs of PCOS women compared to those of control women. Bioinformatic analysis showed that lipid metabolism was significantly activated in GCs from PCOS women. We also found that global methylation level of DNA in GCs from PCOS women was lower than that of control women. Consistent with these findings, further analysis demonstrated that the differentially methylated genes involved in lipid metabolism and steroid synthesis were hypomethylated and there were negative correlations between the gene expression levels and the promoter methylation levels.

Most women (60–80%) with PCOS have hyperandrogenism [1] and excessive circulating androgens that are mostly from the ovary. Therefore, some physician scientists surmise that abnormal steroidogenesis might be the primary pathogenesis of PCOS [16]; however, such a mechanism needs to be further investigated. GCs around the oocyte are closely associated with the development of the female gamete in the ovary [17] and are involved in steroid synthesis and metabolism [18]. Therefore, profiling the gene expression pattern of GCs and performing deep analysis on the genes related to lipid and steroid metabolism are significant contributions to the field.

GCs from 110 unrelated women with PCOS and 119 normal ovulating women with the comparable age were selected to minimize the influences of age on epigenetic modifications [19]. Cases enrolled in this study showed the main characteristics of PCOS: hyperandrogenism, ovulatory dysfunction, and increased number of antral follicles.

Global profiling of gene expression in target organs with RNA-seq is continuously leading to the establishment of key molecules that potentially participate in the pathophysiology of various diseases. However, due to the high cost, this method is not frequently used as microarrays currently. In a previous study, Kaur et al. employed microarray analysis to identify DEGs in GCs from PCOS and indicated that the DEGs were involved in diabetes, inflammation, cardiovascular diseases, and infertility [20], but few DEGs were related to the major functions of GCs. Crucial for folliculogenesis is GC-oocyte signaling, which relies on free fatty acid beta-oxidation as an energy source for meiosis [21–24]. In our study, 92 DEGs were identified in GCs from PCOS women, and functional analysis showed that 18 DEGs, approximately 20% of all identified DEGs, participated in lipid metabolism. The synthesis of lipid and steroid was significantly activated in the GCs of PCOS women. Increased lipid synthesis in GCs provided steroidal precursor for androgen [25]. Hyperandrogenism, the most constant and prominent diagnostic component of PCOS, is correlated with excess lipid synthesis. The mechanism and causal relationship need to be further explored.

BNIP3 plays a critical function in lipid metabolism [26, 27], and BNIP3 deficiency participates in excess

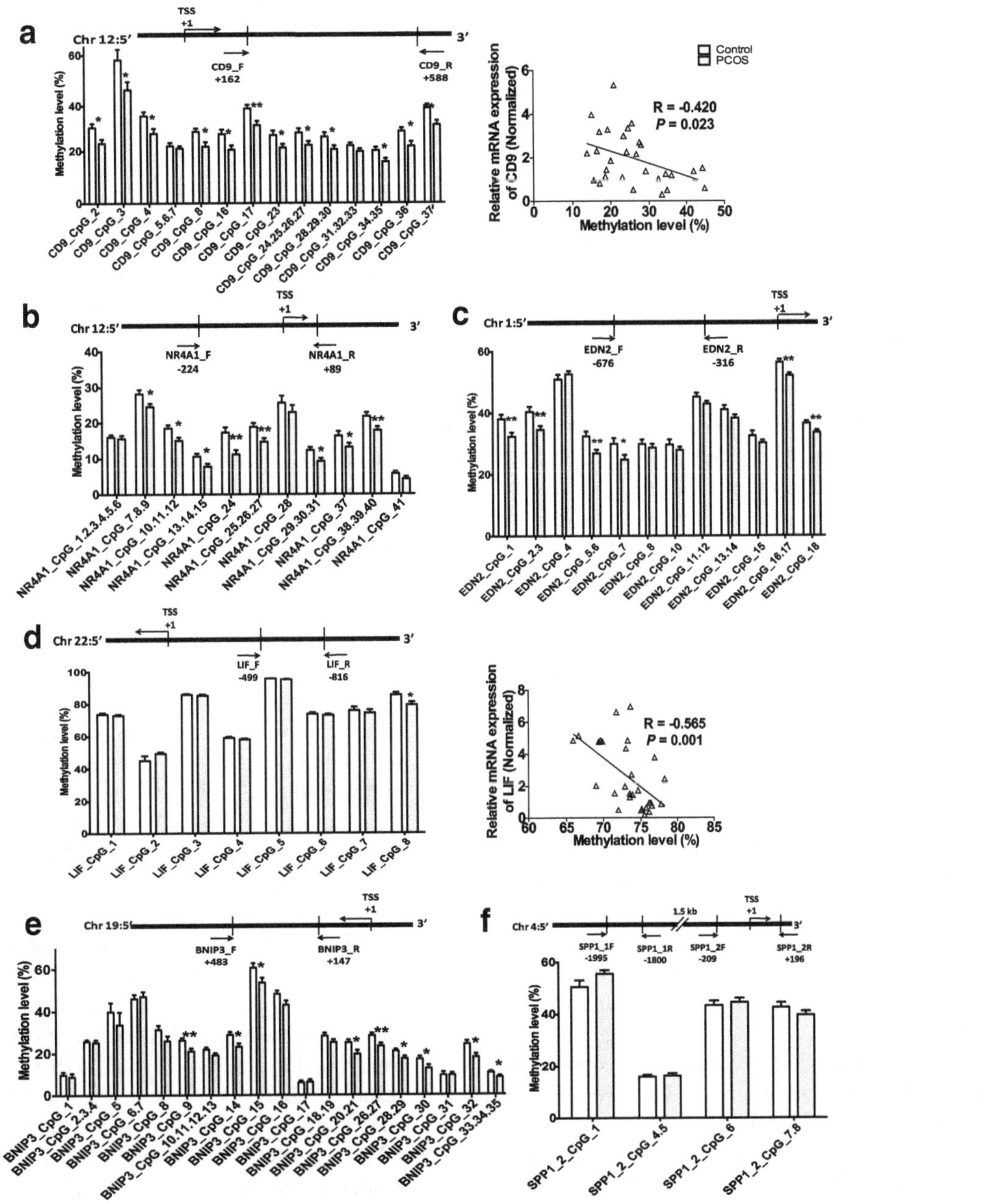

Fig. 5 MassARRAY quantitative methylation analysis of promoter CpG sites of target genes. **a** The schematic diagram of amplicon in the promoter region of CD9 (up). The mean methylation levels for each CpG site of the *CD9* promoter (down). The correlations between *CD9* mRNA expression level and the average CpG site methylation level in the promoter of *CD9* (right). **b** The schematic diagram of amplicon in the promoter region of *NR4A1* (up). The mean methylation levels for each CpG site of the *NR4A1* promoter (down). **c** The schematic diagram of amplicon in the promoter region of *EDN2* (up). The mean methylation levels for each CpG site of the *EDN2* promoter (down). **d** The schematic diagram of amplicon in the promoter region of *LIF* (up). The mean methylation levels for each CpG site of the *LIF* promoter (down). The associations between average methylation level of *LIF* and its expression (right). **e** The schematic diagram of amplicon in the promoter region of *BNIP3* (up). The mean methylation levels for each CpG site of the *BNIP3* promoter (down). **f** The schematic diagram of amplicon in the promoter region of SPP1 (up). The mean methylation levels for each CpG site of the *SPP1* promoter amplified by primer 2 (down). Binding sties for each of the forward and reverse primers are shown as arrows below the diagram. Values are mean ± SE. Thirty-eight GC genomic DNA from controls and 47 GC genomic DNA from PCOS women were analyzed. *P* value is determined by Mann-Whitney *U* test. * represents $P < 0.05$, ** represents $P < 0.01$

lipid accumulation [27]. The decreased expression of BNIP3 in GCs from PCOS women probably results in excessive synthesis of lipid, which provides precursors for the biosynthesis of androgen in follicles, thus participating in hyperandrogenism. BNIP3 is localized to the outer mitochondrial membrane, where it functions in mitophagy and mitochondrial dynamics. BNIP3, binding directly to LC3 and recruiting the growing autophagosome to mitochondria, is also implicated in the induction of autophagy [28], which often leads to cell death and necrosis. The aberrant low expression of BNIP3 in GCs of PCOS women may be involved in apoptotic deficiency of follicular cells from PCOS women [29], which is associated with polycystic ovarian morphology.

NR4A1, a member of orphan nuclear receptors, initiates gene transcription by various stimuli [30]. It has been described to play a role in lipolysis [31] and promote the transcription of key steroidogenic enzymes in ovarian theca cells, thus enhancing the capacity of the ovarian theca cells to produce androgen [29]. Elevated expression of NR4A1 in GCs may also promote the androgen biosynthesis in PCOS women. Furthermore, NR4A1 is also a clock-related gene, which shows a circadian rhythm in different tissues [32, 33]. Disturbed circadian rhythm could be another point-cut for exploring the pathophysiology of PCOS.

PCOS is considered as a complicated disorder and has certain genetic basis [2]. The heritability of this disorder goes beyond simple Mendelian genetics. Epigenetic and environmental factors have been proposed as confounding factors that modulate the phenotype of genetic basis of PCOS [7, 34]. DNA methylation patterns are neither fixed nor consistent among different tissues and have highly spatio-temporal dynamics that require continuous regulation [35–37].

An approximate 25% reduction was observed in the global DNA methylation level of GCs from PCOS compared with matched controls. This hypomethylation of the genome is believed to result in chromosomal and genomic instability [38–40]. Consistent with reduced global methylation levels in GCs from PCOS women, most of the differentially methylated sites of the genes involved in lipid metabolism and steroid synthesis were also hypomethylated. This is the first epigenetic study to investigate whether global DNA methylation is altered in follicular cells in PCOS women compared with matched controls. Although Xu et al. got a negative result about the global DNA methylation status of peripheral blood between the PCOS and control women [41], it was of great significance to evaluate the global DNA methylation level of follicular cells, especially to quantify the methylation level of a specific CpG site. Recently, Wang et al. carried out a genome-wide DNA methylation analysis in PCOS ovaries and identified 7982 differentially methylated CpG sites [14]. Among those sites, 59.8% were hypermethylated and 40.2% were hypomethylated. This result was neither consistent with nor contradictory to our results. The difference between this study and our own could be interpreted in two aspects. Firstly, the collected tissue by Wang et al. was the ovary tissue, not GCs. Secondly, the control ovaries were obtained from cervical cancer patients who were much older (37.00 ± 5.20 years) than the case group (23.33 ± 2.89 years). A major strength of our study was the comparability of the cases and controls, as age has been reported to affect the methylation status [42]. We matched the two groups and tried to exclude the age-associated epigenetic drift that might affect the global DNA methylation level and the CpG site-specific methylation level of target genes.

The causal relationship between the changes in promoter DNA methylation level and differences in gene expression has been well established [43]. In our study, the expression of the DEGs was at least partially negatively correlated with the average methylation level of the CpG sites in the promoter regions of the differentially methylated genes. DNA methylation regulates gene expression via recruitment of transcriptional factors. However, the correlation was compromised in PCOS women, especially for BNIP3. As for LIF, there was only one differentially methylated CpG site; however, the prediction of transcription factors by TFSEARCH (http://diyhpl.us/~bryan/irc/protocol-online/protocol-cache/TFSEARCH.html) and DBD: Transcription factor prediction database (http://www.transcriptionfactor.org/index.cgi) revealed that the differentially methylated CpG site was the binding site for nuclear respiratory factor 2 (NRF-2). NRF-2, as a transcription factor, is involved in the activation of cytochrome oxidase expression and the nuclear control of mitochondrial function [44, 45]. Loss of methylation in this site may result in abnormal recruitment of NRF-2, which would contribute to aberrant gene expression of LIF.

Folate provides methyl groups for the formation of *S*-adenosylmethionine (SAM) [46], the major methyl donor required for DNA methylation [47]. It is well established that folate supplementation can increase global DNA methylation and affect gene expression [48, 49]. Multiple studies have identified increased homocysteine, an indicator of folate deficiency, in women with PCOS [50, 51], and supplementation with folate is useful to increase the beneficial effect of metformin on the vascular endothelium [52]. Considering the role of global DNA hypomethylation in the GCs of PCOS in our study, we speculate that it is advisable to utilize folate to prevent the global loss of methylation for PCOS women, especially for those undergoing IVF procedure. However, prospective study on this subject should be carried out to determine the appropriate dose and administration duration of folate supplementation.

The limitations of this study should be noted. First, the cells collected in this study are derived from IVF procedure and are a mixture of cumulus and mural GCs and macrophages, as well as are predominantly luteinized mural GCs. It is important to further confirm our findings in non-luteinized GCs. Second, the cohort analyzed by RNA-seq is small and should be considered as a pilot study. Finally, though the enrolled subjects in the two groups were of comparable fasting glucose, the PCOS patients had greater BMI and higher fasting insulin levels and HOMA-IR, which indicates obesity and insulin resistance is more prevalent in the enrolled PCOS women. Altered DNA methylation patterns could be a result of PCOS itself or endocrine and metabolic disturbances of the condition [53, 54]. Therefore, it is of significance to analyze the differential methylation status between women with comparable nutrient status or confirm the epigenetic changes after balancing the endocrine or metabolic profiles of PCOS subjects.

Conclusions

In summary, this work represents the first study exploring the DNA methylation alterations in GCs of women with PCOS. Genome-wide or gene-specific DNA methylation aberrations identified in our study may be an inducer of changes in gene expression, thus further disrupting the ovarian microenvironment.

Methods

Patient selection and sample collection

The datasets during and/or analyzed during the current study are available from the corresponding author on reasonable request. The methods in this work were carried out in accordance with the approved guidelines. One hundred ten PCOS patients, diagnosed according to the Rotterdam Consensus (European Society for Human Reproduction and Embryology/American Society for Reproductive Medicine criteria) [55], and 119 infertile women with tubal blockage (serving as controls) seeking in vitro fertilization (IVF) treatment at the Women's Hospital of the School of Medicine of Zhejiang University were recruited. The control women met the following inclusion criteria: (1) age between 22 and 36; (2) both ovaries present, without morphological abnormalities; (3) normal ovarian response; (4) menstrual cycle length range between 26 and 33 days; (5) no structural abnormalities of the uterus and ovaries were found by vaginal ultrasound and/or laparoscopy; (6) no diseases affecting gonadotropin and sex steroid secretion, clearance, or excretion; (7) no signs of hyperandrogenism; and (8) no polycystic ovary morphology. And we excluded anyone whose BMI was greater than 25 from our study. The long agonist protocol for controlled ovarian hyperstimulation (COH) and the collection of FFs and GCs, obtained by follicular aspiration from women undergoing oocyte retrieval for IVF, were performed as previously described [7]. The average follicular diameter used for the analysis of FF is 16 mm, and the minimum follicular diameter used to obtain FF is no less than 14 mm.

Measurement of hormones

Serum fasting glucose levels were measured by glucose oxidase-peroxidase method. The levels of day 3 serum hormones and fasting insulin were measured by chemiluminescence immunoassay (CLIA) in the clinical laboratory of Women's Hospital, School of Medicine, Zhejiang University. TT levels in serum were measured after exaction [56] using CLIA (Roche, Mannheim, Germany). The hormones in FFs were detected by enzyme-linked immunosorbent assay (ELISA), including androstenedione (Abcam, Cambridge, UK), TT (Abcam, Cambridge, UK), sex hormone-binding globulin (SHBG, R&D Systems, Inc. Minneapolis, MN, USA), and insulin (R&D Systems, Inc. Minneapolis, MN, USA). HOMA-IR was calculated using the formula HOMA-IR = [fasting insulin (mIU/L) × fasting glucose (mmol/L)]/22.5 [57]. Free androgen index (FAI) was calculated as the ratio of TT (in nmol/L)/SHBG (in nmol/L) multiplied by 100 [58]. The values in FFs were from the individual follicle from each woman.

Transcriptome library preparation and RNA-seq

Total RNA was extracted using the RNeasy® Mini kit according to the manufacturer's protocol (Qiagen, Hilden, Germany). Total RNA was used to generate the complementary DNA (cDNA) libraries for paired-end sequencing using mRNA-seq Sample Preparation Kit (Illumina). Briefly, 4 μg of total RNA from each sample was used for polyA mRNA selection using polyT oligo--conjugated magnetic beads by two rounds of purification. The cleaved mRNA fragments were reverse transcribed and then converted into double-strand cDNA. Following end repair and A tailing, adapters complementary to sequencing primers were ligated to the ends of DNA fragment. Finally, the ligation products were further purified on 2% agarose gels and 200–250 basepair (bp) fragments were selected for downstream enrichment by 15 cycles of PCR followed by purification using QIAquick PCR purification kit (Qiagen). The libraries were sequenced and quantified with an Illumina HiSeq™ 2000 system.

Mapping of RNA-seq reads using TopHat

After applying quality control check on the raw sequenced reads using the Fast-QC tool (http://www.bioinformatics.babraham.ac.uk/projects/fastqc/) and removing the adaptor sequences, the clean reads were mapped and aligned to the human genome (hg19) using TopHat program (v2.0.6) [59]. TopHat allows multiple alignments per read (up to 20 by default) and a maximum of two mismatches when mapping the reads to the reference. TopHat builds a database of potential splice junctions and confirms these by comparing the previously unmapped reads against the database of putative junctions. The default parameters for the TopHat method were used.

DEG dataset and functional analyses

All genes and transcripts have been assigned a relative coverage rate as measured by fragments per kilobase per million (FPKM). To define genes up- or downregulated between the two groups, the log2 of the proportion between the sum of the FPKM for all gene transcripts and the same sum in control condition was taken as a measure of change in gene expression. The P value was obtained by performing a Fisher exact test (number of reads mapped to the gene and number of reads mapped to all other genes in GCs from PCOS women versus the controls), and the FDR was calculated to correct the P value. The smaller FDR indicates the smaller error in judging the P value. A significant DEG dataset was determined with a fold change (FC) cutoff of 1.5, $P < 0.05$, and FDR < 0.05.

IPA software (Qiagen, Redwood 185 City, CA) was used to identify the top biological functions associated with the DEG dataset, using Fisher's exact test to determine the probability that each biological function assigned to the DEGs is explained by chance alone. Downstream effect analysis was used to predict downstream biological processes and infer their activation state based on the observed gene expression changes in DEG dataset. A z score was calculated and used to infer the activation states ("increased" or "decreased") of implicated biological processes [60].

Reverse transcription and quantitative real-time PCR (qPCR)

Expression level of 15 genes was measured by qPCR in GCs. Total RNA was isolated using the RNAiso™ Reagent, and cDNA was prepared using the PrimeScript™ RT reagent kit with gDNA Eraser. qPCR analysis was carried out to determine the mRNA expression of the related genes using the SYBR® Premix Ex TaqTM (Tli RNaseH Plus) system (TAKARA, Dalian, China) in an Applied Biosystems ViiA™ 7 Real-Time PCR System (ABI, Carlsbad, CA). The amplification thermal cycling conditions were 95 °C for 10 s for one cycle, 95 °C for 5 s, and 60 °C for 30 s, followed by 40 cycles. After PCR, a dissociation curve was constructed at 95 °C for 15 s, 60 °C for 15 s, and 95 °C for 15 s for detection of PCR product specificity. The glyceraldehyde-3-phosphate dehydrogenase (GAPDH) was served as the internal control. Optimal qPCR assay for the gene was amplified using the corresponding primers (listed in Additional file 1: Table S1).

DNA preparation

Genomic DNA from GCs of PCOS patients and controls was isolated using the QIAamp DNA Mini Kit (Qiagen, Hilden, Germany) as recommended by the manufacturer.

Quantification of 5mC

Global methylation of GCs was determined by 5-methylcytosine (5-mC) DNA ELISA kit (Zymo Research, Irvine, CA). One hundred nanogram genomic DNA from GCs was subjected to the quantification of 5-mC, following the manufacturer's instructions. All the samples (or repeats) were loaded with the same amount of DNA in the assay plate. This was followed by the addition of primary (monoclonal antibody specific to 5-mC) and secondary antibody. The absorbance of each sample was read at 405 nm and converted into percentage of 5-mC, according to a standard curve generated by serial dilutions of the 5-mC DNA positive and negative control provided with the kit. The results were taken as average of two independent experiments. This analysis provides the levels of global DNA methylation and not specific to any particular gene.

CT conversion and MassArray EpiTYPER quantitative DNA methylation analysis

Bisulfite conversion of the genomic DNA was performed with the EZ DNA CT Conversion Reagent, Zymo Research Corporation (Irvine, CA, USA) according to the manufacturer's protocol. Quantitative DNA methylation analysis was performed with MassArray EpiTyper (Sequenom, San Diego, CA, USA) as described previously [61]. The promoter regions of the target genes were analyzed. Amplicons cover the regions of the corresponding CpG sites, and the target regions are shown in the corresponding figures. Primers were designed using the online software Epidesigner (http://www.epidesigner.com) shown in Additional file 1: Table S2. The quantitative methylation data for each CpG site or aggregates of multiple CpG sites obtained from MassArray were analyzed on the EpiTYPER software (Sequenom).

Statistical analysis

Statistical analysis is performed using the software SPSS version 19.0 software (SPSS Inc., Chicago, IL, USA). The comparisons between two groups were performed with Student's t test or non-parametric Mann-Whitney U tests. The correlations between mRNA expression levels and CpG site methylation levels of a specific gene were analyzed using Pearson's correlation. $P < 0.05$ was considered statistically significant.

Additional files

Additional file 1: The primer sets used in this study and clinic characteristics of patients used for Transcriptome Sequencing.

Additional file 2: Dataset S1. All genes detected by Transcriptome Sequencing.

Additional file 3: Dataset S2. 92 genes significantly differentially expressed in GCs of PCOS compared with controls.

Additional file 4: Figure S1. MassARRAY Quantitative methylation analysis of the CpG sites in the promoter of target genes. Values are mean ± SE. Eight GC genomic DNA from controls and 8 GC genomic DNA from PCOS women were analyzed. *P* value was determined by Mann-Whitney *U* test. *$P < 0.05$.

Abbreviations

5-mC: 5-Methylcytosine; AFC: Antral follicle count; BMI: Body mass index; CLIA: Chemiluminescence immunoassay; COH: Controlled ovarian hyperstimulation; DEGs: Differentially expressed genes; FAI: Free androgen index; FDR: False discovery rate; FF: Follicular fluid; FPKM: Fragments per kilobase per million; FSH: Follicle-stimulating hormone; GAPHD: Glyceraldehyde-3-phosphate dehydrogenase; GCs: Granulosa cells; HOMA-IR: Homeostasis model assessment of insulin resistance; IPA: Ingenuity Pathway Analysis; IVF: In vitro fertilization; LH: Luteinizing hormone; PCOS: Polycystic ovary syndrome; qPCR: Quantitative polymerase chain reaction; SAM: *S*-Adenosylmethionine; SHBG: Sex hormone-binding globulin; TT: Total testosterone

Acknowledgements

We are greatly indebted to the subjects enrolled in our study and to the medical and paramedical staff of the Women's Hospital of the School of Medicine of Zhejiang University.

Funding

This study was supported by the National Key Research and Development Program of China (2017YFC1001303 to H.-F.H.), the Zhejiang Provincial Natural Science Foundation of China (LQ18H040005 to J.-X.P.), the Natural Science Foundation of China (31471405 to H.-F.H., 81401167 to F.-F.W., 81501276 to Y.-Q.X.), Zhejiang Traditional Chinese Medicine Foundation (2017ZQ020 to J.-X.P.), Zhejiang Project of Medical and Health Research (2017KY462 to J.-X.P.), and Wenzhou Municipal Science and Technology Bureau (CN) (Y20160037 to J.-X.P.).

Authors' contributions

J-XP, H-FH, and J-ZS designed the study. J-XP, Y-JT, F-FW, N-NH, Y-QX, J-YZ, and YL performed the experiment. J-XP, F-FW, YL, FQ, and QM collected and analyzed the data. J-XP, Y-QX, J-YZ, H-FH, and J-ZS wrote the manuscript. JX participated in subject recruitment and sample collection. All authors read and approved the final manuscript.

Competing interests

The authors declare that they have no competing interests.

Author details

[1]The International Peace Maternity and Child Health Hospital, School of Medicine, Shanghai Jiao Tong University, Shanghai 200030, China. [2]The Key Laboratory of Reproductive Genetics, Ministry of Education (Zhejiang University), Hangzhou, Zhejiang 310006, China. [3]Department of Pathology and Pathophysiology, School of Medicine, Zhejiang University, Hangzhou 310058, China. [4]Reproductive Medicine Center, The First Affiliated Hospital of Wenzhou Medical University, Wenzhou 325000, China.

References

1. Norman RJ, Dewailly D, Legro RS, Hickey TE. Polycystic ovary syndrome. Lancet. 2007;370(9588):685–97.
2. Vink J, Sadrzadeh S, Lambalk C, Boomsma D. Heritability of polycystic ovary syndrome in a Dutch twin-family study. The Journal of Clinical Endocrinology & Metabolism. 2006;91(6):2100–4.
3. Govind A, Obhrai MS, Clayton RN. Polycystic ovaries are inherited as an autosomal dominant trait: analysis of 29 polycystic ovary syndrome and 10 control families. J Clin Endocrinol Metab. 1999;84(1):38–43.
4. Kahsar-Miller MD, Nixon C, Boots LR, Go RC, Azziz R. Prevalence of polycystic ovary syndrome (PCOS) in first-degree relatives of patients with PCOS. Fertil Steril. 2001;75(1):53–8.
5. Urbanek M, Legro RS, Driscoll DA, Azziz R, Ehrmann DA, Norman RJ, Strauss JF, Spielman RS, Dunaif A. Thirty-seven candidate genes for polycystic ovary syndrome: strongest evidence for linkage is with follistatin. Proc Natl Acad Sci. 1999;96(15):8573–8.
6. Chen Z-J, Zhao H, He L, Shi Y, Qin Y, Shi Y, Li Z, You L, Zhao J, Liu J. Genome-wide association study identifies susceptibility loci for polycystic ovary syndrome on chromosome 2p16. 3, 2p21 and 9q33. 3. Nat Genet. 2011;43(1):55–9.
7. Qu F, Wang F-F, Yin R, Ding G-L, El-prince M, Gao Q, Shi B-W, Pan H-H, Huang Y-T, Jin M. A molecular mechanism underlying ovarian dysfunction of polycystic ovary syndrome: hyperandrogenism induces epigenetic alterations in the granulosa cells. J Mol Med. 2012;90(8):911–23.
8. Bird A. Perceptions of epigenetics. Nature. 2007;447(7143):396–8.
9. Morgan HD, Santos F, Green K, Dean W, Reik W. Epigenetic reprogramming in mammals. Hum Mol Genet. 2005;14(suppl 1):R47–58.
10. Guo F, Li X, Liang D, Li T, Zhu P, Guo H, Wu X, Wen L, T-P G, Hu B, et al. Active and passive demethylation of male and female pronuclear DNA in the mammalian zygote. Cell Stem Cell. 2014;15(4):447–59.
11. Wang P, Zhao H, Li T, Zhang W, KL W, Li M, Bian YH, Liu HB, Ning YN, Li GY, et al. Hypomethylation of the LH/choriogonadotropin receptor promoter region is a potential mechanism underlying susceptibility to polycystic ovary syndrome. Endocrinology. 2014;155(4):1445–52.
12. Sang Q, Li X, Wang H, Wang H, Zhang S, Feng R, Xu Y, Li Q, Zhao X, Xing Q. Quantitative methylation level of the EPHX1 promoter in peripheral blood DNA is associated with polycystic ovary syndrome. PLoS One. 2014;9(2):e88013.
13. Yu YY, Sun CX, Liu YK, Li Y, Wang L, Zhang W. Promoter methylation of CYP19A1 gene in Chinese polycystic ovary syndrome patients. Gynecol Obstet Inves. 2013;76(4):209–13.
14. Wang X-X, Wei J-Z, Jiao J, Jiang S-Y, D-H Y, Li D. Genome-wide DNA methylation and gene expression patterns provide insight into polycystic ovary syndrome development. Oncotarget. 2014;5(16):6603–10.
15. Pan JX, Zhang JY, Ke ZH, Wang FF, Barry JA, Hardiman PJ, Qu F. Androgens as double-edged swords: induction and suppression of follicular development. Hormones (Athens). 2015;14(2):190–200.
16. Zhang L-H, Rodriguez H, Ohno S, Miller WL. Serine phosphorylation of human P450c17 increases 17, 20-lyase activity: implications for adrenarche and the polycystic ovary syndrome. Proc Natl Acad Sci. 1995;92(23):10619–23.
17. Sen A, Hammes SR. Granulosa cell-specific androgen receptors are critical regulators of ovarian development and function. Mol Endocrinol. 2010;24(7): 1393–403.
18. Adashi EY, CE RESNICK, D'ERCOLE AJ, ME SVOBODA, JJV WYK. Insulin-like growth factors as intraovarian regulators of granulosa cell growth and function. Endocr Rev. 1985;6(3):400–20.
19. Agrawal A, Tay J, Yang G-E, Agrawal S, Gupta S. Age-associated epigenetic modifications in human DNA increase its immunogenicity. Aging (Albany NY). 2010;2(2):93.
20. Kaur S, Archer KJ, Devi MG, Kriplani A, Strauss JF III, Singh R. Differential gene expression in granulosa cells from polycystic ovary syndrome patients with and without insulin resistance: identification of susceptibility gene sets through network analysis. The Journal of Clinical Endocrinology & Metabolism. 2012;97(10):E2016–21.

21. Downs SM, Mosey JL, Klinger J. Fatty acid oxidation and meiotic resumption in mouse oocytes. Mol Reprod Dev. 2009;76(9):844–53.
22. Dunning KR, Cashman K, Russell DL, Thompson JG, Norman RJ, Robker RL. Beta-oxidation is essential for mouse oocyte developmental competence and early embryo development. Biol Reprod. 2010;83(6):909–18.
23. Dunning KR, Anastasi MR, Zhang VJ, Russell DL, Robker RL. Regulation of fatty acid oxidation in mouse cumulus-oocyte complexes during maturation and modulation by PPAR agonists. PLoS One. 2014;9(2):e87327.
24. Valsangkar D, Downs SM. A requirement for fatty acid oxidation in the hormone-induced meiotic maturation of mouse oocytes. Biol Reprod. 2013;89(2):55–64.
25. Miller WL. Molecular biology of steroid hormone synthesis. Endocr Rev. 1988;9(3):295–318.
26. Singh R, Kaushik S, Wang Y, Xiang Y, Novak I, Komatsu M, Tanaka K, Cuervo AM, Czaja MJ. Autophagy regulates lipid metabolism. Nature. 2009; 458(7242):1131–5.
27. Glick D, Zhang W, Beaton M, Marsboom G, Gruber M, Simon MC, Hart J, Dorn GW, Brady MJ, Macleod KF. BNip3 regulates mitochondrial function and lipid metabolism in the liver. Mol Cell Biol. 2012;32(13):2570–84.
28. Zhang J, Ney PA. Role of BNIP3 and NIX in cell death, autophagy, and mitophagy. Cell Death & Differentiation. 2009;16(7):939–46.
29. Das M, Djahanbakhch O, Hacihanefioglu B, Saridogan E, Ikram M, Ghali L, Raveendran M, Storey A. Granulosa cell survival and proliferation are altered in polycystic ovary syndrome. J Clin Endocrinol Metab. 2008; 93(3):881–7.
30. Giguère V. Orphan nuclear receptors: from gene to function 1. Endocr Rev. 1999;20(5):689–725.
31. Maxwell MA, Cleasby ME, Harding A, Stark A, Cooney GJ, Muscat GE. Nur77 regulates lipolysis in skeletal muscle cells EVIDENCE FOR CROSS-TALK BETWEEN THE β-ADRENERGIC AND AN ORPHAN NUCLEAR HORMONE RECEPTOR PATHWAY. J Biol Chem. 2005;280(13):12573–84.
32. Humphries A, Weller J, Klein D, Baler R, Carter DA. NGFI-B (Nurr77/Nr4a1) orphan nuclear receptor in rat pinealocytes: circadian expression involves an adrenergic-cyclic AMP mechanism. J Neurochem. 2004;91(4):946–55.
33. Ishida A, Mutoh T, Ueyama T, Bando H, Masubuchi S, Nakahara D, Tsujimoto G, Okamura H. Light activates the adrenal gland: timing of gene expression and glucocorticoid release. Cell Metab. 2005;2(5):297–307.
34. Pan JX, Wang FF, Liu Y, Meng Q, Sheng JZ, Huang HF. Bisphenol a (BPA) induces abnormal androgen accumulation via androgen-androgen receptor (AR) mediated cyp19a1 transcription inhibition in granulosa cells (GCs). Fertil Steril. 2013;100(3):S13.
35. Bhutani N, Burns DM, Blau HM. DNA demethylation dynamics. Cell. 2011; 146(6):866–72.
36. Schneider E, Pliushch G, El Hajj N, Galetzka D, Puhl A, Schorsch M, Frauenknecht K, Riepert T, Tresch A, Müller AM. Spatial, temporal and interindividual epigenetic variation of functionally important DNA methylation patterns. Nucleic Acids Res. 2010;38(12):3880–90.
37. Deaton AM, Webb S, Kerr AR, Illingworth RS, Guy J, Andrews R, Bird A. Cell type–specific DNA methylation at intragenic CpG islands in the immune system. Genome Res. 2011;21(7):1074–86.
38. Eden A, Gaudet F, Waghmare A, Jaenisch R. Chromosomal instability and tumors promoted by DNA hypomethylation. Science. 2003; 300(5618):455.
39. Matsuzaki K, Deng G, Tanaka H, Kakar S, Miura S, Kim YS. The relationship between global methylation level, loss of heterozygosity, and microsatellite instability in sporadic colorectal cancer. Clin Cancer Res. 2005;11(24):8564–9.
40. Karpf AR, Matsui S-i. Genetic disruption of cytosine DNA methyltransferase enzymes induces chromosomal instability in human cancer cells. Cancer Res. 2005;65(19):8635–9.
41. Xu N, Azziz R, Goodarzi MO. Epigenetics in polycystic ovary syndrome: a pilot study of global DNA methylation. Fertil Steril. 2010;94(2):781–783. e781.
42. Teschendorff AE, West J, Beck S. Age-associated epigenetic drift: implications, and a case of epigenetic thrift? Hum Mol Genet. 2013;22(R1):R7–R15.
43. Jaenisch R, Bird A. Epigenetic regulation of gene expression: how the genome integrates intrinsic and environmental signals. Nat Genet. 2003;33:245–54.
44. Gleyzer N, Vercauteren K, Scarpulla RC. Control of mitochondrial transcription specificity factors (TFB1M and TFB2M) by nuclear respiratory factors (NRF-1 and NRF-2) and PGC-1 family coactivators. Mol Cell Biol. 2005; 25(4):1354–66.
45. Ongwijitwat S, Liang HL, Graboyes EM, Wong-Riley MT. Nuclear respiratory factor 2 senses changing cellular energy demands and its silencing down-regulates cytochrome oxidase and other target gene mRNAs. Gene. 2006; 374:39–49.
46. Shane B. 1 Folate Chemistry and Metabolism. In Lynn B, editor. Folate in health and disease. Boca Raton: CRC Press; 2010. p. 1–24.
47. Bestor TH. The DNA methyltransferases of mammals. Hum Mol Genet. 2000; 9(16):2395–402.
48. Gonda TA, Kim YI, Salas MC, Gamble MV, Shibata W, Muthupalani S, Sohn KJ, Abrams JA, Fox JG, Wang TC. Folic acid increases global DNA methylation and reduces inflammation to prevent Helicobacter-associated gastric cancer in mice. Gastroenterology. 2012;142(4):824–833. e827.
49. Rampersaud GC, Kauwell GP, Hutson AD, Cerda JJ, Bailey LB. Genomic DNA methylation decreases in response to moderate folate depletion in elderly women. Am J Clin Nutr. 2000;72(4):998–1003.
50. de la Calle M, Gallardo T, Diestro MD, Hernanz A, Perez E, Fernandez-Miranda C. Increased homocysteine levels in polycystic ovary syndrome. Medicina clinica. 2007;129(8):292–4.
51. Bayraktar F, Dereli D, Ozgen AG, Yilmaz C. Plasma homocysteine levels in polycystic ovary syndrome and congenital adrenal hyperplasia. Endocr J. 2004;51(6):601–8.
52. Palomba S, Falbo A, Giallauria F, Russo T, Tolino A, Zullo F, Colao A, Orio F. Effects of metformin with or without supplementation with folate on homocysteine levels and vascular endothelium of women with polycystic ovary syndrome. Diabetes Care. 2010;33(2):246–51.
53. Campión J, Milagro FI, Martínez JA. Individuality and epigenetics in obesity. Obesity reviews : an official journal of the International Association for the Study of Obesity. 2009;10(4):383–92.
54. Ma Y, Xia W, Wang DQ, Wan YJ, Xu B, Chen X, Li YY, SQ X. Hepatic DNA methylation modifications in early development of rats resulting from perinatal BPA exposure contribute to insulin resistance in adulthood. Diabetologia. 2013;56(9):2059–67.
55. Rotterdam EA-SPcwg. Revised 2003 consensus on diagnostic criteria and long-term health risks related to polycystic ovary syndrome (PCOS). Hum Reprod. 2004;19(1):41–7.
56. Janse F, Eijkemans MJ, Goverde AJ, Lentjes EG, Hoek A, Lambalk CB, Hickey TE, Fauser BC, Norman RJ. Assessment of androgen concentration in women: liquid chromatography–tandem mass spectrometry and extraction RIA show comparable results. Eur J Endocrinol. 2011;165(6):925–33.
57. Matthews DR, Hosker JP, Rudenski AS, Naylor BA, Treacher DF, Turner RC. Homeostasis model assessment: insulin resistance and beta-cell function from fasting plasma glucose and insulin concentrations in man. Diabetologia. 1985;28(7):412–9.
58. Doi SA, Al-Zaid M, Towers PA, Scott CJ, Al-Shoumer KA. Steroidogenic alterations and adrenal androgen excess in PCOS. Steroids. 2006;71(9):751–9.
59. Trapnell C, Pachter L, Salzberg SL. TopHat: discovering splice junctions with RNA-Seq. Bioinformatics. 2009;25(9):1105–11.
60. Kramer A, Green J, Pollard J Jr, Tugendreich S. Causal analysis approaches in Ingenuity Pathway Analysis. Bioinformatics. 2014;30(4):523–30.
61. Xiang Y, Zhang X, Li Q, Xu J, Zhou X, Wang T, Xing Q, Liu Y, Wang L, He L, et al. Promoter hypomethylation of TIMP3 is associated with pre-eclampsia in a Chinese population. Mol Hum Reprod. 2013;19(3):153–9.

4

Integrative analysis of the epigenetic basis of muscle-invasive urothelial carcinoma

Thomas Sanford[2], Maxwell V. Meng[1], Reema Railkar[2], Piyush K. Agarwal[2] and Sima P. Porten[1*]

Abstract

Background: Elucidation of epigenetic alterations in bladder cancer will lead to further understanding of the biology of the disease and hopefully improved therapies. Our aim was to perform an integrative epigenetic analysis of invasive urothelial carcinoma of the bladder to identify the epigenetic abnormalities involved in the development and progression of this cancer.

Methods: Pre-processed methylation data and RNA-seq data were downloaded from The Cancer Genome Atlas (TCGA) and processed using the R package TCGA-Assembler. An R package MethylMix was used to perform an analysis incorporating both methylation and gene expression data on all samples, as well as a subset analysis comparing patients surviving less than 2 years and patients surviving more than 2 years. Genes associated with poor prognosis were individually queried. Pathway analysis was performed on statistically significant genes identified by MethylMix criteria using ConsensusPathDB. Validation was performed using flow cytometry on bladder cancer cell lines.

Results: A total of 408 patients met all inclusion criteria. There were a total of 240 genes differentially methylated by MethylMix criteria. Review of individual genes specific to poor-prognosis patients revealed the majority to be candidate tumor suppressors in other cancer types. Pathway analysis showed increase in methylation of genes involved in antioxidant pathways including glutathione and NRF2. Genes involved in estrogen metabolism were also hypermethylated while genes involved in the EGFR pathway were found to be hypomethylated. EGFR expression was confirmed to be elevated in six bladder cancer cell lines.

Conclusions: In patients with invasive urothelial carcinoma, we found differential methylation in patients with better and worse prognosis after cystectomy. Differentially methylated genes are involved in many relevant oncologic pathways, including EGFR and antioxidant pathways, that may be a target for therapy or chemoprevention.

Keywords: Epigenetics, Urothelial carcinoma, Integrative analyses

Background

Urothelial carcinoma of the bladder is the eighth most common form of cancer in the USA and the fourth most common type of cancer in men [1]. Although the majority of urothelial carcinoma of the bladder is diagnosed at a non-invasive stage, 30–40% of cases will progress to invade the deeper muscle layer of the bladder [2], at which point the long-term disease-specific survival is 50–70% [3, 4].

Multiple studies have shown that DNA methylation, the process by which a methyl group is added to a cytosine residue of a cytosine-phosphate-guanine (CpG) dinucleotide, plays an important role in the initiation and progression of bladder cancer [5–7]. DNA methylation represents a promising target for therapy since DNA methylation is a reversible process that does not alter the content of DNA [8].

High-throughput methods have been employed in bladder cancer to evaluate the epigenetic alterations involved in the development and progression of this disease [5, 9]. However, many methylation events found to be statistically significant using high-throughput screening methods are not correlated with gene expression changes [10]. There is a need for high-throughput approaches that integrate data across multiple platforms to determine the epigenetic events that are most likely to be involved in bladder cancer [11].

* Correspondence: sima.porten@ucsf.edu
[1]Department of Urology, University of California, Mail code 1695, 550 16th Street, 6th Floor, San Francisco, CA 94143, USA
Full list of author information is available at the end of the article

The Cancer Genome Atlas (TCGA) project demonstrated impressive diversity in both genetic and epigenetic alterations within patients who have muscle-invasive urothelial carcinoma of the bladder [12]. The multiple platforms utilized within TCGA make it possible to perform analyses integrating data from multiple sources to identify specific abnormalities most likely to contribute to oncogenic processes. In this study, we utilized an integrative approach to evaluate the epigenetic processes that may be most important in development and progression of invasive urothelial carcinoma.

Methods

Data acquisition and preprocessing

All data were obtained from bladder cystectomy specimens from The Cancer Genome Atlas Project [13]. Specimen acquisition and processing is described in detail in the original TCGA publication, but briefly: specimens were placed in optimum cutting temperature media and frozen. Normal tissues ($N = 21$) were taken from the cystectomy specimens 2 cm away from tumor. All tumors included in TCGA had less than 50% of variant (non-urothelial) histology.

Methylation was evaluated on the Illumina Infinium HumanMethylation450 platform, which assesses 482,421 CpG sites throughout the genome [14]. Level 3 methylation data were downloaded from the TCGA data portal using the TCGA-Assembler *DownloadMethylationData* function [15]. Level 3 data consist of pre-processed data via TCGA pipelines in the form of beta values, which are a ratio between methylated probe intensities and total probe intensities (https://cancergenome.nih.gov/abouttcga/aboutdata/datalevelstypes). Probe-level data was condensed to a summary beta value for each gene using the *Methylation450_single_value* function in TCGA-Assembler, which calculates the average methylation value for all CpG sites associated with a gene. Level 3 RNA-seq data were also obtained from the TCGA data portal using the TCGA-Assembler function *DownloadRNASeqData*. The functions DGEList and calcNormFactors functions from the edgeR package were used to normalize the data [16]. The *voom* function from the limma package was then used to transform the RNA-seq data for linear modeling [17]. Both tumor tissue and normal tissue were processed in an identical manner.

Clinical data

Clinical data for TCGA patients were obtained via the TCGA data portal. To augment and validate the pathologic data (of which not all variables were complete), pathology reports were downloaded from cbioportal.com for all patients in the TCGA provisional dataset and pathologic data were individually reviewed. All patients included in TCGA had muscle-invasive disease (pT2-T4). Of the 412 patients in the dataset, 408 had complete clinical, gene expression, and methylation data. A total of 101 patients met inclusion criteria for survival of at least 2 years after cystectomy. A total of 142 patients died within 2 years after cystectomy. This left a total of 165 patients with inadequate follow-up to be included in the survival analysis. Clinical data were partitioned into three separate groups for analysis. First, we performed analysis of the entire dataset ($N = 408$). Next, we performed analysis of patients who survived more than 2 years after cystectomy versus patients who died within 2 years of cystectomy.

Integrative analysis

The R package MethylMix was used to perform an analysis integrating methylation data and gene expression (RNA-seq) data [18]. MethylMix is a program designed to identify methylation events that are correlated with gene expression [19]. There are three parts to the MethylMix analysis: first, methylation data are correlated with gene expression data to identify methylation events that results in gene expression changes—only genes passing the correlation filter are selected for further analysis; second, a beta mixture model is used to define a methylation state across a large number of patients, precluding the need for arbitrary thresholds; and third, a Wilcoxon rank sum test is used to compare DNA methylation states in tumor samples versus normal samples [18]. Multiple testing is accounted for using a q value cutoff of 0.05. The end result is a differential methylation (DM) value where a positive DM value signifies hypermethylation and a negative DM value signifies hypomethylation.

Pathway analysis

Pathway analysis was performed with ConsensusPathDB [20]. ConsensusPathDB utilizes a hypergeometric test to evaluate for over-represented pathways based on the imputed gene list. The over-representation analysis function was utilized imputing the HUGO Gene Nomenclature Committee (HGNC) unique identifiers for each gene list. The following pathway databases were selected for our analysis: Inoh, Pid, Biocarta, Netpath, Humancyc, Kegg, Wikipathways, Smpdb, Pharmgkb, Ehmn, and Signalink. We used the default settings: minimum overlap and p value cutoff of 0.01.

Pathway analysis was performed using the gene lists found to be statistically significant by MethylMix. Lists of hypermethylated genes were analyzed separately from lists of hypomethylated genes for the followed groups: all patients, patients who survived at least 2 years after cystectomy, and patients who died within 2 years of cystectomy.

Experimental validation in bladder cancer cell lines

The following bladder cancer cell lines were obtained from ATCC (Manassas, VA, USA): ScaBER (HTB-3), HT1376 (CRL-1472), SW780 (CRL-2169). Dr. David McConkey kindly gifted three additional cell lines UMUC-5, UMUC-1, and 253J (University of Texas, MD Anderson Cancer Center). All the cell lines were grown in the same media, which was minimum essential media (MEM) (Life Technologies) supplemented with 10% fetal bovine serum, 1% penicillin/streptomycin, and 1% GlutaMAX (Life Technologies). The presence of surface EGFR on the cell lines listed above was determined by flow cytometry. For each cell line, a single cell suspension was obtained after trypsinzation ($\sim 1 \times 10^6$ cells/tube), which was incubated in the presence of phycoerythrin(PE)-tagged rat monoclonal antibody to human EGFR (Abcam) or PE-tagged rat IgG2a kappa monoclonal antibody (isotype control; Abcam). The cells were allowed to incubate for 30 min at 4 °C in the antibody solution. We washed the cells to remove all unbound antibody using phosphate-buffered solution. Fluorescence was measured on a FACS Calibur flow cytometer (BD BioSciences).

Statistical analysis

Continuous variables were evaluated using the Student *t* test. Categorical variables were evaluated using chi-squared. *p* value less than 0.05 was considered statistically significant. All analyses were performed using R v 3.3.2. Flow cytometry data were analyzed using FlowJo (Treestar Inc.).

Results

Clinical data

Clinical characteristics are summarized in Table 1 and represent the three groups used for analysis. There was a statistically significant difference between the groups with respect to age, with patients surviving more than 2 years being younger. However, there were no significant differences between the groups for T stage [21].

MethylMix analysis: hypermethylated versus hypomethylated genes by prognostic category

A total of 240 genes were differentially methylated when comparing tumor to normal by MethylMix criteria for all 408 patients. Example of differential methylation of tumor samples compared with normal samples is demonstrated in Fig. 1. Of these genes, 70 genes (29%) were hypermethylated and the remainder of the genes were hypomethylated. When MethylMix analysis was performed on the subset of patients surviving at least 2 years after cystectomy, a total of 266 genes reached statistical significance of which 69 (26%) were hypermethylated. There were a total of 220 significant genes when MethylMix was performed on the cohort of patients who died within 2 years of cystectomy, of which 70 (32%) were hypermethylated (Fig. 2). There was a slightly higher proportion of genes hypermethylated in patients in the worse prognosis group (survive < 2 years) when compared with the group with better prognosis (survive > 2 years), but this difference was not statistically significant ($p = 0.18$).

When the differentially methylated genes in the group that survived more than 2 years were compared with differentially methylated genes in the group that survived less than 2 years, nearly half of the genes (49%) overlapped between the better and worse prognosis cohorts. There were a total of 24 genes (26%) that were uniquely hypermethylated in the worse prognosis group and 23 genes (25%) uniquely hypermethylated in the better prognosis group. When the overlap of hypomethylated genes was evaluated, there was 52% overlap. The proportion of genes unique to the poor-prognosis group in the hypomethylated group was less than the hypermethylated group (13 versus 25%, respectively, $p = 0.02$). Identities of all genes significant by MethylMix are included in Additional file 1: Table S1.

Table 1 Clinical data

Characteristic	Total	Survive > 2 years after surgery	Death < 2 years of surgery	Inadequate follow-up	*p* value
Cohort size	408	101	142	165	
Mean age, years (SD)	68.0 (10.6)	66.2 (10.7)	70.6 (9.5)	69.3 (10.7)	< 0.01
Gender					
Women (%)	106 (26%)	24 (24%)	41 (29%)	51 (31%)	0.45
Men (%)	302 (74%)	77 (76%)	101 (71%)	114 (69%)	
T stage					
pT2	120 (29%)	37 (37%)	24 (17%)	43 (26%)	0.06
pT3	196 (48%)	44 (44%)	76 (54%)	82 (50%)	
PT4	59 (14%)	11 (11%)	29 (20%)	25 (15%)	
NA	33 (8%)	9 (9%)	13 (9%)	15 (9%)	

p value determined by ANOVA for continuous variables and chi-square for categorical variables

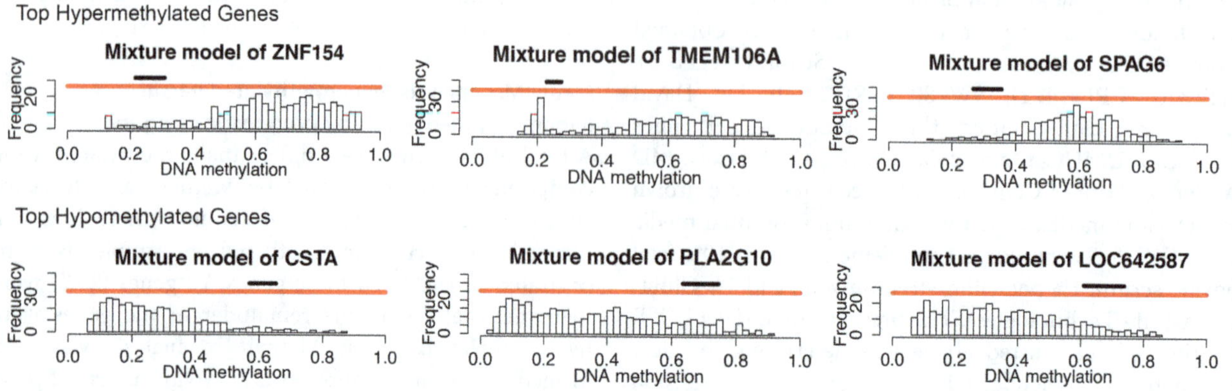

Fig. 1 Summary of top hypermethylated and top hypomethylated genes. The red line demarcates the distribution of methylation in tumor samples and normal samples. The histogram (below red line) demonstrates the distribution of methylation in tumor samples (denoted as beta values where higher beta values represent greater methylation). The horizontal black bar above the red line represents the distribution of methylation values in the normal samples

Evaluation of genes hypermethylated in patients surviving < 2 years

We sought to evaluate the genes hypermethylated in the patients unique to patients surviving less than 2 years to evaluate any potential biologic effect (Additional files 2, 3, and 4). We began by performing a literature search of PubMed for each gene using the terms "[GENE NAME]", "methylation", "cancer." Of the 24 genes unique to patients who died within 2 years of surgery, 19 had been described as being candidate tumor suppressor genes or hypermethylated in various cancer types, including urothelial carcinoma (Table 2). Nine of these genes had been shown to be associated with an aggressive phenotype in prior studies, some in multiple cancer types. Furthermore, some prior studies performed experimental validation of pathway alterations for many of these genes, including the estrogen signaling pathway.

Cumulative effects

While MethylMix describes each gene individually, we also wanted to evaluate the cumulated dose of hypermethylation across genes in any given patient. Thus, we assessed the effect of cumulative methylation changes for the 24 genes unique to patients with poor prognosis. Across the entire matrix of methylation values, the average methylation value (beta value) for normal samples

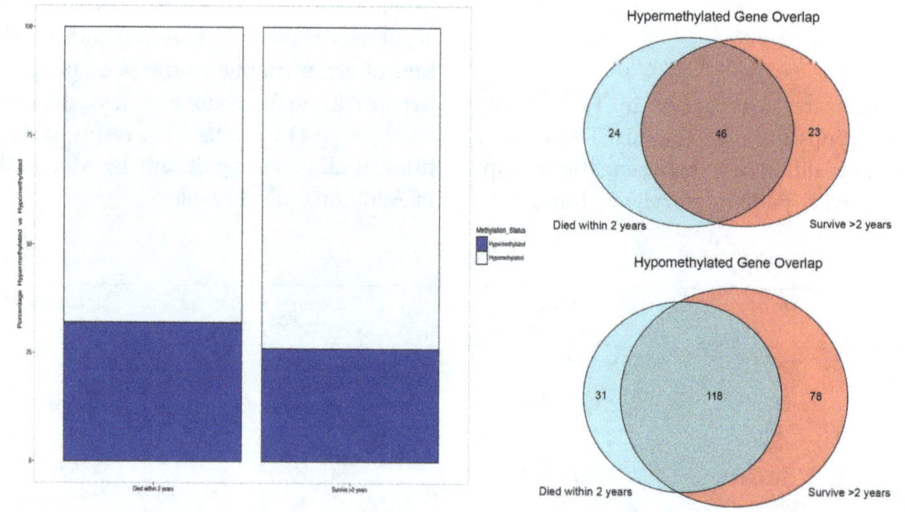

Fig. 2 Of the 220 statistically significant genes for patients who died within 2 years, 32% were hypermethylated. Of the 266 statistically significant genes for patients who survived more than 2 years after cystectomy, 26% were hypermethylated and the remainder of the genes were hypomethylated. For both hypermethylated and hypomethylated genes, the majority of genes were shared by the better and worse prognosis groups. However, there were some genes with unique methylation status between the two groups, and there were more genes uniquely hypermethylated in the group that did not survive 2 years compared with the group that survived at least 2 years ($p = 0.02$). Identities of all genes significant by MethylMix are included in Additional file 1: Table S1

Table 2 Hypermethylated genes by MethylMix criteria unique to patients who survived less than 2 years after cystectomy (references listed in Additional file 3: Table S3)

Gene symbol	Gene name	Chromosome	Associated with aggressive behavior in cancer	Tumor suppressor/ hypermethylated in cancer	Altered pathways	Cancer types
CXCL6	C-X-C motif chemokine liqand 6	4q13.3		[44]		Ovarian cancer [44]
ZFP42	ZFP42 zinc finger protein	4q35.2			Sox2, NOTCH/ STAT3 [45]	Human embryonic stem cell marker [45]
PITX1	Paired-like homeodomain 1	5q31.1	[46, 47]			Kidney cancer [46] Hepatocellular cancer [47]
RSPH9	Radial spoke head 9 homolog	6p21.1	[48]	[49]		*Bladder cancer* [50] Hepatocellular cancer
HIST1H3E	Histone cluster 1 H3 family member e	6p22.2	[51]			Glioma [51]
SP8	Sp8 transcription factor	7p21.2			Wnt/B-Catenin [52]	
TAC1	Tachykinin precursor 1	7q21-q22	[46, 53, 54]	[55]		Head/neck cancer [53] Colorectal cancer [54, 55] Esophageal cancer [46]
PON3	Paraoxonase 3	7q21.3		[56, 57]		Bladder cancer [56] Prostate cancer [57]
ABF1	Musculin (activated B cell factor 1)	8q13.3		[58]		Lymphoma [58]
FOXE1	Forkhead box E1	9q22	[59]	[60]	Estrogen signaling [61]	Colorectal carcinoma [59] Cutanous squamous cell cancer [60] Thyroid cancer [62]
CCDC67	Deuterosome assembly protein 1	11q21	[63]	[64]		Thyroid carcinoma [63] Gastric carcinoma [64]
ALX1	ALX homeobox 1	12q21.31	[65]	[66]	Snail [67]	Breast cancer [66] Non-small cell lung cancer [65] Ovarian cancer [67]
SLC6A15	Solute carrier family 6 member 15	12q21.31		[68, 69]		Colorectal carcinoma [68, 69]
EID3	EP300 interacting inhibitor of differentiation 3	12q23.3		[70]		Colorectal cancer [70]
NKX2-8	NK2 homeobox 8	14q13.3	[71]	[72, 73]	NF-KB [72], MEK/ERK [71]	*Bladder cancer* [71] Cervical cancer [73] Esopheageal cancer [72]
DIO3	Deiodinase, iodothyronine type III	14q32		[74, 75]		Lung cancer [74] Hematologic malignancies [75]
FOXC2	Forkhead box C2	16q24.1		[76]	MPK/AKT	Breast cancer [76]
HSPB6	Heat shock protein family B (small) member 6	19q13.13	[77]			Melanoma [77]
ZNF382	Zinc finger protein 382	19q13.13		[78]	NF-kB [79]	Esophageal cancer [78]

for these genes was 0.23, whereas the average methylation value for tumor samples was 0.39 ($p < 0.01$). Figure 3 is a heatmap of the methylation values of all patients with survival of less than 2 years with poor prognosis genes selected. This heatmap demonstrates patients who survive less than 2 years may have hypermethylation of multiple genes associated with hypermethylation in various cancer types and/or poor prognosis.

Pathway analysis

Figure 4 is a graphical representation of pathways enriched for genes significant by MethylMix criteria in the analysis that included all 408 patients. There were unique pathways represented by analysis of hypermethylated and hypomethylated genes. For hypermethylated genes, pathways involved in management of free radicals were found to be significant—both the glutathione and

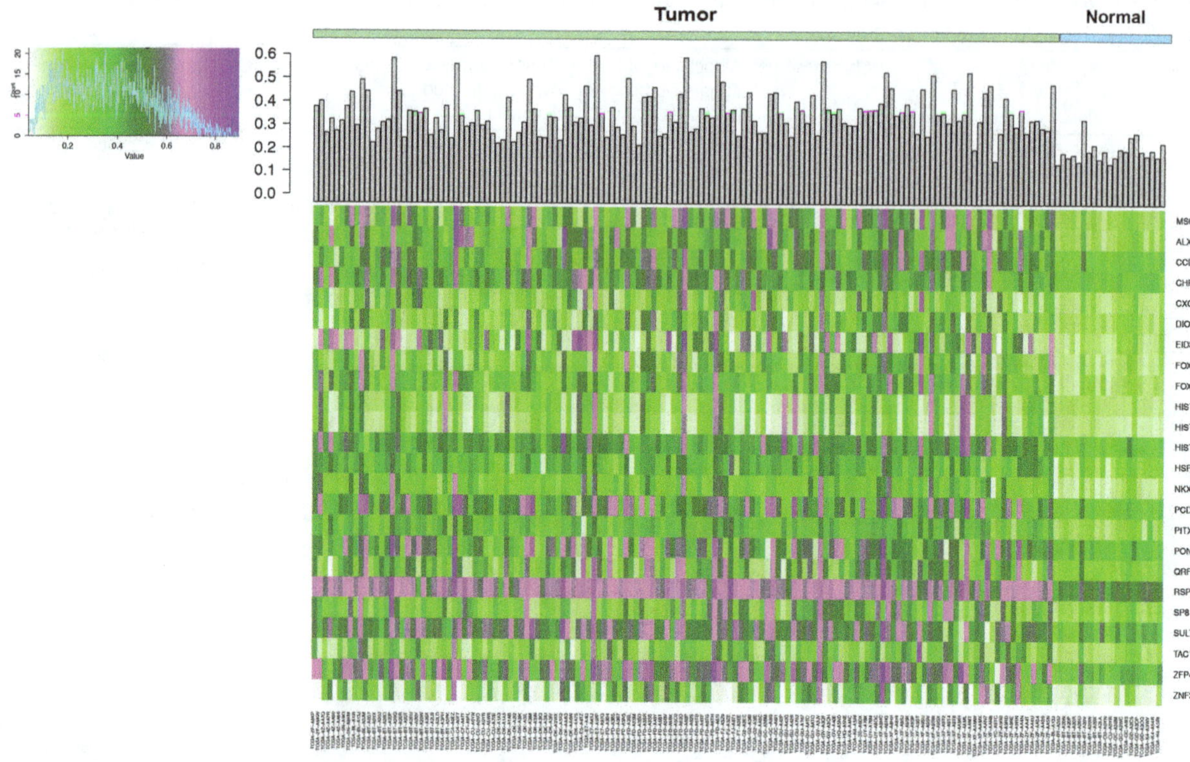

Fig. 3 Heatmap of methylation values (beta values) for 24 genes uniquely hypermethylated in patients who survived less than 2 years after cystectomy. The gray bar histogram represents the mean beta value across all genes for each patient

NRF2 pathways are key antioxidant pathways [6]. The estrogen metabolism pathway was also enriched in hypermethylated genes. The chemical carcinogenesis pathway was also hypermethylated, consistent with the relationship between bladder cancer and environmental exposures such as tobacco smoking and cyclic amines [22]. The most notable hypomethylated pathway was the EGFR1 pathway, a well-known oncogene that has been shown to be over-expressed in multiple cancer types [23]. Genes in the cyclophosphamide pathway were found to be hypomethylated—this agent can have significant effects on the urothelium causing hemorrhagic cystitis as well as delayed malignancy. There were also multiple pathways involved in fatty acid metabolism. Additional file 2: Table S2 lists detailed pathway analysis results by methylation status and patient group.

Flow cytometry confirms the presence of EGFR

There was a substantial amount of EGFR in all six cell lines tested, reflecting hypomethylation (Fig. 5). There was a mean increase of 83-fold over isotype control. The mean intensity for isotype control was 81.7 (range 12.5–154) while the EGFR mean intensity was 6816 (range 1544–11,222), *t* test p value < 0.01 (Fig. 5).

Discussion

Epigenetic changes and modifications are an important part of carcinogenesis and subsequent tumor progression [24, 25]. Of the various epigenetic mechanisms, DNA methylation has been most studied and is classically associated with gene silencing via hypermethylation of CpG islands located in promoter regions of tumor suppressor genes. DNA hypomethylation has also been implicated in the development of cancer and likely results in genome rearrangement and chromosomal instability. Alterations in DNA methylation may be involved in the development of urothelial carcinoma of the bladder, with abnormalities identified in the normal urothelium of those who later develop frank cancer [5]. However, the methylation status of specific genes has been shown to be associated with worse prognosis [9, 10, 26], indicating that epigenetic changes may also be involved in tumor progression.

The earliest studies demonstrating the role of methylation in the development of urothelial carcinoma demonstrated a relationship between adverse clinical outcomes and the methylation state of promoters of specific genes known to be involved in the development of cancer [6, 7, 27]. These gene-specific studies demonstrated the relationship between increased methylation of specific gene promoters and grade [27], stage [28],

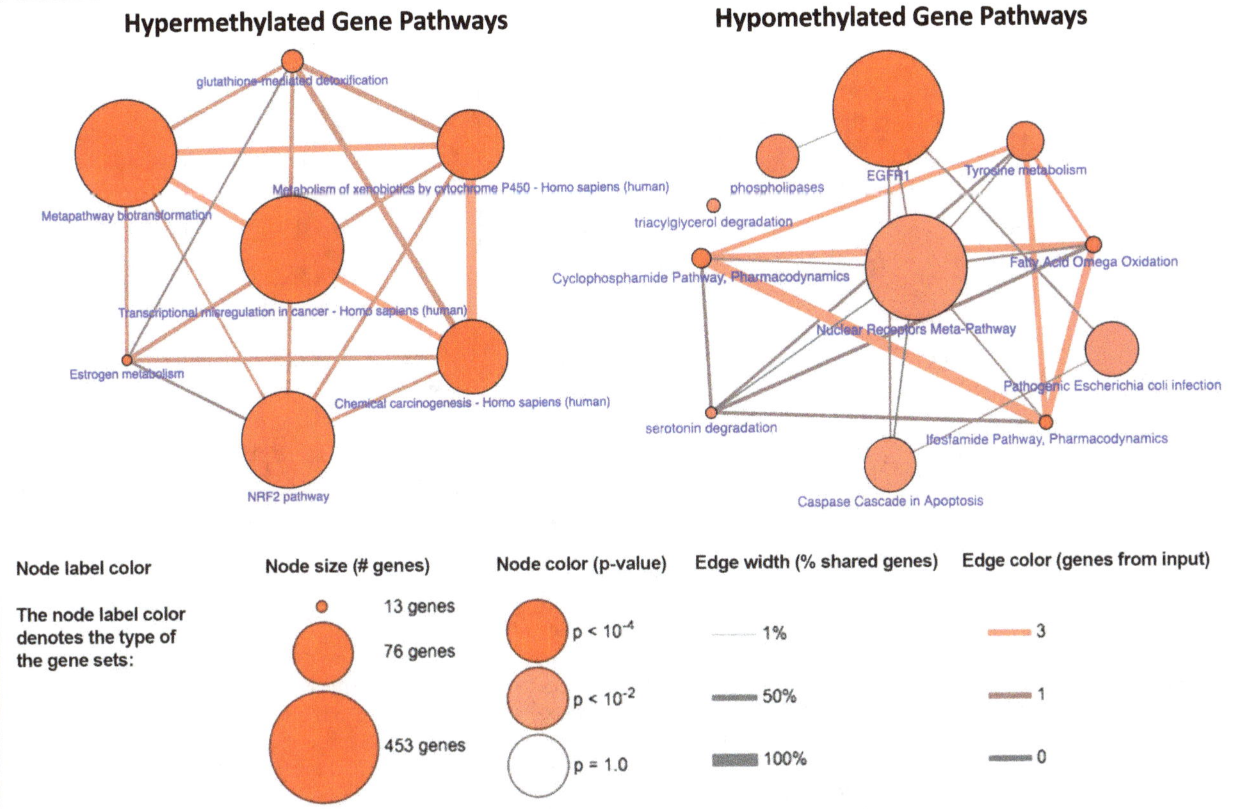

Fig. 4 Select pathways enriched for genes hypermethylated and hypomethylated by MethylMix criteria in the analysis including all patients in the TCGA cohort. The full list of pathways is included in Additional file 2: Table S2

and progression [7]. In addition to hypermethylation of specific genes, there was also evidence of an association between hypermethylation of multiple genes (characterized by a methylation index) and increased cancer aggressiveness [27].

The widespread use of high-throughput arrays created an opportunity to discover new genes involved in the epigenetic regulation of carcinoma [9, 29–31]. We sought to further elucidate the role and importance of methylation in bladder cancer by applying an integrative analysis tool to The Cancer Genome Atlas Project [32]. Although the TCGA has revealed the remarkable diversity of genetic alterations in bladder cancer, with only lung cancer harboring more mutations per megabase, it is clear that not all identified abnormalities contribute to the development of urothelial cancer, as many events deemed abnormal using high-throughput screening may have no biologic effect [33]. Fan et al. evaluated the relationship between methylation status in the promotor of 90 genes and RNA expression in six tissue types and found no correlation between methylation status and gene expression [34]. In bladder cancer, Lauss et al. demonstrated only 8% of methylated genes had an effect on gene expression [10]. When using high-throughput methodology with 450,000 probes, there is a need to distinguish the epigenetic alterations that act as effectors of the malignant phenotype from "passenger" alterations with no biologic effect. Thus, we used a model-based tool (MethylMix) to identify those genes with aberrant methylation and linked these data to RNA-seq data reflecting gene expression. This tool has been shown to produce results consistent with other methods of integrative analysis but also to produce unique findings [19]. The marriage of these complementary "omics" may aid in revealing biologically and clinically relevant information [11].

Our study corroborates findings from prior studies. We found increases in methylation of specific genes were associated with more aggressive disease [27, 35, 36], and we found a slightly greater proportion of genes being hypermethylated in the group who survived at least 2 years when compared to the group that died within 2 years of surgery. Although there was some overlap in statistically significant genes between patients with better versus worse survival, there were 24 genes that were unique to the group with worse survival. While the evaluation of these genes showed the majority were candidate tumor suppressor genes in a variety of cancers, this is the first time most of

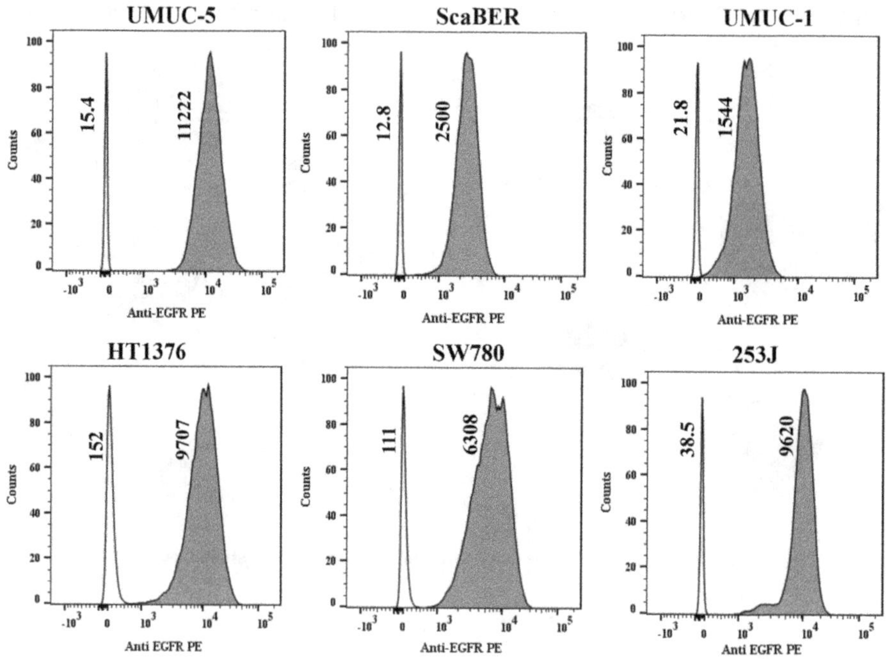

Fig. 5 Flow cytometry analysis demonstrating expression of EGFR on the cell surface of various cell lines. The curve shaded gray represents binding of rat monoclonal antibody to human EGFR tagged with phycoerythrin (PE). The curve without shading (white) represents binding of an isotype control, which in the case was a PE-tagged monoclonal rat IgG2a kappa. The vertically written numbers next to each peak represent median fluorescence intensity for isotype control and anti-EGFR PE. For all cell lines tested (UMUC1, UMUC5, Scaber, HT1376, SW780, and 253 J), there was substantial EGFR expression compared with isotype control

these genes have been associated with bladder cancer. This provides validation of the methodology and also provides an opportunity to evaluate the effect of cumulative methylation events. As a proof of principle, we show that many patients had hypermethylation of multiple poor-prognosis genes, suggesting that there may be many combinations of hypermethylation events that can lead to poor prognosis.

Our pathway analysis provided an opportunity to evaluate the gene lists produced by integrative analysis of all three patient groups, which is unique to our study. In examining all patients, one interesting finding from our pathway analysis was the enrichment of hypermethylated genes involved in antioxidant pathways. Genes involved in both glutathione-mediated detoxification as well as the nuclear factor (erythroid-derived)-like 2 (NRF2) pathway were statistically significantly hypermethylated, and both are integral in the cellular defense against oxidative stress. Glutathione is the most plentiful intracellular antioxidant and is a key component of redox-dependent regulation [37]. NRF2 is a transcription factor that serves as a key regulator in the cellular response to oxidative stress via induction of genes involved in the response to oxidative stress and xenobiotics, including those that regulate glutathione [38]. Deficiency of NRF2 has been shown to contribute to the development of cancer. In mice, knockout of the NRF2 gene increased susceptibility to formation of invasive bladder tumors in response to administration of a carcinogen [39].

In addition, there were two other notable findings. First, our pathway analysis enriched for hypermethylation of genes involved in the metabolism of estrogen. This is consistent with evidence for the role of estrogens in bladder cancer and suggests a basis for the observed clinical differences in the prevalence of bladder cancer between men and women. Shen et al. demonstrated that higher expression of estrogen receptor beta was associated with increasing stage and grade [40], and anti-estrogen compounds have been shown to inhibit the growth of bladder cancer cell lines [40, 41]. Targeting this pathway with anti-estrogens may have a therapeutic role in specific patients [42]. A second interesting observation was enrichment of hypomethylated genes associated with the epidermal growth factor receptor (EGFR) pathway. We were able to validate the presence of a substantial amount of EGFR on six bladder cancer cell lines. However, further validation of our findings is needed on independent cohorts.

Methylation is an attractive investigative tool for the study of aggressive cancer given that methylation is a reversible process. In myelodysplastic syndrome and AML, demethylating agents have been shown to have some effectiveness [43]. In this study, our integrative approach supports the findings of others showing that hypermethylation of specific genes is associated with aggressive urothelial carcinoma. The findings of this work may have application in the prevention of new disease and the reduction of disease recurrence in those with existing disease.

Conclusions

Taken together, our integrative approach to identify biologically active methylation events has demonstrated anomalies in methylation in invasive urothelial carcinoma. Genes involved in oncologically relevant pathways including EGFR were found to be hypomethylated. We found a substantial increase in methylation in pathways involved in the management of free radicals including NRF2 and glutathione. It appears that multiple of genes with tumor suppressor activity may be associated with overall poor prognosis.

Abbreviations

TCGA: The Cancer Genome Atlas Project

Acknowledgements

None.

Funding

None.

Authors' contributions

TS performed the statistical analysis and the lead author in the manuscript preparation. MVM is the co-lead author on the study design and assisted in the manuscript preparation and revisions. PKA input on the design of the study and assisted in the manuscript preparation and revisions. RR performed the cell line-based experiments and assisted in the manuscript preparation and revisions. SPP is the co-lead author on the study design, assisted in the manuscript preparation and revisions, and the corresponding author. All authors read and approved the final manuscript.

Competing interests

The authors declare that they have no competing interests.

Author details

[1]Department of Urology, University of California, Mail code 1695, 550 16th Street, 6th Floor, San Francisco, CA 94143, USA. [2]Urologic Oncology Branch, Center for Cancer Research, National Cancer Institute, Building 10—Hatfield CRC, Room 2-5952, Bethesda, MD 20892-1210, USA.

References

1. Siegel RL, Miller KD, Jemal A. Cancer statistics, 2015. CA Cancer J Clin. 2015; 65:5–29.
2. Rübben H, Lutzeyer W, Fischer N, Deutz F, Lagrange W, Giani G. Natural history and treatment of low and high risk superficial bladder tumors. J Urol. 1988;139:283–5.
3. Ghoneim MA, Abdel-Latif M, El-Mekresh M, Abol-Enein H, Mosbah A, Ashamallah A, et al. Radical cystectomy for carcinoma of the bladder: 2,720 consecutive cases 5 years later. J Urol. 2008;180:121–7.
4. Dalbagni G, Genega E, Hashibe M, Zhang ZF, Russo P, Herr H, et al. Cystectomy for bladder cancer: a contemporary series. J Urol. 2001;165:1111–6.
5. Wolff EM, Chihara Y, Pan F, Weisenberger DJ, Siegmund KD, Sugano K, et al. Unique DNA methylation patterns distinguish noninvasive and invasive urothelial cancers and establish an epigenetic field defect in premalignant tissue. Cancer Research American Association for Cancer Research. 2010;70:8169–78.
6. Catto JWF, Azzouzi A-R, Rehman I, Feeley KM, Cross SS, Amira N, et al. Promoter hypermethylation is associated with tumor location, stage, and subsequent progression in transitional cell carcinoma. J Clin Oncol. 2005;23: 2903–10.
7. Yates DR, Rehman I, Abbod MF, Meuth M, Cross SS, Linkens DA, et al. Promoter hypermethylation identifies progression risk in bladder cancer. Clin Cancer Res. 2007;13:2046 53.
8. Ning B, Li W, Zhao W, Wang R. Targeting epigenetic regulations in cancer. Acta Biochim Biophys Sin Shanghai. 2016;48:97–109.
9. Reinert T, Modin C, Castano FM, Lamy P, Wojdacz TK, Hansen LL, et al. Comprehensive genome methylation analysis in bladder cancer: identification and validation of novel methylated genes and application of these as urinary tumor markers. Clin Cancer Res American Association for Cancer Research. 2011;17:5582–92.
10. Lauss M, Aine M, Sjödahl G, Veerla S, Patschan O, Gudjonsson S, et al. DNA methylation analyses of urothelial carcinoma reveal distinct epigenetic subtypes and an association between gene copy number and methylation status. Epigenetics. 2012;7:858–67.
11. Wang KS, Liu X. Integrative analysis of genome-wide expression and methylation data. J Biom Biostat. 2013;
12. Robertson AG, Kim J, Al-Ahmadie H, Bellmunt J, Guo G, Cherniack AD, et al. Comprehensive molecular characterization of muscle invasive bladder cancer. Cell. 2017;171(3):540–56.
13. Cancer Genome Atlas Research Network. Comprehensive molecular characterization of urothelial bladder carcinoma. Nature. 2014;507:315–22.
14. Bibikova M, Barnes B, Tsan C, Ho V, Klotzle B, Le JM, et al. High density DNA methylation array with single CpG site resolution. Genomics. 2011;98:288–95.
15. Zhu Y, Qiu P, Ji Y. TCGA-Assembler: open-source software for retrieving and processing TCGA data. Nat Meth. 2014;11:599–600.
16. Robinson MD, McCarthy DJ, Smyth GK. edgeR: a Bioconductor package for differential expression analysis of digital gene expression data. Bioinformatics. 2009;26:139–40.
17. Ritchie ME, Phipson B, Wu D, Hu Y, Law CW, Shi W, et al. limma powers differential expression analyses for RNA-sequencing and microarray studies. Nucleic Acids Res. 2015;43:e47.
18. Gevaert O. MethylMix: an R package for identifying DNA methylation-driven genes. Bioinformatics. 2015;31:1839–41.
19. Gevaert O, Tibshirani R, Plevritis SK. Pancancer analysis of DNA methylation-driven genes using MethylMix. Genome Biol. 2015;16:17.
20. Kamburov A, Wierling C, Lehrach H, Herwig R. ConsensusPathDB—a database for integrating human functional interaction networks. Nucleic Acids Res. 2009;37:D623–8.
21. Welty C, Sanford T, Wright J, Carroll P, Meng M, Porten S. PD41-10 the impact of tumor stage on cancer specific survival in patients with node positive urothelial cancer of the bladder. J Urol. 2015;193:e843–4.
22. Malats N, Real FX. Epidemiology of bladder cancer. Hematol Oncol Clin North Am. 2015;29:177–89–vii.
23. Black PC, Agarwal PK, CPN D. Targeted therapies in bladder cancer—an update. Urologic Oncology: Seminars and Original Investigations. 2007;25:433–8.
24. Sharma P, Sharma R, Vijay M, Tiwari P, Goel A, Kundu A. Emphysematous pyelonephritis: our experience with conservative management in 14 cases. Urol Ann. 2013;5:157.
25. Kanwal R, Gupta S. Epigenetic modifications in cancer. Clin Genet. 2012;81: 303–11.
26. Kim Y-J, Yoon H-Y, Kim JS, Kang HW, Min B-D, Kim S-K, et al. HOXA9, ISL1and ALDH1A3methylation patterns as prognostic markers for nonmuscle invasive bladder cancer: array-based DNA methylation and expression profiling. Int J Cancer. 2013;133:1135–42.
27. Jarmalaite S, Jankevicius F, Kurgonaite K, Suziedelis K, Mutanen P, Husgafvel-Pursiainen K. Promoter hypermethylation in tumour suppressor genes shows association with stage, grade and invasiveness of bladder cancer. Oncology. 2008;75:145–51.
28. Catto JWF, Yates DR, Rehman I, Azzouzi AR, Patterson J, Sibony M, et al. Behavior of urothelial carcinoma with respect to anatomical location. J Urol. 2007;177:1715–20.
29. Chihara Y, Kanai Y, Fujimoto H, Sugano K, Kawashima K, Liang G, et al. Diagnostic markers of urothelial cancer based on DNA methylation analysis. BMC Cancer. 4 ed. 2013;13:275.

30. Kandimalla R, van Tilborg AAG, Kompier LC, Stumpel DJPM, Stam RW, Bangma CH, et al. Genome-wide analysis of CpG island methylation in bladder cancer identified TBX2, TBX3, GATA2, and ZIC4 as pTa-specific prognostic markers. Eur Urol. 2012;61:1245–56.
31. Marsit CJ, Houseman EA, Christensen BC, Gagne L, Wrensch MR, Nelson HH, et al. Identification of methylated genes associated with aggressive bladder cancer. PLoS One. 2010;5:e12334.
32. Network TCGAR. Comprehensive molecular characterization of urothelial bladder carcinoma. Nature Nature Publishing Group. 2014;507:315–22.
33. Kandoth C, McLellan MD, Vandin F, Ye K, Niu B, Lu C, et al. Mutational landscape and significance across 12 major cancer types. Nature. 2013;502: 333–9.
34. Fan S, Zhang X. CpG island methylation pattern in different human tissues and its correlation with gene expression. Biochem Biophys Res Commun. 2009;383:421–5.
35. Dhawan D, Hamdy FC, Rehman I, Patterson J, Cross SS, Feeley KM, et al. Evidence for the early onset of aberrant promoter methylation in urothelial carcinoma. J Pathol. 2006;209:336–43.
36. Brait M, Begum S, Carvalho AL, Dasgupta S, Vettore AL, Czerniak B, et al. Aberrant promoter methylation of multiple genes during pathogenesis of bladder cancer. Cancer Epidemiol Biomarkers Prev American Association for Cancer Research. 2008;17:2786–94.
37. Kalinina EV, Chernov NN, Novichkova MD. Role of glutathione, glutathione transferase, and glutaredoxin in regulation of redox-dependent processes. Biochemistry Moscow. 2015;79:1562–83.
38. Motohashi H, Yamamoto M. Nrf2-Keap1 defines a physiologically important stress response mechanism. Trends Mol Med. 2004;10:549–57.
39. Iida K, Itoh K, Kumagai Y, Oyasu R, Hattori K, Kawai K, et al. Nrf2 is essential for the chemopreventive efficacy of oltipraz against urinary bladder carcinogenesis. Cancer Res. 2004;64:6424–31.
40. Shen SS, Smith CL, Hsieh J-T, Yu J, Kim IY, Jian W, et al. Expression of estrogen receptors-alpha and -beta in bladder cancer cell lines and human bladder tumor tissue. Cancer. 2006;106:2610–6.
41. Hoffman KL, Lerner SP, Smith CL. Raloxifene inhibits growth of RT4 urothelial carcinoma cells via estrogen receptor-dependent induction of apoptosis and inhibition of proliferation. Horm Cancer. 2013;4:24–35.
42. Dellagrammaticas D, Bryden AA, Collins GN. Regression of metastatic transitional cell carcinoma in response to tamoxifen. J Urol. 2001;165:1631.
43. Issa J-PJ, Roboz G, Rizzieri D, Jabbour E, Stock W, O'Connell C, et al. Safety and tolerability of guadecitabine (SGI-110) in patients with myelodysplastic syndrome and acute myeloid leukaemia: a multicentre, randomised, dose-escalation phase 1 study. Lancet Oncol. 2015;16:1099–110.
44. Menendez L, Walker D, Matyunina LV, Dickerson EB, Bowen NJ, Polavarapu N, et al. Identification of candidate methylation-responsive genes in ovarian cancer. Mol Cancer. 2007;6:10.
45. Xu J, Sylvester R, Tighe AP, Chen S, Gudas LJ. Transcriptional activation of the suppressor of cytokine signaling-3 (SOCS-3) gene via STAT3 is increased in F9 REX1 (ZFP-42) knockout teratocarcinoma stem cells relative to wild-type cells. J Mol Biol. 2008;377:28–46.
46. Wei J-H, Haddad A, Wu K-J, Zhao H-W, Kapur P, Zhang Z-L, et al. A CpG-methylation-based assay to predict survival in clear cell renal cell carcinoma. Nat Commun. 2015;6:8699.
47. Calvisi DF, Ladu S, Conner EA, Seo D, Hsieh J-T, Factor VM, et al. Inactivation of Ras GTPase-activating proteins promotes unrestrained activity of wild-type Ras in human liver cancer. J Hepatol. 2011;54:311–9.
48. Yoon H-Y, Kim Y-J, Kim JS, Kim Y-W, Kang HW, Kim WT, et al. RSPH9 methylation pattern as a prognostic indicator in patients with non-muscle invasive bladder cancer. Oncol. Rep. Spandidos Publications. 2016;35:1195–203.
49. Yamada N, Yasui K, Dohi O, Gen Y, Tomie A, Kitaichi T, et al. Genome-wide DNA methylation analysis in hepatocellular carcinoma. Oncol Rep. 2016;35: 2228–36.
50. Schneider BP, Gray RJ, Radovich M, Shen F, Vance G, Li L, Jiang G, Miller KD, Gralow JR, Dickler MN, Cobleigh MA, Perez EA, Shenkier TN, Vang Nielsen K, Müller S, Thor A, Sledge GW Jr, Sparano JA, Davidson NE, Badve SS. Prognostic and predictive value of tumor vascular endothelial growth factor gene amplification in metastatic breast cancer treated with paclitaxel with and without bevacizumab; results from ECOG 2100 trial. Clin Cancer Res. 2013;19(5):1281-9. https://doi.org/10.1158/1078-0432.CCR-12-3029.
51. Zhang Z, Tang H, Wang Z, Zhang B, Liu W, Lu H, et al. MiR-185 targets the DNA methyltransferases 1 and regulates global DNA methylation in human glioma. Mol Cancer BioMed Central. 2011;10:124.
52. Kennedy MW, Chalamalasetty RB, Thomas S, Garriock RJ, Jailwala P, Yamaguchi TP. Sp5 and Sp8 recruit β-catenin and Tcf1-Lef1 to select enhancers to activate Wnt target gene transcription. Proc Natl Acad Sci U S A. 2016;113:3545–50.
53. Misawa K, Mochizuki D, Imai A, Endo S, Mima M, Misawa Y, et al. Prognostic value of aberrant promoter hypermethylation of tumor-related genes in early-stage head and neck cancer. Oncotarget. Impact Journals. 2016;7: 26087–98.
54. Tham C, Chew M, Soong R, Lim J, Ang M, Tang C, et al. Postoperative serum methylation levels of TAC1 and SEPT9 are independent predictors of recurrence and survival of patients with colorectal cancer. Cancer. 2014;120: 3131–41.
55. Liu Y, Tham CK, Ong SYK, Ho KS, Lim JF, Chew MH, et al. Serum methylation levels of TAC1. SEPT9 and EYA4 as diagnostic markers for early colorectal cancers: a pilot study. Biomarkers. 2013;18:399–405.
56. Kitchen MO, Bryan RT, Emes RD, Glossop JR, Luscombe C, Cheng KK, et al. Quantitative genome-wide methylation analysis of high-grade non-muscle invasive bladder cancer. Epigenetics. 2016;11:237–46.
57. Shui IM, Wong C-J, Zhao S, Kolb S, Ebot EM, Geybels MS, et al. Prostate tumor DNA methylation is associated with cigarette smoking and adverse prostate cancer outcomes. Cancer. 2016;122:2168–77.
58. Ushmorov A, Leithäuser F, Ritz O, Barth TFE, Möller P, Wirth T. ABF-1 is frequently silenced by promoter methylation in follicular lymphoma, diffuse large B-cell lymphoma and Burkitt's lymphoma. Leukemia. 2008;22:1942–4.
59. Sugimachi K, Matsumura T, Shimamura T, Hirata H, Uchi R, Ueda M, et al. Aberrant methylation of FOXE1 contributes to a poor prognosis for patients with colorectal cancer. Ann Surg Oncol. 2016;
60. Venza I, Visalli M, Tripodo B, De Grazia G, Loddo S, Teti D, et al. FOXE1 is a target for aberrant methylation in cutaneous squamous cell carcinoma. Br J Dermatol. 2010;162:1093–7.
61. Park E, Gong E-Y, Romanelli MG, Lee K. Suppression of estrogen receptor-alpha transactivation by thyroid transcription factor-2 in breast cancer cells. Biochem Biophys Res Commun. 2012;421:532–7.
62. Landa I, Ruiz-Llorente S, Montero-Conde C, Inglada-Pérez L, Schiavi F, Leskelä S, et al. The variant rs1867277 in FOXE1 gene confers thyroid cancer susceptibility through the recruitment of USF1/USF2 transcription factors. PLoS Genet. 2009;5:e1000637.
63. Yin DT, Xu J, Lei M, Li H, Wang Y, Liu Z, et al. Characterization of the novel tumor-suppressor gene CCDC67 in papillary thyroid carcinoma. Oncotarget Impact Journals. 2016;7:5830–41.
64. Park S-J, Jang H-R, Kim M, Kim J-H, Kwon O-H, Park J-L, et al. Epigenetic alteration of CCDC67 and its tumor suppressor function in gastric cancer. Carcinogenesis. 2012;33:1494–501.
65. Sandoval J, Mendez-Gonzalez J, Nadal E, Chen G, Carmona FJ, Sayols S, et al. A prognostic DNA methylation signature for stage I non-small-cell lung cancer. J Clin Oncol. 2013;31:4140–7.
66. de Groot JS, Pan X, Meeldijk J, van der Wall E, van Diest PJ, Moelans CB. Validation of DNA promoter hypermethylation biomarkers in breast cancer—a short report. Cell Oncol (Dordr) Springer Netherlands. 2014;37:297–303.
67. Yuan H, Kajiyama H, Ito S, Yoshikawa N, Hyodo T, Asano E, et al. ALX1 induces snail expression to promote epithelial-to-mesenchymal transition and invasion of ovarian cancer cells. Cancer Research. American Association for Cancer Research. 2013;73:1581–90.
68. Kim Y-H, Lee HC, Kim S-Y, Yeom YI, Ryu KJ, Min B-H, et al. Epigenomic analysis of aberrantly methylated genes in colorectal cancer identifies genes commonly affected by epigenetic alterations. Ann Surg Oncol. 2011;18:2338–47.
69. Mitchell SM, Ross JP, Drew HR, Ho T, Brown GS, Saunders NFW, et al. A panel of genes methylated with high frequency in colorectal cancer. BMC Cancer BioMed Central. 2014;14:54.
70. Ashktorab H, Daremipouran M, Goel A, Varma S, Leavitt R, Sun X, et al. DNA methylome profiling identifies novel methylated genes in African American patients with colorectal neoplasia. Epigenetics. 2014;9:503–12.
71. Yu C, Zhang Z, Liao W, Zhao X, Liu L, Wu Y, et al. The tumor-suppressor gene Nkx2.8 suppresses bladder cancer proliferation through upregulation of FOXO3a and inhibition of the MEK/ERK signaling pathway. Carcinogenesis Oxford University Press. 2012;33:678–86.

72. Lin C, Song L, Gong H, Liu A, Lin X, Wu J, et al. Nkx2-8 downregulation promotes angiogenesis and activates NF-κB in esophageal cancer. Cancer Research. American Association for Cancer Research. 2013;73:3638–48.
73. Steenbergen RD, Ongenaert M, Snellenberg S, Trooskens G, van der Meide WF, Pandey D, Bloushtain-Qimron N, Polyak K, Meijer CJ, Snijders PJ, Van Criekinge W. Methylation-specific digital karyotyping of HPV16E6E7-expressing human keratinocytes identifies novel methylation events in cervical carcinogenesis. J Pathol. 2013;231(1):53-62. https://doi.org/10.1002/path.4210.
74. Molina-Pinelo S, Salinas A, Moreno-Mata N, Ferrer I, Suarez R, Andrés-León E, et al. Impact of DLK1-DIO3 imprinted cluster hypomethylation in smoker patients with lung cancer. Oncotarget. 2016;
75. Martin-Subero JI, Ammerpohl O, Bibikova M, Wickham-Garcia E, Agirre X, Alvarez S, et al. A comprehensive microarray-based DNA methylation study of 367 hematological neoplasms. PLoS One. 2009;4:e6986.
76. Lindqvist BM, Wingren S, Motlagh PB, Nilsson TK. Whole genome DNA methylation signature of HER2-positive breast cancer. Epigenetics. 2014;9:1149–62.
77. Koga Y, Pelizzola M, Cheng E, Krauthammer M, Sznol M, Ariyan S, et al. Genome-wide screen of promoter methylation identifies novel markers in melanoma. Genome Res. 2009;19:1462–70.
78. Ma K, Cao B, Guo M. The detective, prognostic, and predictive value of DNA methylation in human esophageal squamous cell carcinoma. Clin Epigenetics BioMed Central. 2016;8:43.
79. Cheng Y, Geng H, Cheng SH, Liang P, Bai Y, Li J, et al. KRAB zinc finger protein ZNF382 is a proapoptotic tumor suppressor that represses multiple oncogenes and is commonly silenced in multiple carcinomas. Cancer Res. 2010;70:6516–26.

5

Overexpression of *UHRF1* promotes silencing of tumor suppressor genes and predicts outcome in hepatoblastoma

Alexander Beck[1†], Franziska Trippel[1†], Alexandra Wagner[1], Saskia Joppien[1], Max Felle[2], Christian Vokuhl[3], Thomas Schwarzmayr[4,5], Tim M. Strom[4,5], Dietrich von Schweinitz[1], Gernot Längst[2] and Roland Kappler[1*]

Abstract

Background: Hepatoblastoma (HB) is the most common liver tumor of childhood and occurs predominantly within the first 3 years of life. In accordance to its early manifestation, HB has been described to display an extremely low mutation rate. As substitute, epigenetic modifiers seem to play an exceptional role in its tumorigenesis, which holds promise to develop targeted therapies and establish biomarkers for patient risk stratification.

Results: We examined the role of a newly described protein complex consisting of three epigenetic regulators, namely E3 ubiquitin-like containing PHD and RING finger domain 1 (UHRF1), ubiquitin-specific-processing protease 7 (USP7), and DNA methyltransferase 1 (DNMT1), in HB. We found the complex to be located on the promoter regions of the pivotal HB-associated tumor suppressor genes (TSGs) *HHIP*, *IGFBP3*, and *SFRP1* in HB cells, thereby leading to strong repression through DNA methylation and histone modifications. Consequently, knockdown of *UHRF1* led to DNA demethylation and loss of the repressive H3K9me2 histone mark at the TSG loci with their subsequent transcriptional reactivation. The observed growth impairment of HB cells upon *UHRF1* knockdown could be attributed to reduced expression of genes involved in cell cycle progression, negative regulation of cell death, LIN28B signaling, and the adverse 16-gene signature, as revealed by global RNA sequencing. Clinically, overexpression of *UHRF1* in primary tumor tissues was significantly associated with poor survival and the prognostic high-risk 16-gene signature.

Conclusion: These findings suggest that UHRF1 is critical for aberrant TSG silencing and sustained growth signaling in HB and that *UHRF1* overexpression levels might serve as a prognostic biomarker and potential molecular target for HB patients.

Keywords: UHRF1, Hepatoblastoma, DNMT1, USP7, Histone methylation, DNA methylation, Epigenetic silencing, Tumor suppressor genes, Biomarker

Background

Hepatoblastoma (HB) is the most common liver tumor of childhood, with the majority of cases occurring in children under the age of 3 years [1]. Over the last four decades, advances in treatment protocols comprising chemotherapy and surgery drastically improved outcome of HB patients from a 30% to a roughly 80% overall survival rate [2]. However, there is still a relevant subgroup of high-risk patients presenting with distant metastasis, vascular invasion, advanced tumor stages, or unfavorable histology, whose outcome remains poor [3, 4]. In recent years, molecular markers have been shown to improve HB risk stratification and the effort to find robust markers that can predict outcome in HB patients continues [5, 6].

Molecularly, the development of this aggressive embryonal tumor remains largely unknown. Exome sequencing of primary HB revealed a surprisingly low mutation rate of only 2.9 mutations per tumor on average, and

* Correspondence: roland.kappler@med.uni-muenchen.de
†Equal contributors
[1]Department of Pediatric Surgery, Dr. von Hauner Children's Hospital, Ludwig-Maximilians-University Munich, Lindwurmstr. 2a, 80337 Munich, Germany
Full list of author information is available at the end of the article

there is evidence that epigenetic dysregulation plays a key role in HB development and progression [7]. Aberrant epigenetic silencing of tumor suppressor genes (TSGs) and overexpression of epigenetic regulators of gene silencing such as histone deacetylases (HDACs) appear to be important drivers of this disease [8]. In particular, the silencing of the TSGs hedgehog-interacting protein (*HHIP*), insulin-like growth factor-binding protein 3 (*IGFBP3*), and secreted frizzled-related protein 1 (*SFRP1*) have been shown to deregulate pivotal pathways of embryonic development, thus promoting HB pathogenesis [9, 10]. While there is evidence that DNA methylation and repressive histone modifications are responsible for aberrant silencing of those genes, the molecular mechanisms through which those epigenetic changes are conveyed and maintained remain largely elusive.

We recently discovered a protein complex that is involved in aberrant DNA methylation and repression of TSGs in a human colon adenocarcinoma cell line [11]. The complex comprises three subunits, namely DNA methyltransferase 1 (DNMT1), ubiquitin-specific-processing protease 7 (USP7), and E3 ubiquitin-like containing PHD and RING finger domain 1 (UHRF1) (Fig. 1a). Those three proteins are capable of forming a trimeric repression complex through their specific binding domains and carry out distinct functions within the complex. DNMT1 effectively methylates DNA on CpG islands and maintains DNA methylation patterns throughout the cell cycle [12, 13]. USP7 has been shown to enhance DNMT1 function and to stabilize UHRF1 levels by preventing its degradation [11]. While UHRF1 has no chromatin or DNA methylation activities itself, it functions as a crucial guide for DNMT1 and USP7 by binding to both via its SET- and RING-associated (SRA) domain. Through this domain, UHRF1 is also capable of recognizing hemi-methylated DNA, thereby recruiting the complex to hemi-methylated CpGs and maintaining DNA methylation throughout the genome [14].

Furthermore, UHRF1 is involved in histone modification, as it recognizes the repressive histone H3 lysine 9 methylation mark (H3K9me2) via its tandem tudor domain (TTD), thus facilitating the maintenance of this mark and the formation of heterochromatin [15, 16]. UHRF1 is also able to form a complex with HDAC1, another facilitator of histone-driven gene repression [17]. Because of this dynamic crosstalk between histone and DNA modifications, UHRF1 occupies a unique role when it comes to long-term silencing of genes [18].

Overexpression and dysregulation of UHRF1 are common features in a variety of human malignancies, and UHRF1-mediated silencing of TSGs appears to drive tumorigenesis in a disease-specific context [19]. In fact, UHRF1 is so widely overexpressed in solid tumors that it has been suggested as a universal biomarker for cancer [20]. However, the challenge lies in deciphering the disease-specific context in which UHRF1 conveys its oncogenic properties.

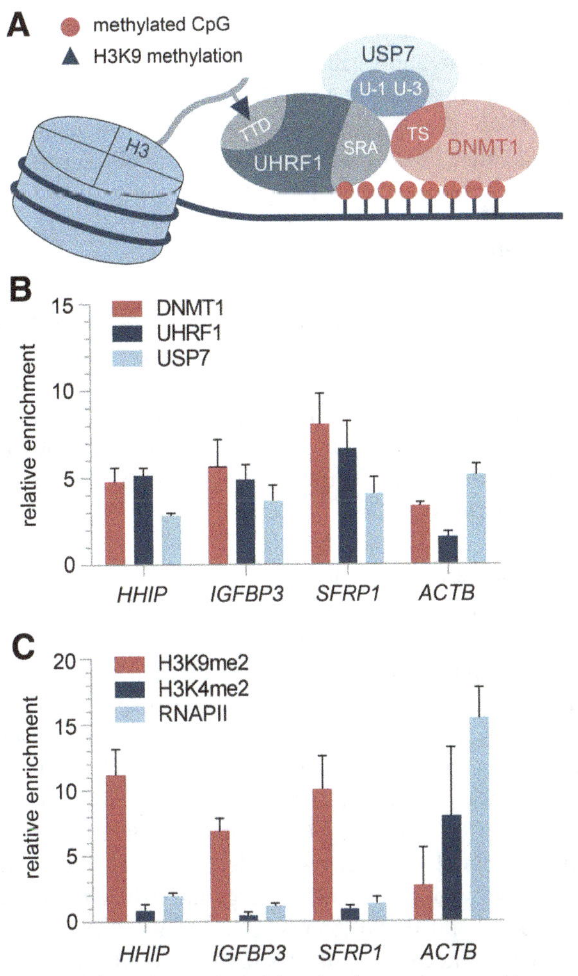

Fig. 1 **a** Schematic overview of the trimeric complex comprising UHRF1, USP7, and DNMT1. Involved protein interactions and protein domains according to Felle et al. are shown [11]. **b**, **c** Chromatin immunoprecipitation (ChIP) was performed with HUH6 cells and the indicated antibodies. The average of two independent ChIP experiments for **b** DNMT1, UHRF1, and USP7 as well as **c** H3K9me2, H3K4me2, and RNAPII is shown. Standard deviations, genes of interest, and antibodies used for ChIP are indicated. The enrichment of specific IP versus IgG background is plotted

Here, we show the trimeric UHRF1 complex to be located on the promoter regions of *HHIP*, *IGFBP3*, and *SFRP1* in HB cells, thereby leading to strong repression of those pivotal HB-associated TSGs through DNA methylation and histone modifications. Knockdown of *UHRF1* results in demethylation of promoter regions, loss of the repressive H3K9me2 mark, and subsequent re-expression of the abovementioned TSGs in HB cells. Furthermore, we show that *UHRF1* knockdown facilitates proliferation impairment and global transcriptional changes in HB cells. Finally, we reveal overexpression of *UHRF1* in primary HB to be associated with poor patient outcome and established risk stratification criteria. These findings suggest that UHRF1 is critical for aberrant TSG silencing and sustained growth signaling in HB and that *UHRF1* expression levels might serve as a prognostic biomarker for HB patients.

Methods

Patients

A total of 40 liver tumor specimens were obtained from pediatric patients undergoing surgical resection in our department. Matching normal liver was available from seven patients. Written informed consent was obtained from each patient, and the study protocol was approved by the Committee of Ethics of the Ludwig Maximilian University of Munich.

Cell culture and transfection

The human hepatoblastoma cell lines HUH6 (Japanese Collection of Research Bioresources, JCRB, Osaka, Japan), HepT1 (provided by Dr. T. Pietsch), and HepG2 (ATCC, Manassas, USA) were cultured under standard conditions in RPMI 1640 growth media (Invitrogen, Carlsbad, CA, USA), supplemented with 10% fetal calf serum, 100 U/mL penicillin, and 100 µg/mL streptomycin at 37 °C in a 5% CO_2 incubator. For knockdown experiments, 2×10^6 cells were electroporated for 10 ms at 350 V with either siRNA targeting *UHRF1* (siRNA #s26553, Applied Biosystems, Darmstadt, Germany) or appropriate negative control siRNA (siGENOMEN non targeting siRNA #1, Thermo Scientific, Karlsruhe, Germany) in a final concentration of 80 pmol.

RNA isolation, reverse transcription, and qRT-PCR

Total RNA was isolated 48 h after transfection using TriReagent (Sigma-Aldrich, Steinheim, Germany) according to the manufacturer's instructions. Two micrograms of total RNA was reverse transcribed into cDNA using random hexamer primer (Roche Diagnostics, Penzberg, Germany) and SuperScriptII Reverse Transcriptase (Invitrogen, Karlsruhe, Germany). PCR amplifications on the Master cycler ep gradient (Eppendorf, Hamburg, Germany) using iTaq-SYBR Green-Supermix (Bio-Rad, Hercules, CA) were performed in doublets as described previously [21]. The following primer pairs (5′-> 3′ orientation) were used: UHRF1, CTCCACGTC-CAGGCCG, TGGAGTTCATCTGGACCACG; HHIP, TGTACATCATTCTTGGTGATGGG, AGCCGTAGCA CTGAGCCTGT; IGFBP3, GTCCAAGCGGGAGACA-GAATAT, CCTGGGACTCAGCACATTGA; SFRP1, CA TGACGCCGCCCAAT, GATGGCCTCAGATTTCAAC TCG; and TBP, GCCCGAAACGCCGAATAT, CCGTG GTTCGTGGCTCTCT. Data were normalized to the expression level of the housekeeping gene TATA-Box-binding protein (TBP). For calculation of the relative mRNA expression level, the ΔΔCT method was used and expressed as fold change relative to the corresponding control sample [22].

Western blot analysis

Forty-eight hours after transfection, cells were harvested with ice-cold lysis buffer (0.2 M KCl, 0.03 M Tris, pH 7.25) containing proteinase inhibitor cocktail (Roche Diagnostics). Lysates were boiled in equal volumes of loading buffer (125 mM Tris-HCl, pH 6.8, 4% SDS, 20% glycerol, and 10% ß-mercaptoethanol), and 20 µg of protein was separated in a 8–12% gradient Tris-glycine gradient gel (Novex, San Diego, CA, USA) under reducing conditions and transferred to nitrocellulose membranes (GE Healthcare, Piscataway, USA). Afterwards, membranes were blocked at room temperature with PBS containing 0.1% Tween and 5% non-fat dry milk to block non-specific binding for 2 h. Membranes were incubated with primary antibodies (rabbit anti-human ß-actin, Cell Signaling Technology, Danvers, USA; mouse anti-human UHRF1, generously provided by Dr. C. Bronner, Institute of Genetics and Molecular and Cellular Biology, Strasbourg, France) at 4 °C overnight, followed by a 1-h incubation with the corresponding secondary antibodies (goat anti-rabbit-HRP and goat anti-mouse-HRP, both Dako Cytomation, Hamburg, Germany) at room temperature. For chemiluminescent detection, the ECL Plus Western detection kit (GE Healthcare) was used. Protein bands were detected by autoradiography using the high-performance autoradiography Hyperfilm™ MP (GE Healthcare).

Methylation-specific polymerase chain reaction (MSP)

Genomic DNA was extracted by phenol/chloroform after proteinase K treatment. Two micrograms of purified genomic DNA was used for bisulfite-mediated conversion of unmethylated cytosine using the Epitec Bisulfite Kit (Qiagen, Hilden, Germany). For MSP, bisulfite-treated DNA was amplified with primers specific for the methylated (M) and unmethylated (U) promoter region of either the *HHIP* (from − 230 to − 87 bp upstream of the transcriptional start site), the *IGFBP3* (from − 180 to − 13 bp upstream of the transcriptional start site), or the *SFRP1* (from + 36 to + 175 bp downstream of the transcriptional start site) gene. As a control for MSP, we used in vitro methylated genomic DNA that has been treated for 4 h with 40 U CpG methyltransferase (M. SssI), NEBuffer2 (10×), and SAM (1:20) at 37 °C, followed by heat inactivation for 20 min at 65 °C. For MSP, we used 1 U hot start Taq polymerase (Thermo Scientific, Schwerte, Germany), 1× hot start Taq buffer, 2 mM dNTPs, 1.5 mM $MgCl_2$, 100 ng bisulfite-treated DNA, and 500 nM of the following forward and reverse primers (5′-> 3′ orientation) and annealing temperatures: HHIP-M-F, AGTAGTCGGGTATGTTCG GAATTTTC and HHIP-M-R, GAACCTTCGAAACCAAC CTCG at 53 °C; IGFBP3-M-F, GCGAGTTTCGAGTTG TACGTTTTC and IGFBP3-M-R, GCCGACCGCTATATA AAAACCG at 61 °C; SFRP1-M-F, TTTGTAGTTTTCGGA GTTAGTGTCGC and SFRP1-M-R, CGACCCTCGACC TACGATCG at 58 °C; HHIP-U-F, TTGTAGTAGTTGGG TAGTTTTGGAATTTTT and HHIP-U-R, AAACCTTAA AACCAACCTCAAAA at 53 °C; IGFBP3-U-F, TTGGG TGAGTTTTGAGTTGTATGTTTTT and IGFBP3-U-R, AAACACACCAACCACTATATAAAAACCAAA at 61 °C; and SFRP1-U-F, TTTTGTAGTTTTTGGAGTTAGTGTT GTGTG and SFRP1-U-R, CAATAACAACCCTCAACCTA CAATCAA at 58 °C. MSP primer design was accomplished using Methyl Primer Express (Applied Biosystems) using the following criteria: CpG percentage > 55%, observed/expected CpG > 65%, and CpG length > 300 bp. MSP reactions were carried out at the following conditions: hot start at 94 °C for 4 min, followed by 38 cycles of 94 °C for 30 s, gene-specific annealing temperature (see above) for 30 s, 72 °C for 45 s, and final extension at 72 °C for 10 min. One percent agarose gel electrophoresis was performed to visualize DNA amplicons.

Pyrosequencing

For pyrosequencing, 100 ng bisulfite-treated DNA was first amplified in a PCR reaction, using 1 U hot start Taq polymerase (Thermo Scientific), 1× hot start Taq buffer, 2 mM dNTPs, 1.5 mM $MgCl_2$, 100 ng bisulfite-treated DNA, and 500 nM of the following forward and reverse primers (5′-> 3′ orientation) and annealing temperatures: HHIP-F, GGGAGGAGAGAGGAGTTT and HHIP-R, AACCAACCTCCAAAATACTAAACC at 55 °C; IGFBP3-F, TGGTTTTTTGAGATTTAAATGTAAGTTAGA and IGFBP3-R, ATCACCCCAATCACTCCTA at 57 °C; SFRP1-F, GGAGTTAGAGATTAGTTTGGTTAATATGG and SFRP1-R, AAAAACCTAAATCATACTTACAACC at 54 °C; and LINE1-F and LINE1-R (assay X58075, Qiagen) at 55 °C. PCR reactions were run at 95 °C for 4 min and 45 cycles of 95 °C for 20 s, gene-specific annealing temperature (see above) for 20 s, and 72 °C for 30 s. PCR products were sequenced with the corresponding sequencing primers HHIP-Seq, TTTAGGATTGAGTTTTTGTT TTAAG; IGFBP3-Seq, TTGGGTTATTTAGGTTTTATAT AG; and SFRP1-Seq, GGTAAGAGGTTGTAATTTTAG TTAT using PyroMark Gold Q24 reagents (Qiagen).

Chromatin immunoprecipitation (ChIP)

8.0×10^6 HUH6 cells were transfected with siRNA against *UHRF1* or corresponding non-target siRNA and subsequently seeded in 15-cm plates. After 48 h, the protein-DNA complexes were cross-linked with 1% formaldehyde for 10 min. The cross-linked reaction was quenched with Glycine Stop-Fix Solution for 5 min. Cell lysis, enzymatic digest (5 min), chromatin immunoprecipitation with 2 μg of antibody against di-methylated H3K4, di-methylated H3K9, RNA-Pol2 (all from Active Motif, La Hulpe, Belgium), and mouse IgG (Santa Cruz, Heidelberg, Germany), respectively, as well as final elution, cross-link reversal, and proteinase K digestion, were performed according to the manufacturer's protocol (catalog no. 53009, Active Motif). Chromatin samples were subjected to a DNA clean-up step using the QIAquick PCR Purification kit (QIAGEN). Real-time PCR was performed on purified DNA from each of the ChIP reactions using primer pairs for loci of the promoter region of the *HHIP* gene, the *IGFBP3* gene, the *SFRP1* gene, and the *ACTB* gene. Primer pairs used in this study were the following: HHIP_ChIP_F, TTCCCACCTCCT ACGGCC and HHIP_ChIP_R, TCCTCTCTCCTCCCC GCTT; IGFBP3_ChIP_F, GCTCCCTGAGACCCAAA TGTAA and IGFBP3_ChIP_R, GCTCGGCATTCGTG TGTACC; SFRP1_ChIP_F, ACGCCGTGATCCATTC CC and SFRP1_ChIP_R, CGGCTCAACACCCCTTAA AAA; and ACTB_ChIP_F, GCCAACGCCAAAACT CTCC and ACTB_ChIP_R, CAGTGCAGCATTTTT TTACCCC.

Cell viability assay

To assess cell proliferation, a 3-(4,5-dimethyl-2-thiazolyl)-2,5-diphenyl-2*H*-tetrazolium bromide (MTT)-based protocol was used. Directly after electroporation, cells were seeded at a density of 2500 (HUH6 and HepT1) or 5000 (HepG2) cells per well in a 96-well format (Nunc, Wiesbaden, Germany) in 100 μL RPMI medium. Ten microliters of MTT labeling agent (5 mg/mL, Sigma) was added to each well and incubated at 37 °C for 4 h. One hundred microliters of a SDS-HCl solution was added to each well and mixed thoroughly. Microplate was incubated overnight at 37 °C in a humidified chamber. The absorbance of this colorimetric reaction was quantified on the GENios reader (Tecan, Männedorf, Switzerland) by measuring at a wavelength of 595 nm.

Cell migration assay

Transfected HB cells were seeded into 12-well plates and grown to complete confluency. A wound of approximately 1 mm was inflicted to cell monolayers with a pipette tip. The wells were washed with PBS to remove detached cells and incubated at 37 °C for a maximum time of 120 h. Images were taken every 24 h after scratching, and the wound widths were measured with ImageJ (Rasband, W.S., ImageJ, US National Institutes of Health, Bethesda, MD, USA).

RNA sequencing

Total RNA of siUHRF1 and control transfected HUH6 cells was quality checked and quantitatively measured using the RNA 6000 nanokit on a 2100 Bioanalyzer (Agilent Technologies, Santa Clara, CA, USA). Coding transcriptomes were enriched from 1 μg total RNA in solution with TruSeq non-stranded RNA v2 kits (Illumina, San Diego, CA, USA) and sequenced as 100 bp paired-end runs on a HiSeq2500 system (Illumina) generating 35–79 million mapped reads. The STAR aligner v 2.4.2a [23] with modified parameter settings (–twopassMode=Basic) is used for split-read alignment against the human genome assembly hg19 (GRCh37) and UCSC knownGene annotation. To quantify the number of reads mapping to annotated genes, we use HTseq-count v0.6.0 [24]. The R Bioconductor package DESeq2 [25] with modified standard settings (no fold-change shrinkage) is used to investigate differences in gene expression.

Gene set enrichment analysis

Enrichment analysis of gene ontology and hallmark gene sets was performed by using the top 1000 differentially expressed genes of the RNA sequencing results as input for the latest version of the Molecular Signatures Database (MSigDB) developed by the Broad Institute [26]. Gene sets were selected by statistical significance ($p <$ 0.05) and the calculated representation factor. The representation factor is the number of overlapping genes divided by the expected number of overlapping genes drawn from two independent groups. A representation factor > 1 indicates more overlap than expected of two independent groups, and a representation factor < 1 indicates less overlap than expected.

Statistical analysis

Data were expressed as mean ± standard deviation or ±standard error of the mean and statistically subjected to Student's unpaired t test. Kaplan-Meier estimates of specific survival time in the various groups were compared using the log-rank Mantel-Cox test. Gene expression correlation was performed with GraphPad Prism version 6.0 using Spearman's rank correlation. A level of $p < 0.05$ was considered to be significant.

Results

UHRF1 repression complex binds to HB-specific TSG promoter regions

We used chromatin immunoprecipitations (ChIP) to identify enrichment of the UHRF1 repression complex (Fig. 1a) on chromatin of HB cells. We found all three complex partners, namely UHRF1, DNMT1, and USP7, to be enriched on the promoter regions of the HB-specific TSGs *HHIP*, *IGFBP3*, and *SFRP1* (Fig. 1b). Furthermore, ChIP analysis of the repressive H3K9me2 and activating H3K4me2 histone marks showed enrichment of H3K9me2, while H3K4me2 was not detected (Fig. 1c). The enrichment for RNA polymerase II (RNAPII) was negligible, indicating very low or no active transcription of those genes. Subsequent methylation-specific polymerase chain reaction (MSP) revealed hypermethylated promoter regions of those three genes (Fig. 2a). Quantitative mRNA analysis of *HHIP*, *IGFBP3*, and *SFRP1* confirmed the virtual silencing of gene expression (Fig. 2b). In sharp contrast, the housekeeping gene *ACTB* did not show any enrichment for UHRF1 and the repressive H3K9me2 mark, but high levels of H3K4me2 and RNAPII, which was accompanied by an unmethylated promoter and a high transcriptional activity. These data suggest that the trimeric UHRF1 repression complex might play a crucial role in deep silencing of the TSGs *HHIP*, *IGFBP3*, and *SFRP1* in HB via combined epigenetic mechanisms, comprising repressive histone modification and DNA methylation.

***UHRF1* knockdown leads to re-expression of TSGs through epigenetic modifications**

To evaluate the effect of *UHRF1* depletion in HB cells, we performed knockdown experiments, which resulted in a strong reduction of *UHRF1* both on the mRNA and the protein level (Fig. 3a, b). Depletion of *UHRF1* led to a significant re-expression of *HHIP* and *IGFBP3* (Fig. 3c). While the re-expression of *SFRP1* was not significant,

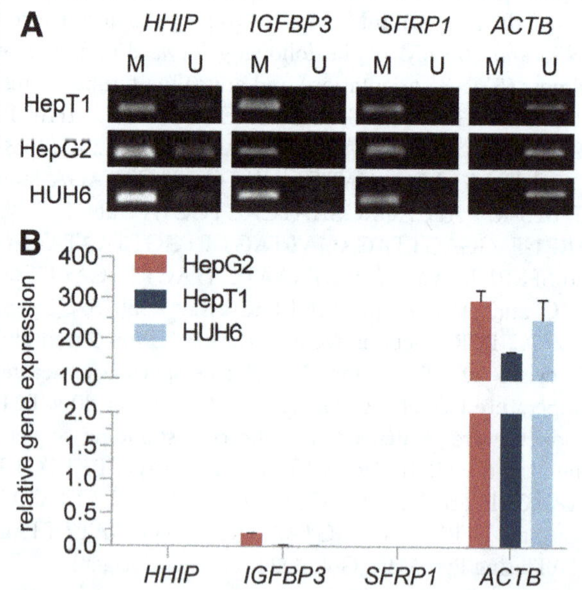

Fig. 2 a Methylation status (U, unmethylated; M, methylated) of the *HHIP*, *IGFBP3*, *SFRP1*, and *ACTB* promoter region was determined for the indicated cell lines by MSP. Representative images of MSP experiments are shown. **b** Relative expression levels of indicated genes compared to the *TBP* housekeeping gene in three liver tumor cell lines are given. The average of three independent experiments is shown

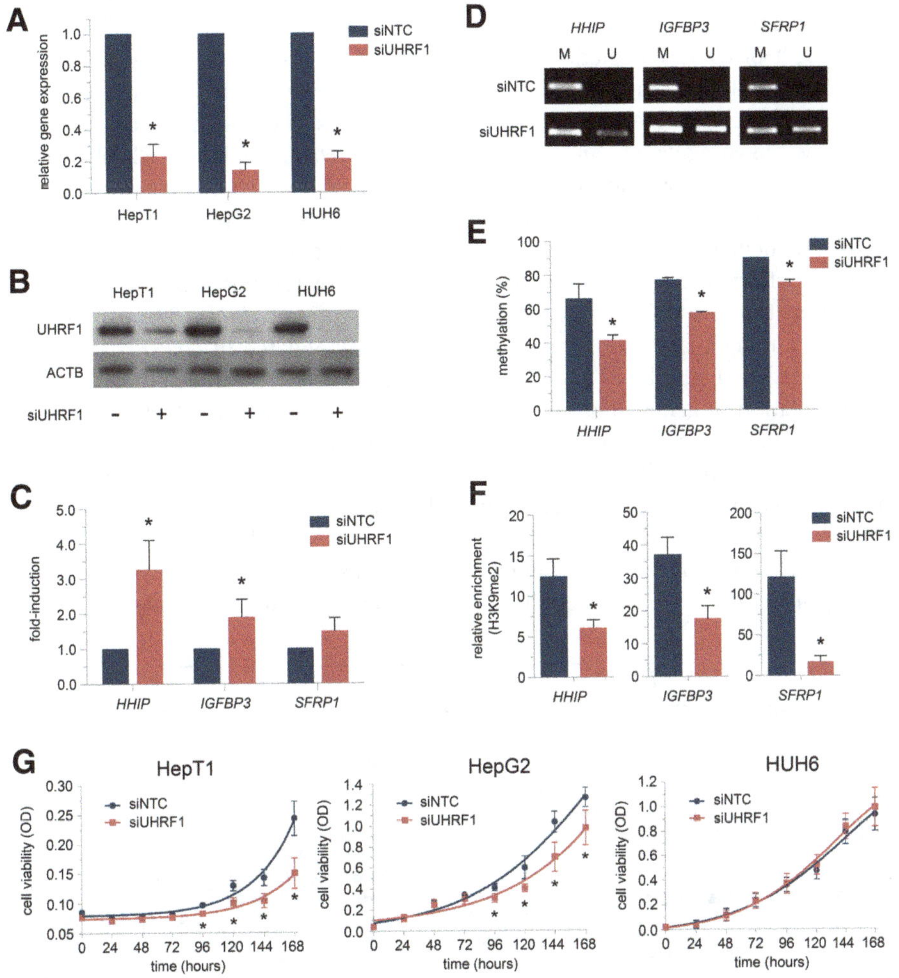

Fig. 3 a Knockdown of *UHRF1* in indicated cell lines. Relative gene expression in cells transfected with siRNA against *UHRF1* compared to negative control (siNTC) after 48 h is shown. Data represents average of three independent experiments. **b** Western blot analysis of HepT1, HepG2, and HUH6 cells 48 h after *UHRF1* knockdown. **c** Relative expression levels of indicated genes in HUH6 cells 48 h after *UHRF1* knockdown compared to negative control. The average of three independent experiments is shown. **d** Methylation status (U, unmethylated; M, methylated) of the *HHIP*, *IGFBP3*, and *SFRP1* promoter region 48 h after *UHRF1* knockdown was determined by MSP in HUH6 cells. Representative images of MSP experiments are shown. **e** Pyrosequencing results of promoter regions of indicated genes in HUH6 cells 48 h after *UHRF1* knockdown of three independent experiments are shown. **f** ChIP analyses in HUH6 cells 48 h after *UHRF1* knockdown. The relative enrichment of H3K9me2 at the indicated gene promoter regions is shown. **g** Cell viability of HepG2, HepT1, and HUH6 cells as evaluated by MTT assay at the indicated time points after *UHRF1* knockdown. Values represent means ± standard deviation of three independent experiments performed in duplicates. Statistical significance of all experiments was calculated using *t* test ($p < 0.05$)

we still observed an increase of *SFRP1* expression upon *UHRF1* knockdown. To further elucidate the role of the *UHRF1* repression complex, we performed MSP upon knockdown of *UHRF1*, *USP7*, and *DNMT1*, respectively. *UHRF1* knockdown led to a significant demethylation of DNA on the indicated TSG promoter regions (Fig. 3d). Quantification of those differentially methylated loci by pyrosequencing revealed a methylation decrease of 25, 20, and 15% for *HHIP*, *IGFBP3*, and *SFRP1*, respectively, upon *UHRF1* knockdown (Fig. 3e). This decrease in methylation correlates well with the strength of TSG re-expression. In addition, *UHRF1* knockdown also led to loss of the repressive H3K9me2 mark at those loci (Fig. 3f). *USP7* knockdown had no significant effect on the epigenetic marks regulating those genes and also did not result in gene reactivation (data not shown). To investigate the effect of those epigenetic changes and the re-expression of TSGs on HB cell proliferation, we performed viability assays over the course of 1 week following the knockdown. *UHRF1*-depleted HB cells showed a significant growth reduction in two out of three cell lines over time (Fig. 3g). This data suggests a combined derepressive effect of *UHRF1* knockdown on TSGs by alleviating repressive DNA and histone modifications, leading to a subsequent growth inhibition in HB cells.

RNA sequencing reveals HB-specific transcriptional changes upon *UHRF1* knockdown

In order to assess the effect of *UHRF1* depletion on the transcriptome, we performed RNA sequencing of HB cells upon *UHRF1* knockdown. As expected, we found *UHRF1* to be strongly downregulated and known UHRF1-repressed target genes [27–29] to be upregulated after *UHRF1* knockdown, thus emphasizing the significance of our RNA sequencing results (Fig. 4a).

To evaluate the general effect of *UHRF1* depletion in HB cells, we then used the top 1000 differentially expressed genes as input for the analysis of gene ontology and hallmark gene sets (Fig. 4b). The analysis showed significant upregulation of genes involved in the promotion of cell differentiation and development as well as cell adhesion. Genes involved in the p53 pathway were also significantly upregulated, indicating activation of this tumor suppressive pathway upon *UHRF1* knockdown. Conversely, *UHRF1* depletion led to significant downregulation of genes involved in epithelial-mesenchymal transition (EMT), cell cycle progression, and negative regulation of cell death. In order to evaluate the functional effect of downregulated EMT genes of *UHRF1*-depleted HUH6 cells, we performed cell migration assays in the identical cell line upon *UHRF1* knockdown. *UHRF1*-depleted cells showed a markedly slower cell migration compared to their control-transfected counterparts (Fig. 4e).

In recent years, LIN28B has been shown to play a pivotal role in HB initiation and progression [30]. Interestingly, we found *LIN28B* and its downstream targets to be downregulated in *UHRF1*-depleted HB cells (Fig. 4c). In agreement with this finding, we detected upregulation of *LET7* species, which are commonly suppressed by LIN28B in HB.

In HB, a prognostic 16-gene classifier has been established that discriminates between two subclasses of tumors, the so-called C1 subclass that is associated with early tumor stage and favorable patient outcome and the C2 subclass that is linked to metastases, vascular

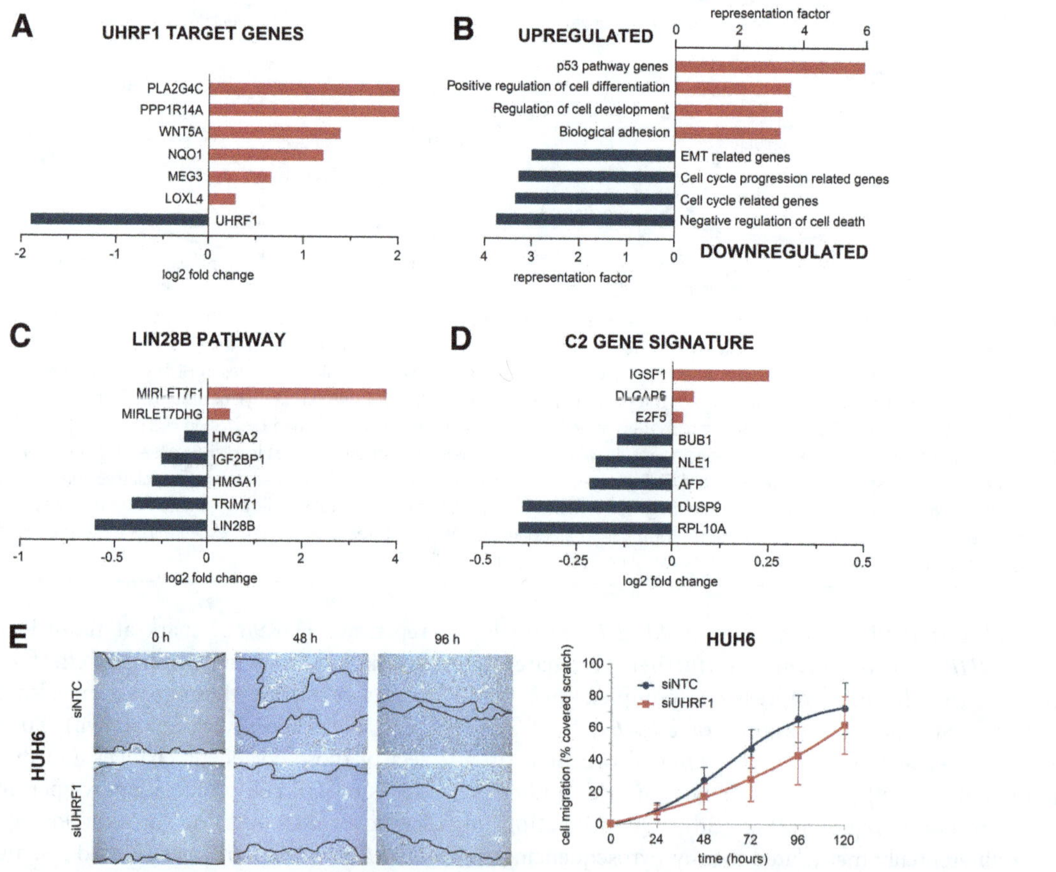

Fig. 4 RNA sequencing results upon *UHRF1* knockdown in HUH6 cells. Log_2 fold change of **a** known UHRF1 target genes, **c** genes related to the LIN28B pathway, and **d** genes highly expressed in the adverse C2 gene signature. **b** Significant enrichment of up- or downregulated genes within the indicated gene ontology and hallmark gene sets. Enrichment is indicated by the corresponding representation factor of each gene set. **e** Scratch assay. Representative images of HUH6 cells transfected with siRNA against *UHRF1* migrating into a cell-free space at 0, 48, and 96 h compared to negative control (siNTC). Quantitative evaluation of scratch closure shows the mean values of two independent experiments

invasion, advanced tumor stage, and poor prognosis [5]. Since HB cell lines initially showed the adverse C2 expression signature, we looked for changes in the eight genes that exhibit high expression levels within the C2 signature. Notably, five of those genes were downregulated upon *UHRF1* depletion (Fig. 4d), indicating a shift towards the favorable C1 signature, which is associated with low expression levels of those genes. Real-time qPCR analysis confirmed the downregulation of C2- and LIN28B-associated genes upon *UHRF1* knockdown (Additional file 1: Figure S1). These findings suggest a more global role of *UHRF1* in HB that goes well beyond the activation of only a few TSGs.

UHRF1 overexpressed in high-risk HB

When we investigated the expression levels of all three subunits of the trimeric repression complex, we found only *UHRF1* to be overexpressed in primary tumor samples and HB cell lines when compared to normal liver tissue (Fig. 5a). Overexpression of *UHRF1* has been reported in a variety of human malignancies and is often predictive for higher tumor stages and poor patient outcome [20]. Indeed, we found that high *UHRF1* expression levels were significantly associated with poor survival in HB patients (Fig. 5b). Of note, when comparing *UHRF1* expression levels with previously published expression levels of the tumor suppressor gene *HHIP* [21] in primary tumor tissues and the three cell lines, we also found a significant inverse correlation of both genes (Fig. 5c, inset).

Interestingly, we also found tumors exhibiting the high-risk C2 signature to be significantly associated with high expression levels of *UHRF1* (Fig. 5c). Consequently, patients with vascular tumor invasion, the unfavorable embryonal histology, metastases, large PRETEXT IV, and multifocal tumors predominantly had high expression of *UHRF1*. These data suggest that, consistent with findings in other solid tumors, *UHRF1* expression might be a prognostic marker for patients suffering from HB.

Discussion

Genetically, HB is a very simple tumor with one of the lowest mutation rates ever reported for any malignancy [31]. Characterizing HB by its genetic events has only

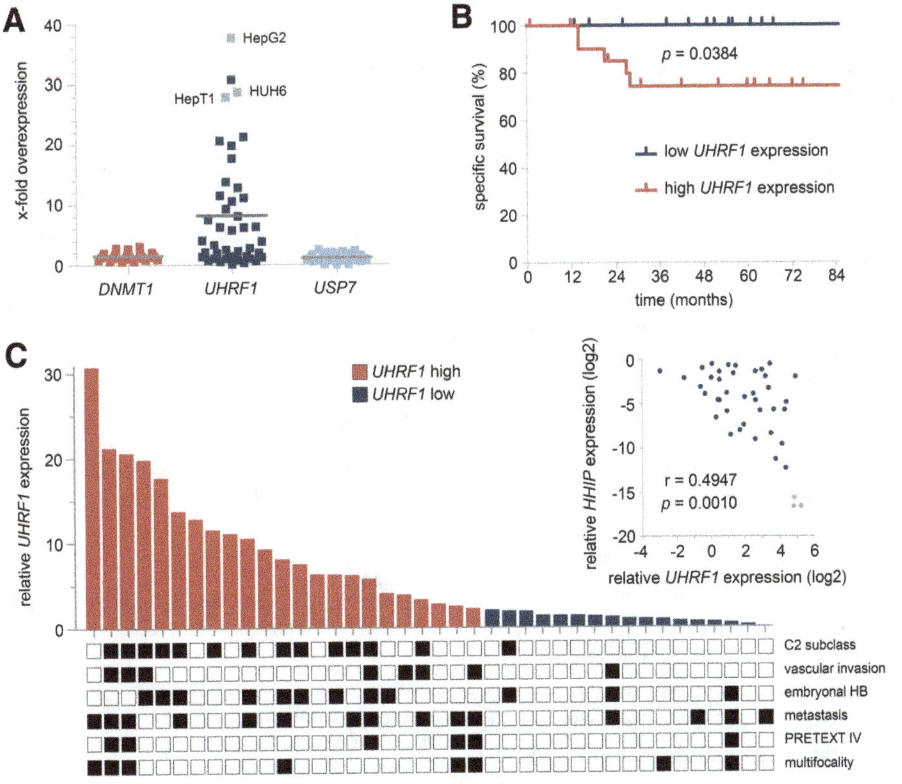

Fig. 5 a The relative expression of *DNMT1*, *UHRF1*, and *USP7* in 40 primary HB and three HB cell lines (depicted in gray) compared to the mean of seven normal liver tissues are given. **b** Overall survival was calculated as time from diagnosis to death of the disease and is plotted for 40 HB patients. Statistical significance was calculated using the Mantel-Cox test. **c** Individual *UHRF1* expression levels of 40 primary HBs are shown with the occurrence of important clinicopathological characteristics depicted as black boxes below. Inset: Expression levels of *UHRF1* and *HHIP* in primary tumor tissues (dark blue dots) and tumor cell lines (light blue dots) were plotted against each other, and Spearman's rank correlation was performed

limited significance when it comes to risk stratification and treatment selection. In addition, genetic mutations do not explain HB tumorigenesis sufficiently and previous studies made clear that epigenetic phenomena play a key role in HB development [10, 32].

While a number of epigenetic events, such as silencing of TSGs in HB, have been described in the past, the underlying molecular mechanisms remain largely unknown. Here, we identified a trimeric repression complex that is located at HB-specific TSG sites and is capable of conveying strong transcriptional repression of those genes by combined histone and DNA modification. Knockdown of *UHRF1*, which appears to be the critical subunit of the trimeric complex, leads to histone and DNA demethylation, re-expression of TSGs, and growth inhibition in HB cells. Reduced viability upon knockdown might be a result of the downregulation of genes involved in cell cycle progression and the negative regulation of cell death. UHRF1 has been shown to be a negative regulator of the p53 tumor suppressor pathway, and growth inhibition in HB cells might be augmented by the activation of this pathway following *UHRF1* depletion [33]. Knockdown-related upregulation of genes involved in cell differentiation and development might be a combined effect of p53 activation and the re-expression of TSGs that are capable of blocking aberrant growth signaling in HB cells. Notably, *UHRF1* knockdown led to downregulation of the HB-initiating LIN28B pathway and induced a shift towards the more favorable C1 signature. It also led to the upregulation of genes involved in cell adhesion and downregulation of EMT-related genes, thus promoting a more anti-metastatic phenotype. Our results strongly indicate that *UHRF1* represents an interesting molecular target for novel treatment strategies in HB.

As epigenetic aberrations are potentially reversible, a number of epigenetic therapy approaches have been developed in the last few years, some of which have shown great promise in the treatment of cancer [34]. In fact, we have recently shown that HDAC inhibition constitutes a potential epigenetic treatment option for high-risk HB patients [8]. Targeting *UHRF1* in HB holds the potential to further improve patient outcome, while reducing doses and toxicities of untargeted chemotherapeutic agents. Notably, the first in vitro studies of newly discovered *UHRF1* inhibitors have shown encouraging results in several cancer cell lines [35–38].

Furthermore, *UHRF1* overexpression seems to be a common feature in many malignancies and has therefore been suggested as a universal biomarker for cancer [20, 39–41]. Our systematic expression analysis of a large set of primary HB uncovered *UHRF1* overexpression to be a potential high-risk feature of HB, as high *UHRF1* expression levels were significantly correlated with poor survival in HB patients. Moreover, the C2 subtype of the 16-gene signature that has been shown to predict poor prognosis in HB was also significantly associated with high *UHRF1* expression.

Conclusions

Collectively, our findings suggest that UHRF1 is critical for aberrant epigenetic modifications and sustained growth signaling in HB. The unique capability of UHRF1 to convey repressive DNA and histone modifications highlights its potential to induce deep TSG silencing and other oncogenic events. UHRF1 therefore constitutes a promising target for novel therapeutic approaches in HB patients. Its overexpression in patients with high-risk features makes UHRF1 also a strong candidate for a prognostic biomarker in HB.

Abbreviations

ACTB: Beta actin; ChIP: Chromatin immunoprecipitation; CpG: Cytosine-phospho-guanine; DNMT1: DNA methyltransferase 1; EMT: Epithelial-mesenchymal transition; H3K4me2: Histone 3 lysine 4 di-methylation; H3K9me2: Histone 3 lysine 9 di-methylation; HB: Hepatoblastoma; HDAC: Histone deacetylase; HHIP: Hedgehog-interacting protein; IGFBP3: Insulin-like growth factor-binding protein 3; LIN28B: Lin-28 homolog B; MSP: Methylation-specific polymerase chain reaction; p53: Tumor protein p53; RNAPII: RNA polymerase II; SFRP1: Secreted frizzled-related protein; SRA: SET- and RING-associated; TSG: Tumor suppressor gene; TTD: Tandem tudor domain; UHRF1: E3 ubiquitin-like containing PHD and RING finger domain 1; USP7: Ubiquitin specific-processing protease 7

Acknowledgements

We are grateful to F. Promoli for the technical assistance, Dr. C. Bronner for generously providing the mouse anti-human UHRF1 antibody, and Dr. T. Pietsch for supplying us with the HepT1 cell line.

Funding

This work was supported by grants of the Bettina Bräu Foundation, Munich, Germany, and the Gänseblümchen-Voerde Foundation, Voerde, Germany (to RK).

Authors' contributions

AB, FT, AW, SJ, and MF performed the experiments and analyzed data. CV and DvS provided the patient materials and clinical data and interpreted the patient data. TS and TMS set up the RNA sequencing analysis tool and generated the data. GL contributed to the design and interpretation of experiments. AB and RK prepared the manuscript and figures. RK designed and supervised the study. All authors read and approved the final manuscript.

Competing interests
The authors declare that they have no competing interests.

Author details
[1]Department of Pediatric Surgery, Dr. von Hauner Children's Hospital, Ludwig-Maximilians-University Munich, Lindwurmstr. 2a, 80337 Munich, Germany. [2]Department of Biochemistry III, University Regensburg, Regensburg, Germany. [3]Institute of Paidopathology, Pediatric Tumor Registry, Christian-Albrecht's-University Kiel, Kiel, Germany. [4]Institute of Human Genetics, Helmholtz Zentrum München, Neuherberg, Germany. [5]Institute of Human Genetics, Technische Universität München, Munich, Germany.

References

1. Zimmermann A. The emerging family of hepatoblastoma tumours: from ontogenesis to oncogenesis. Eur J Cancer. 2005;41:1503–14.
2. Czauderna P, Lopez-Terrada D, Hiyama E, Haberle B, Malogolowkin MH, Meyers RL. Hepatoblastoma state of the art: pathology, genetics, risk stratification, and chemotherapy. Curr Opin Pediatr. 2014;26:19–28.
3. Meyers RL, Maibach R, Hiyama E, Haberle B, Krailo M, Rangaswami A, Aronson DC, Malogolowkin MH, Perilongo G, von Schweinitz D, et al. Risk-stratified staging in paediatric hepatoblastoma: a unified analysis from the Children's Hepatic tumors International Collaboration. Lancet Oncol. 2017; 18:122–31.
4. Zsiros J, Maibach R, Shafford E, Brugieres L, Brock P, Czauderna P, Roebuck D, Childs M, Zimmermann A, Laithier V, et al. Successful treatment of childhood high-risk hepatoblastoma with dose-intensive multiagent chemotherapy and surgery: final results of the SIOPEL-3HR study. J Clin Oncol. 2010;28:2584–90.
5. Cairo S, Armengol C, De Reynies A, Wei Y, Thomas E, Renard CA, Goga A, Balakrishnan A, Semeraro M, Gresh L, et al. Hepatic stem-like phenotype and interplay of Wnt/beta-catenin and Myc signaling in aggressive childhood liver cancer. Cancer Cell. 2008;14:471–84.
6. Sumazin P, Chen Y, Trevino LR, Sarabia SF, Hampton OA, Patel K, Mistretta TA, Zorman B, Thompson P, Heczey A, et al. Genomic analysis of hepatoblastoma identifies distinct molecular and prognostic subgroups. Hepatology. 2017;65:104–21.
7. Eichenmüller M, Trippel F, Kreuder M, Beck A, Schwarzmayr T, Häberle B, Cairo S, Leuschner I, von Schweinitz D, Strom TM, Kappler R. The genomic landscape of hepatoblastoma and their progenies with HCC-like features. J Hepatol. 2014;61:1312–20.
8. Beck A, Eberherr C, Hagemann M, Cairo S, Haberle B, Vokuhl C, von Schweinitz D, Kappler R. Connectivity map identifies HDAC inhibition as a treatment option of high-risk hepatoblastoma. Cancer Biol Ther. 2016;17:1168–76.
9. Regel I, Eichenmüller M, Joppien S, Liebl J, Häberle B, Müller-Höcker J, Vollmar A, von Schweinitz D, Kappler R. IGFBP3 impedes aggressive growth of pediatric liver cancer and is epigenetically silenced in vascular invasive and metastatic tumors. Mol Cancer. 2012;11:9.
10. Tomlinson GE, Kappler R. Genetics and epigenetics of hepatoblastoma. Pediatr Blood Cancer. 2012;59:785–92.
11. Felle M, Joppien S, Nemeth A, Diermeier S, Thalhammer V, Dobner T, Kremmer E, Kappler R, Langst G. The USP7/Dnmt1 complex stimulates the DNA methylation activity of Dnmt1 and regulates the stability of UHRF1. Nucleic Acids Res. 2011;39:8355–65.
12. Hermann A, Gowher H, Jeltsch A. Biochemistry and biology of mammalian DNA methyltransferases. Cell Mol Life Sci. 2004;61:2571–87.
13. Freitag M, Selker EU. Controlling DNA methylation: many roads to one modification. Curr Opin Genet Dev. 2005;15:191–9.
14. Bostick M, Kim JK, Esteve PO, Clark A, Pradhan S, Jacobsen SE. UHRF1 plays a role in maintaining DNA methylation in mammalian cells. Science. 2007; 317:1760–4.
15. Karagianni P, Amazit L, Qin J, Wong J. ICBP90, a novel methyl K9 H3 binding protein linking protein ubiquitination with heterochromatin formation. Mol Cell Biol. 2008;28:705–17.
16. Bronner C, Fuhrmann G, Chedin FL, Macaluso M, Dhe-Paganon S. UHRF1 links the histone code and DNA methylation to ensure faithful epigenetic memory inheritance. Genet Epigenet. 2009;2010:29–36.
17. Unoki M, Nishidate T, Nakamura Y. ICBP90, an E2F-1 target, recruits HDAC1 and binds to methyl-CpG through its SRA domain. Oncogene. 2004;23: 7601–10.
18. Hashimoto H, Horton JR, Zhang X, Cheng X. UHRF1, a modular multi-domain protein, regulates replication-coupled crosstalk between DNA methylation and histone modifications. Epigenetics. 2009;4:8–14.
19. Alhosin M, Omran Z, Zamzami MA, Al-Malki AL, Choudhry H, Mousli M, Bronner C. Signalling pathways in UHRF1-dependent regulation of tumor suppressor genes in cancer. J Exp Clin Cancer Res. 2016;35:174.
20. Ashraf W, Ibrahim A, Alhosin M, Zaayter L, Ouararhni K, Papin C, Ahmad T, Hamiche A, Mely Y, Bronner C, Mousli M. The epigenetic integrator UHRF1: on the road to become a universal biomarker for cancer. Oncotarget. 2017; 8:51946–62.
21. Eichenmüller M, Gruner I, Hagl B, Häberle B, Müller-Höcker J, von Schweinitz D, Kappler R. Blocking the hedgehog pathway inhibits hepatoblastoma growth. Hepatology. 2009;49:482–90.
22. Pfaffl MW. A new mathematical model for relative quantification in real-time RT-PCR. Nucleic Acids Res. 2001;29:e45.
23. Dobin A, Davis CA, Schlesinger F, Drenkow J, Zaleski C, Jha S, Batut P, Chaisson M, Gingeras TR. STAR: ultrafast universal RNA-seq aligner. Bioinformatics. 2013;29:15–21.
24. Anders S, Pyl PT, Huber W. HTSeq—a python framework to work with high-throughput sequencing data. Bioinformatics. 2015;31:166–9.
25. Love MI, Huber W, Anders S. Moderated estimation of fold change and dispersion for RNA-seq data with DESeq2. Genome Biol. 2014;15:550.
26. Subramanian A, Tamayo P, Mootha VK, Mukherjee S, Ebert BL, Gillette MA, Paulovich A, Pomeroy SL, Golub TR, Lander ES, Mesirov JP. Gene set enrichment analysis: a knowledge-based approach for interpreting genome-wide expression profiles. Proc Natl Acad Sci. 2005;102:15545–50.
27. Jung HJ, Byun HO, Jee BA, Min S, Jeoun UW, Lee YK, Seo Y, Woo HG, Yoon G. The ubiquitin-like with PHD and ring finger domains 1 (UHRF1)/DNA methyltransferase 1 (DNMT1) axis is a primary regulator of cell senescence. J Biol Chem. 2017;292:3729–39.
28. Abu-Alainin W, Gana T, Liloglou T, Olayanju A, Barrera LN, Ferguson R, Campbell F, Andrews T, Goldring C, Kitteringham N, et al. UHRF1 regulation of the Keap1-Nrf2 pathway in pancreatic cancer contributes to oncogenesis. J Pathol. 2016;238:423–33.
29. Zhuo H, Tang J, Lin Z, Jiang R, Zhang X, Ji J, Wang P, Sun B. The aberrant expression of MEG3 regulated by UHRF1 predicts the prognosis of hepatocellular carcinoma. Mol Carcinog. 2016;55:209–19.
30. Nguyen LH, Robinton DA, Seligson MT, Wu L, Li L, Rakheja D, Comerford SA, Ramezani S, Sun X, Parikh MS, et al. Lin28b is sufficient to drive liver cancer and necessary for its maintenance in murine models. Cancer Cell. 2014;26:248–61.
31. Vogelstein B, Papadopoulos N, Velculescu VE, Zhou S, Diaz LA Jr, Kinzler KW. Cancer genome landscapes. Science. 2013;339:1546–58.
32. Aguiar TFM, Carneiro TN, da Costa CML, Rosenberg C, da Cunha IW, Krepischi ACV. The genetic and epigenetic landscapes of hepatoblastomas. Applied Cancer Research. 2017;37:20.
33. Ma J, Peng J, Mo R, Ma S, Wang J, Zang L, Li W, Fan J. Ubiquitin E3 ligase UHRF1 regulates p53 ubiquitination and p53-dependent cell apoptosis in clear cell renal cell carcinoma. Biochem Biophys Res Commun. 2015;464:147–53.
34. Yoo CB, Jones PA. Epigenetic therapy of cancer: past, present and future. Nat Rev Drug Discov. 2006;5:37–50.
35. Ding G, Chen P, Zhang H, Huang X, Zang Y, Li J, Li J, Wong J. Regulation of ubiquitin-like with plant homeodomain and RING finger domain 1 (UHRF1) protein stability by heat shock protein 90 chaperone machinery. J Biol Chem. 2016;291:20125–35.
36. Seo JS, Choi YH, Moon JW, Kim HS, Park S-H. Hinokitiol induces DNA demethylation via DNMT1 and UHRF1 inhibition in colon cancer cells. BMC Cell Biol. 2017;18:14.
37. Walker DA, Wyhs N, Giovinazzo H, Yegnasubramanian S, Nelson WG. Abstract 5390: development of a high-throughput screening assay to identify UHRF1 inhibitors via time-resolved fluorescence resonance energy transfer (TR-FRET). Cancer Res. 2014;74:5390.

38. Unoki M, Brunet J, Mousli M. Drug discovery targeting epigenetic codes: the great potential of UHRF1, which links DNA methylation and histone modifications, as a drug target in cancers and toxoplasmosis. Biochem Pharmacol. 2009;78:1279–88.
39. Sidhu H, Capalash N. UHRF1: the key regulator of epigenetics and molecular target for cancer therapeutics. Tumour Biol. 2017;39:1010428317692205.
40. Zhou L, Shang Y, Jin Z, Zhang W, Lv C, Zhao X, Liu Y, Li N, Liang J. UHRF1 promotes proliferation of gastric cancer via mediating tumor suppressor gene hypermethylation. Cancer Biol Ther. 2015;16:1241–51.
41. Liu X, Ou H, Xiang L, Li X, Huang Y, Yang D. Elevated UHRF1 expression contributes to poor prognosis by promoting cell proliferation and metastasis in hepatocellular carcinoma. Oncotarget. 2017;8:10510–22.

6

Combined inhibition of BET proteins and class I HDACs synergistically induces apoptosis in urothelial carcinoma cell lines

Alexander S. Hölscher, Wolfgang A. Schulz, Maria Pinkerneil, Günter Niegisch and Michèle J. Hoffmann*

Abstract

Background: New efficient therapies for urothelial carcinoma (UC) are urgently required. Small-molecule drugs targeting chromatin regulators are reasonable candidates because these regulators are frequently mutated or deregulated in UC. Indeed, in previous work, Romidepsin, which targets class I histone deacetylases (HDAC), efficiently killed UC cells, but did not elicit canonical apoptosis and affected benign urothelial cells indiscriminately. Combinations of HDAC inhibitors with JQ1, an inhibitor of bromodomain-containing acetylation reader proteins like BRD4, which promote especially the transcription of pro-tumorigenic genes, have shown efficacy in several tumor types. We therefore investigated the effects of combined Romidepsin and JQ1 treatment on UC and benign urothelial control cells.

Results: JQ1 alone induced cell cycle arrest, but only limited apoptosis in eight UC cell lines with strongly varying IC_{50} values between 0.18 and 10 μM. Comparable effects were achieved by siRNA-mediated knockdown of BRD4. Romidepsin and JQ1 acted in a synergistic manner across all UC cell lines, efficiently inhibiting cell cycle progression, suppressing clonogenic growth, and inducing caspase-dependent apoptosis. Benign control cells were growth-arrested without apoptosis induction, but retained long-term proliferation capacity. In UC cells, anti-apoptotic and oncogenic factors Survivin, BCL-2, BCL-XL, c-MYC, EZH2 and SKP2 were consistently downregulated by the drug combination and AKT phosphorylation was diminished. Around the transcriptional start sites of these genes, the drug combination enhanced H3K27 acetylation, but decreased H3K4 trimethylation. The cell cycle inhibitor CDKN1C/$p57^{KIP2}$ was dramatically induced at mRNA and protein levels. However, Cas9-mediated CDKN1C/$p57^{KIP2}$ knockout did not rescue UC cells from apoptosis.

Conclusion: Our results demonstrate significant synergistic effects on induction of apoptosis in UC cells by the combination treatment with JQ1 and Romidepsin, but only minor effects in benign cells. Thus, this study established a promising new small-molecule combination therapy approach for UC.

Keywords: BET inhibitor, JQ1, HDACi, Romidepsin, Bladder cancer, Apoptosis

Background

For more than 30 years, chemotherapy of invasive urothelial carcinoma has been based on combinations of cisplatin with other cytotoxic drugs. This treatment is moderately efficacious and limited by frequent development of resistance and toxicity in the often elderly patients. Novel drugs targeting growth factor receptors or signal transduction pathways have so far not yielded significant benefits in clinical trials and have therefore not been introduced into clinical practice. Intriguingly, among all cancer types, urothelial carcinoma appears to have the highest prevalence of mutations in chromatin regulator proteins, including various components of the trithorax-like histone-modifying and SWI/SNF1 chromatin remodeling protein complexes [1]. It is therefore reasonable to assume that epigenetic inhibitors represent an alternative approach to chemotherapy of urothelial carcinoma.

Many epigenetic inhibitors target the activity of enzymes modifying histones or DNA. For instance, HDAC inhibitors (HDACi) interfere with the enzymatic activity of histone deacetylases and are considered good drug candidates. Our previous comprehensive analysis of expression of different HDACs isoenzymes in UC and their suitability as therapeutic targets revealed HDAC class I

* Correspondence: Michele.Hoffmann@hhu.de
Department of Urology, Medical Faculty, Heinrich-Heine-University, Duesseldorf, Moorenstr. 5, 40225 Duesseldorf, Germany

enzymes as the best targets for HDACi in UC therapy [2]. Drugs targeting specific class I HDACs like Romidepsin, Givinostat, or 4SC-202 most efficiently inhibited cell proliferation and caused cell death in UC cells. Despite their efficacy, these compounds do not seem optimal for treatment of UC on their own, because cell death occurred only partly by apoptosis and proliferation of benign urothelial control cells was also efficiently blocked [3, 4]. We therefore investigated the combination of Romidepsin with the BET inhibitor JQ1, which has been proposed to synergize with HDACi in several cancer types and to induce a canonical apoptotic response [5–8]. In pancreatic adenocarcinoma, the synergism was ascribed to several interacting mechanisms, encompassing inhibition of AKT signaling, increased STAT3 phosphorylation, and prominent induction of the CDK inhibitor $p57^{KIP2}$ [8].

JQ1 is the best characterized representative of a novel class of compounds which blocks binding of chromatin proteins by targeting domains recognizing histone modifications. JQ1 specifically targets the bromodomains of transcriptional coactivators like "bromodomain and extra-terminal" (BET) proteins, especially BRD proteins, and appears to be particularly effective in cancers dependent on MYC transcription factors, which are not well druggable by other means [9]. The best studied BET protein BRD4 has been shown to be overexpressed in UC tissues [10] correlating with grade, progression towards metastatic disease, and poor overall survival [11]. As an epigenetic reader of acetylation marks at histone tails, BRD4 functions as a scaffold protein linking chromatin remodeling and transcriptional regulation to cell cycle progression. A newly discovered histone acetyltransferase activity for H3K122 further contributes to chromatin decompaction and transcription activation [12]. Inhibition of BRD4 in particular disrupts super enhancers and represses the oncogenes *c-MYC* and *EZH2* [13, 14]. A pioneer study by Wu et al. on BRD4 in UC revealed its upregulation in cancer tissues and inhibition of cell proliferation by JQ1 in two related UC cell lines, T24 and EJ [10]. Knockdown of *BRD4* likewise inhibited proliferation of these UC cell lines. The authors ascribe these effects to inhibition of *c-MYC* and subsequent downregulation of *EZH2*.

In the present study, we therefore investigated whether JQ1 exerts antineoplastic effects on a broader range of UC cell lines which cover the heterogeneity of urothelial carcinoma more comprehensively. Indeed, its efficacy varied between the cell lines, and JQ1 neither suppressed clonogenic growth nor elicited pronounced apoptosis consistently. The combination of JQ1 with Romidepsin however displayed strong synergies in tumor cell growth suppression and apoptosis induction across all cell lines; concomitantly, histone acetylation was broadly enhanced. As in pancreatic adenocarcinoma cells, $p57^{KIP2}$ emerged as one factor synergistically responding to the combination treatment. Surprisingly, however, $p57^{KIP2}$ knockout rather enhanced apoptosis in UC cells.

Methods

Cell culture, transfections, drug exposure

BRD4 expression, effects of siRNA-mediated knockdown, and drug exposure were studied in a range of urothelial carcinoma cell lines (UCCs) representing the heterogeneity of urothelial carcinoma, namely, VM-Cub1, RT-112, T24, 5637, UM-UC-3, HT-1376, 639-V, BFTC-905, J-82, and SW-1710. All cell lines were regularly authenticated by STR profiling and checked for mycoplasm contamination. As normal cell controls, we used the normal urothelial cell lines HBLAK [15] and TERT-NHUC, a culture of primary urothelial cells (NHUC) [16], and benign immortalized fetal kidney HEK-293 cells.

UCCs and HEK-293 cells were cultured in DMEM GlutaMAX-I (Gibco, Darmstadt, Germany) supplemented with 4.5 g/l D-glucose, pyruvate, and 10% FBS (Biochrom, Berlin, Germany). HBLAK cells were cultured in CnT-Prime Epithelial Culture Medium (CELLnTEC, Bern, Switzerland). TERT-NHUC cells were cultured in keratinocyte serum-free medium (Gibco) supplemented with 0.35 μg/ml *N*-epinephrine and 0.33 mg/ml hydrocortisone. NHUC were cultured in keratinocyte serum-free medium (Gibco) supplemented with penicillin/streptomycin, EGF, and BPE. Primary urothelial carcinoma cultures were established from fresh transurethral resectates and cultured in Epilife Medium (Gibco) supplemented with 0.5 ng/ml EGF, 25 μg/ml BPE, 1% nonessential amino acids (Invitrogen, Darmstadt, Germany), 1% ITS mix (Invitrogen), 3 mM glycine, and 10% fibroblast-conditioned medium on a collagen IV matrix [17]. All cells were cultured at 37 °C and 5% CO_2.

For siRNA-mediated knockdown, cells cultured in six-well plates were transfected with 8 nM BRD4 ON-TARGET plus BRD4 siRNA-SMART pool (L-004937-00-0005, Dharmacon, Freiburg, Germany) or ON-Target plus Control pool (D-001810-10-05, Dharmacon) using Lipofectamine RNAiMAX (Life Technologies, Darmstadt, Germany) and assayed 48, 72, or 120 h post-transfection.

For BRD4 overexpression, cells were transfected with p6344 pcDNA4-TO-HA-Brd4FL (Addgene plasmid #31351) [18] or empty vector (pcDNA4-TO) using X-tremeGENE 9 DNA Transfection Reagent (Roche, Penzberg, Germany).

Romidepsin and (+)-JQ1 were purchased from Selleck Chemicals (Munich, Germany) and dissolved in DMSO. Control cells were treated with DMSO only. Drugs were added 24 h after cell seeding. Pan-Caspase inhibitor Q-VD-Oph (SML0063, Sigma Aldrich, Hamburg, Germany) was dissolved in DMSO and used at 30 μmol/l.

Drug concentrations for combination treatments were adjusted for each cell line since IC_{50} values for both compounds varied strongly (Table 1 upper part).

Determination of viability

Viability of cells treated with JQ1 was measured after 72 h by 3-(4,5-dimetylthiazol-2-yl)-2,5-diphenyltetrazolium bromide dye reduction assay (MTT, Sigma Aldrich). Viability of cells after siRNA-mediated BRD4 knockdown or treatment with Q-VD-Oph was measured via total cellular ATP using CellTiter-Glo Assay (Promega, Mannheim, Germany).

Calculation of IC_{50} values and drug synergy

For determination of IC_{50} values, JQ1 was added in defined concentration ranges. For determination of drug synergy, JQ1 and Romidepsin were used in fixed dose ratios. For each cell line, individual dose ratios were chosen based on the IC_{50} of the individual drugs (Table 1 upper part). For each cell line, at least five different combinations of concentrations were applied and then analyzed by the Chou-Talalay method using CompuSyn software [19]. The final cell line-dependent concentrations for the 48-h combination treatment used for subsequent analyses are given in Table 1 (lower part).

Table 1 Treatment doses for single and combined treatment. Eight UCCs, two immortalized benign urothelial cells (TERT-NHUC, HBLAK), primary urothelial cells (NHUC), and HEK-293 cells were treated with JQ1 at a fixed range of concentrations. Cell viability was measured by MTT- assay 72 h later. IC_{50} values for each cell line were determined (upper part). Cell viability results were used according to the Chou-Talalay method to determine doses for the combination treatment with synergistic effects for each investigated cell line. The respective doses were applied for further functional characterization for 48 h (lower part)

Urothelial carcinoma cell lines		Control cell lines	
	JQ1 IC_{50} [µmol/l]		JQ1 IC_{50} [µmol/l]
VM-Cub1	0.18	TERT-NHUC	0.4
RT-112	0.19	HBLAK	0.4
T24	0.23	NHUC	0.26
5637	0.39	HEK-293	0.26
UM-UC-3	2.6		
HT-1376	5.2		
639-V	6.8		
BFTC-905	10		
JQ1 + Romidepsin combination doses			
	JQ1 [µmol/l]		Romidepsin [nmol/l]
Vm-Cub1	0.22		2.2
UM-UC-3	1		2
T24	0.22		2.2
639-V	1.8		1.6
HBLAK	0.4		0.89

Colony-forming assay and Giemsa staining

For colony-forming assays, cells were seeded into six-well plates at a density of 1000 cells/well 48 h post drug treatment and either 48, 72, or 120 h post-siRNA transfection. After 10–15 days, cells were fixed in methanol and stained with Giemsa (Merck, Darmstadt, Germany).

Flow cytometry

Cell cycle analyses were performed 48 h after treatment with individual drugs or their combinations and 48, 72, and 120 h post-siRNA transfections. Detached cells in supernatant and attached cells were collected and stained with buffer containing 50 µg/ml propidium iodide, 0.1% sodium citrate, and 0.1% Triton X-100 for 1 h at room temperature. To assess apoptotic cell death and necrosis, cells were incubated with Annexin V-FITC (31490013, Immunotools, Friesoythe, Germany), Annexin V binding buffer, and propidium iodide at 2 µg/ml. Flow cytometry was done using the MACSQuant Analyzer (Miltenyi Biotech, Bergisch Gladbach, Germany) and MACSQuantify software as previously described [20].

RNA isolation, cDNA synthesis, and qRT-PCR

Total mRNA was isolated using the Qiagen RNeasy Mini Kit (Qiagen, Hilden, Germany) according to the manufacturer's protocol. cDNA synthesis was performed using the QuantiTect Reverse Transcription Kit (Qiagen) with an extended incubation time of 30 min at 42 °C. qRT-PCR was performed using the QuantiTect SYBR Green RT-PCR Kit (Qiagen) and self-designed primers for the target genes and the reference gene *TBP* (TATA-box-binding protein) on the LightCycler 96 PCR platform (Roche). The primers used are listed in Additional file 1.

Western blot analyses

Total cellular protein was extracted by lysis for 30 min on ice in RIPA buffer containing 150 mmol/l NaCl, 1% Triton X-100, 0.5% deoxycholate, 1% Nonidet P-40, 0.1% SDS, 1 mmol/l EDTA, 50 mmol/l TRIS (pH 7.6), protease inhibitor cocktail (10 µl/ml, Sigma Aldrich), and phosphatase inhibitor (10 µl/ml, Sigma Aldrich). Protein concentrations were determined by bicinchoninic acid protein assay (ThermoFisher Scientific, Darmstadt, Germany). Proteins were separated in SDS-PAGE gels and then wet-blotted to polyvinylidene difluoride (PVDF) membranes (Merck Millipore, Darmstadt, Germany). Membranes were blocked by 5% non-fat dry milk or BSA in TBS-T (150 mmol/l NaCl, 10 mmol/l TRIS, pH 7.6 and 0.1% TWEEN-20), washed several times, and then incubated with primary antibodies at 4 °C overnight. After several washings with TBS-T, membranes were incubated with horseradish peroxidase-conjugated secondary antibody at room temperature for 1 h. Membranes were then developed using Super Signal West Femto (ThermoFisher Scientific) or Western Bright Quantum (Biozym, Hessisch Oldendorf, Germany). α-tubulin was used as a loading control. Antibodies are listed in Additional file 1.

Extraction and analysis of histones

Histones were acid-extracted according to a published protocol [21]. One microgram of each sample was used for Western blot analysis with 15% SDS-PAGE gels and PVDF membranes (Merck Millipore) as described above using antibodies listed in Additional file 1. Histone H3 was used as a histone loading control.

Chromatin immunoprecipitation

ChIP-IT™ Express Kit (#53008, Active Motif, La Hulpe, Belgium) was used according to the manufacturer's instructions. Rabbit Gamma Globulins (#31887, Invitrogen) served as a background control. Quantitative real-time PCR was used to determine enrichment of indicated gene regions at their transcriptional start site (TSS) as well as 2 kb upstream and downstream of each TSS. For a list of antibodies and primers, see Additional file 1.

Generation of $p57^{KIP2}$ knockout cells by gene editing

Cells were transfected by X-tremeGENE 9 DNA transfection reagent (Roche, Penzberg, Germany) with p57 Double Nickase Plasmid (sc-400444-NIC-2, Santa Cruz Biotechnology, Heidelberg, Germany) encoding a GFP marker, puromycin resistance, and two different sgRNAs targeting *CDKN1C* exon 1 and D10A mutant Cas9 (Nickase). Double Nickase control Plasmid (sc-437281) with non-targeting sgRNAs was used as a control. GFP expression allowed monitoring of transfection efficiency. Transfected cells were selected with 0.5 μg/ml puromycin for 5 days before single-cell seeding into 96-well plates. Genomic DNA was extracted from single-cell clones using QIAamp DNA Mini Kit (Qiagen). An amplicon spanning the sgRNA binding sites was amplified using HotStarTaq polymerase (Qiagen); PCR products were cloned into PCR4-TOPO TA Vector (450030, Invitrogen) and Sanger-sequenced. Mutant sequences were compared to the NCBI *CDKN1C* reference sequence (NG_008022.1). Successful knockout of $p57^{KIP2}$ was verified by Western blot analysis.

Results

Knockdown of BRD4 exerts antineoplastic effects on UCCs

Since BRD4 is considered the most important target of the BET inhibitor JQ1 in various cancers, we evaluated BRD4 protein expression in a series of UCCs compared to the benign urothelial control cell lines HBLAK, TERT-NHUC, and NHUC (Fig. 1a). BRD4 was expressed in all tested UCCs at variable levels, in some UCCs more strongly than in the normal controls.

Next, we investigated by siRNA-mediated knockdown how dependent different UCCs are on BRD4 function and whether effects of siRNA knockdown differed from that by pharmacological inhibition in the same cell line. VM-Cub1 and UM-UC-3 cells were chosen for their very different phenotypes and have had been extensively characterized for their response to HDACi previously [3, 4]. As shown below, they were also differentially sensitive to JQ1 (Table 1 upper part). Efficient knockdown of BRD4 protein was confirmed at 48, 72, and 120 h post-transfection. Expression of c-MYC, a common target of BRD4, was strongly decreased in VM-Cub1 cells 120 h post-transfection, but not in UM-UC-3 (Fig. 1b).

Cell viability decreased following BRD4 knockdown in a time-dependent manner in both cell lines (Fig. 1c). Concordantly, clonogenic growth was significantly suppressed (Fig. 1d; $p \leq 0.01$). Changes in cell cycle distribution intensified over time; VM-Cub1 cells became arrested in G0/G1, whereas UM-UC-3 cells accumulated in G2/M (Fig. 1e). Only minor increases in subG1 fractions were observed.

UCCs differ in sensitivity to pharmacological BET inhibition

Next, we investigated the dose response of eight different UCCs, including VM-Cub1 and UM-UC-3, to JQ1. JQ1 diminished viability in all cell lines, but they clearly fell into two groups, with low and high sensitivity. Calculated IC_{50} values were below 0.5 μM in the first group, but well above 1 μM in the second group (Table 1). Notably, at the highest concentration of JQ1 (25 μM) tested, a sizeable fraction of cells survived the treatment. This fraction correlated only partially with the respective IC_{50}, indicating that JQ1 alone acted rather in a cytostatic fashion. No correlation was seen between sensitivity to JQ1 and BRD4 protein expression or any other previously investigated characteristics of the cell lines. Benign control cells generally responded to low concentrations of JQ1 (IC_{50} 0.26–0.4 μM).

BET inhibitor JQ1 and class I HDAC inhibitor Romidepsin synergistically inhibit UCC proliferation and clonogenic growth

Cell viability results from dose-response curves for JQ1, and Romidepsin were used to generate combination index plots (Fa/CI-Plots; fraction affected/combination index; Fig. 2a) by the Chou-Talalay method [19]. Strong synergisms ($CI < 1$) were detected for all four UCCs at effect rates (Fa; percentage of dead cells) from 0.2 (T24) to 0.4 (UM-UC-3). Synergies intensified with increasing effect rates. Intriguingly, the strongest synergies were seen in the less JQ1-sensitive 639-V and UM-UC-3 cells.

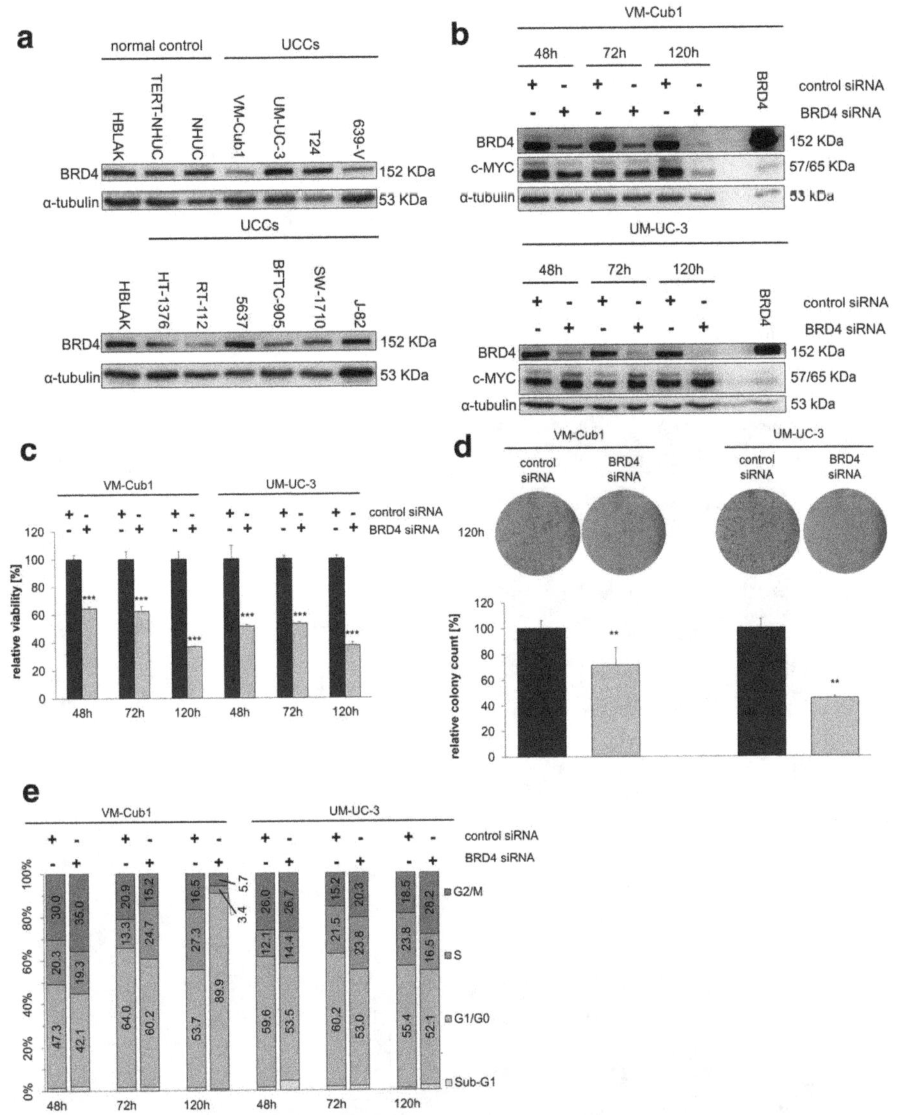

Fig. 1 Effects of BRD4 knockdown on urothelial carcinoma cell lines. **a** Western blot analysis of BRD4 expression in 10 UCCs compared to the benign urothelial control cell lines HBLAK, NHUC, and NHUC-TERT. α-tubulin served as a loading control. **b** Western blot analysis of BRD4 and c-MYC expression after siRNA-mediated knockdown of BRD4 in VM-Cub1 and UM-UC-3 cells. Cells transfected with BRD4 expression plasmid served as a positive control, with 3 μg instead of 20 μg protein loaded. **c** Relative viability of VM-Cub1 and UM-UC-3 cells after BRD4 knockdown for 48, 72, and 120 h compared to treatment with control siRNA. Relative viability is displayed on the ordinate in percent of the control cells treated with non-targeting siRNA. Differences between control and targeting siRNA were analyzed using Student's *t* test (***$p \leq 0.001$). **d** Clonogenicity assays of VM-Cub1 and UM-UC-3 cells after BRD4 knockdown for 120 h and results of quantification (**$p \leq 0.01$). **e** Flow cytometric cell cycle analysis of VM-Cub-1 and UM-UC-3 cells after BRD4 knockdown for 48, 72, or 120 h. Percentages of cells in the respective cell cycle phase are given

Similarly, primary cancer cell cultures established from patient tissues responded strongly towards combined treatment resulting in strong synergies (Additional file 2). In contrast, only a limited synergy of the combined treatment was seen with benign HBLAK cells (Fig. 2a).

Next, we compared the effects of single and combined treatment on cell proliferation and apoptosis. Dosages for the combined treatment were chosen from synergistic combinations and mostly below individual agent IC_{50}s (Table 1). Single treatment with JQ1 alone diminished clonogenic growth of the more sensitive VM-Cub1 cells (Fig. 2b), whereas the less sensitive UM-UC-3 cells readily formed colonies. Clone formation by benign HBLAK cells was rather unaffected. Next, we evaluated the combination of JQ1 and Romidepsin in two more (VM-Cub1 and T24) and two less (UM-UC-3 and 639-V) JQ1-sensitive UCCs and in HBLAK as a benign urothelial control. The combination treatment synergistically suppressed long-term proliferation

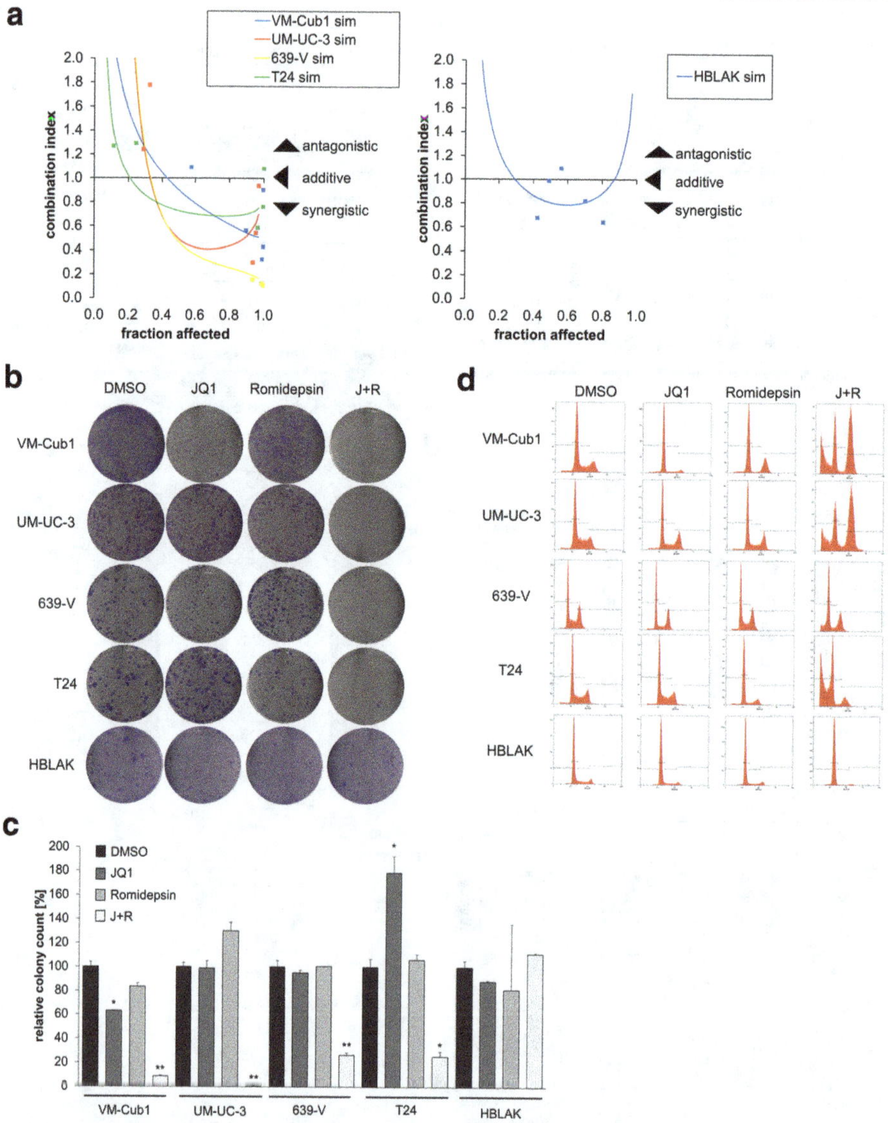

Fig. 2 Effects of combined treatment with JQ1 and Romidepsin on proliferation and clonogenic growth of UCCs. **a** Combination index (CI/Fa) plots for the combination of JQ1 and Romidepsin. Cell viability was measured at five constant dose ratio experimental data points by ATP assay after 72-h treatment. CI plots were then generated using CompuSyn software. CI < 1 indicates synergism. Benign HBLAK cells were compared to four UCCs. **b** Clonogenicity assay following treatment for 48 h with JQ1, Romidepsin, or both compounds compared to DMSO as indicated in Table 1 (lower part). **c** Quantification of colony counts from clonogenicity assays. Differences between control and treated cells were analyzed using Student's *t* test (** $p \leq 0.01$, * $p \leq 0.05$). **d** Flow cytometric cell cycle analyses following the indicated treatment for 48 h in four different UCCs and in HBLAK cells. See Additional file 3 for cell numbers in the respective cell cycle phases

of all four UCCs (at least 4-fold compared to DMSO; Fig. 2b, c), much more strongly than each inhibitor alone at the same doses (at least 3.5-fold compared to single treatments; Fig. 2b, c). Remarkably, no significant inhibition of clonogenic growth was observed in HBLAK cells.

To characterize the cellular effects of the drug combination in more detail, we performed cell cycle analysis by flow cytometry. Treatment with JQ1 alone led to accumulation of cells in the G0/G1-phase and a decreased S-phase fraction in most UCCs (Fig. 2d, Additional file 3), except in UM-UC-3, where an increased G2/M fraction was observed. The subG1 fraction increased slightly in several, albeit not in all UCCs. HBLAK cells were likewise arrested in G0/G1, with decreased S-phase fraction, but no increased subG1 fraction. Cell cycle distribution changes after treatment with JQ1 were very similar to those after BRD4 knockdown (see Fig. 1e). Likewise, UCCs responded towards single treatment with Romidepsin by accumulating in G0/G1 or G2/M (Fig. 2d) in accord with our previous results [4].

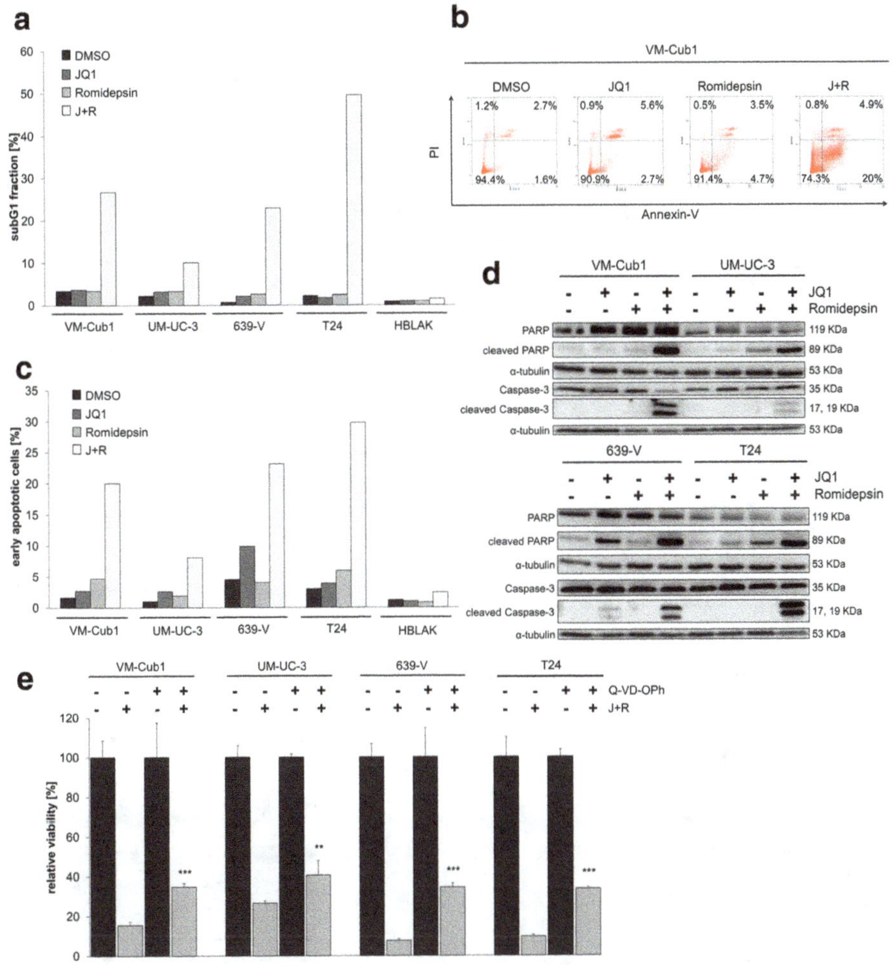

Fig. 3 Induction of apoptotic cell death by combined treatment with Romidepsin and JQ1. **a** Increase of subG1 fraction by combination treatment as determined by flow cytometry. **b** Flow cytometric analysis of UCCs with indicated treatment (Table 1 lower part) after combined staining with PI and Annexin V. Percentages of viable (lower left), early (lower right), or late (upper right) apoptotic and necrotic (upper left) VM-Cub1 cells subsequent to indicated treatments. **c** Percentage of early apoptotic cells as measured by Annexin V staining for all UCCs and HBLAK control cells are displayed in bar graphs for the respective treatment. **d** PARP and Caspase-3 cleavage 48 h after treatment assessed by Western blot analysis. **e** Four UCCs received the combination treatment with or without the Pan-Caspase inhibitor Q-VD-Oph at 30 μmol/l. All cells received the same concentration of DMSO. Cell viability displayed on the ordinate was measured by ATP assay after 48 h. Differences between J + R treatment and J + R treated plus Caspase inhibitor were analyzed using Student's *t* test (***$p \leq 0.001$, **$p \leq 0.01$)

In contrast, combination treatment resulted consistently in a strong increase of the subG1 fraction across all four UCCs (Fig. 3a), whereas the number of S-phase cells was reduced dramatically, indicating cell cycle inhibition and cell death (Fig. 2d, Additional file 3). Although the cell lines reacted rather uniformly in so far, they differed in the cell cycle phase, in which they became arrested. Whereas VM-Cub1 and UM-UC-3 cells showed a strong G2/M increase with decreased G0/G1 cells, 639-V and T24 cells displayed an increased G0/G1 fraction (Fig. 2d, Additional file 3). HBLAK cells arrested in G0/G1 with a remarkable decrease of the S-phase and G2/M fractions. Notably, the combination induced a subG1 fraction much more prominently than either agent on its own in UCC, but not in HBLAK cells (Fig. 3a).

Combination treatment causes apoptotic cell death

The increased subG1 fractions and according morphological changes in cell morphology indicated that combination treatment elicited pronounced apoptosis. Concordantly, the number of early apoptotic cells determined by Annexin V staining (Fig. 3b, c and Additional file 4) as well as cleaved Caspase 3 and cleaved PARP were significantly enhanced (Fig. 3d). These markers of apoptosis were not or only weakly induced by either a single drug treatment. Of note, induction of apoptosis was less pronounced in UM-UC-3 compared to the other UCCs. Moreover, cytotoxicity of the combination treatment was partly prevented by the Pan-Caspase inhibitor Q-VD-Oph in all four UCCs (Fig. 3e) indicating that the combination treatment efficiently elicited caspase-dependent apoptosis.

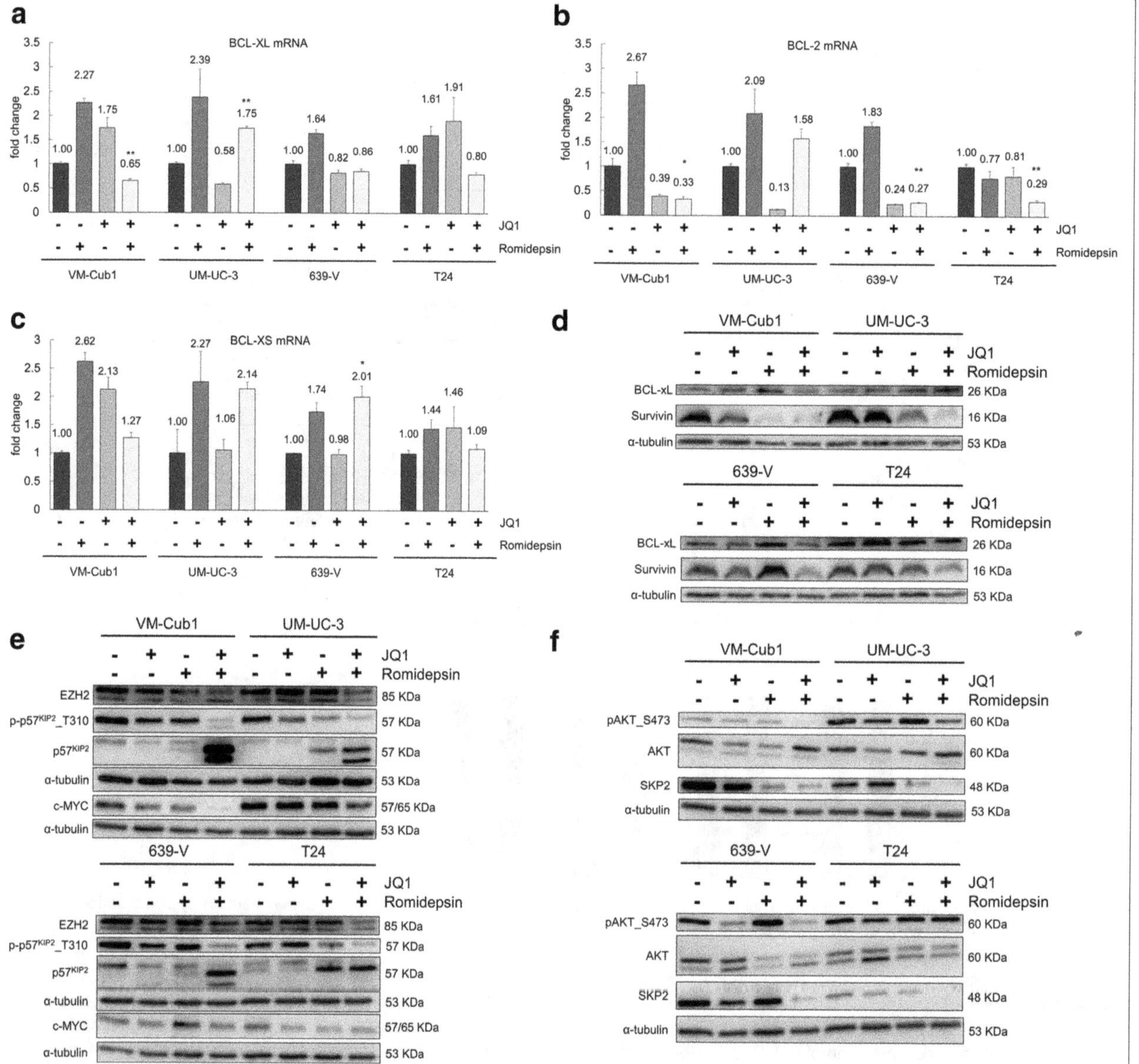

Fig. 4 Changes in expression of apoptotic regulators and cellular signaling after combined treatment with Romidepsin and JQ1. Relative mRNA expression levels of antiapoptotic *BCL-XL* (**a**) and *BCL-2* (**b**) and proapoptotic *BCL-XS* (**c**). mRNA levels were measured by qRT-PCR and normalized to the expression of *TBP*. Fold change compared to DMSO control 48 h after treatment is displayed on the ordinate. Differences between combination treatment samples and untreated controls were analyzed using Student's *t* test (**$p \leq 0.01$, *$p \leq 0.05$). **d** Protein expression of antiapoptotic BCL-XL and Survivin after combination treatment for 48 h assessed by Western blot. **e** Protein expression of c-MYC, EZH2, $p57^{KIP2}$, and phospho-$p57^{KIP2}$ (Thr310) assessed by Western blot analysis. **f** Phosphorylated AKT (S473) and expression of AKT and SKP2 was detected by Western blot analysis

Concurringly, mRNA expression of the antiapoptotic regulators BCL-XL (Fig. 4a) and BCL-2 (Fig. 4b) was diminished by combination treatment in UCCs, again with the exception of UM-UC-3. Expression of BCL-XS was either increased or remained unchanged (Fig. 4c). Similarly, the antiapoptotic BCL-XL and Survivin proteins were generally downregulated by the combination treatment (Fig. 4d). These anti-apoptotic proteins were not consistently downregulated by either single agent and in some cases actually induced. Thus, in contrast to single drug treatments, combined treatment led to stronger and more consistent downregulation of antiapoptotic regulators. This downregulation was less pronounced in UM-UC-3, presumably accounting for the weaker apoptotic response in this cell line.

Expression of c-MYC and EZH2, which have previously been identified as targets of BRD4 knockdown and JQ1 treatment mediating cell cycle arrest and apoptosis [10], were likewise clearly diminished following combined treatment (Fig. 4e).

JQ1 and Romidepsin synergistically induce p57^{KIP2} by various mechanisms

Since the cell cycle regulator protein p57^{KIP2} (encoded by the *CDKN1C* gene, hereafter p57) had been reported to mediate synergistic induction of apoptosis by combined HDAC and BET inhibition in pancreatic ductal adenocarcinoma [8], we evaluated its expression in four UCCs after treatment. p57 mRNA was induced between 17-fold (T24) and up to 1000-fold (VM-Cub1) by combination treatment. It was also induced regularly, but to a smaller extent, by Romidepsin, but not consistently by JQ1 (Additional file 5). Western blot analysis revealed a double band around the predicted molecular weight, of which especially the lower band was strongly induced by the combination treatment (Fig. 4e). The upper band likely reflects a phosphorylated isoform generated by active AKT protein kinase which is destined to degradation via a SKP2-containing E3 ubiquitin ligase complex. Accordingly, a (T310) phospho-specific p57 antibody demonstrated loss of phosphorylated p57 following combination treatment, indicating accumulation of the more stable unphosphorylated p57 protein (Fig. 4e).

Accordingly, active pAKT was diminished in three of four cell lines by JQ1 single treatment, but particularly strongly by combined treatment (Fig. 4f). SKP2 expression, too, was strongly downregulated in all four cell lines by the combination treatment. VM-Cub1 cells displayed the strongest induction of p57 protein and mRNA and the most pronounced decrease in its negative regulators c-MYC, pAKT, and SKP2. Conversely, T24 cells displayed the weakest increase of p57 protein and pAKT levels remaining unchanged. These findings suggest that, in addition to increased transcription of *CDKN1C*, stabilization of p57 contributes to its accumulation. Of note, reduced activity of AKT by combined treatment is likely to diminish pro-survival signaling in UCCs by other pathways as well.

STAT3 activation may also be involved in regulation of cell cycle progression and anti-apoptotic response and had been reported to be inactivated by combined HDAC and BET inhibition in pancreatic ductal adenocarcinoma [8]. However, we neither observed significant changes in STAT3 phosphorylation nor expression after combined treatment with JQ1 and Romidepsin (Additional file 6).

Gene editing of *p57^{KIP2}* in UCC

To investigate to which extent p57 contributes to apoptosis induction by combined treatment in UCCs, we generated VM-Cub1 *p57* knockout clones by CRISPR/Cas9-mediated gene editing. In contrast to the parental cells, p57 protein remained undetectable in cell clones with successful knockout even after combined treatment (Fig. 5a). Surprisingly, however, *p57* knockout did not rescue the cells from induction of cell death; viability was instead further decreased (Fig. 5b) and cleaved PARP was enhanced (Fig. 5a). Colony formation assays displayed concurring results (Fig. 5c), as did cell cycle analysis. Double treatment of *p57* knockout cells disrupted the cell cycle completely, and the majority of cells died rapidly (Fig. 5d, Additional file 3).

Combination treatment strongly increases histone acetylation around transcriptional start sites

To follow the effects of the drug combination on the chromatin level, we analyzed changes in histone acetylation. Overall, acetylation of histones H3 and H4 increased after treatment with Romidepsin alone, but was further enhanced by combination treatment (Fig. 6a). We further analyzed H3K27 acetylation and H3K4 trimethylation, which are established markers for active transcription, around the transcriptional start sites of six genes affected by the drug combination using chromatin immunoprecipitation (ChIP). ChIP results for acetylated H3K27 revealed a broad and strongly enhanced enrichment of acetylation after combined treatment encompassing at least 2 kb upstream of the transcriptional start site (TSS) to 2 kb downstream of the TSS of all six investigated genes (Fig. 6b). By comparison, treatment with Romidepsin alone did not significantly increase H3K27 acetylation compared to DMSO controls. Strikingly, H3K4 trimethylation was increased at the TSS of BCL2, *CDKN1C*/p57, and SKP2 genes after treatment with JQ1 alone, but decreased, mostly significantly, at the TSS of genes downregulated by the combination treatment.

Discussion

In this study, we examined the efficacy of a combination treatment with small-molecule inhibitors of chromatin regulators in urothelial carcinoma cell lines. In previous studies, we had identified HDAC class I-specific inhibitors like Romidepsin to be the most efficient HDAC inhibitors in UC. However, as this treatment did not induce apoptosis straightforwardly and did not appear particularly selective for tumor cells, we searched for a second drug for an improved combination therapy [2, 4]. Here, we combined Romidepsin with the BET inhibitor JQ1, which had been proposed to synergize with HDACi in several cancer types and to induce a canonical apoptotic response [22]. To our knowledge, the particular combination of Romidepsin and JQ1 has only been investigated by Jostes et al. in testicular cancer cell lines. These authors reported about reduced tumor burden even at lower and less frequent doses in xenograft experiments [6]. Other studies to date applied mainly pan-HDAC inhibitors like panobinostat or SAHA [23–25].

The results of our current study clearly demonstrate a significant synergistic effect on cell proliferation and

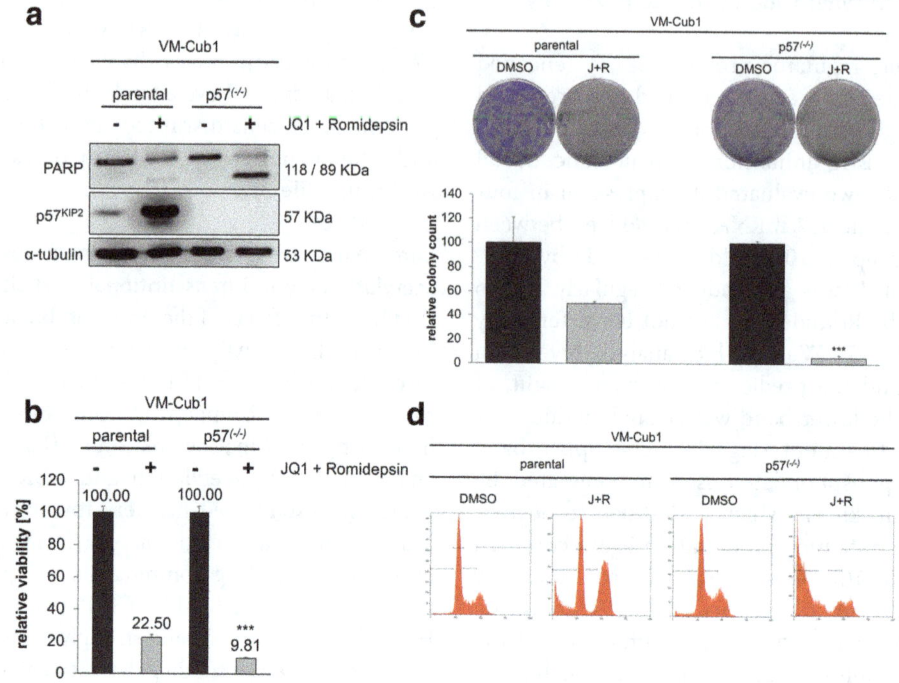

Fig. 5 Effect of *p57*^{KIP2} gene knockout on induction of apoptosis by combination treatment. **a** Protein expression of p57 and PARP1 in parental and knockout VM-Cub1 cells with or without combination treatment. **b** Relative viability of VM-Cub1 parental and *p57* knockout cells after combination treatment. Differences between samples with combination treatment of parental and knockout cells were analyzed using Student's *t* test (***$p \leq 0.001$). **c** Examples of clonogenicity assay, with quantified colony counts (***$p \leq 0.001$) and **d** cell cycle analysis for the indicated cells following combined inhibitor treatment. See Additional file 3 for cell numbers in the respective cell cycle phases

prominent apoptotic cell death for the combination of the BET protein inhibitor JQ1 and the HDAC class I-specific inhibitor Romidepsin. As UC cells are quite resistant to apoptosis induction under many conditions, we were especially interested in characterizing these cellular effects.

A pioneer study on the efficacy of single treatment with JQ1 alone in two related UC cell lines (T24 and EJ) provided first direct evidence that UC cells may be dependent on BRD4 [10]. shRNA mediated knockdown in the respective cells, decreased cell viability in a time-dependent manner (72 h), and induced cell cycle arrest in G0/G1 phase. In addition, in vivo tumor growth was reduced by BRD4 inhibition in a xenograft mouse model. We also found BRD4 overexpressed in some of the 12 investigated UC cell lines compared to benign urothelial cells, but overexpression was not uniformly observed, indicating that T24 may not be representative for all UC cell lines. Indeed, in our study, siRNA-mediated knockdown of BRD4 in both VM-Cub1 and UM-UC-3 cells resulted in a time-dependent reduction of cell viability and long-term proliferation, but the cells responded differentially with respect to cell cycle arrest. VM-Cub1 cells displayed the expected arrest in G0/G1, whereas UM-UC-3 arrested in G2/M. In many further functional assays, we likewise observed that UM-UC-3 cells responded differently or less efficiently, e.g., with regard to induction of apoptosis. Similar heterogeneity of BRD4 expression and response to BRD4 inhibition may occur in cancer patients due to the pronounced heterogeneity of urothelial carcinoma. This prompted us to characterize the response of UC towards single and combined treatment more comprehensively across different cell lines.

Indeed, our investigations on the cellular effects of pharmacological BRD4 inhibition in eight UC cell lines chosen to represent the heterogeneity of urothelial carcinoma demonstrated that the previously reported results on T24 [10] cannot be simply extended to all UC cell lines. Instead, dose-response curves for JQ1 in eight UC cell lines demonstrated that they could be clearly classified into two groups with low and high sensitivity and that not all UCCs are as sensitive as T24. The differential sensitivity was not related to BRD4 protein expression or any other obvious characteristics of the cell lines and remains to be further investigated.

Like T24 in the study by Wu et al. [10], most cell lines accumulated in G0/G1 following treatment with IC_{50} doses of JQ1 (0.18–6.8 μM), but UM-UC-3 accumulated in G2/M. At these doses, we detected only a slight increase of the subG1-fraction. Comparable results were reported for colon cancer and medulloblastoma cells, which arrested in G0/G1 after treatment with

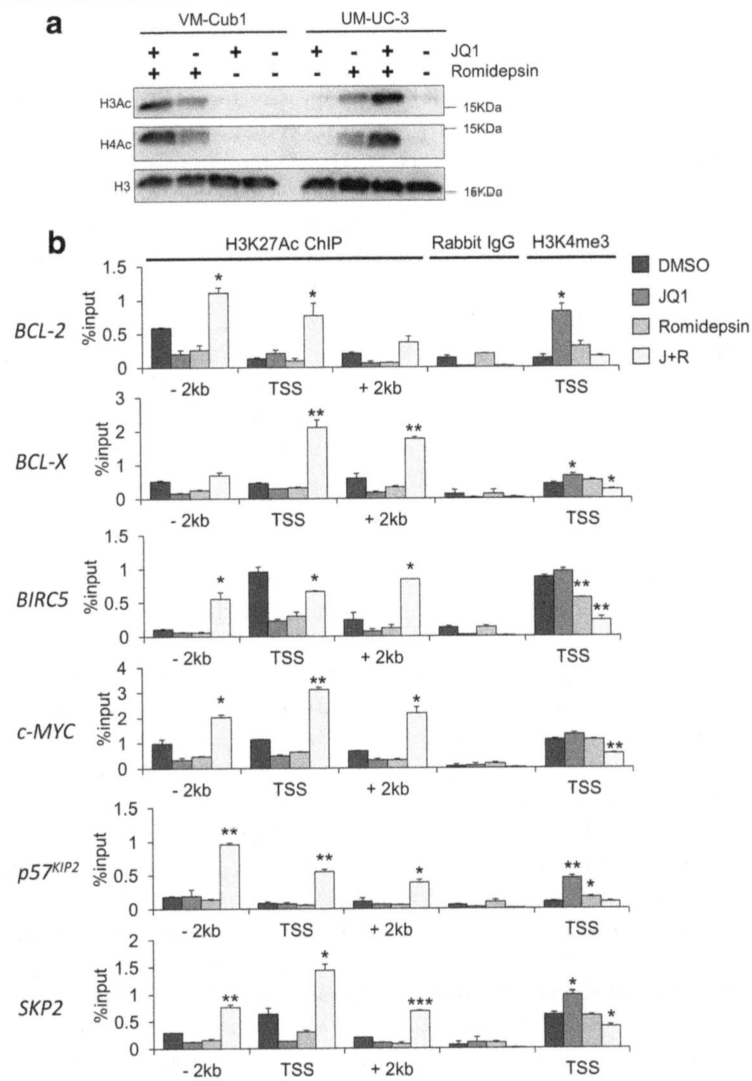

Fig. 6 Changes in histone modifications elicited by combination treatment. **a** Changes in H3 and H4 acetylation were detected after single and combined treatment in VM-Cub1 and UM-UC-3 cells by acid histone extraction and Western blot analysis. Total histone 3 served as a loading control. **b** Chromatin immunoprecipitation analysis of H3K27 acetylation at transcriptional start sites (TSS) as well as 2 kb upstream (− 2 kb) and 2 kb downstream (+2 kb) of *BCL-2*, *BCL2L1/BCL-X*, *BIRC5/Survivin*, *c-MYC*, *CDKN1C/p57* and *SKP2 genes* after single and combined treatment of VM-Cub1 cells. Immunoprecipitated DNA amounts measured by qPCR for each condition are expressed as percentage of input DNA. Additionally, H3K4 trimethylation was analyzed at the TSS of the same genes. Rabbit IgG served as a background control. Differences between samples with combination treatment and DMSO treated cells were analyzed using Student's *t* test (***$p \leq 0.001$, **$p \leq 0.01$, *$p \leq 0.05$)

0.1–0.5 μM JQ1 [14, 26]. However, in contrast to various other cancer cell types, JQ1 treatment alone neither significantly inhibited long-term proliferation of UCCs nor induced significant apoptosis suggesting that UC cells are generally less sensitive towards JQ1 than other tumor types [8, 14, 24, 27] and recover over time. Benign urothelial cells also arrested at rather low concentrations, but no apoptosis was observed and long-term proliferation ability was retained.

Using the Chou-Talalay method [19], we determined doses for the combined treatment with JQ1 and Romidepsin with synergistic effects on cell viability at doses mostly lower than the IC_{50} concentrations of either single treatment. Importantly, all UC cell lines, including those with low sensitivity to JQ1 alone like UM-UC-3 and 639-V, as well as primary tumor cultures, responded strongly to the combination treatment. The combination of JQ1 with Romidepsin was clearly more efficacious in inhibiting proliferation of UCCs than JQ1 alone. Moreover, the combination elicited apoptosis much more efficiently than either JQ1 or Romidepsin. Benign control cells were strikingly less affected suggesting that the combined treatment might achieve a higher tumor specificity with lower toxic side effects for normal cells than single treatment with Romidepsin [4]. Accordingly, long-term proliferation was not affected in HBLAK cells, but was very strongly diminished in all cancer cell lines, again irrespective of their sensitivity towards JQ1 alone. The cell cycle was heavily disturbed, and we observed very strongly increased subG1 fractions as well as high numbers of early apoptotic cells subsequent to combination treatment in UCCs, but not in benign HBLAK cells. Similar synergistic effects on proliferation and apoptosis have been reported in pancreatic cancer, neuroblastoma, and AML cells by combination treatment using JQ1 with the pan-HDAC inhibitors SAHA (vorinostat) or panobinostat [8, 23, 24] and in melanoma cells by panobinostat and BET inhibitor I-BET151 [7]. Borbeley et al. also combined the class I-specific inhibitor mocetinostat with JQ1 for treatment of breast cancer cells [27]. Interestingly, normal melanocytes, embryonic fibroblasts, and normal hematopoietic progenitor cells were spared from apoptosis similar to HBLAK cells, again emphasizing the increased tumor specificity of the combination [7, 23, 24].

Molecular biomarkers and application of the caspase-inhibitor Q-VD-OPh confirmed that the combination treatment, other than treatment with either inhibitor alone, efficiently induced canonical caspase-dependent apoptosis in UC cells. Similar changes in apoptosis-related proteins were found in pancreatic cancer [8], neuroblastoma [23], melanoma [7], and AML cells [24]. Anti-apoptotic proteins like BCL-2 may be induced by activated STAT3 [25, 28], and in pancreatic adenocarcinoma cells, the combination of JQ1 and SAHA diminished STAT3 phosphorylation to downregulate BCL-2 [8]. However, in UC cells, we observed neither diminished phosphorylation nor decreased expression of STAT3, again indicating that the mechanisms mediating cellular effects may differ between cancer entities. Accordingly, gene expression profiles following treatment with BETi and HDACi drug combination in studies on different cancer cell types each describe hundreds of differentially expressed genes, with limited overlap, but converging on a cellular response resulting in cell cycle arrest and apoptosis [23, 27]. These relatively uniform ultimate cellular effects thus appear to be driven by cell type-dependent transcriptional programs.

In addition, suppression of AKT-mediated survival signaling is likely to contribute to the observed cell death. Diminished AKT kinase activity may especially contribute to the dramatic overexpression of $p57^{KIP2}$ via stabilization of the protein following decreased phosphorylation priming for SKP2-mediated degradation [29, 30], as especially non-phosphorylated $p57^{KIP2}$ accumulated. SKP2 itself was as well strongly diminished by the treatment, presumably further contributing to p57 accumulation. In accordance with other studies reporting $p57^{KIP2}$ as a prominent factor induced in treated cells [6, 8], we found both its mRNA and protein strongly elevated.

The function of p57 with regard to regulation of apoptosis is controversial. Obviously, p57 can prevent or promote apoptosis dependent on the cellular context [31]. Promotion of apoptosis may occur by p57 translocation into mitochondria to trigger the intrinsic apoptotic pathway [32]. In pancreatic cancer cells, depletion of *p57* by shRNA decreased apoptotic markers induced by JQ1 and SAHA combination treatment; Cas9-mediated knockout of *Cdkn1c* in mice significantly diminished apoptosis of combination-treated animals [8]. In an analogous approach, we generated *p57* knockout UC cells by gene editing. Intriguingly, this knockout did not rescue the cells from apoptosis induced by combination treatment. This finding underlines the context-dependent function of p57 on the one hand. On the other hand, it supports again the idea that compounds like JQ1 targeting general transcriptional regulators do rarely act through their effect on a single gene but elicit broad effects on the transcriptome which are cell type-dependent due to the respective transcriptional programs [5]. For instance, in other studies, suppression of c-MYC was proposed to be the central event mediating effects in the treated cells, but forced overexpression of this supposedly crucial target gene failed to rescue all phenotypes [5]. In this respect, we note that downregulation of c-MYC was observed in all UCCs treated with the drug combination, but that its extent varied.

Recent publications have suggested a mechanism for the downregulation of oncogenic and anti-apoptotic factors like c-MYC or BCL-2 after combined treatment with HDAC and BET inhibitors [23, 33]. HDAC inhibitor treatment induces histone hyperacetylation, as also observed in UC cells. Genes undergoing hyperacetylation of H3K27 within a 5 kb region around their transcriptional start site by this treatment appear to become particularly dependent on binding of BET proteins like BRD4 to their regulatory regions, including enhancers, to promote gene transcription. Accordingly, genes activated by HDAC inhibitor treatment were reported to be enriched for BRD4 [33]. Abolishment of BRD4 binding by JQ1 then leads to their transcriptional inactivation. This mechanism has been proposed for combined treatment with 4SC-202, Entinostat, or mocetinostat [27, 33], all of which predominantly target class I HDAC isoenzymes, similar to Romidepsin. Indeed, Romidepsin alone resulted also in activation of anti-apoptotic factors like BCL-2 and BCL-X in UC cells, suggesting that this mechanism also applies in our experimental setting. Accordingly, ChIP analysis revealed broad H3K27 hyperacetylation around the transcriptional start sites of all investigated genes after combined treatment, which would render them sensitive to transcriptional repression by JQ1. Consequently, H3K4 trimethylation, a marker for transcriptionally active genes, was significantly reduced at the TSS of four genes down-regulated by combination treatment in UC cells. Notably, Mishra et al. [33] reported globally increased H3K4me3 at the TSS of genes upon treatment with the HDAC inhibitor 4SC-202, which—different from Romidepsin—additionally inhibits the LSD1 histone demethylase.

Conclusions

In conclusion, we have demonstrated that the combination of JQ1 and Romidepsin exerts strong synergistic antineoplastic effects on urothelial carcinoma cells. Due to the strong synergy, the applied doses were well below the IC_{50} doses of the single treatments and affected benign control cells only mildly. UC cells are often particularly resistant towards induction of caspase-dependent apoptosis [34]. Therefore, this novel combination treatment constitutes a promising approach for a small-molecule therapy of UC with reduced toxic side effects to normal cells.

Additional files

Additional file 1: Information on primer sequences and antibodies. Sequence information and amplicon sizes for qRT-PCR and ChIP qPCR primers as well as product information and dilution of applied antibodies are given.

Additional file 2: Data on synergistic effects on cell viability of primary cancer cells by combined treatment with Romidepsin and JQ1. (a), (b) Relative viability of primary cultures 1 and 2 established from primary tumor tissue of two different patients after single or combined treatment for 48 h. Relative viability is displayed on the ordinate in percent of the control cells treated with DMSO. (c) Primary culture 2 was used for an extended dose response curve analysis after 24 h to perform Chou-Talalay calculations (***$p \leq 0.001$, **$p \leq 0.01$, *$p \leq 0.05$). (d) Combination index (CI/Fa) plot for the combination of JQ1 and Romidepsin. Cell viability was measured at five constant dose ratio experimental data points by ATP assay for primary culture 2. CI plots were then generated using CompuSyn software. CI < 1 indicates synergism.

Additional file 3: Detailed flow cytometry results from cell cycle analysis. Displayed are percentages of cells in the indicated cell cycle phase as measured by flow cytometric cell cycle analyses following the indicated treatment for 48 h in four different UCCs and in HBLAK cells (Fig. 2d) or in VM-Cub1 knockout cells (Fig. 5d). (PDF 177 kb)

Additional file 4: Data on induction of apoptotic cell death by combined treatment with Romidepsin and JQ1. Induction of apoptotic cell death by combined treatment with Romidepsin and JQ1. Flow cytometric analysis of UCCs with indicated treatment after combined staining with PI and Annexin V. Percentages of viable (lower left), early (lower right), or late (upper right) apoptotic and necrotic (upper left) VM-Cub1 cells subsequent to indicated treatments.

Additional file 5: Data on expression changes of of $p57^{KIP2}$ mRNA by combination treatment in UC cells. Relative mRNA expression levels of $p57^{KIP2}$ mRNA after single and combined treatment with Romidepsin and JQ1. mRNA levels were measured by qRT-PCR and normalized to the expression of TBP. Fold change compared to DMSO control 48 h after treatment is displayed on the ordinate.

Additional file 6: Data on STAT3 activation and expression after combination treatment in UC cells. Phosphorylated and total STAT3 protein was detected by Western blot analysis in four UC cell lines cells after indicated treatment. α-tubulin served as an additional loading control.

Abbreviations

BET: Bromodomain and extra-terminal; CI: Combination index; Fa: Fraction affected; HDAC: Histone deacetylase; HDACi: HDAC inhibitor; NHUC: Primary normal human urothelial cells; PVDF: Polyvinylidene difluoride; TSS: Transcriptional start site; UC: Urothelial carcinoma; UCC: Urothelial carcinoma cell

Acknowledgements

The authors thank Julia Lachner and Ananda A. Jaguva Vasudevan for the help with some experiments and Marija Lenzen for the technical assistance.

Funding

AH was supported by a fellowship of the Duesseldorf School of Oncology (funded by the Comprehensive Cancer Centre Duesseldorf/Deutsche Krebshilfe and the Medical Faculty Heinrich-Heine-University Duesseldorf). MP and GN were supported by a grant of the Deutsche Forschungsgemeinschaft (NIE 1398/1-1).

Authors' contributions

WAS, MJH, and GN designed the study. AH, MP, and MJH performed the experiments and analyzed and interpreted the data. AH, MJH, WAS, and GN wrote the manuscript. Project administration and funding acquisition was done by WAS, MJH, and GN. All authors read and approved the final manuscript.

Competing interests

The authors declare that they have no competing interests.

References

1. Cancer Genome Atlas Research Network. Comprehensive molecular characterization of urothelial bladder carcinoma. Nature. 2014;507:315–22.
2. Pinkerneil M, Hoffmann MJ, Schulz WA, Niegisch G. HDACs and HDAC inhibitors in urothelial carcinoma—perspectives for an antineoplastic treatment. Curr Med Chem. 2017;24:4151-65. epub
3. Pinkerneil M, Hoffmann MJ, Kohlhof H, Schulz WA, Niegisch G. Evaluation of the therapeutic potential of the novel isotype specific HDAC inhibitor 4SC-202 in urothelial carcinoma cell lines. Target Oncol. 2016;11:783–98.
4. Pinkerneil M, Hoffmann MJ, Deenen R, Kohrer K, Arent T, Schulz WA, et al. Inhibition of class I histone deacetylases 1 and 2 promotes urothelial carcinoma cell death by various mechanisms. Mol Cancer Ther. 2016;15:299–312.
5. Bhadury J, Nilsson LM, Muralidharan SV, Green LC, Li Z, Gesner EM, et al. BET and HDAC inhibitors induce similar genes and biological effects and synergize to kill in Myc-induced murine lymphoma. Proc Natl Acad Sci U S A. 2014;111:E2721–30.
6. Jostes S, Nettersheim D, Fellermeyer M, Schneider S, Hafezi F, Honecker F, et al. The bromodomain inhibitor JQ1 triggers growth arrest and apoptosis in testicular germ cell tumours in vitro and in vivo. J Cell Mol Med. 2016;21:1300–14.
7. Heinemann A, Cullinane C, Paoli-Iseppi R, Wilmott JS, Gunatilake D, Madore J, et al. Combining BET and HDAC inhibitors synergistically induces apoptosis of melanoma and suppresses AKT and YAP signaling. Oncotarget. 2015;6:21507–21.
8. Mazur PK, Herner A, Mello SS, Wirth M, Hausmann S, Sanchez-Rivera FJ, et al. Combined inhibition of BET family proteins and histone deacetylases as a potential epigenetics-based therapy for pancreatic ductal adenocarcinoma. Nat Med. 2015;21:1163–71.
9. Posternak V and Cole MD. Strategically targeting MYC in cancer [version 1; referees: 2 approved]. F1000Research 2016, 5(F1000 Faculty Rev):408 (doi: https://doi.org/10.12688/f1000research.7879.1).
10. Wu X, Liu D, Tao D, Xiang W, Xiao X, Wang M, et al. BRD4 regulates EZH2 transcription through upregulation of C-MYC and represents a novel therapeutic target in bladder cancer. Mol Cancer Ther. 2016;15:1029–42.
11. Yan Y, Yang F-Q, Zhang H-M, Li J, Li W, Wang G-C, et al. Bromodomain 4 protein is a predictor of survival for urothelial carcinoma of bladder. Int J Clin Exp Pathol. 2014;7:4231–8.
12. Devaiah BN, Case-Borden C, Gegonne A, Hsu CH, Chen Q, Meerzaman D, et al. BRD4 is a histone acetyltransferase that evicts nucleosomes from chromatin. Nat Struct Mol Biol. 2016;23:540–8.

13. L-l F, Tian M, Li X, Li J-j, Huang J, Ouyang L, et al. Inhibition of BET bromodomains as a therapeutic strategy for cancer drug discovery. Oncotarget. 2015;6:5501–16.
14. Venkataraman S, Alimova I, Balakrishnan I, Harris P, Birks DK, Griesinger A, et al. Inhibition of BRD4 attenuates tumor cell self-renewal and suppresses stem cell signaling in MYC driven medulloblastoma. Oncotarget. 2014;5:2355–71.
15. Hoffmann MJ, Koutsogiannouli E, Skowron MA, Pinkerneil M, Niegisch G, Brandt A, et al. The new immortalized uroepithelial cell line HBLAK contains defined genetic aberrations typical of early stage urothelial tumors. Bladder Cancer (Amsterdam, Netherlands). 2016;2:449–63.
16. Swiatkowski S, Seifert H-H, Steinhoff C, Prior A, Thievessen I, Schliess F, et al. Activities of MAP-kinase pathways in normal uroepithelial cells and urothelial carcinoma cell lines. Exp Cell Res. 2003;282:48–57.
17. Koch A, Hatina J, Rieder H, Seifert HH, Huckenbeck W, Jankowiak F, et al. Discovery of TP53 splice variants in two novel papillary urothelial cancer cell lines. Cell Oncol (Dordr). 2012;35:243–57.
18. Rahman S, Sowa ME, Ottinger M, Smith JA, Shi Y, Harper JW, et al. The Brd4 extraterminal domain confers transcription activation independent of pTEFb by recruiting multiple proteins, including NSD3. Mol Cell Biol. 2011;31:2641–52.
19. Chou TC, Talalay P. Quantitative analysis of dose-effect relationships: the combined effects of multiple drugs or enzyme inhibitors. Adv Enzym Regul. 1984;22:27–55.
20. Isono M, Hoffmann MJ, Pinkerneil M, Sato A, Michaelis M, Cinatl J, et al. Checkpoint kinase inhibitor AZD7762 strongly sensitises urothelial carcinoma cells to gemcitabine. J Exp Clin Cancer Res. 2017;36:1.
21. Shechter D, Dormann HL, Allis CD, Hake SB. Extraction, purification and analysis of histones. Nat Protoc. 2007;2:1445–57.
22. Conery AR, Centore RC, Spillane KL, Follmer NE, Bommi-Reddy A, Hatton C, et al. Preclinical anticancer efficacy of BET bromodomain inhibitors is determined by the apoptotic response. Cancer Res. 2016;76:1313–9.
23. Shahbazi J, Liu PY, Atmadibrata B, Bradner JE, Marshall GM, Lock RB, et al. The bromodomain inhibitor JQ1 and the histone deacetylase inhibitor panobinostat synergistically reduce N-Myc expression and induce anticancer effects. Clin Cancer Res. 2016;22:2534–44.
24. Fiskus W, Sharma S, Qi J, Valenta JA, Schaub LJ, Shah B, et al. Highly active combination of BRD4 antagonist and histone deacetylase inhibitor against human acute myelogenous leukemia cells. Mol Cancer Ther. 2014;13:1142–54.
25. Zeng H, Qu J, Jin N, Xu J, Lin C, Chen Y, et al. Feedback activation of leukemia inhibitory factor receptor limits response to histone deacetylase inhibitors in breast cancer. Cancer Cell. 2016;30:459–73.
26. Zhang C, Su Z-Y, Wang L, Shu L, Yang Y, Guo Y, et al. Epigenetic blockade of neoplastic transformation by bromodomain and extra-terminal (BET) domain protein inhibitor JQ-1. Biochem Pharmacol. 2016;117:35–45.
27. Borbely G, Haldosen LA, Dahlman-Wright K, Zhao C. Induction of USP17 by combining BET and HDAC inhibitors in breast cancer cells. Oncotarget. 2015;6:33623–35.
28. Ray S, Zhao Y, Jamaluddin M, Edeh CB, Lee C, Brasier AR. Inducible STAT3 NH2 terminal mono-ubiquitination promotes BRD4 complex formation to regulate apoptosis. Cell Signal. 2014;26:1445–55.
29. Lo H-W. Akt destabilizes p57 (Kip2): Akt at the converging crossroad? Cell Cycle (Georgetown, Tex). 2013;12:870–1.
30. Kamura T, Hara T, Kotoshiba S, Yada M, Ishida N, Imaki H, et al. Degradation of p57Kip2 mediated by SCFSkp2-dependent ubiquitylation. Proc Natl Acad Sci U S A. 2003;100:10231–6.
31. Besson A, Dowdy SF, Roberts JM. CDK inhibitors: cell cycle regulators and beyond. Dev Cell. 2008;14:159–69.
32. Vlachos P, Nyman U, Hajji N, Joseph B. The cell cycle inhibitor p57(Kip2) promotes cell death via the mitochondrial apoptotic pathway. Cell Death Differ. 2007;14:1497–507.
33. Mishra VK, Wegwitz F, Kosinsky RL, Sen M, Baumgartner R, Wulff T, et al. Histone deacetylase class-I inhibition promotes epithelial gene expression in pancreatic cancer cells in a BRD4- and MYC-dependent manner. Nucleic Acids Res. 2017;45:6334–49.
34. Knievel J, Schulz WA, Greife A, Hader C, Lubke T, Schmitz I, et al. Multiple mechanisms mediate resistance to sorafenib in urothelial cancer. Int J Mol Sci. 2014;15:20500–17.

7

A multiplatform approach identifies miR-152-3p as a common epigenetically regulated onco-suppressor in prostate cancer targeting *TMEM97*

João Ramalho-Carvalho[1,2,3,11], Céline S. Gonçalves[4,5], Inês Graça[1], David Bidarra[1], Eva Pereira-Silva[1], Sofia Salta[1], Maria Inês Godinho[6], Antonio Gomez[2,12], Manel Esteller[2,7,8], Bruno M. Costa[4,5], Rui Henrique[1,9,10†] and Carmen Jerónimo[1,10*†]

Abstract

Background: Prostate cancer (PCa) is a major cause of morbidity and mortality in men worldwide. MicroRNAs are globally downregulated in PCa, especially in poorly differentiated tumors. Nonetheless, the underlying mechanisms are still elusive. Herein, using combined analysis of microRNAs expression and genomewide DNA methylation, we aimed to identify epigenetically downregulated microRNAs in PCa.

Results: We found that miR-152-3p was underexpressed in PCa and that lower expression levels were associated with promoter hypermethylation in accordance with TCGA dataset analysis. Functional in vitro assays suggest that miR-152-3p suppresses cell viability and invasion potential, whereas it promotes cell cycle arrest at S and G2/M phases. Additionally, miR-152-3p expression was associated with longer disease-free survival in PCa patients from TCGA. Finally, *TMEM97*, which is overexpressed in PCa, was identified as a novel miR-152-3p target gene.

Conclusions: Our findings demonstrate the advantages of using a combinatory approach to identify microRNAs downregulated due to aberrant promoter methylation. MiR-152-3p downregulation and promoter methylation was found to be prevalent in primary PCa, which impairs its role in control of cell viability, cell cycle regulation and invasion.

Keywords: miR-152-3p, Prostate cancer, Cell cycle, DNA methylation, CRISPR, *TMEM97*

Background

MicroRNAs (miRNAs) are a class of small (~ 22-nucleotide) RNAs that mediate post-transcriptional gene silencing by guiding Argonaute (AGO) proteins to target mRNAs [1, 2], either by repressing translation or by promoting destabilization [3]. Target guidance and specificity is mainly determined by nucleotides at positions 2–7 of the miRNA (the seed-sequence) [4]. Such mechanisms are critical for homeostasis maintenance, both under physiological conditions and in cell's response to environment alterations, including stress signals [5]. Thus, a vast number of biological processes are subject to miRNA-dependent regulation, encompassing cell proliferation, signaling, differentiation, stress response, DNA repair, cell adhesion and motility, inflammation, cell survival, senescence, and apoptosis [1]. Interestingly, miRNA's expression, processing, and functional output are also stringently controlled [6]. Indeed, miRNAs' expression and activity are tightly spatially and temporally regulated, and its disruption has been extensively linked to human disease, including the development of cancer and metastasis formation [1, 7]. Globally, miRNAs are mostly downregulated in cancer, including that of the prostate [1]. Multiple mechanism are known to induce miRNA deregulation, including epigenetic alterations,

* Correspondence: carmenjeronimo@ipoporto.min-saude.pt; cljeronimo@icbas.up.pt
†Equal contributors
[1]Cancer Biology & Epigenetics Group – Research Center (CI-IPOP), Portuguese Oncology Institute of Porto (IPO Porto), F Bdg, 1st floor, Rua Dr António Bernardino de Almeida, 4200-072 Porto, Portugal
[10]Department of Pathology and Molecular Immunology, Institute of Biomedical Sciences Abel Salazar– University of Porto (ICBAS-UP), Porto, Portugal
Full list of author information is available at the end of the article

aberrant transcription factors binding (e.g., p53, MYC), miRNA biogenesis machinery disruption, RNA editing, post-transcriptional RNA modifications, Argonaute loading, and RNA decay [7, 8].

Prostate cancer (PCa) is the most common non-cutaneous cancer worldwide in men, and a leading cause of cancer-related death in developed countries [9]. Multiple factors, comprising age, family history, genetic susceptibility and ethnicity, contribute to the high incidence of PCa [10]. Owing to its complexity and heterogeneity, and despite extensive studies, the molecular mechanisms that drive prostatic carcinogenesis are still far from complete understanding. Because miRNAs regulate a wide range of signaling pathways that are frequently deregulated in PCa, this class of noncoding RNAs might be of critical relevance for tumor development and progression. Thus, its study may provide novel insights into PCa biology and afford innovative tools for patient management, aiding in diagnosis and prognosis assessment, as well as the identification of new therapeutic targets [11].

Methods

Aim

Here, we attempted to discover new epigenetically regulated miRNA loci in PCa using a combinatory approach that compared miRNAs expression profiling with DNA methylation patterns. The candidate microRNAs were subsequently validated in two large patient cohorts, which included ours and that of TCGA; in vitro assays were performed to characterize their role in cancer cell biology, and in silico analysis, followed by in vitro validation, allowed for the identification of relevant target mRNAs. Overall, our data extends current knowledge about epigenetic deregulation and biological significance of miRNAs in prostate carcinogenesis. A flow chart depicting the different steps followed in this study is provided in Additional file 1: Figure S1. All methods were performed in accordance with the relevant guidelines and regulations both for tissue samples and in vitro assays.

Patient and samples

PCa tissue samples (n = 100) from patients diagnosed and primarily treated with radical prostatectomy at Portuguese Oncology Institute of Porto, Portugal, were prospectively collected. Fourteen normal prostate tissue (MNPT) samples, of peripheral zone of prostates without PCa, from patients submitted to radical cystoprostatectomy due to bladder cancer, served as controls. All specimens, promptly frozen at – 80 °C, were cut for nucleic acid extraction. For routine histopathological examination, formalin-fixed and paraffin-embedded (FFPE) fragments were also collected. Relevant clinical data was retrieved from clinical charts. This study was approved by the institutional ethics committee [Comissão de Ética para a Saúde- Instituto Português de Oncologia do Porto Francisco Gentil, EPE (CES-IPOPFG-EPE 215/013)]. Moreover, in compliance with the Helsinki Declaration and after CES approval, informed consent was obtained for all patients previously to surgery. Additionally, a Cohort of patients available at TCGA were included for validation. The clinical and pathological data of both cohorts of patients (IPO Porto's cohort and TCGA's cohort) included in this study is reported in Table 1.

PCa cell lines and demethylation treatment

Prostate cell lines, LNCaP, 22RV1, DU145, PC-3 (malignant), and RWPE (benign) were used for in vitro studies. LNCaP and 22Rv1 cells were grown in RPMI 1640, whereas DU145 and PC-3 cells were maintained in MEM and 50% RPMI-50% F-12 medium, while RWPE was cultured in Keratinocyte-SFM, containing human recombinant Epidermal Growth Factor 1-53 and Bovine Pituitary Extract (GIBCO, Invitrogen, Carlsbad, CA, USA), respectively. HEK293Ta were maintained in DMEM. All basal culture media were supplemented with 10% fetal bovine serum and 1% penicillin/streptomycin (GIBCO, Invitrogen, Carlsbad, CA, USA). Cells were maintained in an incubator at 37 °C with 5% CO_2. All cell lines were G-banding karyotyped (for validation) and routinely tested for *Mycoplasma spp.* contamination (PCR Mycoplasma Detection Set, Clontech Laboratories).

Table 1 Clinical and pathological data of the patients included in this study

(A) IPO Porto's cohort		
Clinicopathological features	MNPT	PCa
Patients, *n*	14	100
Median age, years (range)	65 (49–80)	65 (49–75)
PSA (ng/mL), median (range)	n.a.	8.45 (3.5–23)
pT2	n.a.	60 (60%)
pT3	n.a.	40 (40%)
< 7	n.a.	36 (36%)
= 7	n.a.	58 (58%)
> 7	n.a.	6 (6%)
(B) TCGA's cohort		
Clinicopathological Features	NAT	PCa
Patients, n	52	497
Median age, years (range)	61 (43–72)	61 (41–78)
pT2	29 (56%)	189 (38%)
pT3	21 (40%)	292 (59%)
pT4	2 (4%)	10 (2%)
< 7	5 (10%)	45 (9%)
= 7	40 (77%)	248 (50%)
> 7	7 (13%)	204 (41%)

MNPT morphologically normal prostate tissue, *PCa* prostate cancer, *NAT* normal adjacent tissue, *n.a.* not applicable
(A) IPO Porto's cohort (B) TCGA's cohort

One micromolar of the DNA methyltransferases inhibitor 5-aza-2-deoxycytidine (5-Aza-CdR; Sigma-Aldrich, Schnelldorf, Germany) was used for DNA demethylation. Cells were harvested and RNA extracted after 72-h exposure to the demethylating agent.

Nuclei acid extraction and bisulfite conversion

DNA was extracted from fresh frozen tissue samples and cell lines using phenol: chloroform (Sigma). RNA was isolated using TRIzol (Invitrogen, Carlsbad, CA, USA) according to the manufacturer's instructions.

Bisulfite conversion of genomic DNA (1000 ng) was accomplished using EZ DNA Methylation Kit (Zymo Research), following the manufacturer's instructions.

sgRNA cloning

Complementary single-stranded oligos (Additional file 1: Table S1) were phosphorylated and annealed by combining 100 μM oligos, 1× T4 PNK Buffer, 1 mM ATP, 5 U T4 PNK and incubating the reaction at 37 °C/30 min, 95 °C/ 5 min followed by a ramp down to 25 °C at 5 °C/min. Annealed oligos were diluted at 1:100 in sterile water and ligated to plasmid vector lentiCRISPRv2 (gift from Feng Zhang (Addgene plasmid #52961)) using the following parameters: 50 ng BsmBI (Fermentas) digested plasmid, 1 μl diluted oligo duplex, 1× Ligation Buffer (Roche), and 5 U T4 DNA Ligase (Roche) incubated at RT/30 min. The ligation reactions were used to transform highly competent *Escherichia coli* cells according to the manufacturer's protocol [12]. Transformation mixtures were plated in LB-agar plates. After colony selection, they grew in liquid LB and plasmid DNA was harvested using PureLink HiPure Plasmid Maxiprep Kit (Invitrogen, Carlsbad, CA, USA). The resulting DNA was then subjected to Sanger sequencing to confirm the correct either the orientation and sequence of each sgRNA.

Lentivirus production, purification, and transduction

To produce lentivirus, 4×10^6 HEK293T cells per sgRNA were seeded in ten 100-mm dishes 1 day before transfection. For each dish, we diluted 10 μg of plasmid DNA (corresponding to individual sgRNA), 3.5 μg of pVSV-G, 5 μg of pMDL RRE, and 2.5 μg of pRSV-REV in 450 μl of 0.1× TE/H2O, added 50 μl of CaCl2 and incubated 5 min at RT. Plasmid DNA was precipitated by adding 500 μl 2× HBS to the solution while vortexing at full speed. The precipitate was added immediately to the plate and the cells were incubated for 14 h at 37 °C, after which the medium was refreshed. Lentivirus-containing supernatants were collected 60 h post-transfection, filtered through a 0.45-μm membrane (Milipore Steriflip HV/PVDF) and stored at − 80 °C. Cell lines were infected with lentivirus supernatants supplemented with 8 μg/ml polybrene (Sigma). At 24 h post-infection, medium was replaced and cells were selected with 2 μg/ml puromycin (Gibco). Antibiotic selection was stopped as soon as no surviving cells remained in the no-transduction control plate.

PCR and sanger sequencing

Genomic DNA ($\sim 1 \times 10^5$ cells) from cloned cells was isolated with DNeasy Blood and Tissue kit (Qiagen). PCR reactions were carried out with 500 ng of genomic DNA using Phusion DNA polymerase (Thermo Scientific) according to the manufacturer's instructions. The PCR products were run in a gel and purified using the Agarose Gel DNA Extraction Kit (Roche). The primer pairs spanning the target site (covering around 500 bp for each cutting site) are listed in the Additional file 1: Table S1. Purified PCR samples (50 ng) were prepared for sequencing using 4 μl of BigDye terminator v3.1 (Applied Biosystems) and 5 pM primer in final volume of 20 μl. PCR program: 1 min at 96 ° C (1×), followed by 30 s at 96 °C, 15 s at 50 °C, and 4 min at 60 °C (30×), and finishing with 1 min incubation at 4 °C (1×). Samples were analyzed in an Applied Biosystems 3730xl DNA Analyser. The quantitative assessment of CRISPR-Cas9 genome editing was done using a freely available online software—TIDE [13]. Specifically, using Sanger sequencing reactions (sgRNA NT, sgTMEM97#1.1, sgTMEM97#1.2, sgTMEM97#2.1 and sgTMEM97#2.2), insertions/deletions (indels) and editing efficacy was assessed by TIDE software [13]. For that, the chromatogram sequence files of respectively the control sample (i.e., transduced with the sgRNA NT) and the test sample (i.e., transduced with the target sgRNA) were analyzed. As output, the quantitative spectrum of indels around the cut site was obtained [13].

MicroRNA expression profiling

MiRNAs expression was assessed in ten PCa and four MNPT using microRNA Ready-to-Use PCR Human Panel (I + II) v2.R (Exiqon, Vedbaek, Denmark), comprising 752 miRNAs as previously described [14, 15]. Extracted RNAs were submitted to cDNA synthesis using miRCURY LNA Universal RT microRNA PCR (Exiqon, Vedbaek, Denmark) following the manufacturer's instructions. Data were analyzed using the comparative Ct method, and the median value was calculated for reference genes' expression normalization. MiRNAs with fold change of − 1.5 in PCa compared with MNPT were considered downregulated.

MicroRNA's promoter methylation analysis in prostate tissues

All DNA samples were assessed for integrity, quantity, and purity by electrophoresis in a 1.3% agarose gel, picogreen quantification, and nanodrop measurements. All samples were randomly distributed into 96-well plates. Bisulfite conversion of 500 ng of genomic DNA was performed using the EZ DNA Methylation Kit (Zymo Research) following the manufacturer's instructions. Two hundred nanograms of bisulfite-converted DNA was used for hybridization on the HumanMethylation450 BeadChip (Illumina). Briefly, samples were whole-genome amplified followed by enzymatic end-point fragmentation, precipitation, and resuspension. The resuspended samples were hybridized onto the BeadChip for 16 h at 48 °C, then washed. A single nucleotide extension with labeled dideoxynucleotides was performed, and repeated rounds of staining were applied with a combination of labeled antibodies differentiating between biotin and DNP.

HumanMethylation450 BeadChip data were processed using Bioconductor minfi package [16]. The "Illumina" procedure that mimics the method of GenomeStudio (Illumina) was performed, including background correction and normalization considering the first array of the plate as reference. Probes with one or more single nucleotide polymorphisms (SNPs) with a minor allele frequency (MAF) > 1% (1000 Genomes) in the first 10 bp of the interrogated CpG were removed. The methylation level (β value) for each of the 485,577 CpG sites was calculated as the ratio between the methylated probe intensity and the overall intensity (sum of methylated and unmethylated probe intensities) multiplied by 100. After normalization step, probes mapped within X and Y chromosomes were removed. All analyses were performed in human genome version 19 (hg19), and data was deposited in GEO repository under accession number GSE52955.

TCGA dataset analysis

Data on miRNA expression and clinical information (when available) from PCa and matched normal tissue samples was retrieved from The Cancer Genome Atlas (TCGA) database. The mRNA expression data from samples hybridized at University of North Carolina, Lineberger Comprehensive Cancer Center, using Illumina HiSeq 2000 mRNA Sequencing version 2, were downloaded from data matrix including 494 miRNA-Seq, 496 RNA-Seq, and 498 Methylation Array for PCa samples and 52 matched normal adjacent tissue samples (NAT). To prevent duplicates, when there was more than one portion per patient, median values were used. The provided value was pre-processed and normalized according to "level 3" specifications of TCGA. Clinical data of each patient was provided by Biospecimen Core Resources (BCRs). Data is available for download through https://gdc-portal.nci.nih.gov/projects/TCGA-PRAD.

Real-time quantitative PCR (RT-qPCR)

MiR-152-3p transcript levels were assessed using TaqMan MicroRNA Assay (assay ID: 000475; Applied Biosystems) and normalized with RNU48 (assay ID: 001006; Applied Biosystems).

Real-time quantitative PCR analysis was performed using gene-specific primers and normalized using *GUSB* housekeeping gene (Additional file 1: Table S1). Specific-miRNA cDNA was obtained using TaqMan MicroRNA Reverse Transcription Kit from Applied Biosystems (Foster City, CA, USA). Total cDNA synthesis was performed using high-capacity cDNA Reverse Transcription Kit (Applied Biosystems, Foster City, CA, USA).

NOL4 and *TMEM97* mRNA levels were confirmed in the same group of tissue samples previously indicated. A total of 300 ng was reverse transcribed and amplified using TransPlex® Whole Transcriptome Amplification Kit (Sigma-Aldrich®, Schnelldorf, Germany) with subsequent purification using QIAquick® PCR Purification Kit (QIAGEN, Hilden, Germany), according to the manufacturer's instructions. Expression levels were evaluated using TaqMan® Gene Expression Assays (Applied Biosystems, Foster City, CA, USA), and GUSB was used as a reference gene for normalization.

The expression of each gene or small RNA was obtained using the formula: Relative expression = (Target gene mean quantity/Reference gene mean quantity). Ratios were then multiplied by 1000 for easier tabulation. Each plate included multiple non-template controls, and serial dilutions (× 10) of a cDNA obtained from human prostate RNA (Carlsbad, CA, USA) were used to construct a standard curve for each plate. All experiments were run in triplicates (Additional file 1: Table S1).

DNA methylation analysis

DNA methylation analysis was performed by quantitative methylation PCR (qMSP) using KAPA SYBR FAST qPCR Kit (Kapa Biosystems, MA, USA) and pyrosequencing. All reactions were run in triplicates in 384-well plates using Roche LightCycler 480 II, with *β-actin* (*ACTB*) as internal reference gene for normalization. Primer sequences (Additional file 1: Table S1) were designed using Methyl Primer Express 1.0 and purchased from Sigma-Aldrich (St. louis, MO, USA).

For pyrosequencing, specific sets of primers for PCR amplification and sequencing were designed using a specific software pack (PyroMark assay design version 2.0.01.15). Primer sequences were designed, when possible, to hybridize with CpG-free sites to ensure methylation-independent amplification. PCR was performed under standard conditions with biotinylated primers, and the PyroMark Vacuum Prep Tool (Biotage, Uppsala, Sweden) was used to prepare single-stranded PCR products, according to the manufacturer's instructions. Pyrosequencing reactions and methylation quantification were performed in a PyroMark Q96 System version 2.0.6 (Qiagen, Hilden, Germany) using appropriate reagents and recommended protocols (Additional file 1: Table S1).

Pre-miR transfections

To overexpress miR-152-3p, synthetic, commercially available, miRNAs' precursors (pre-miR-152-3p, ID: PM12269; pre-miR-NC, ID: AM17110; Ambion, Carlsbad, CA, USA) were transfected at 30 nM. Transfections were performed using Oligofectamine (Invitrogen, Carlsbad, CA, USA), per manufacturer's instructions.

Viability assay

Cell viability was evaluated by MTT assay. Briefly, PCa cells were seeded onto 96-well flat-bottomed culture plates, allowed to adhere overnight later (number of cells plated before transfection: LNCaP: 10000 cells/well; PC3: 3000 cells/well), and transfected 24 h later. At each time point, 0. 5 mg/ml of MTT reagent [3-(4, 5dimethylthiazol-2-yl)-2, 5-diphenyl-tetrazolium bromide] was added to each well, and the plates were incubated in the dark for 1 h at 37 °C. Formazan crystals were then dissolved in DMSO and absorbance was read at 540 nm in a microplate reader (FLUOstar Omega, BMG Labtech, Offenburg, Germany), subtracting the background, at 630 nm. The number of cells was calculated using the formula: [(OD experiment x Number of cells at day 0)/Mean OD at day 0]. Three replicates were performed for each condition and at least three independent experiments were carried out.

GFP-competitive proliferation assay

LNCaP cells were infected with sgRNAs targeting the exon 1 or exon 2 of *TMEM97*. Separately, we generated polyclonal LNCaP cells stably expressing GFP using pLX304-GFP30 (gift from David Root; Addgene plasmid # 25890). GFP expressing cells were mixed in a 1:3 ratio with cells containing individual sgRNAs. The percentage of GFP-expressing cells was assessed by flow cytometry at the beginning of the experiment ($T = 0$) and every 72 h onwards ($T = 3$d; $T = 6$d, and $T = 9$d). For each condition, 10,000 events were recorded. The cells were measured on a BD FACSCalibur cytometer (BD Biosciences, San Jose, CA, USA) and analyzed using FlowJo software.

Apoptosis evaluation

Evaluation of apoptosis was performed using APOPercentage apoptosis assay kit (Biocolor Ltd., Belfast, Northern Ireland) according to the manufacturer's instructions. PCa cells were seeded onto 24-well plates (LNCaP: 50000 cells/well, and PC3: 30000 cells/well) and 24 h later were transfected. Apoptotic cells were assessed at the end of the day 3, in a FLUOstar Omega microplate reader at 550 nm and the background subtracted at 620 nm. The results were normalized to number of viable cell obtained in the MTT assay according to the following formula (OD of apoptosis assay at 72 h/ OD of MTT at 72 h).

Cell cycle analysis

Cell cycle distribution of LNCaP and PC3 cells was determined by flow cytometry. Briefly, 72 h after transfections, 5×10^5 harvested cells were fixed overnight at 4 °C with 70% cold ethanol. After cold PBS washing, cells were re-suspended in staining Propidium Iodide Solution (Cytognos S.L, Salamanca, Spain) and incubated for 30 min at room temperature. All cells were then measured on a Cytomics FC500 flow cytometer (Beckman Coulter, Fullerton, CA, USA) and analyzed using Modfit LT (Verity Software House, Inc., Topshan, Maine, USA).

Cell invasion assay

Cell invasion was determined using BD BioCoat Matrigel Invasion Chamber (BD Biosciences, Franklin Lakes, NJ, USA). Briefly, 5×10^4 cells/mL of LNCaP or PC3 cells were added to the upper chamber. Both cell lines were transfected for 72 h with miRNA molecules, after which, the non-invading cells were removed with cotton swabs from the upper side of the membrane. The membrane bottom containing invading cells was fixed in methanol, washed in PBS, and stained with DAPI (Vector Laboratories, Burlingame, CA). All the invading cells were counted under a fluorescent microscope. PC3 cell line invasion capability was quantified upon trans-well matrigel invasion assays ($n = 3$ for each sample) comparing pre-miR-152-3p to pre-miR-NC cells. Error bars in all panels indicate standard deviation, unless otherwise specified.

Transcriptomic evaluation of altered genes following miR-152-3p manipulation

Cells (LNCaP: 400000 cells/well, and PC3: 150000 cells/well) were plated in 6-well, in the day before transfection. Cells were collected 72 h post transfection and RNA was extracted and used as template for cDNA synthesis. RT-qPCR was performed as previously described and data analyzed according to the comparative Ct method [17].

Gene expression microarrays

RNA was extracted from tissue samples using TRIzol (Invitrogen by Life Technologies, Carlsbad, CA), as previously described [18], and 1 μg of RNA was processed into cDNA and hybridized to Affymetrix GeneChip Human Exon 1.0 ST arrays, following the manufacturer's recommendations [19]. The Affymetrix Expression Console v1.1 software was used to obtain exon-level robust multi-array average (RMA)-normalized expression values for the core probe sets only. The data is freely available in GEO repository under accession number GSE42954.

Luciferase assay

A reporter plasmid containing a binding site at NOL4 or TMEM97 3′UTR for miR-152-3p (GeneCopoeia, Rockville, MD, USA) was co-transfected into HEK293Ta cells using Lipofectamine 2000 transfection reagent (Invitrogen, Carlsbad, CA, USA). Thirty nanomolars of synthetic pre-miRNA was used. Luciferase activity was assessed with the Secrete-Pair™ Dual Luminescence Assay Kit (GeneCopoeia, Rockville, MD, USA) according to the manufacturer's instructions. The ratio of luminescence intensities (RLU, Relative Light Unit) of the GLuc (Gaussia luciferase) over SEAP (secreted Alkaline Phosphatase) was obtained as follows: GLuc/SEAP, for each triplicate.

Statistical analysis

Non-parametric tests (Kruskal-Wallis and Mann-Whitney *U* test) were used for group comparisons analysis for both expression and methylation levels for the two patient cohorts (IPO's and TCGA) and for the in vitro assays. Correlations between expression levels and methylation were evaluated by Spearman's correlation test. Data are shown as mean ± s.d., unless otherwise specified. Student's *t* test was used for invasion assays. To evaluate the prognostic value of mir152 and *TMEM97* expression in PCa patients from the TCGA dataset, univariable (Log-rank test) and multivariable (Cox regression) analyses of disease-free survival were performed, where putative confounding effects (Gleason score and patients' age) were considered. Disease-free survival was calculated from the date of the radical prostatectomy to the date of relapse, or date of last follow-up or death if relapse-free. For the purposes of survival analyses, high gene expression was considered for samples within the 90th percentile (10% of samples with highest gene expression values). All statistical tests were two-sided. All experiments were run in triplicate. Statistical analysis was carried out using Graph Pad Prism version 5 and IBM SPSS statistics version 22. Significance level was set at $p < 0.05$.

Results

Identification of hypermethylated and downregulated microRNAs in prostate cancer

Global miRNA expression was assessed using microRNA Ready-to-Use PCR Human Panel (I + II) v2.0 (Exiqon, Vedbaek, Denmark). To identify differentially expressed miRNAs in PCa, compared to morphologically normal prostate tissue (MNPT), 740 miRNAs were profiled in 10 PCa tissues and 4 MNPT [20]. Using a cutoff value of log fold change < – 1.5, 39 miRs were found downregulated in PCa compared to MNPT (Additional file 1: Table S2 and Figure S1). From these miRNAs, 10 were selected for validation in a larger and independent dataset (miR-10a, miR-23b, miR-27b, miR-135b, miR-143, miR-152-3p, miR-187, miR-204, miR-205, miR-221), i.e., the miRNAseq expression data from PCa patients and matched normal samples deposited in The Cancer Genome Atlas (TCGA) ($n = 326$ and $n = 52$, respectively) (Fig. 1a–c and Additional file 1: Figure S2).

We also determined global differences in DNA methylation in the prostate tissues [21]. This cohort was composed of 5 MNPT and 25 PCa. DNA samples were hybridized on the Infinium DNA methylation BeadChip platform (Illumina), which analyzes more than 450,000 CpG sites in the genome [22]. After normalization, we filtered out poor-quality probes and those containing single nucleotide polymorphisms (SNPs; > 1%) [23] and copy number variations (CNV; > 5%) in the detection sequence. Following these filters, DNA methylation profiling disclosed 38 hypermethylated promoter regions in known miRNA regions, three of which were further validated in TCGA dataset (Additional file 1: Table S2 and Figure S3).

Because gene expression and DNA promoter methylation correlate with gene regulatory activity status, we merged the results of the two analytical platforms (expression by Exiqon platform and methylation profiling by Illumina) to identify miRNAs with decreased expression associated with promoter hypermethylation in PCa. From this combined analysis, 5 miRNAs emerged as simultaneously downregulated and hypermethylated in PCa: miR-10a, miR-23b, miR-27b, miR-34c, and miR-152-3p (Fig. 1a; Additional file 1: Table S2, highlighted in blue). In TCGA dataset, the common microRNAs were confirmed to be downregulated in primary PCa compared to noncancerous prostate tissues (Fig. 1b), but miR-34c showed no statistical significance. Moreover, and except for miR-10a, all displayed significantly lower expression in PCa in comparison with matched non-cancerous prostate tissues (Fig. 1c). Because miRNA's promoter methylation status was available at TCGA database, these data were also retrieved and it confirmed our finding of increased methylation indexes in these miR's obtained with the Infinium 450 K DNA methylation profiling platform (Fig. 1d). Then, we focused our study on miR-152-3p as it fulfilled the criteria for downregulation associated with promoter hypermethylation in PCa. Remarkably, we had already suggested that miR-152-3p was regulated by DNA methylation in PCa [21, 24], confirming previous published findings [25, 26] which support the observations that miR-152-3p is a common epigenetically regulated miRNA in PCa.

MiR-152-3p expression and promoter methylation analysis in prostate cells

MiR-152-3p is located at chromosome 17q21.32, within an intronic region of *COPZ2*. Data from the 450 K array revealed that 9 probes targeting this locus were differentially methylated (Fig. 2a). The cg05850656 and cg24389730 showed the highest β values (0.55 and 0.53). These probes map to TSS200-Body for miR-152-3p-*COPZ2* locus. To further validate these findings, miR-152-3p (Fig. 2b) and *COPZ2* (Fig. 2c) expression levels were assessed in our cohort of prostatic tissues (PCa = 100 and MNPT = 14) and

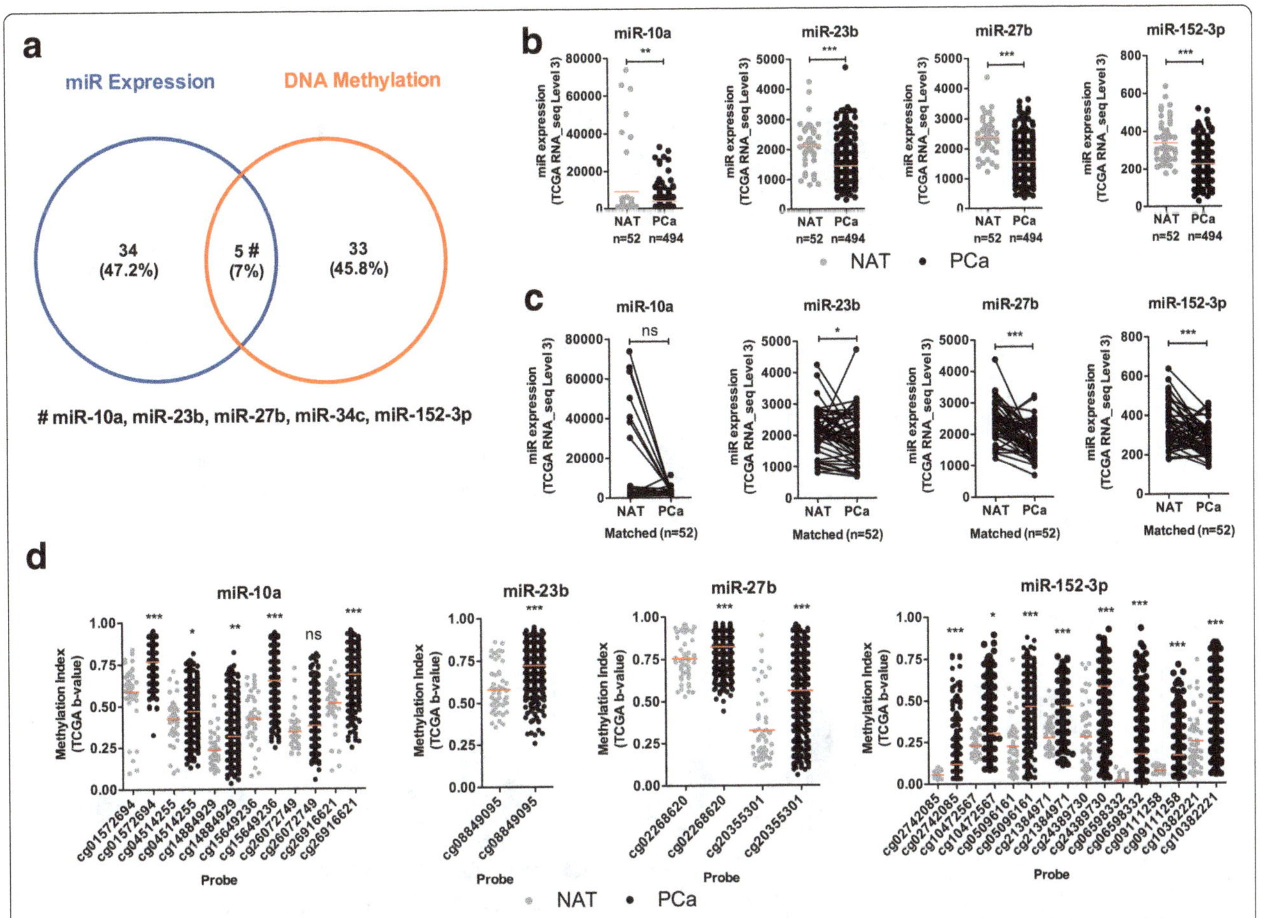

Fig. 1 Identification of miRNAs downregulated by DNA methylation in prostate cancer, using a combinatorial approach. **a** Venn diagram of the intersection of the miR expression (Exiqon) versus DNA methylation (Infinium HumanMethylation450 BeadChip) for miRNA promoters. Intersection is shown for the downregulated miRNAs and hypermethylated miRNAs. The five common miRNAs based on expression level and DNA methylation in PCa tissues are miR-10a, miR-23b, miR-27b, miR-34c, and miR-152-3p. **b** Independent validation using the TCGA Prostate RNA-seq cohort for miR-10a, miR-23b, miR-27b, and miR-152-3p in PCa samples compared to NAT samples. **c** MiRNA expression analysis of 52 matched normal and PCa samples pairs using TCGA cohort. Except for miR-10a, all miRs were significantly downregulated in PCa. **d** DNA methylation levels (β-Values) for each probe in specific miRNA loci, comparing normal and PCa samples using TCGA Prostate 450 K cohort. Overall, DNA methylation gain (hypermethylation) was found in PCa samples. NAT: Normal Adjacent Tissue; PCa: Prostate Cancer; Mann-Whitney *U* test: *$p < 0.05$, **$p < 0.01$, ***$p < 0.001$

downregulation of both in PCa compared to MNPT was confirmed ($p < 0.0001$ and $p = 0.0022$, respectively).

In both patients' cohorts, miR-152-3p and *COPZ2* expression levels were inversely and significantly correlated with methylation levels in PCa samples ($p = -0.444$, $p < 0.0001$, and $p = -0.435$, $p < 0.0001$ for IPO Porto cohort; $p = -0.331$, $p < 0.0001$ and $p = -0.561$, $p < 0.0001$, TCGA Cohort, respectively).

Pyrosequencing analysis demonstrated that the promoter shared by miR-152-3p and *COPZ2* was aberrantly methylated in PCa (Fig. 2d; $p < 0.0001$).

In LNCaP, DU 145, and PC3 cells, miR-152-3p and *COPZ2* expression levels were also significantly lower than those found on RWPE cells, which are benign epithelial prostate cells (Figs. 2e, f), whereas promoter methylation levels followed the opposite trend, specifically for the latter two cell lines—LNCaP and PC3 (Fig. 2g). These findings suggest that miR-152-3p is transcribed in parallel with its host gene, *COPZ2*. Exposure of PCa cells to demethylating agent 5-Aza-2-deoxycytidine (5-Aza-CdR) caused a 38 and 67% reduction in *COPZ2*-miR-152-3p promoter methylation levels, in LNCaP ($p = 0.0411$) and PC3 cells ($p = 0.0043$), respectively (Fig. 2h). Nonetheless, the impact in gene expression differed as miR-152-3p re-expression was observed in both cell lines (LNCaP, FC: 1.75; and PC3, FC: 1.94) (Fig. 2i), whereas *COPZ2* transcript levels were only significantly restored in PC3 cells (FC: 3.98) (Fig. 2j).

MiR-152-3p attenuates malignant phenotype in vitro

Using in vitro assays, we found that miR-152-3p overexpression significantly decreased cell viability in both LNCaP and PC3 cells (Fig. 3a, d) and promoted a significant accumulation of cells in S and G2/M phases (Fig. 3b, e). Accordingly, at transcriptional level, both cell lines displayed a significant

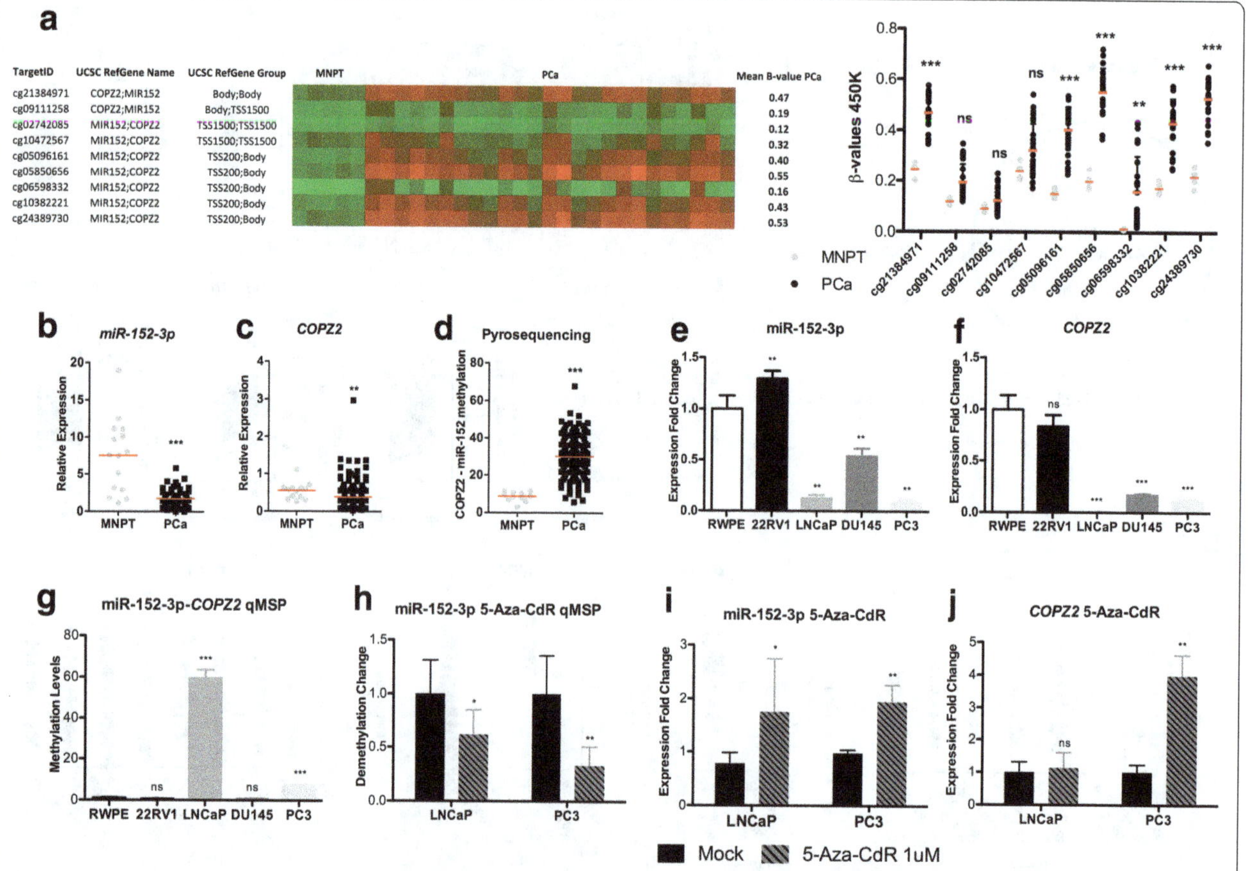

Fig. 2 *COPZ2*-miR-152-3p transcriptional unit's DNA methylation and expression validation in IPO Porto's cohort of prostate samples. **a** HumanMethylation450 BeadChip data for miR-152-3p locus, showing a significant increase in cg21384971, cg05096161, cg05850656, cg06598332, cg10382221, and cg24389730. **b** Significant miR-152-3p downregulation in PCa ($n = 100$) compared to morphologically normal prostate tissues (MNPT, $n = 14$), as determined by RT-qPCR ($p < 0.0001$). **c** Significantly decreased *COPZ2* transcript levels in PCa samples ($p = 0.0022$). **d** *COPZ2*-miR-152-3p promoter hypermethylation in PCa samples determined by pyrosequencing (p = < 0.0001). **e** MiR-152-3p expression levels in PCa cell lines compared to benign RWPE cells [expression (E):1] assessed by RT-qPCR. Expression is significantly lower in LNCaP (E ~ 0.13), DU145 (E ~ 0.54) and PC3 (E ~ 0.09) cells. **f** Significantly lower *COPZ2* expression levels by RT-qPCR in LNCaP (E ~ 0.005), DU145 (E ~ 0.17) and PC3 (E ~ 0.12) cells compared to RWPE (E 1). **g** Prostate cell lines' DNA methylation profiling. LNCaP (FC of methylation levels: ~ 59) and PC3 (FC: ~ 7) cells showed increased miR152-*COPZ2* promoter hypermethylation compared to RWPE (FC: 1), 22RV1 and DU145 cells. **h** A 72-h 5-Aza-CdR exposure, associated with significant decrease in promoter methylation levels of the transcriptional unit *COPZ2*-miR-152-3p in LNCaP (decreased ~ 40%) and PC3 (decreased ~ 68%) cells. LNCaP and PC3 cells miR-152-3p (**i**) and *COPZ2's* (**j**) expression levels following 72-h exposure to 5-Aza-CdR associated with increased miR-152-3p expression levels (FC:1.75; 1.95, respectively) and *COPZ2* (FC:1.12; 3.98, respectively). Error bars represent the s.d. for three biological replicates. Mann-Whitney *U* test: $*p < 0.05$, $**p < 0.01$, $***p < 0.001$. β values range from 0 to 1 and were determined by the ratio of the methylated probe intensity and the overall intensity (sum of methylated and unmethylated probe intensities). MNPT: Morphologically Normal Prostate Tissue; PCa: Prostate Cancer; 5-Aza-CdR: 5-aza-2-deoxycytidine

decrease of several cell cycle regulators (Fig. 3c, f). Conversely, miR-152-3p's mimic transfection associated with increased apoptosis in LNCaP ($p = 0.0286$) and PC3 ($p = 0.0286$) cells (Fig. 3g; Additional file 1: Figure S4). These results were further supported by the significantly reduced NF-kB expression in both PCa cell lines, as well as significantly increased *CASP3* expression levels, although only in PC3 transfected cells (Fig. 3h, i). Moreover, miR-152-3p overexpression significantly reduced PC3 invasion ability in PC3 cells ($p = 0.0286$; Fig. 3j) and associated with specific epithelial–mesenchymal transition genes' downregulation. Indeed, along with *TWIST* and *VIM* downregulation, *MAPK1*, *SMAD4*, and *STAT3* were significantly downregulated after miR-152-3p restored expression in both LNCaP and PC3 cells (Fig. 3k, l).

miR-152-3p targets *NOL4* and *TMEM97*

Because the previous results suggested that miR-152-3p was an onco-suppressor, we sought to identify its targets for post-transcriptional regulation, using a combination of multiple in silico target prediction tools (putative targets must contain at least one miRNA response element (MRE)) (Additional file 1: Table S3) and a publicly available gene expression dataset. Among the 329 genes

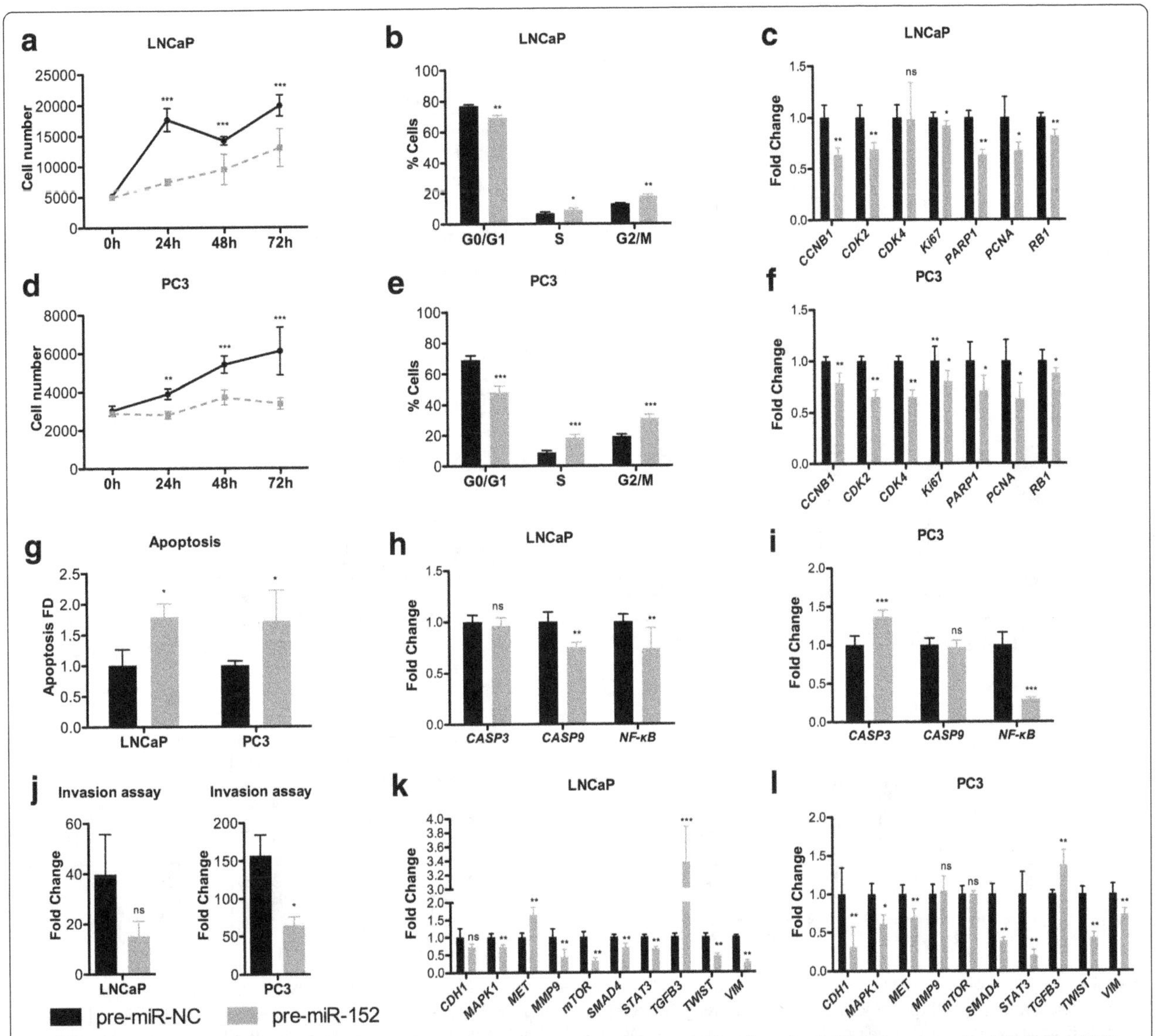

Fig. 3 miR-152-3p overexpression associated with attenuated malignant features in LNCaP and PC3 cells. **a, d** miR-152-3p overexpression in LNCaP and PC3 cells significantly decreased cell viability compared to pre-miR-NC transfected cells (MTT assay at 24, 48, and 72 h). **b, e** Cell cycle arrest at S and G2/M phases was depicted for LNCaP and PC3 cells overexpressing miR-152-3p (cytometry analysis was performed 72 h after transfection). **c, f** Reduced transcription levels of several cell cycle-promoting genes in miR-152-3p overexpressing LNCaP and PC3 cells. **g** MiR-152-3p overexpression associated with significant increase in apoptosis compared to cells transfected with negative control miRNA. **h, i** Apoptosis-related genes' expression levels were deregulated in PCa miR-152-3p overexpressing cells. Significantly reduced *NF-kB* levels were found in both miR-152-3p overexpressing cell lines. **j** MiR-152-3p forced expression in LNCaP and PC3 cells associated with a significant decrease number of cells invading through the Matrigel coated Boyden chamber assay. **k, l** Transcriptional deregulation of EMT and invasion-related genes in miR-152-3p transfected LNCaP and PC3. Differential *MET, mTOR and MMP9S* results suggest cell-specific gene regulation. *TGFB3* overexpression and EMT markers *STAT3, TWIST*, or *VIM* decrease was shared by both miR-152-3p overexpressing cells. Error bars represent the s.d. for three biological replicates. Mann-Whitney U-test: $^{*}p < 0.05$, $^{**}p < 0.01$, $^{***}p < 0.001$

predicted as miR-152-3p targets in silico, only six—*BEND4, ELOVL2, NOL4, OAS2, SLC7A11*, and *TMEM97*—disclosed a gene expression log fold change > 1.5 in PCa samples ($n = 368$) analyzed by GeneChip Human Exon ST Array (Fig. 4a). Moreover, forced expression of miR-152-3p caused a significant downregulation of *BEND4, ELOVL2*, and *TMEM97* in LNCaP cells (Fig. 4b), whereas in PC3 cells, only *NOL4* transcript levels significantly diminished following miR-152-3p's overexpression (Fig. 4c). LNCaP cells overexpressing miR-152-3p exposed to 5-Aza-CdR showed significantly reduced *TMEM97* expression levels (Fig. 4d), and *NOL4* was downregulated in PC3 cells (Fig. 4e).

To further confirm the biological significance of our previous findings, *NOL4* and *TMEM97* expression levels were assessed in two independent cohorts of PCa patients (from our institution and from TCGA). Remarkably, we found that *TMEM97* and *NOL4* expression levels were

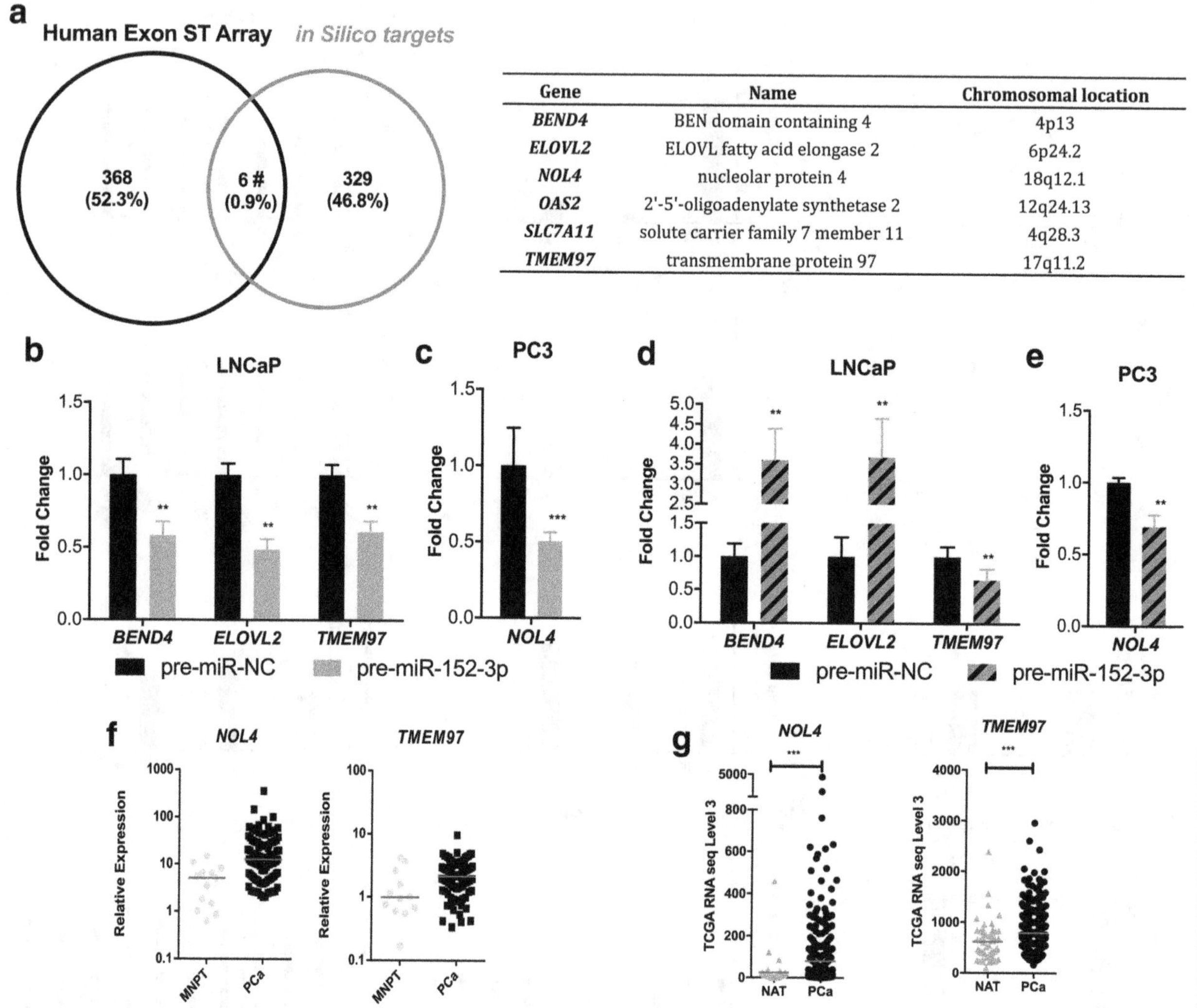

Fig. 4 Identification of putative targets of miR-152-3p in PCa cell lines. **a** Genes selected for validation in our experimental settings: combining in silico prediction targets with genome-wide expression using GeneChip® Human Exon ST Array. **b** MiR-152-3p overexpression in LNCaP cells associated with significant decreased levels of *BEND4* (~ 40%), *ELOVL2* (52%) and *TMEM97* (40%) as determined by RT-qPCR. **c** PC3 miR-152-3p's transfected cells displayed significantly decreased *NOL4* expression (approximately 50%). **d, e** Effect of 5-Aza-CdR treatment in the selected target genes transcript levels in LNCaP revealed *TMEM97* downregulation (up to 35%), whereas in PC3 cells it associated with significantly decreased *NOL4* transcript levels (– 30%). *NOL4* and *TMEM97* upregulation in PCa tissues. **f** Significantly higher *NOL4* and *TMEM97* expression in PCa tissue samples ($n = 100$) compared with morphologically normal prostate tissue ($n = 14$), determined by RT-qPCR. **g** Expression levels in TCGA Prostate by RNA-seq cohort (NAT: $n = 52$; PCa: $n = 497$). MNPT: Morphologically Normal Prostate Tissue; NAT: Normal Adjacent Tissue; PCa: Prostate Cancer. Error bars represent the s.d. for three biological replicates. Mann-Whitney U-test: *$p < 0.05$, **$p < 0.01$, ***$p < 0.001$

significantly upregulated in PCa cases from both cohorts, compared to normal prostate tissues ($p = 0.0132$ and $p = 0.0004$, respectively, in IPO Porto's cohort; $p < 0.0001$ and $p < 0.0001$, respectively, in TCGA cohort; Fig. 4f, g).

TMEM97 knockdown decreases cell proliferation

Since both *NOL4* and *TMEM97* 3′UTRs contain a MRE for miR-152-3p (Fig. 5a, left panel), the functional interaction between miR-152-3p and *NOL4*, on the one hand, and *miR-152-3p* and *TMEM97*, on the other hand, was investigated using luciferase assays. Interestingly, a 30% reduction ($p = 0.0022$) in luciferase activity for the *TMEM97* MRE was found, although only a 10% decrease was depicted for the *NOL4* MRE (Fig. 5a, right panel).

Thus, we tested 4 individual sgRNAs designed to target *TMEM97*. We validated the candidate sgRNAs with a competitive proliferation assay. LNCaP cells were transduced with the indicated sgRNAs and allowed to proliferate for 9 days. No clonal selection was performed; thus, cells' population not only comprises a pool of homozygous/heterozygous mutants, but also unmutated cells (Additional file 1: Figure S5).

CRISPR-Cas9-mediated knockout of *TMEM97* with four different sgRNAs (sgTMEM97 exon#1 and exon#2) in

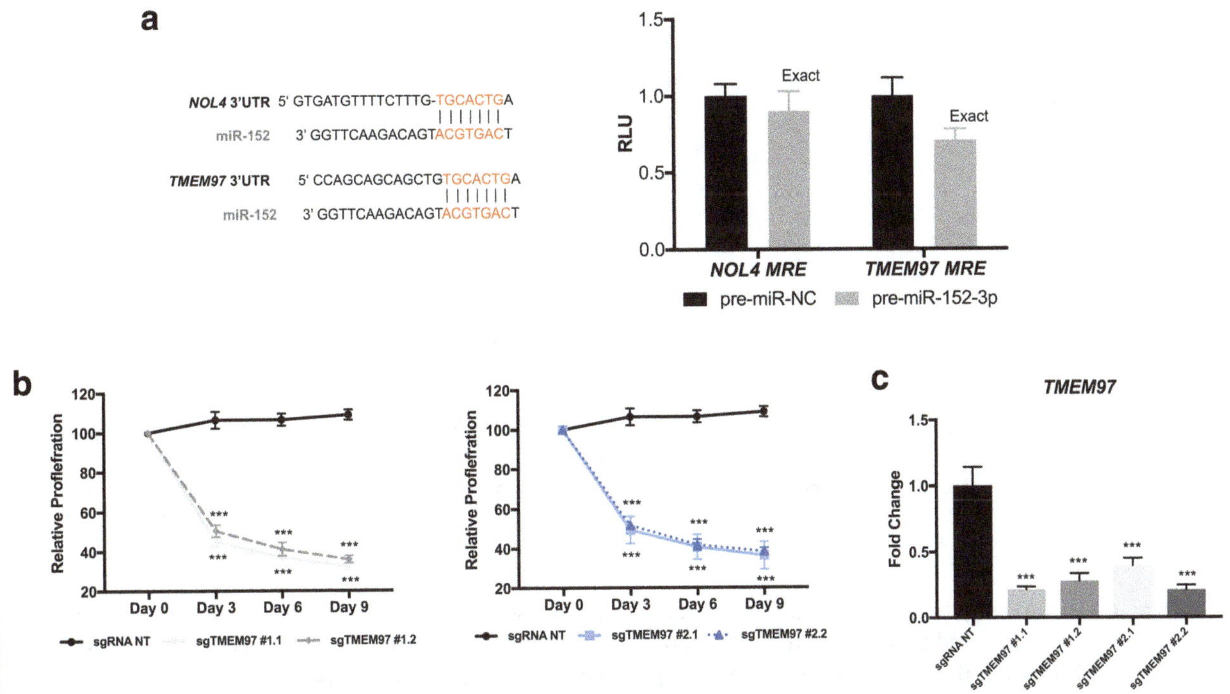

Fig. 5 *NOL4* and *TMEM97* are miR-152-3p targets **a** Schematic representation of the miR-152-3p's MRE in *NOL4* and *TMEM97*. Luciferase activity in HEK293Ta cells co-transfected with reporter constructs containing *NOL4* MRE or *TMEM97* MRE and either pre-miR-152-3p or pre-miR-NC. **b** Validation of candidate sgRNAs for *TMEM97* by a competitive proliferation assay in LNCaP cells. **c** SgRNA NT indicates a nontargeting. GFP levels were measured by flow cytometry. Values are normalized to day 0 ($T = 0$). 3'UTR: 3' Untranslated Region; MRE: miRNA response element Mann-Whitney U test: *$p < 0.05$, **$p < 0.01$, ***$p < 0.001$

LNCaP cells resulted in a significant decrease in proliferation (Fig. 5b). Remarkably, all four sgRNAs significantly diminished *TMEM97* mRNA levels (Fig. 5c), probably due to nonsense-mediated decay [27]. Cas9-nuclease activity generates DNA double-strand breaks that result in deletions and insertions at the vicinity of the sgRNA recognition site. We examined the range of deletions/insertions caused by each sgRNA targeting *TMEM97* (Additional file 1: Figure S5). All the sgTMEM97 caused on-target indels, with a percentage ranging from 42.3–79.2%.

Overall, the sgRNAs targeting *TMEM97* mimicked the restoration of miR-152, suggesting that this gene is required for LNCaP cells growth.

miR-152, *TMEM97*, and *NOL4* clinical potential in PCa

Lastly, to further evaluate the biological significance of the previous findings in primary PCa, the prognostic value of miR-152, *NOL4*, and *TMEM97* expression levels was assessed in both PCa patients' cohorts. Although, no associations were found in IPO Porto's cohort, in TCGA's cohort, higher miR-152-3p expression levels (90th percentile) predicted longer disease-free survival in univariable analysis (Log-rank test $p = 0.004$; Fig. 6a) and in multivariable Cox regression analysis adjusted for patients' age and Gleason score (HR = 0.228, $p = 0.012$; Table 2). However, *TMEM97* or *NOL4* expression levels did not significantly associate with PCa patients' outcome (Fig. 6b, c, Table 2).

Discussion

MiRNAs are key players in cellular differentiation and homeostasis, being involved in regulation of transcriptional programs through the elimination of aberrant transcripts and suppression of random fluctuations in transcript copy number [28]. Thus, its deregulation impairs cellular homeostasis and is involved in the emergence of several pathologies, including PCa.

In this study, we aimed to extend current knowledge on the impact of epigenetic deregulation of miRNAs expression in PCa. For that purpose, we used a combined analysis that allowed the identification of downregulated and aberrantly methylated microRNAs. Interestingly, only 8% of downregulated miRNAs in PCa tissues were found to be simultaneously aberrantly methylated. Thus, promoter hypermethylation does not seem to be a prevalent mechanism underlying microRNA downregulation in this cancer model, and other causes, whether genetic [29], epigenetic [30] or microenvironment-related (e.g., abnormal AR signaling [31]), are likely to be more frequent. Notwithstanding, we have recently shown that aberrant microRNA promoter methylation might constitute a clinically useful tool for PCa detection and prognostication [24]. Although the number of candidate microRNAs was small, the combined approach used in this study seems to be more robust and efficient than each strategy (i.e., micro-RNA expression analysis and differential methylation mapping) alone,

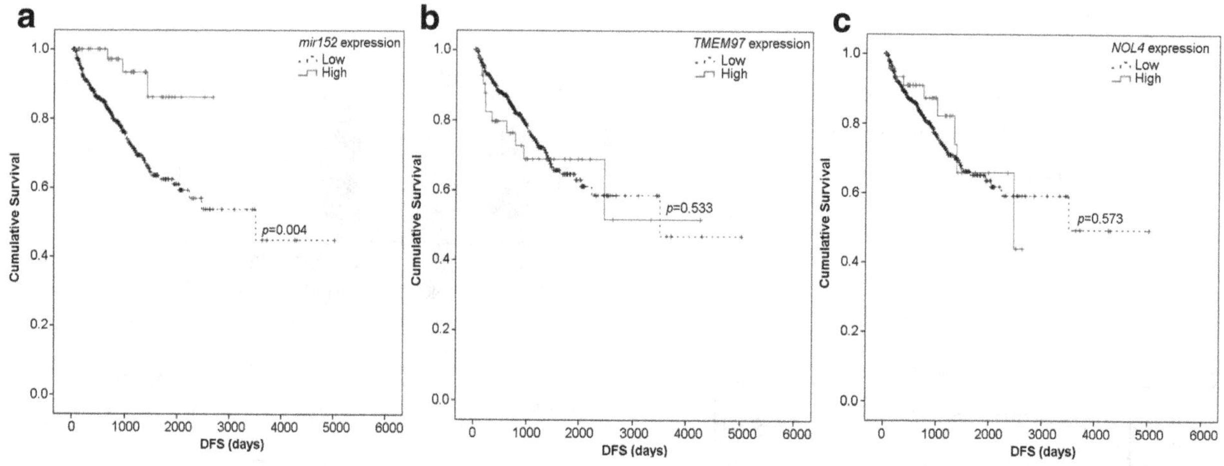

Fig. 6 miR-152-3p is valuable prognostic biomarker in PCa. **a–c** Disease-free survival analyses were performed in PCa patients from the TCGA dataset. **a** High miR-152-3p expression levels significantly associated with longer disease-free survival ($p = 0.004$; Log-rank test). **b** *TMEM97* and **c** *NOL4* expression do not present prognostic value

considering the significantly higher proportion of validated candidates obtained compared to previous studies from our group [15, 21]. Moreover, the results also validate this approach as it confirmed previous reports on miR-23b and miR-27b (members of the cluster miR-23b/27b/24-1) downregulation associated with promoter methylation in PCa [32–34]. Remarkably, two novel microRNAs within this category were found—miR-10a and miR-152-3p—although only the latter was validated in two independent datasets.

Interestingly, several miRNAs, including miR-135b, miR-143, miR-187, miR-204, miR-205 and miR-221 that were commonly downregulated in the Exiqon expression dataset, were also downregulated in TCGA dataset. In contrast, the number of putatively downregulated microRNAs due to aberrant DNA methylation found in the HumanMethylation450 BeadChip and validated in TCGA dataset was much smaller. Thus, our data indicate that miRNA expression's profiling is more likely to identify bona fide miRNA deregulated due to promoter methylation compared to DNA methylation profiling, as aberrant DNA methylation might not indicate effective transcriptional silencing. Nevertheless, DNA methylation profiling might be particularly suitable for integrative analytic approaches [35].

Because miR-152-3p fulfilled the criteria for methylation-associated downregulation and it had not been previously reported in PCa, we sought to investigate its role in prostate carcinogenesis. Our study indicates that miR-152-3p is a sense-oriented intronic miRNA that forms a transcriptional unit (TU) with the respective host gene, *COPZ2*, being processed as part of the host gene mRNA [36, 37]. Globally, aberrant promoter methylation associated with simultaneous downregulation of *COPZ2*-miR152 expression. This further supports that host gene promoter methylation status is, indeed, associated with miRNAs deregulation, as previously suggested [26]. Nonetheless, the results of 5-Aza-CdR exposure in LNCaP suggest that this is not the only mechanism regulating *COPZ2*-miR152 expression, and we are tempted to speculate whether an independent promoter might be located upstream in the host gene, as reported for other genes [38, 39].

MiR-152-3p promoter methylation has also been reported in endometrial cancer [40] and in MLL-rearranged infant acute lymphoblastic leukemia [41]. In accordance with previous reports, our results also suggest an onco-suppressor function for miR-152-3p in PCa. Indeed, in non-small cell lung cancer miR-152-3p suppressed cell proliferation, colony formation, migration and invasion [42], in endometrial cancer miR-152-3p restored expression prevented tumor cell growth both in vitro and in vivo [40], and in ovarian cancer miR-152-3p was suggested to contribute to cisplatin resistance in vitro and in vivo through direct *DNMT1* targeting [43]. Moreover, in the TCGA PCa cohort, *DNMT1* upregulation associated with miR-152 promoter hypermethylation (Pearson's = 0.12, $p = 0.0236$), although with limited statistical significance [26]. Interestingly, in prostatectomy samples, lower miR-152-3p expression levels were previously significantly associated with higher risk for biochemical recurrence, although only in univariable analysis [44]. Concordantly, our study shows miR-152-3p has prognostic value, although only in the TCGA cohort. Daniunaite et al. showed, using Kaplan-Meier analysis, that mir-152 promoter hypermethylation had a significant negative impact on BCR-free survival [26]. However, in a recent study aiming at PCa early detection, miR-152-3p expression did not discriminate PCa patients from the matched healthy controls in plasma samples [45]. Moreover, *TMEM97* and *NOL4* expression levels did not associate with patients' prognosis in both cohorts.

In vitro functional assays demonstrated that miR-152-3p controls cell viability in PCa cells acting as S and G2/

Table 2 Disease-free survival analysis by Cox regression in TCGA patients

DFS	Multivariable analysis		
	HR	95% CI for HR	*p* value
mir152			
mir152 expression level[a]	*0.228*	*0.072–0.722*	*0.012*
Age	0.999	0.970–1.028	0.928
Gleason Score[b]			
6			*< 0.0001*
7	5.528	0.754–40.536	0.093
8	*11.104*	*1.455–84.709*	*0.020*
9	*23.559*	*3.247–170.946*	*0.002*
10	*24.146*	*1.502–388.242*	*0.025*
TMEM97			
TMEM97 expression level[a]	1.007	0.550–1844	0.980
Age	1.000	0.971–1.029	0.978
Gleason Score[b]			
6			*< 0.0001*
7	5.369	0.732–39.373	*0.098*
8	*10.978*	*1.438–83.790*	*0.002*
9	*23.087*	*3.179–167.641*	*0.005*
10	30.812	2.786–340.785	0.978
NOL4			
NOL4 expression level[a]	0.778	0.392–1.545	0.473
Age	1.000	0.972–1.029	0.979
Gleason Score[b]			
6			*< 0.0001*
7	5.309	0.724–38.935	0.101
8	*10.967*	*1.438–83.629*	*0.021*
9	*22.911*	*3.158–166.213*	*0.002*
10	*31.102*	*2.811–344.117*	*0.005*

p value significant when $p < 0.05$
HR hazard ratio, *CI* confidence interval.
[a]Reference group: high expression level
[b]Reference group: Gleason Score 6

M cell-cycle transitions regulator, in both cell lines tested, but more expressively PC3 cells. However, these effects might be cell-context dependent. In line with functional assays' results, miR-152-3p overexpression associated with different specific transcript alterations depending on the tested cell line. Our results indicate that miR-152-3p fine-tunes the expression of several genes involved in the MAPK/ERK, TFG-Beta, JAK–STAT3 and EMT pathways. Thus, our data not only supports that miR-152-3p is a promising molecular target that inhibits PCa cell cycle and invasion [25, 46], but also demonstrates its role in apoptosis regulation. Since these biological processes are critical for cancer progression, a major role for miR-152-3p in PCa progression might be anticipated.

To better understand the role of miR-152-3p, we attempted to identify putative targets. In silico analysis followed by validation in two independent patient cohorts indicated *NOL4* (nucleolar protein 4) and *TMEM97* (transmembrane protein 97) as miR-152-3p targets. Although no information is available for the role of *NOL4* in cancer, *TMEM97* has been shown to be upregulated in several malignancies, including glioma [47] as well as colorectal [48] and ovarian [49] cancers. Interestingly, in glioma cells, *TMEM97* depletion inhibited cancer cell growth and metastasis formation, in parallel with deregulation of EMT-related genes. In our model, *TMEM97* disruption decreased LNCaP proliferation, further suggesting its involvement in cell growth. Remarkably, increased *TMEM97* expression correlated with shorter survival in glioma [47], ovarian [49], non-small cell lung [50], and colorectal [48] cancer patients. Moreover, *TMEM97* cytoplasmic expression has been positively correlated with *PCNA* expression [48], which acts as a scaffold to recruit proteins involved in DNA replication or DNA repair, being required for post-replication repair [51]. Remarkably, in our study, miR-152-3p overexpression associated with *PCNA* downregulation in both cell lines. Therefore, since *TMEM97* might be functionally associated with *PCNA* [52], it might suggest that both are controlled by miR-152-3p. Concerning other previously reported miR-152-3p's targets, we were not able to confirm DNMT1 as a miR-152-3p's direct target [25, 43, 53].

Conclusions

In conclusion, this study uncovered novel miRNAs downregulated by aberrant DNA methylation, including a transcriptional unit formed by *COPZ2*-miR-152-3p. Furthermore, it was demonstrated that miR-152-3p downregulation is a common feature in PCa, favoring the acquisition and development of the malignant traits, as in vitro miR-152-3p's restored expression attenuated PCa cell phenotype, by impairment of cell viability, cell cycle progression and invasion, through targeting of several genes involved in critical cancer-related pathways.

Additional file

Additional file 1: Supplementary information. Table S1 Primers and TaqMan assays used in this study; Table S2 microRNAs selected for evaluation in TCGA dataset; Table S3 Putative miR-152 target genes determined by multiple in silico prediction tools; Figure S1 Flow chart depicting the different steps followed to ascertain downregulated miRNAs in PCa; Figure S2 Representative examples of downregulated microRNAs at the TCGA cohort from the initial microRNA profiling by Exiqon; Figure S3 Representative examples of microRNAs downregulated at the TCGA cohort derived from the DNA methylation mapping by 450 K Illumina's array; Figure S4 Efficiency of miR-152 mimic's transfection in PCa cell lines; Figure S5 TIDE analysis of deletions/insertions caused by each sgRNA targeting TMEM97.

Abbreviations

5-Aza-CdR: 5-Aza-2-deoxycytidine; AGO: Argonaute; CNV: Copy Number Variations; FFPE: Formal-Fixed and Paraffin-Embedded; MAF: Minor Allele Frequency; miRNAs: microRNAs; MNPT: Morphologically Normal Prostate Tissue; NAT: Normal Adjacent Tissue; *NOL4*: Nucleolar Protein 4; PCa: Prostate Cancer; qMSP: quantitative Methylation Specific PCR; SNP: Single Nucleotide Polymorphisms; *TMEM97*: Transmembrane Protein 7

Acknowledgements

The authors are grateful to the Departments of Urology and Laboratory Medicine of the Portuguese Oncology Institute of Porto for their collaboration.

Funding

This study was funded by research grants from Research Center of Portuguese Oncology Institute of Porto (FB-GEBC-27 and 19-CI-IPOP-2016). JR-C and CSG are supported by FCT- Fundação para a Ciência e Tecnologia PhD fellowships (SFRH/BD/71293/2010 and SFRH/BD/92786/2013), SS is supported by a PhD fellowship IPO/ESTIMA-1 NORTE-01-0145-FEDER-000027, and IG is a research fellow from the strategic funding of FCT (PCT: PEst- UID/DTP/00776/2013 and COMPETE: POCI-01-0145-FEDER-006868). BMC is funded by FCT-Fundação para a Ciência e a Tecnologia (IF/00601/2012). The funders had no role in study design, data collection and analysis, decision to publish, or preparation of the manuscript.

Authors' contributions

JR-C, RH, and CJ conceived and designed the experiments. JR-C, IG, DB, EPS, SS, and MIG performed the experiments. JR-C, CSG, IG, AG, BMC, RH, and CJ analyzed the data. CSG, MIG, ME, BMC, RH, and CJ contributed reagents/material/analysis. All authors read and approved the final manuscript.

Competing interests

The authors declare that they have no competing interests.

Author details

[1]Cancer Biology & Epigenetics Group – Research Center (CI-IPOP), Portuguese Oncology Institute of Porto (IPO Porto), F Bdg, 1st floor, Rua Dr António Bernardino de Almeida, 4200-072 Porto, Portugal. [2]Cancer Epigenetics and Biology Program, Bellvitge Biomedical Research Institute, Barcelona, Catalonia, Spain. [3]Biomedical Sciences Graduate Program, Institute of Biomedical Sciences Abel Salazar– University of Porto (ICBAS-UP), Porto, Portugal. [4]Life and Health Sciences Research Institute (ICVS), School of Medicine, University of Minho, Campus de Gualtar, Braga, Portugal. [5]ICVS/3B's - PT Government Associate Laboratory, Braga/Guimarães, University of Minho, Campus de Gualtar, Braga, Portugal. [6]Department of Immunology, Portuguese Oncology Institute of Porto, Porto, Portugal. [7]Institucio Catalana de Recerca i Estudis Avançats (ICREA), Barcelona, Catalonia, Spain. [8]Physiological Sciences Department, School of Medicine and Health Sciences, University of Barcelona (UB), Barcelona, Catalonia, Spain. [9]Department of Pathology, Portuguese Oncology Institute of Porto, Porto, Portugal. [10]Department of Pathology and Molecular Immunology, Institute of Biomedical Sciences Abel Salazar– University of Porto (ICBAS-UP), Porto, Portugal. [11]Present Address: Division of Oncogenomics, Netherlands Cancer Institute, Plesmanlaan 121, 1066 CX Amsterdam, the Netherlands. [12]Present Address: Gene Regulation, Stem Cells and Cancer Programme, Centre for Genomic Regulation (CRG), The Barcelona Institute of Science and Technology, Barcelona, Spain.

References

1. Ramalho-Carvalho J, Fromm B, Henrique R, Jeronimo C. Deciphering the function of non-coding RNAs in prostate cancer. Cancer Metastasis Rev. 2016;35:235–62.
2. Fromm B, Billipp T, Peck LE, Johansen M, Tarver JE, King BL, Newcomb JM, Sempere LF, Flatmark K, Hovig E, Peterson KJ. A uniform system for the annotation of vertebrate microRNA genes and the evolution of the human microRNAome. Annu Rev Genet. 2015;49:213–42.
3. Jonas S, Izaurralde E. Towards a molecular understanding of microRNA-mediated gene silencing. Nat Rev Genet. 2015;16:421–33.
4. Lewis BP, Shih IH, Jones-Rhoades MW, Bartel DP, Burge CB. Prediction of mammalian microRNA targets. Cell. 2003;115:787–98.
5. Vidigal JA, Ventura A. The biological functions of miRNAs: lessons from in vivo studies. Trends Cell Biol. 2015;25:137–47.
6. Ha M, Kim VN. Regulation of microRNA biogenesis. Nat Rev Mol Cell Biol. 2014;15:509–24.
7. Adams BD, Kasinski AL, Slack FJ. Aberrant regulation and function of microRNAs in cancer. Curr Biol. 2014;24:R762–76.
8. Lujambio A, Lowe SW. The microcosmos of cancer. Nature. 2012;482:347–55.
9. Siegel RL, Miller KD, Jemal A. Cancer statistics, 2016. CA Cancer J Clin. 2016; 66:7–30.
10. Cancer Genome Atlas Research N. The molecular taxonomy of primary prostate Cancer. Cell. 2015;163:1011–25.
11. Fabris L, Ceder Y, Chinnaiyan AM, Jenster GW, Sorensen KD, Tomlins S, Visakorpi T, Calin GA. The potential of MicroRNAs as prostate Cancer biomarkers. Eur Urol. 2016;70:312–22.
12. Korkmaz G, Lopes R, Ugalde AP, Nevedomskaya E, Han R, Myacheva K, Zwart W, Elkon R, Agami R. Functional genetic screens for enhancer elements in the human genome using CRISPR-Cas9. Nat Biotechnol. 2016; 34:192–8.
13. Brinkman EK, Chen T, Amendola M, van Steensel B. Easy quantitative assessment of genome editing by sequence trace decomposition. Nucleic Acids Res. 2014;42:e168.
14. Costa-Pinheiro P, Ramalho-Carvalho J, Vieira FQ, Torres-Ferreira J, Oliveira J, Goncalves CS, Costa BM, Henrique R, Jeronimo C. MicroRNA-375 plays a dual role in prostate carcinogenesis. Clin Epigenetics. 2015;7:42.
15. Pires-Luis AS, Vieira-Coimbra M, Ferreira MJ, Ramalho-Carvalho J, Costa-Pinheiro P, Antunes L, Dias PC, Lobo F, Oliveira J, Graca I, et al. Prognostic significance of MST1R dysregulation in renal cell tumors. Am J Cancer Res. 2016;6:1799–811.
16. Aryee MJ, Jaffe AE, Corrada-Bravo H, Ladd-Acosta C, Feinberg AP, Hansen KD, Irizarry RA. Minfi: a flexible and comprehensive Bioconductor package for the analysis of Infinium DNA methylation microarrays. Bioinformatics. 2014;30:1363–9.
17. Schmittgen TD, Livak KJ. Analyzing real-time PCR data by the comparative C(T) method. Nat Protoc. 2008;3:1101–8.
18. Vieira FQ, Costa-Pinheiro P, Ramalho-Carvalho J, Pereira A, Menezes FD, Antunes L, Carneiro I, Oliveira J, Henrique R, Jeronimo C. Deregulated expression of selected histone methylases and demethylases in prostate carcinoma. Endocr Relat Cancer. 2014;21:51–61.
19. Paulo P, Ribeiro FR, Santos J, Mesquita D, Almeida M, Barros-Silva JD, Itkonen H, Henrique R, Jeronimo C, Sveen A, et al. Molecular subtyping of primary prostate cancer reveals specific and shared target genes of different ETS rearrangements. Neoplasia. 2012;14:600–11.
20. Ramalho-Carvalho J, Martins JB, Cekaite L, Sveen A, Torres-Ferreira J, Graca I, Costa-Pinheiro P, Eilertsen IA, Antunes L, Oliveira J, et al. Epigenetic disruption of miR-130a promotes prostate cancer by targeting SEC23B and DEPDC1. Cancer Lett. 2017;385:150–9.
21. Ramalho-Carvalho J, Graca I, Gomez A, Oliveira J, Henrique R, Esteller M, Jeronimo C. Downregulation of miR-130b~301b cluster is mediated by aberrant promoter methylation and impairs cellular senescence in prostate cancer. J Hematol Oncol. 2017;10:43.
22. Sandoval J, Heyn H, Moran S, Serra-Musach J, Pujana MA, Bibikova M, Esteller M. Validation of a DNA methylation microarray for 450,000 CpG sites in the human genome. Epigenetics. 2011;6:692–702.
23. Genomes Project C, Abecasis GR, Altshuler D, Auton A, Brooks LD, Durbin RM, Gibbs RA, Hurles ME, McVean GA. A map of human genome variation from population-scale sequencing. Nature. 2010;467:1061–73.
24. Torres-Ferreira J, Ramalho-Carvalho J, Gomez A, Menezes FD, Freitas R, Oliveira J, Antunes L, Bento MJ, Esteller M, Henrique R, Jeronimo C. MiR-193b promoter methylation accurately detects prostate cancer in urine sediments and miR-34b/c or miR-129-2 promoter methylation define subsets of clinically aggressive tumors. Mol Cancer. 2017;16:26.
25. Theodore SC, Davis M, Zhao F, Wang H, Chen D, Rhim J, Dean-Colomb W, Turner T, Ji W, Zeng G, et al. MicroRNA profiling of novel African American and

Caucasian prostate Cancer cell lines reveals a reciprocal regulatory relationship of miR-152 and DNA methyltranferase 1. Oncotarget. 2014;5:3512–25.
26. Daniunaite K, Dubikaityte M, Gibas P, Bakavicius A, Rimantas Lazutka J, Ulys A, Jankevicius F, Jarmalaite S. Clinical significance of miRNA host gene promoter methylation in prostate cancer. Hum Mol Genet. 2017;26:2451–61.
27. Popp MW, Maquat LE. Leveraging rules of nonsense-mediated mRNA decay for genome engineering and personalized medicine. Cell. 2016;165:1319–22.
28. Ebert MS, Sharp PA. Roles for microRNAs in conferring robustness to biological processes. Cell. 2012;149:515–24.
29. Bonci D, Coppola V, Musumeci M, Addario A, Giuffrida R, Memeo L, D'Urso L, Pagliuca A, Biffoni M, Labbaye C, et al. The miR-15a-miR-16-1 cluster controls prostate cancer by targeting multiple oncogenic activities. Nat Med. 2008;14:1271–7.
30. Jiang X, Hu C, Arnovitz S, Bugno J, Yu M, Zuo Z, Chen P, Huang H, Ulrich B, Gurbuxani S, et al. miR-22 has a potent anti-tumour role with therapeutic potential in acute myeloid leukaemia. Nat Commun. 2016;7:11452.
31. Kroiss A, Vincent S, Decaussin-Petrucci M, Meugnier E, Viallet J, Ruffion A, Chalmel F, Samarut J, Allioli N. Androgen-regulated microRNA-135a decreases prostate cancer cell migration and invasion through downregulating ROCK1 and ROCK2. Oncogene. 2015;34:2846–55.
32. Goto Y, Kojima S, Nishikawa R, Enokida H, Chiyomaru T, Kinoshita T, Nakagawa M, Naya Y, Ichikawa T, Seki N. The microRNA-23b/27b/24-1 cluster is a disease progression marker and tumor suppressor in prostate cancer. Oncotarget. 2014;5:7748–59.
33. Rice MA, Ishteiwy RA, Magani F, Udayakumar T, Reiner T, Yates TJ, Miller P, Perez-Stable C, Rai P, Verdun R, et al. The microRNA-23b/-27b cluster suppresses prostate cancer metastasis via huntingtin-interacting protein 1-related. Oncogene. 2016;35:4752–61.
34. Majid S, Dar AA, Saini S, Arora S, Shahryari V, Zaman MS, Chang I, Yamamura S, Tanaka Y, Deng G, Dahiya R. miR-23b represses proto-oncogene Src kinase and functions as methylation-silenced tumor suppressor with diagnostic and prognostic significance in prostate cancer. Cancer Res. 2012; 72:6435–46.
35. Heyn H. Quantitative trait loci identify functional noncoding variation in Cancer. PLoS Genet. 2016;12:e1005826.
36. Berezikov E. Evolution of microRNA diversity and regulation in animals. Nat Rev Genet. 2011;12:846–60.
37. Kim YK, Kim VN. Processing of intronic microRNAs. EMBO J. 2007;26:775–83.
38. Isik M, Korswagen HC, Berezikov E. Expression patterns of intronic microRNAs in Caenorhabditis elegans. Silence. 2010;1:5.
39. Martinez NJ, Ow MC, Reece-Hoyes JS, Barrasa MI, Ambros VR, Walhout AJ. Genome-scale spatiotemporal analysis of Caenorhabditis elegans microRNA promoter activity. Genome Res. 2008;18:2005–15.
40. Tsuruta T, Kozaki K, Uesugi A, Furuta M, Hirasawa A, Imoto I, Susumu N, Aoki D, Inazawa J. miR-152 is a tumor suppressor microRNA that is silenced by DNA hypermethylation in endometrial cancer. Cancer Res. 2011;71:6450–62.
41. Stumpel DJ, Schotte D, Lange-Turenhout EA, Schneider P, Seslija L, de Menezes RX, Marquez VE, Pieters R, den Boer ML, Stam RW. Hypermethylation of specific microRNA genes in MLL-rearranged infant acute lymphoblastic leukemia: major matters at a micro scale. Leukemia. 2011;25:429–39.
42. Su Y, Wang Y, Zhou H, Lei L, Xu L. MicroRNA-152 targets ADAM17 to suppress NSCLC progression. FEBS Lett. 2014;588:1983–8.
43. Xiang Y, Ma N, Wang D, Zhang Y, Zhou J, Wu G, Zhao R, Huang H, Wang X, Qiao Y, et al. MiR-152 and miR-185 co-contribute to ovarian cancer cells cisplatin sensitivity by targeting DNMT1 directly: a novel epigenetic therapy independent of decitabine. Oncogene. 2014;33:378–86.
44. Lichner Z, Fendler A, Saleh C, Nasser AN, Boles D, Al-Haddad S, Kupchak P, Dharsee M, Nuin PS, Evans KR, et al. MicroRNA signature helps distinguish early from late biochemical failure in prostate cancer. Clin Chem. 2013;59: 1595–603.
45. Chen H, Liu H, Zou H, Chen R, Dou Y, Sheng S, Dai S, Ai J, Melson J, Kittles RA, et al. Evaluation of plasma miR-21 and miR-152 as diagnostic biomarkers for common types of human cancers. J Cancer. 2016;7:490–9.
46. Zhu C, Li J, Ding Q, Cheng G, Zhou H, Tao L, Cai H, Li P, Cao Q, Ju X, et al. miR-152 controls migration and invasive potential by targeting TGFalpha in prostate cancer cell lines. Prostate. 2013;73:1082–9.
47. Qiu G, Sun W, Zou Y, Cai Z, Wang P, Lin X, Huang J, Jiang L, Ding X, Hu G. RNA interference against TMEM97 inhibits cell proliferation, migration, and invasion in glioma cells. Tumour Biol. 2015;36:8231–8.
48. Moparthi SB, Arbman G, Wallin A, Kayed H, Kleeff J, Zentgraf H, Sun XF. Expression of MAC30 protein is related to survival and biological variables in primary and metastatic colorectal cancers. Int J Oncol. 2007;30:91–5.
49. Yang S, Li H, Liu Y, Ning X, Meng F, Xiao M, Wang D, Lou G, Zhang Y. Elevated expression of MAC30 predicts lymph node metastasis and unfavorable prognosis in patients with epithelial ovarian cancer. Med Oncol. 2013;30:324.
50. Han KY, Gu X, Wang HR, Liu D, Lv FZ, Li JN. Overexpression of MAC30 is associated with poor clinical outcome in human non-small-cell lung cancer. Tumour Biol. 2013;34:821 5.
51. Svetlova MP, Solovjeva LV, Nikiforov AA, Chagin VA, Lehmann AR, Tomilin NV. Staurosporine-sensitive protein phosphorylation is required for postreplication DNA repair in human cells. FEBS Lett. 1998;428:23–6.
52. Grinchuk OV, Motakis E, Kuznetsov VA. Complex sense-antisense architecture of TNFAIP1/POLDIP2 on 17q11.2 represents a novel transcriptional structural-functional gene module involved in breast cancer progression. BMC Genomics. 2010;11 Suppl 1:S9.
53. Xu Q, Jiang Y, Yin Y, Li Q, He J, Jing Y, Qi YT, Xu Q, Li W, Lu B, et al. A regulatory circuit of miR-148a/152 and DNMT1 in modulating cell transformation and tumor angiogenesis through IGF-IR and IRS1. J Mol Cell Biol. 2013;5:3–13.

8

Integrated analyses of multi-omics reveal global patterns of methylation and hydroxymethylation and screen the tumor suppressive roles of HADHB in colorectal cancer

Yimin Zhu[1†], Hanlin Lu[2,3†], Dandan Zhang[4], Meiyan Li[2], Xiaohui Sun[1], Ledong Wan[4], Dan Yu[4], Yiping Tian[4], Hongchuan Jin[5], Aifen Lin[6], Fei Gao[2,3*] and Maode Lai[4,7*]

Abstract

Background: DNA methylation is an important epigenetic modification, associated with gene expression. 5-Methylcytosine and 5-hydroxymethylcytosine are two epigenetic hallmarks that maintain the equilibrium of epigenetic reprogramming. Disequilibrium in genomic methylation leads to carcinogenesis. The purpose of this study was to elucidate the epigenetic mechanisms of DNA methylation and hydroxymethylation in the carcinogenesis of colorectal cancer.

Methods: Genome-wide patterns of DNA methylation and hydroxymethylation in six paired colorectal tumor tissues and corresponding normal tissues were determined using immunoprecipitation and sequencing. Transcriptional expression was determined by RNA sequencing (RNA-Seq). Groupwise differential methylation regions (DMR), differential hydroxymethylation regions (DhMR), and differentially expressed gene (DEG) regions were identified. Epigenetic biomarkers were screened by integrating DMR, DhMR, and DEGs and confirmed using functional analysis.

Results: We identified a genome-wide distinct hydroxymethylation pattern that could be used as an epigenetic biomarker for clearly differentiating colorectal tumor tissues from normal tissues. We identified 59,249 DMRs, 187,172 DhMRs, and 948 DEGs by comparing between tumors and normal tissues. After cross-matching genes containing DMRs or DhMRs with DEGs, we screened seven genes that were aberrantly regulated by DNA methylation in tumors. Furthermore, hypermethylation of the HADHB gene was persistently found to be correlated with downregulation of its transcription in colorectal cancer (CRC). These findings were confirmed in other patients of colorectal cancer. Tumor functional analysis indicated that HADHB reduced cancer cell migration and invasiveness. These findings suggested its possible role as a tumor suppressor gene (TSG).

Conclusion: This study reveals the global patterns of methylation and hydroxymethylation in CRC. Several CRC-associated genes were screened with multi-omic analysis. Aberrant methylation and hydroxymethylation were found to be in the carcinogenesis of CRC.

Keywords: DNA methylation, DNA hydroxymethylation, Sequencing, Colorectal cancer, Epigenetic

* Correspondence: flys828@gmail.com; lmp@zju.edu.cn
†Equal contributors
[2]BGI-Shenzhen, Shenzhen 518083, China
[4]Key Laboratory of Disease Proteomics of Zhejiang Province and Department of Pathology, School of Medicine, Zhejiang University, Hangzhou 310058, China
Full list of author information is available at the end of the article

Background

Cancer is a disease driven by the accumulation of genetic mutations [1] and the disruption of epigenetic regulation [2]. Epigenetic modifications are associated with gene expression [3, 4]. DNA methylation, such as methylation of cytosine to 5-methylcytosine (5-mC), is catalyzed de novo and maintained by DNA methyltransferases (DNMTs) [5, 6], and this methylation is preserved through cell division [7, 8]. The aberrant regulation of DNA methylation, such as global hypomethylation or regional hypermethylation, has consistently reported as an important epigenetic hallmark of cancers, including colorectal cancer [8, 9]. For example, hypermethylation of CpG islands in the promoter regions and in exon 1 represses or even silences the transcriptional expression of tumor suppressor genes (TSG) and promotes carcinogenesis.

In addition to DNA methylation, DNA hydroxymethylation (5-hmC) is another important epigenetic hallmark for cancers. 5-hmC is synthesized from 5-mC by ten-eleven translocation (TET) proteins [10, 11]. TET proteins further oxidize 5-hmC into 5-formylcytosine and 5-carboxylcytosine. An unmethylated cytosine is restored by the removal of the carboxyl group from 5-carboxylcytosine by the enzyme thymine-DNA glycosylase (TDG). Therefore, 5-hmC is regarded as an intermediate during active demethylation and is believed to help maintain the equilibrium of epigenetic reprogramming [12–16]. Despite this, 5-hmC has been observed as a stable epigenetic modification, especially in the cancer genome, where reduced levels have been previously reported [17, 18].

Although there is a significant amount of data regarding the global distribution of 5-mC in colorectal cancer, there is a great need for examining both 5-mC and 5-hmC simultaneously. Because of their resistance to bisulfite conversion, 5mC and 5hmC cannot be distinguished from each other using only bisulfite sequencing data [19]. In order to understand the role of DNA demethylation, a series of techniques have been developed to accurately differentiate cytosine methylation states, including hMeDIP-seq, oxBS-seq, and TAB-seq [14, 20, 21]. Compared to enrichment steps, methods like oxBS-seq and TAB-seq require an immense amount of sequencing and are very costly. In the present study, we collected tumors and the corresponding adjacent normal tissues from six colorectal cancer patients, then determined the levels of genome-wide DNA methylation by methylated DNA immune-precipitation sequencing (MeDIP-seq) and hydroxymethylation by hydroxymethylated DNA immunoprecipitation sequencing (hMeDIP-seq). Their transcriptional expression was determined using RNA-seq. We found a distinct genome-wide hydroxymethylation pattern that could be used as an epigenetic biomarker for differentiating colorectal tumor tissues from normal tissues. Furthermore, hypermethylation of the hydroxyacyl-CoA dehydrogenase trifunctional multi-enzyme complex subunit beta gene (HADHB) was persistently found to be correlated with its transcriptional downregulation in colorectal cancer (CRC). The differences in methylation, hydroxymethylation, and transcriptional expression of HADHB between cancerous and normal tissues were confirmed in additional colorectal cancer patients. To further validate these findings, we performed functional analyses and found that the overexpression of HADHB clearly reduced cancer cell migration and invasiveness. These results suggest that HADHB could play the role of a TSG. In brief, this study provided valuable data for the screening of epigenetic biomarkers and for elucidating the epigenetic mechanisms of carcinogenesis in colorectal cancer.

Methods

Tissue collection and preparation

Colorectal tumor samples, as well as the corresponding adjacent normal tissues (5 cm away from the edge of the tumor), were surgically collected and then preserved in liquid nitrogen. The genomic DNA and RNA of each sample were extracted using Qiagen's DNA and RNA extraction kits, respectively. The study protocols were approved by the research ethics committees of Zhejiang University School of Medicine (2012-1-012) and BGI-Shenzhen (NO. BGI-IRB 15060). All participants signed the written informed consent form.

Library construction and data analysis of RNA-seq

The total RNA samples were first treated with DNase I to degrade any possible DNA contamination. The mRNA was then enriched using oligo (dT) magnetic beads and mixed with a fragmentation buffer to be fragmented into approximately 200-bp fragments. First-strand cDNA synthesis was performed using random hexamers. Buffer, dNTPs, RNase H, and DNA polymerase I were added to synthesize the second strand. The double-stranded cDNA was purified with magnetic beads. End preparation and 3′-end addition of the nucleotide adenine (A) were performed. Finally, sequencing adaptors were ligated to the fragments. The fragments were enriched by PCR amplification. During the QC step, the Agilent 2100 Bioanalyzer and ABI StepOnePlus Real-Time PCR System were used to qualify and quantify the DNA library. The library products were then sequenced with the Illumina HiSeq 2000.

The levels of gene expression level and the differentially expressed genes were analyzed using the method described by Audic and Claverie [22]. Levels of gene expression were calculated using the reads per kilobase million (RPKM) method. In cases where more than one transcript was found for a gene, the longest read was used to calculate its expression level and coverage. The RPKM values were then used directly to compare gene expression differences between the tumor and the normal samples. The significantly differentially expressed genes (DEG) were determined at a threshold false discovery rate (FDR) ≤ 0.05 and the absolute value of log2-ratio ≥ 0.585.

Library construction and data analysis of MeDIP-seq and hMeDIP-seq

Prior to immunoprecipitation, 5 µg of genomic DNA was sonicated to a mean fragment size of 200 bp, followed by end repair with the addition of deoxyadenosine (dA) and adaptor ligation, according to the Illumina Paired-End protocol. MeDIP-Seq and hMeDIP-Seq libraries were constructed, as described in a previous study [23]. The libraries were sequenced using the Illumina HiSeq analyzer, according to the manufacturer's instructions. After base calling, low-quality reads were omitted, and the clean reads were aligned to the UCSC human reference genome hg19 using SOAP2 (Version 2.21). Mismatches of no more than two bases were allowed in the alignment.

Identification of DMR and DhMR between tumors and corresponding normal tissues

Identification of groupwise differential methylation regions (DMR) and differential hydroxyl-methylation regions (DhMR) was performed using a sliding windows strategy along the entire genome, as described in our previous study [24]. This strategy identified DMR and DhMR between tumors and the corresponding normal tissues, based on a threshold of $P < 0.05$ and at least five CG sites.

Functional enrichment analysis for DMRs and DhMR in promoters

Functional enrichment analysis was performed by Gene Ontology (GO) and pathway analysis using the DAVID (Database for Annotation, Visualization, and Integrated Discovery) web server (http://david.abcc.ncifcrf.gov). Genes with DMRs, DhMR in promoters, and DEG were mapped to their respective human orthologs, and the lists were submitted to DAVID for enrichment analysis to determine any significant overrepresentation of GO biological processes (GO-BP), molecular functions (GO-MF), and KEGG-pathway categories. For all analyses, the known, full-length genes were set as the background, and the *P* values (EASE score), indicating the significance of the overlap between various gene sets, were calculated using Benjamini-corrected modified Fisher's exact test. Only GO-BP, GO-MF, or KEGG-pathway terms with *P* values less than 0.05 were considered significant and listed as differentially expressed.

Quantitative PCR of HADHB expression

Total RNA was isolated from cells using TRIzol (Invitrogen, USA). The concentration of RNAs was measured and normalized using a spectrophotometer (Eppendorf, Hamburg, Germany). Reverse transcription was performed using a PrimeScript RT reagent kit (Perfect Real Time) and real-time PCR was performed using the SYBR Premix Ex Taq (Tli RNaseH Plus), both from TaKaRa Biotechnology Co., Ltd. (Dalian, China). The following PCR primers were used to amplify HADHB: 5′-ACACTGTCACCATGGCTTGT -3′ (forward) and 5′-CTGGCCAGAAGCAATCAAG -3′ (reverse). For GAPDH, the following primers were used: 5′-ACCACAGTCCATGC-CATCAC-3′ (forward) and 5′-TCCACCACCCTGTTGCTG TA-3′ (reverse). GAPDH was used as the reference gene. The Ct values of the samples were calculated, and the relative levels of HADHB mRNA were analyzed by the $2^{-\Delta\Delta Ct}$ method.

Cell culture and plasmid construction

Human colorectal carcinoma cell lines, HT29 and HCT8, were obtained from the American Type Culture Collection (ATCC). HT29 and HCT8 were maintained in liquid nitrogen and incubated in 5% CO_2 at 37 °C in a PRMI1640 medium with 10% fetal bovine serum (FBS).

The pcDNA3.1 (+) vector was sliced using restriction enzymes Xhol1 and Bamh1. First-strand cDNA was synthesized using the HiScript® 1st Strand cDNA Synthesis Kit (Vazyme biotech co., Ltd., Suzhou, China). The complete coding sequence of HADHB was PCR-amplified with the following primers: 5″–CTTGGTACCGAGCTCGGATC CATGAC TATCTTGACTTACCCCTTTAAAA–3′ (forward) and 5′–CCCTCTAGATGCATGCTCG A GTTATT TTGGATAAGCTTCCACTATCAT–3″ (reverse). The PCR product was then inserted into the linearized pcDNA3.1 to perform recombination cloning using the ClonExpress II one-step cloning kit (Vazyme Biotech Co., Ltd.). The recombined products were verified by DNA sequencing and transfected using Lipfectamine™2000, according to the manufacturer's instructions. The efficiency of overexpression was validated using qRT-PCR and western blot analyses.

RNA interference analysis

Small interfering RNA (siRNA) against HADHB and a negative control siRNA were purchased from Shanghai Genepharma Co. Ltd. (Shanghai, China). The anti-HADHB siRNA sequence was 5`-GCACAGUGACAG-CUGCAAATT-3`, which was not homologous to any other human DNA sequence. HT29 and HCT8 cells were cultured in six-well plates in antibiotic-free DMEM for 48 h and transfected using the PowerFect™ siRNA Transfection Reagent (SigmaGen) according to the manufacturer's instructions. The efficiency of knockdown was determined by qRT-PCR and western blot analyses.

Western blot analysis

Cells were extracted using a RIPA lysis buffer and prepared according to the standard procedure. Proteins were extracted using 12% SDS-PAGE and transferred onto nitrocellulose membranes. The membranes were blocked with 5% skimmed milk in TBS-Tween 20 for 2 h before being incubated overnight with primary antibodies at 4 °C. They were then incubated with secondary antibodies at 20 °C for nearly 1 h. After extensive washing in TBST, the protein level was measured using the Odyssey system (Li-COR, Lincoln, NE, USA). The loading was monitored by GAPDH. Primary antibodies were directed against HADHB (Abcam, 1:1000) and GAPDH (Santa Cruz, CA, USA, 1:5000).

Cell counting kit-8 (CCK-8) assay

Cells were plated in 96-well plates (1×10^3 cells/well) with 100 μl of the medium. The absorbance at 450 nm was measured to estimate the relative number of viable cells after culturing with 10 μl of CCK-8 reagent, which was purchased from Boster Biological Technology Co., Ltd. (Wuhan, China). The analysis was performed in three replicate wells for each sample and repeated for three times.

Cell migration and invasion assays

Transwell 24-well Boyden chambers (8-μm pores; Costar, Corning, NK, USA) were used to measure cell migration and invasion according to the manufacturer's protocol. For studying migration, cells (1×10^5) in 200 μl of a serum-free medium were seeded on the upper chamber, and 600 μl of a complete medium containing 10% FBS was added to the lower chamber as a chemoattractant. After incubation at 37 °C for 20 h (HCT8 cells) and 96 h (HT29 cells), the non-migratory cells were removed with cotton swabs. Cells on the lower surface of the membrane were fixed in 4% paraformaldehyde and stained with crystal violet solution. The number of invading cells was counted in five randomly selected fields using an inverted microscope equipped with a digital camera at × 40 magnification.

For the cell invasion assay, 2×10^5 cells were seeded in the upper chamber, which had been coated with 50 μL Matrigel basement membrane matrix (BD Biosciences, USA), followed by incubation for 16 h (HCT8 cells) and 96 h (HT29 cells).

Results

Generation and characterization of CRC methylome and hydroxymethylome

Six patients with colorectal cancer, three with rectal cancer, and three with colon cancer were recruited for this study. The characteristics of these patients are summarized in Additional file 1: Table S1, including gender, age, and pathological types. Primary tumor tissue samples and their adjacent normal tissues were collected after surgery. We applied MeDIP-seq and hMeDIP-seq technologies to examine whole-genome DNA methylation and hydroxymethylation patterns, respectively, for all 12 DNA samples. MeDIP-seq and hMeDIP-seq technologies allow for the highly efficient enrichment of methylated and hydroxymethylated DNA fragments [25] using antibodies against methylated and hydroxymethylated cytosines, respectively. On average, 120.1 and 117.9 million paired-end reads, 50 bp in length, were generated from MeDIP-seq and hMeDIP-seq, respectively. Of these reads, 116.0 (96.63%) and 114.2 (96.88%) million clean reads were aligned to the human reference genome hg19. After removing the ambiguously mapped reads, we acquired 99.7 (83.03%) million and 104.7 (87.32%) million uniquely aligned reads, reaching an average depth coverage of 3.49 and 3.71 for DNA methylation and hydroxymethylation, respectively (Additional file 1: Table S2 and Additional file 2: Figure S1). To enable pair-wise comparisons across different samples, we used reads per million (RPM) as a measure of the methylation and hydroxymethylation levels in a genomic region in order to normalize the data.

We first characterized the global patterns of methylome and hydroxymethylome by correlating their read depths with the number of different genomic elements. In general, both DNA methylation and hydroxymethylation were positively correlated with the number of repeat sequences, gene number, SNP number, and GC content, both in the tumors and adjacent normal tissues (Fig. 1). No significant correlation was found between chromosome length and ratio of observed and expected number of CpGs (CpG O/E), although similar patterns of methylation and hydroxymethylation were observed in relation to GC content. High levels of hydroxymethylation and methylation were found in the regions of high GC content of approximately 50 to 60% (Additional file 3: Figure S2). Furthermore, uneven distribution of methylation and hydroxymethylation was found in the features of chromosomes in tumors and normal tissues, especially at transcriptional start sites (TSS) and CpG islands (CGIs), where there were lower levels. In contrast, CGI shores (regions that flank CGIs with less CG density) showed higher levels of methylation and hydroxymethylation than other genomic elements. The highest level of methylation, but not hydroxymethylation, was observed in short interspersed elements (SINEs), which are highly repetitive sequences (Additional file 4: Figure S3). These findings indicated that the distribution of both 5-mC and 5-hmC was closely dependent on the characteristics of the genomic sequences (Fig. 1, Additional file 1: Table S3), which were consistent with previous studies [23, 25].

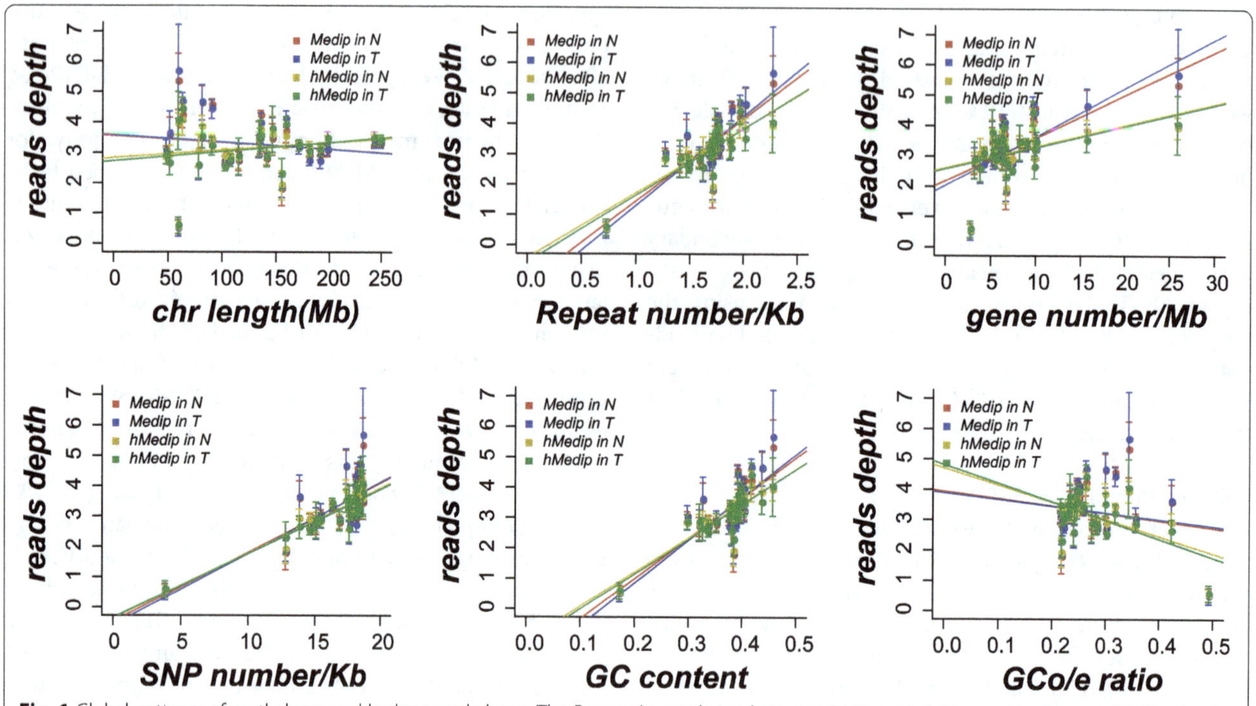

Fig. 1 Global patterns of methylome and hydroxymethylome. The Pearson's correlation between DNA methylation and hydroxymethlation levels and features of autosomes (chromosomes 1–12) and sex chromosomes X and Y. The read depth was plotted against the length, repeat density, gene density, SNP density, GC content, and CpGo/e ratio of the individual chromosome. The line represents linear regression. Different colors represent the different modifications in tumor and normal tissues (red is Medip in normal tissue, blue is Medip in tumor tissue, gold is hMedip in normal tissue, and green is hMedip in tumor tissue)

Positive correlation between global methylation and hydroxymethylation levels

The whole genome was divided into 0.5-kb windows, and the levels of 5-mC and 5-hmC were classified into different groups, according to the RPMs of MeDIP and hMeDIP, respectively. The correlations between methylation and hydroxymethylation are shown in Additional file 5: Figure S4. The levels of methylation were positively correlated with those of hydroxymethylation in tumors (Pearson's correlation coefficient $r = 0.9630$, $P = 2.843e{-}12$) and normal tissues (Pearson's correlation coefficient $r = 0.9686$, $P = 6.115e{-}13$). These results were consistent with previous results from mouse hippocampus [26], human brain [27], and pancreatic cancer [28]. As 5-hmC is believed to be an intermediate compound in the oxidation reaction of 5-mC, this finding suggests that methylated regions may be constantly undergoing reprogramming, depending on the cell type. For different cell populations, the hotspot of epigenomic reprogramming may vary. For instance, in neurons and stem cells, 5-mC usually co-localizes with heterochromatin, whereas 5-hmC co-localizes with euchromatin [29–31]. In the current CRC study, we found that, when comparing tumors with normal tissues (slope of fitted line = 0.234), the gradient response of hydroxymethylation against methylation was lower in tumor tissues (0.178) (Additional file 5: Figure S4). This result suggested that tumor tissues in CRC display a global reduction in 5-hmC compared to normal tissues like the majority of cancers [32–35].

Distinct global pattern of hydroxymethylome, but not methylome, in CRC

In addition to the correlation coefficient difference between 5-mC and 5-hmC, we also observed variations in the average levels of the two types of DNA modifications, when comparing tumors and normal tissues. For instance, compared to normal tissues, tumor tissues showed higher than average levels of DNA methylation in TSSs, promoters, exons, transcriptional end sites (TES), CpG islands, CGI shores, and SINEs, but lower than average hydroxymethylation levels in exons, introns, gene bodies, SINEs, TESs, enhancers, and CGI shores (Additional file 4: Figure S3). Additionally, higher inter-individual variations in tumors were suggested for methylation and hydroxymethylation levels in nearby TSSs and TES [28], as indicated by the comparisons of standard deviations (SD) between tumors and normal tissues ($P < 0.001$, paired t test) (Additional file 6: Figure S5). These results suggested that the potential dysregulation of epigenetic modifications could lead to large-scale latent instability, which might cause carcinogenesis.

Based on these observations, we used principal component analysis to infer the inter-group global patterns of methylome and hydroxymethylome, using the RPM of 0.5-kb windows across the whole genome. The global methylation pattern of tumor tissues and normal tissues could not be clearly differentiated (Fig. 2a). In contrast, a clear separation between the tumors and normal tissues was observed in the principal component analysis (PCA) of hydroxymethylation, indicating distinct patterns of the hydroxymethylome in tumors, compared to normal tissues (Fig. 2b). Therefore, a global change in the hydroxymethylome can be considered as a key characteristic of CRC. Gilat et al. also found that global levels of 5-hmC could distinguish between colon tumors and normal colon tissue adjacent to the tumor based on the levels [36]. Bhattacharyya et al. [28] reported a similar discovery in pancreatic cancer, in which they found that the distribution pattern of 5-hmC samples were strikingly different from those of normal cells.

Pair-wise comparison revealing extensive DhMRs and DMRs in CRC

Next, we applied a sliding-window strategy to identify differentially methylated regions (DMRs) and differentially hydroxymethylated regions (DhMRs) in tumors and normal corresponding normal tissues, in order to reveal key genomic regions with significant DNA methylation and hydroxymethylation changes during carcinogenesis. Based on the threshold of $P < 0.05$ and at least five CG sites, we obtained 59,249 DMRs and 187,172 DhMRs (Fig. 2c). The representative differential regions of DMR (Fig. 2d, right) and DhMRs (Fig. 2d, left) were presented. Most DMRs and DhMRs were more frequently distributed (observed/expected ratio > 1) in promoter regions, exons, enhancers, and repeat sequences, such as LTRs, LINEs, and SINEs. Unlike DMRs, DhMRs were also frequently distributed in TES regions (Additional file 7: Figure S6). Aberrant methylations or hydroxymethylations in promoter regions were less frequent than those in other regions, consistent with previous observations in cancer

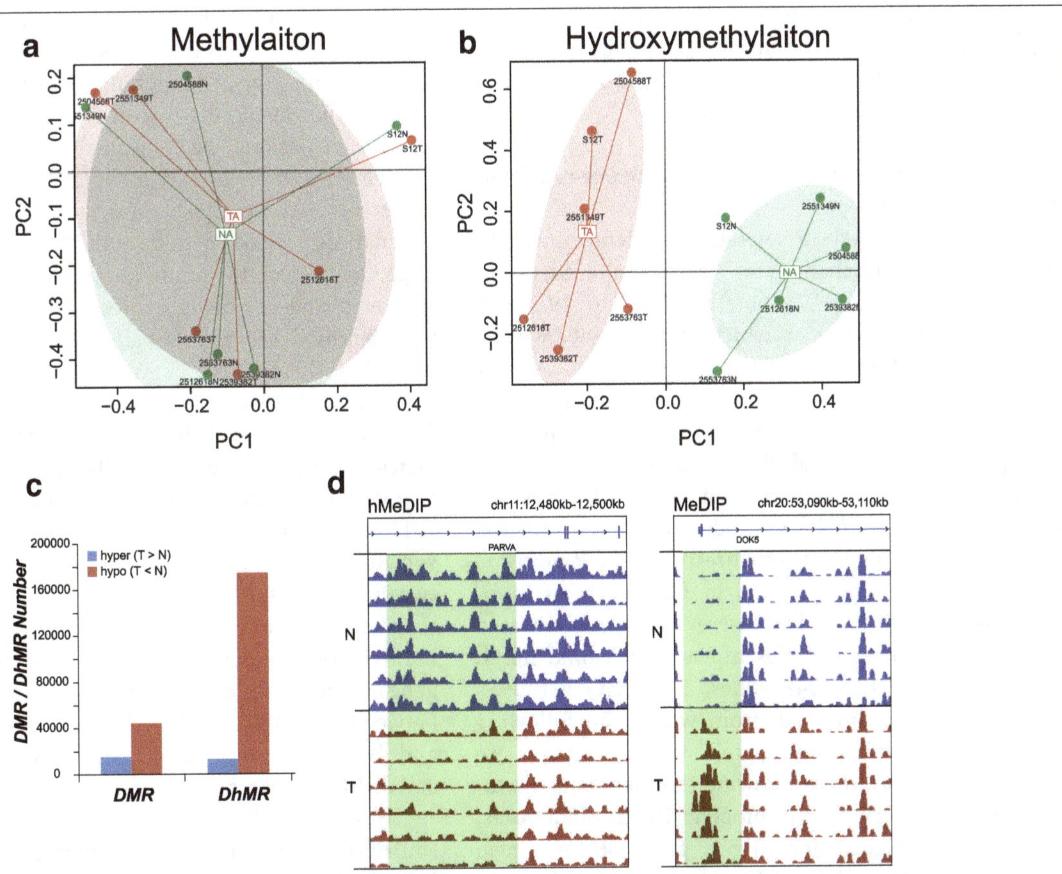

Fig. 2 Different distributions of methylation and hydroxymethylation. **a**, **b** Principal component (PC) analysis based on methylation and hydroxymethylation levels for 0.5-kb tiles across 6 normal and tumor tissue samples. Coloring indicates classification of samples into subgroups. The red area denotes tumor tissues and the green area means normal tissue. **c** A large number of regions of differential hydroxymethylation (DhMRs) and methylation (DMRs) occur in colorectal cancer. Regions that gain a mark ("hyper-") are represented by blue bars, whereas losses ("hypo-") are red. **d** Visualization of DMRs (left) and DhMRs (right) patterns across all normal and tumor tissues (blue and red bars in the box). Boxed regions with green are candidate DMRs or DhMRs

[25]. Despite this, aberrant DNA modifications within promoters were most likely correlated with altered gene expressions [37, 38]. Therefore, we provided further annotation to the genes with DMRs or DhMRs. Because the gene promoter is the most important regulatory element in the genome and the aberration of methylation and hydroxymethylation in this region may be associated with carcinogenesis, we focused on the genes with DMRs and/or DhMRs in the promoter. We obtained 1699 and 7864 genes containing DMRs and DhMRs in the promoter, respectively. The lists of these genes are presented in Additional file 1: Table S4 and Table S5, respectively. KEGG analysis was performed with the WebGestalt tool (http://www.webgestalt.org). We found 49 significant pathways enriched in genes containing DMRs and 170 containing DhMRs, respectively. The top five methylation-enriched functional pathways were neuroactive ligand-receptor interactions, tight junctions, pathways in cancer, long-term depression, and Chagas disease. Pathways with enriched DhMRs included glycosylphosphatidylinositol (GPI)-anchor biosynthesis, African trypanosomiasis (sleeping sickness), tyrosine metabolism, tryptophan metabolism, and shigellosis (Additional file 1: Table S6).

CRC transcriptome profiling reveals epigenetics-regulated gene expression changes

We also performed RNA-seq to determine the transcriptome-wide changes in CRC, compared to adjacent normal tissues. We obtained 14.0 to 19.2 million reads per sample, of which 96.5 to 99.2% were clean data. Most of these clean reads (91.4% - 94.1%) could be uniquely aligned to the human reference genome hg19, and 45.0–61.2% were mapped to RefSeq genes (Additional file 1: Table S7). The expression levels were measured in terms of reads per kilobase per million (RPKM) and were used to further analysis. Based on a strict threshold (FDR-adjusted $P < 0.05$ and fold change > 1.5 in four or more samples), 948 significant DEGs were identified between the cancer and the normal samples (Additional file 1: Table S8). From these 948 genes, 12 KEGG pathways were found to be enriched, from which the following top five categories were found to be relevant to tumorigenesis: cell cycle, purine metabolism, metabolic pathways, ribosome biogenesis in eukaryotes, and ribosomes (Additional file 1: Table S6). We also cross-matched these DEG KEGG pathways with those previously identified to be enriched in DMR- and DhMR-containing genes; we found that metabolic pathways, purine metabolism, and axon guidance were shared features in these groups (Additional file 8: Figure S7).

We then correlated the expression levels of all genes with levels of methylation or hydroxymethlation in their promoter regions (TSS ± 500 bp) and gene bodies (Fig. 3a, b). Gene expression levels in tumors and normal tissues were negatively correlated with promoter methylation, but positively correlated with gene body methylation, which has been reported in previous genome-wide analyses [28, 39]. A similar positive correlation was observed for hydroxymethylation in the gene body, although no clear correlation was observed in promoter regions. When we classified the associated genes into genes with high and low expression levels, the highly expressed genes displayed significantly lower levels of promoter methylation, but significantly higher levels of hydroxymethylation in the gene body (Fig. 3c, d). These results suggest that many DEGs could be potentially regulated by promoter methylation or gene body hydroxymethylation.

Integrated analyses identifying DEGs aberrantly regulated by DNA methylation in tumors

In order to identify the DEGs that were aberrantly regulated by DNA modifications in tumors, we cross-matched the genes containing DMRs or DhMRs with DEGs. Considering the role of 5-hmC as an intermediate of demethylation, we reasoned that the genes with hypermethylation and hypohydroxymethylation in promoters would be most stably repressed within a cell population, while genes with hypomethylation and hyper-hydroxymethylation in promoters would have a greater chance of being expressed. With this reasoning, we identified seven genes that contained both DMRs and DhMRs. These seven genes were HIGD1A, AHCYL2, IL11RA, CHL1, SEMA6D, BIRC3, and HADHB (Additional file 1: Table S9). Among these genes, the methylation of HIGD1A and CHL1 has been reported in common tumors. Expressions of SEMA6D, IL11RA, and BIRC3 genes have been reported to be associated with tumors; however, no association between colorectal cancer and methylation has been reported. There have been no reports on tumors or methylation associated with HADHB or AHCYL2 genes. Thus, we are the first to report associations between HADHB and AHCYL2 genes and tumors and between the methylation of SEMA6D, IL11RA, and BIRC3 genes and tumors.

HADHB as a potential tumor suppressor gene aberrantly repressed by promoter hypermethylation in CRC

Importantly, we identified one DEG, HADHB, which showed hypermethylation and hypohydroxymethylation with significantly downregulated expression in CRC (Additional file 9: Figure S8). To confirm that the expression level of the HADHB gene was associated with

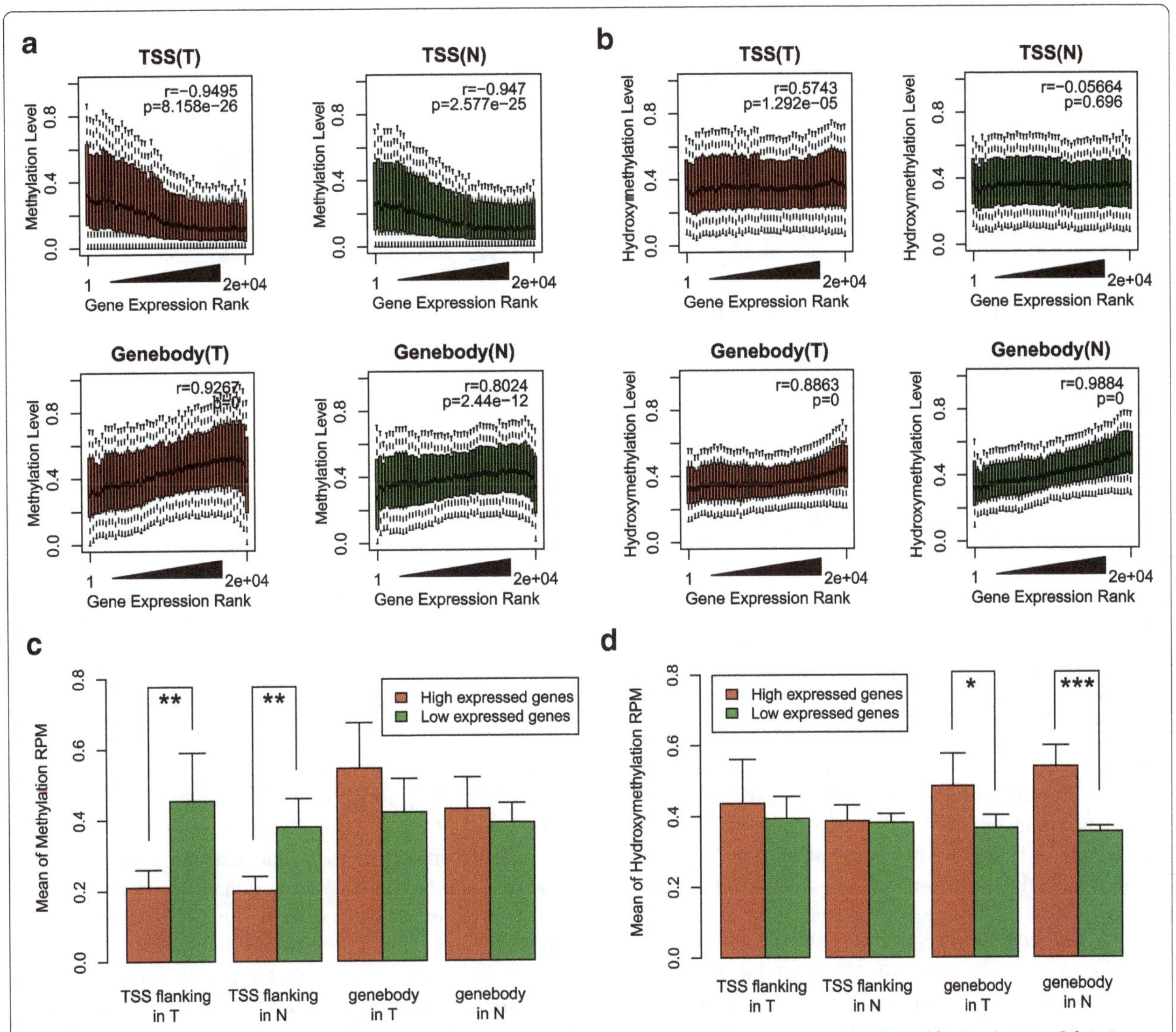

Fig. 3 Association between epigenomic modification and gene expression. **a**, **b** Correlations between epigenomic modification (**a** is 5-mC, **b** is 5-hmC) and gene expression in TSS (defined as − 500 bp to + 500 bp across TSS) and genebody respectively. For Medip, there is a clear anti-correlation of gene expression in TSS and a positive correlation in the genebody. For hMedip, only positive correlations in the genebody can be observed. **c** 5-mC is enriched in the TSS flanking region (defined as − 500 bp to + 500 bp across TSS) of lowly expressed genes in both despite normal and tumor tissues. **d** 5-hmC is enriched in the genebody region of highly expressed genes in both normal and tumor tissues

its methylation and hydroxymethylation levels in a larger population, we collected 15 additional pairs of samples from colorectal tumors and their adjacent normal tissues. The methylation and hydroxymethylation levels were determined with MeDIP and hMeDIP, respectively, followed by real-time PCR to determine the expression level of HADHB (Additional file 6). We also collected the expression data for HADHB from The Cancer Genome Atlas (TCGA) (http://cancergenome.nih.gov/) and the Gene Expression Omnibus (GEO) (http://www.ncbi.nlm.nih.gov/geo/) databases. We found the expression levels of HADHB in tumor tissues (0.18 ± 0.15) were significantly lower than those in normal tissues (0.32 ± 0.24) ($P = 0.025$) (Fig. 4a). This result was consistent with the findings from data of GEO (Fig. 4b), TCGA sequencing (Fig. 4c), and TCGA array (Fig. 4d). Compared to normal tissues, tumor tissues had higher levels of methylation (0.74 ± 0.19 vs 0.17 ± 0.068) (Fig. 4e) and lower levels of hydroxymethylation (2.58 ± 1.97 vs 3.48 ± 1.52) (Fig. 4f). These results indicate that lower levels of HADHB expression in tumor tissues are associated with higher levels of methylation and lower levels of hydroxymethylation. This is consistent with the results of genome-wide sequencing analyses of methylation and hydroxymethylation. The HADHB gene may be a potential tumor suppressor gene, whose expression is modified by methylation and reduced by hydroxymethylation.

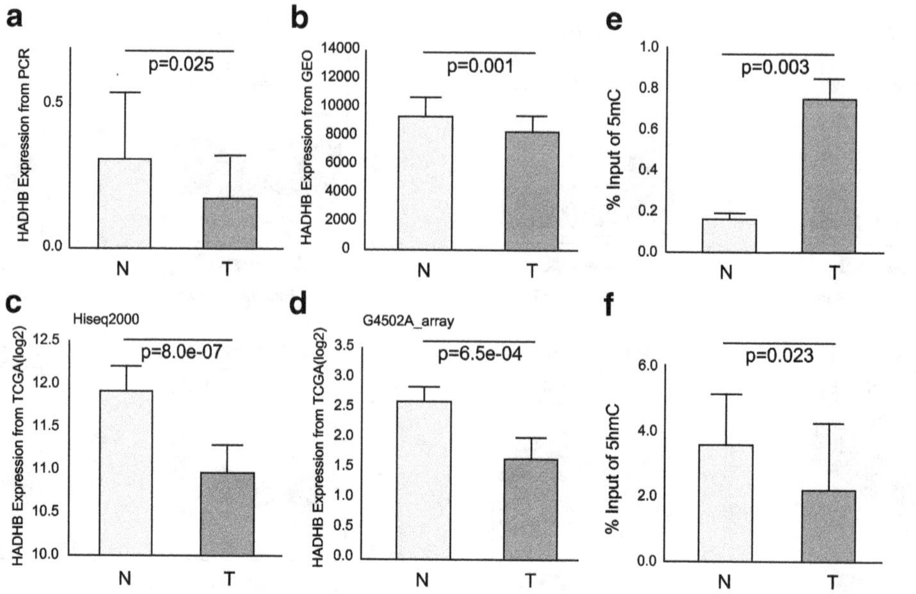

Fig. 4 Expression and epigenetic modification validation of HADHB in additional samples and public functional genomics data. **a** Expression level of HADHB determined by real-time PCR in 15 additional pairs of colorectal tumors and their adjacent normal tissues. **b** Expression data of HADHB from the GEO database. **c, d** Expression level of HADHB from the TCGA database. The results derived from different platform (**c** is Hiseq200 and **d** is G450 array) are shown respectively. **e, f**, Methylation and hydroxymethylation levels were determined by real-time PCR in 15 additional pairs of colorectal tumors and their adjacent normal tissues

To evaluate the potential contribution of the HADHB gene to tumorigenesis, we further performed gene knockdown and overexpression experiments in colorectal cancer cell lines. After evaluating the expression levels of HADHB in seven cell lines using reverse transcriptase PCR (RT-PCR) and western blot analyses, we selected the HCT-8 cell line for HADHB overexpression and the HT-29 cell line for HADHB knockdown, in which HADHB expression was the lowest and highest, respectively (Fig. 5a). Our results showed that the expression of HADHB efficiently decreased in the HADHB-knockdown HT-29 cell line and increased in the HADHB-overexpressed HT-8 cell line, compared with that in the normal cell lines (Fig. 5b). In the subsequent characterization of cell capacity, we found that knockdown and overexpression of HADHB had no effect on cell growth (Fig. 5c). Interestingly, the migration and invasion of cells were significantly reduced in cells overexpressing HADHB. In contrast, HADHB knockdown caused enhanced migration and invasion (Fig. 5d).

Taken together, these functional experiments support the hypothesis that HADHB is a potential tumor suppressor gene, which can reduce tumor cell invasiveness and migration, suggesting that silencing HADHB may contribute to colorectal oncogenesis and progression.

Discussion

DNA methylation has become a promising biological marker of cancer risk, diagnosis, and prognosis. DNA methylation in the promoter can repress or silence gene expression. Therefore, 5-mC is usually considered the "fifth base" of DNA. The discovery of hydroxymethylation, often considered to be the sixth base of DNA, has increased the complexity of methylation research. While 5-hmC is mostly believed to be an intermediate of the demethylation process catalyzed by the TET enzyme, many studies have shown that the TET enzyme and 5-hmC act as regulatory factors. Therefore, genome-wide analyses of DNA methylation and hydroxymethylation, which are important epigenetic biomarkers, will help reveal aberrantly regulated tumor suppressor genes that may be involved in carcinogenesis.

Bisulfite treatment-based sequencing technologies cannot distinguish between these two types of epigenetic modifications. Methods like oxBS-seq and TAB-seq require an immense amount of sequencing and are costly. Instead, immunoprecipitation by methylation and hydroxymethylation-specific antibodies, combined with next-generation sequencing, can be used to determine genome-wide methylation and hydroxymethylation. In this study, we applied MeDIP-seq, hMeDIP-seq, and RNA-seq for a thorough screening of the epigenome and transcriptome of colorectal tumors.

Previous studies have revealed that aberrant methylation and hydroxymethylation in cancers occur in either specific or global genomic regions [2, 8, 15]. Therefore, by comparing the distribution of methylation and hydroxymethylation between tumors and normal tissues, this

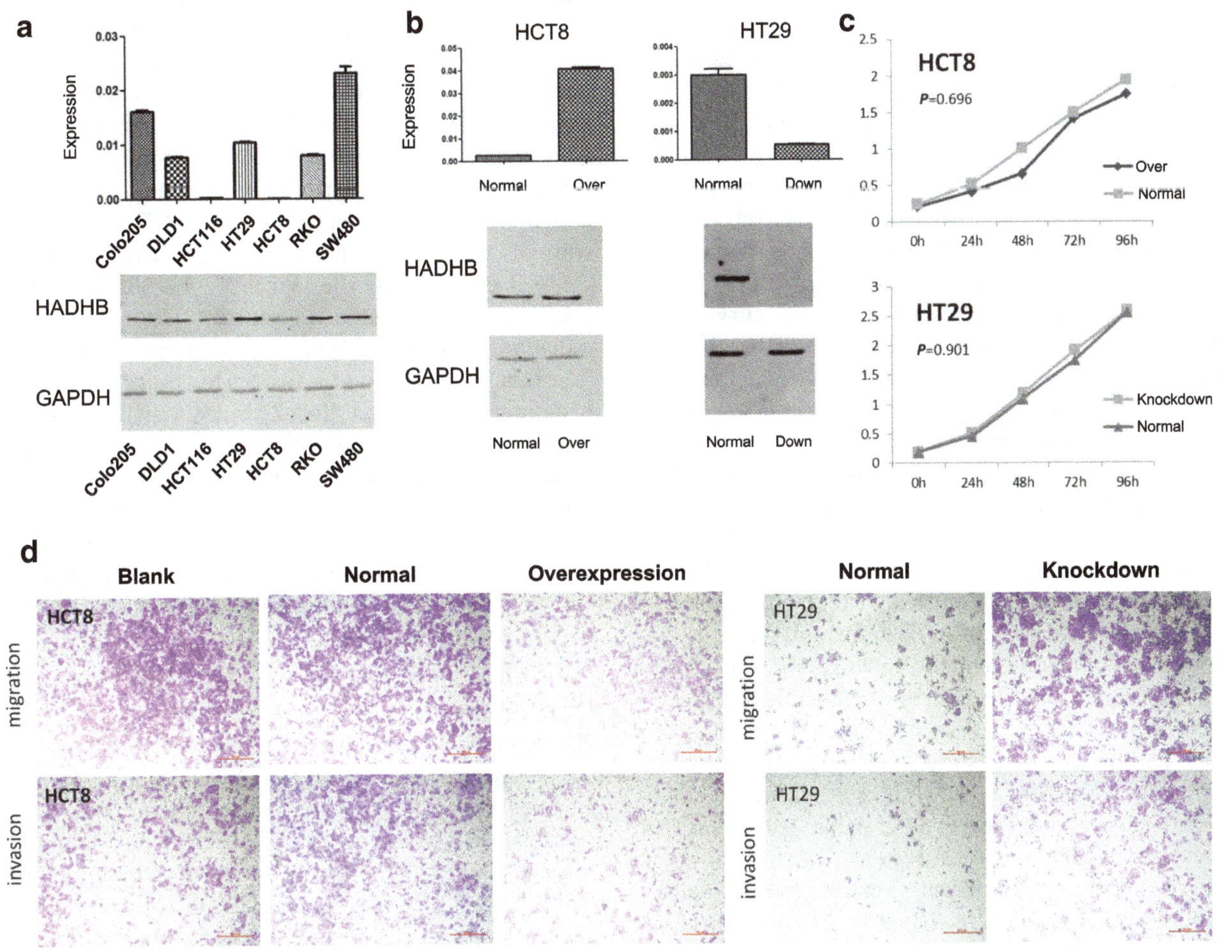

Fig. 5 Functional experiments of HADHB on CRC cell line. **a** Transcriptional and translational levels of HADHB in seven cell lines detected by RT-PCR and western blot. **b** HADHB expression in knockdown and overexpression cell lines of HT29 and HCT8. **c** Cell growth curves in the knockdown and overexpression cell lines of HT29 and HCT8. **d** Cells migration and invasion in the knockdown and overexpression cell lines of HT29 and HCT8

study provides valuable data for screening epigenetic biomarkers. Our results showed distinct hydroxymethylome, but not methylome, global methylation patterns in CRCs and their adjacent normal tissues, using PCA. Specifically, divergent hypohydroxymethylation regions were more often located in gene bodies, TESs, enhancers, LTRs, LINEs, and SINEs. Overall, genomic methylation correlated with hydroxymethylation. However, these two modifications do not usually coexist on the DNA [25, 31]. 5-mC usually co-localizes in the heterochromatin, whereas 5-hmC has been found to co-localize in the euchromatin [29, 30]. It can be inferred that euchromatin-specific conversion of 5-mC to 5-hmC is regulated by a combination of cell cycle-dependent chromatin decompensation events and Tet enzyme instability [29]. Our genome-wide study suggested that 5-hmC is a stable potential predictive biomarker for CRC.

Although we did not observe distinct global methylation patterns, we did observe a higher frequency of divergently methylated regions, when comparing tumors and normal tissues, specifically in CGIs, promoters, exons, enhancers, LTRs, LINEs, and SINEs. Previous studies have confirmed that promoter hypermethylation might cause reduced gene expression and contribute to carcinogenesis, including colorectal cancer [25, 39, 40]. Based on genome-wide, pair-wise comparative analyses of tumors and the corresponding normal tissues, 170 significant pathways were found to be enriched in 7864 genes with DhMRs, 49 pathways in 1699 genes with DMRs, and 12 pathways in 948 DEGs. Among these pathways, metabolic pathways, purine metabolism, and axon guidance were overlapped. This suggests that these pathways may be involved in the carcinogenesis of colorectal cancer.

By linking the divergent regions with gene expression, we identified 26 DEGs with both DMRs and DhMRs. Seven genes in which DEGs contained both DMRs and DhMRs were identified (Additional file 1: Table S9):

HADHB, HIGD1A, AHCYL2, IL11RA, CHL1, SEMA6D, and BIRC3. The methylation of five genes (AHCYL2, IL11RA, SEMA6D, BIRC3, and HADHB) was associated with tumors, and four genes (IL11RA, CHL1, SEMA6D, and BIRC3) were associated with colorectal cancer. HIGD1A, hypoxia-inducible gene domain 1A, is a mitochondrial protein and a positive regulator of cytochrome c oxidase, which is regulated by hypoxia-inducible factor-1α (HIF1α) [41]. During glucose deprivation, HIGD1A regulates oxygen consumption, ROS production, and AMPK activity to modulate cell survival and tumor growth [41]. The promoter of the HIGD1A gene is differentially methylated in human cancers, preventing its hypoxic induction. This protein is also a potential marker of metabolic stress in vivo and is frequently observed in diverse pathological states such as myocardial infarction, hypoxic-ischemic encephalopathy (HIE), and different cancers [42, 43]. AHCYL2 (adenosyl-homocysteinase like 2) is highly homologous to IRBIT, which regulates ion-transporting proteins. It may also be a potential regulator of NBCe1-B in mammalian cells [44]. However, its function remains unclear. CHL1 (cell adhesion molecule), which encodes a member of the L1 family of neural cell adhesion molecules, is essential for brain development and is involved in signal transduction pathways. It has been found to play an important role in carcinogenesis and cancer progression. He et al. had found that CHL1 was downregulated in human breast cancer and was associated with lower-grade tumors [45]. This downregulation is mediated by DNA methylation. Therefore, CHL1 may be a putative tumor suppressor gene in breast cancer and other common cancers [45–47]. Interleukin 11 receptor subunit alpha (IL11RA), a stromal cell-derived cytokine, is overexpressed in patients with human osteosarcoma and advanced breast cancer with bone metastasis. Additionally, amplification was detected at 9p13.3, where the IL11RA gene is located. Some primary gastric adenocarcinoma samples (19.1%) were found to have an increased copy number of IL11RA [48]. Semaphorin 6D (SEMA6D) has been previously implicated in immune responses, heart development, and neurogenesis. SEMA6D has been reported to be highly expressed in vascular epithelial cells in gastric cancer; it was also positively correlated with the expression of vascular endothelial growth factor receptor 2 (VEGFR2). Therefore, SEMA6D may be associated with tumor angiogenesis [49, 50]. The HADHB gene encodes the beta subunit of a mitochondrial trifunctional protein that catalyzes the last three steps of mitochondrial beta-oxidation of long-chain fatty acids. Mutations in the HADHB gene have been associated with mitochondrial trifunctional protein deficiency [51, 52]. HADHB interacts with estrogen receptor alpha and affects beta-oxidation activity [53]. Hypermethylation in the HADHB gene was found in hepatocellular carcinoma [54]. The baculoviral IAP repeat, which contains the 3 apoptosis inhibitor 2 (BIRC3) and encodes a member of the IAP family of proteins, has multi-biological functions. It not only regulates caspases and apoptosis, but also modulates inflammatory signaling and immunity, mitogenic kinase signaling and cell proliferation, and cell invasion and metastasis. Overexpression of BIRC3 is associated with glioma progression and aggression and chronic and acute B cell lymphocytic leukemia [55, 56]; it is also a predictor of therapeutic resistance to treatment with irradiation, doxorubicin, and temozolomide [57, 58].

In this study, we used a two-stage strategy to confirm hypermethylation and hypohydroxymethylation of the promoter region of the HADHB gene, which exhibited significantly decreased expression in CRC. The functional studies indicated that HADHB might act as a tumor suppressor gene. Therefore, our findings implicated HADHB as a potential biomarker for the diagnosis and treatment of CRC, especially for alleviating and controlling cancer progression.

Conclusions

To summarize, this study characterized global patterns of methylome and hydroxymethylome and found a genome-wide distinct hydroxymethylation pattern that could be used to differentiate between tumor tissues and normal tissues. We screened 59,249 DMRs, 187,172 DhMRs, and 948 significant DEGs. After integrating genome-wide expression with genome-wide patterns of DNA methylation and hydroxymethylation, we identified 7 genes that were aberrantly regulated by DNA methylation in tumors and were possibly associated with carcinogenesis of colorectal cancer. We confirmed that HADHB could be a novel tumor suppressor gene.

Additional files

Additional file 1: Table S1. The basic characteristics of six patients of colorectal cancer. **Table S2**. Summary of MeDIP-seq and hMeDIP-seq data production. **Table S3**. Pearson's product-moment correlation for the levels of DNA methylation and DNA hydroxymethylation with the elements in chromosome. **Table S4**. Differentially methylated regions (DMRs) in promoters. **Table S5**. Differentially hydroxymethylated regions (DhMRs) in promoters. **Table S6**. The top 10 pathways enriched in DMRs, DhMRs and DEG. **Table S7**. Summary of RNA-seq data production. **Table S8**. Differentially expressed genes (DEGs) in 6 pairs of samples. **Table S9**. The list of 7 genes of which DEGs contained both DMRs and DhMRs.

Additional file 2: Figure S1. Coverage and depth of reads for MeDIP-seq and hMeDIP-seq. CpG sites coverage with different sequencing depth are presented. MeDIP-seq data are shown at the top and hMeDIP-seq data are shown at the bottom. Different colors indicate tumor and normal samples.

Additional file 3: Figure S2. Methylation and hydroxymethylation levels distribution against GC content(%) and CpG o/e ratio. Higher levels of hydroxymethylation were found in the regions of GC content around

55% - 65% and CpG O/E ratio of 1.14-1.15. The regions with a GC content around 45% - 55% had a higher methylation level.

Additional file 4: Figure S3. Methylation and hydroxymethylation levels distribution in different types of genomic elements. Normal is shown by green, and tumor is shown by red. TSS: transcriptional start sites; TES: transcriptional end sites; CGI: CpG islands; LTR: long terminal repeat; SINE: short interspersed nuclear elements; LINE: long interspersed nuclear elements. *, $P < 0.05$, **, $P < 0.01$ and ***, $P < 0.001$

Additional file 5: Figure S4. Correlation between 5-mC and 5-hmC in normal (left) and tumor (right) samples. The whole genome was divided into 0.5 kb windows and the levels of 5-mC and 5-hmC were classified into different groups according to the RPMs of Medip and hMedip, respectively.

Additional file 6: Figure S5. Mean profiles with standard deviation (SD) over TSS and TES regions. 4-kb regions were divided in 80 bins from 5′ to 3′ end, and the mean RPM values (with SD) within each bin for each modification type was determined (5-mC left, 5-hmC right). Additionally, SD distribution are be shown at bottom left in each region.

Additional file 7: Figure S6. Distribution of DMRs and DhMRs in different types of genomic elements.

Additional file 8: Figure S7. Gene functional pathways of DMR, DhMR and DEG. Three pathway, metabolic pathways, purine metabolism and axon guidance, overlapped pathways among DMR, DhMR and DEG.

Additional file 9: Figure S8. Visualization of DMRs (bottom) and DhMRs (top) in HADHB. DMR and DhMR are denoted by the green box.

Abbreviations

5-hmC: Hydroxyl-methylation; 5-mC: 5-Methylcytosine; CGI: CpG islands; CRC: Colorectal cancer; DEG: Differentially expressed genes; DhMR: Differential hydroxyl-methylation regions; DMR: Differential methylation regions; DNMT: DNA methyltransferase; FDR: False discovery rate; hMeDIP-seq: Hydroxyl-methylation by hydroxymethylated DNA immunoprecipitation sequencing; LINE: Long interspersed nuclear elements; LTR: Long terminal repeat; MeDIP-seq: Methylated DNA immune-precipitation sequencing; RPKM: Reads per kilobase million; SINE: Short interspersed nuclear elements; TDG: Thymine-DNA glycosylase; TES: Transcriptional end sites; TET: Ten-eleven translocation; TSG: Tumor suppressor gene; TSS: Transcriptional start sites

Acknowledgements

None.

Funding

This work was supported by the grants from the 111 Project (B13026), Major program of Zhejiang Province (2012C13014-3), BGI-Shenzhen and the Agricultural Science and Technology Innovation Program (ASTIP) of China, Science and Technology Project of Shenzhen (JSGG20160427104724699), Zhejiang Provincial Program for the Cultivation of High-level Innovative Health talents, and the Fundamental Research Funds for Central Universities.

Authors' contributions

MDL and YMZ designed and supervised the study; FG, YMZ, DDZ, XHS, LDW, DY, YPT, and HLL performed the experiments and analyzed the data. FG and YMZ wrote parts of the manuscript. AFL, MYL, and HCJ collected samples and data from CRC patients. MDL, FG, and YMZ discussed the results. All authors read and approved the final manuscript.

Competing interests

The authors declare that they have no competing interests.

Author details

[1]Department of Epidemiology and Biostatistics, School of Public Health, Zhejiang University, Hangzhou 310058, China. [2]BGI-Shenzhen, Shenzhen 518083, China. [3]Agricultural Genomics Institute at Shenzhen, Chinese Academy of Agricultural Sciences, Shenzhen 518120, China. [4]Key Laboratory of Disease Proteomics of Zhejiang Province and Department of Pathology, School of Medicine, Zhejiang University, Hangzhou 310058, China. [5]Laboratory of Cancer Biology, Provincial Key Lab of Biotherapy in Zhejiang, Sir Runrun Shaw Hospital, Medical School of Zhejiang University, Hangzhou, China. [6]Human Tissue Bank/Medical Research Center, Taizhou Hospital of Zhejiang Province, Wenzhou Medical University, Linhai, Zhejiang 317000, China. [7]Department of Pathology, School of Medicine, Zhejiang University, 866 Yuhangtang Road, Zhejiang, Hangzhou 310058, China.

References

1. Hanahan D, Weinberg RA. Hallmarks of cancer: the next generation. Cell. 2011;144(5):646–74.
2. Goel A, Boland CR. Epigenetics of colorectal cancer. Gastroenterology. 2012; 143(6):1442–60. e1441
3. Dawson MA, Kouzarides T. Cancer epigenetics: from mechanism to therapy. Cell. 2012;150(1):12–27.
4. You JS, Jones PA. Cancer genetics and epigenetics: two sides of the same coin? Cancer Cell. 2012;22(1):9–20.
5. Liao J, Karnik R, Gu H, Ziller MJ, Clement K, Tsankov AM, Akopian V, Gifford CA, Donaghey J, Galonska C, et al. Targeted disruption of DNMT1, DNMT3A and DNMT3B in human embryonic stem cells. Nat Genet. 2015;47(5):469–78.
6. Hamidi T, Singh AK, Chen T. Genetic alterations of DNA methylation machinery in human diseases. Epigenomics. 2015;7(2):247–65.
7. Huidobro C, Fernandez AF, Fraga MF. The role of genetics in the establishment and maintenance of the epigenome. Cell Mol Life Sci. 2013; 70(9):1543–73.
8. Bergman Y, Cedar H. DNA methylation dynamics in health and disease. Nat Struct Mol Biol. 2013;20(3):274–81.
9. Lichtenstein AV. Cancer: evolutionary, genetic and epigenetic aspects. Clin Epigenetics. 2010;1(3-4):85–100.
10. Kinney SR, Pradhan S. Ten eleven translocation enzymes and 5-hydroxymethylation in mammalian development and cancer. Adv Exp Med Biol. 2013;754:57–79.
11. Tan L, Shi YG. Tet family proteins and 5-hydroxymethylcytosine in development and disease. Development. 2012;139(11):1895–902.
12. Uysal F, Akkoyunlu G, Ozturk S. Dynamic expression of DNA methyltransferases (DNMTs) in oocytes and early embryos. Biochimie. 2015; 116:103–13.
13. Spruijt CG, Gnerlich F, Smits AH, Pfaffeneder T, Jansen PW, Bauer C, Munzel M, Wagner M, Muller M, Khan F, et al. Dynamic readers for 5-(hydroxy)methylcytosine and its oxidized derivatives. Cell. 2013;152(5):1146–59.
14. Ficz G, Branco MR, Seisenberger S, Santos F, Krueger F, Hore TA, Marques CJ, Andrews S, Reik W. Dynamic regulation of 5-hydroxymethylcytosine in mouse ES cells and during differentiation. Nature. 2011;473(7347):398–402.
15. Yoshioka H, Minamizaki T, Yoshiko Y. The dynamics of DNA methylation and hydroxymethylation during amelogenesis. Histochem Cell Biol. 2015;144(5):471–8.
16. Sontag LB, Lorincz MC, Georg Luebeck E. Dynamics, stability and inheritance of somatic DNA methylation imprints. J Theor Biol. 2006;242(4):890–9.
17. Kudo Y, Tateishi K, Yamamoto K, Yamamoto S, Asaoka Y, Ijichi H, Nagae G, Yoshida H, Aburatani H, Koike K. Loss of 5-hydroxymethylcytosine is accompanied with malignant cellular transformation. Cancer Sci. 2012;103(4):670–6.
18. Kraus TF, Globisch D, Wagner M, Eigenbrod S, Widmann D, Munzel M, Muller M, Pfaffeneder T, Hackner B, Feiden W, et al. Low values of 5-hydroxymethylcytosine (5hmC), the "sixth base," are associated with anaplasia in human brain tumors. Int J Cancer. 2012;131(7):1577–90.
19. Jin SG, Kadam S, Pfeifer GP. Examination of the specificity of DNA methylation profiling techniques towards 5-methylcytosine and 5-hydroxymethylcytosine. Nucleic Acids Res. 2010;38(11):e125.
20. Booth MJ, Branco MR, Ficz G, Oxley D, Krueger F, Reik W, Balasubramanian S. Quantitative sequencing of 5-methylcytosine and 5-hydroxymethylcytosine at single-base resolution. Science. 2012;336(6083):934–7.
21. Yu M, Hon GC, Szulwach KE, Song CX, Zhang L, Kim A, Li X, Dai Q, Shen Y, Park B, et al. Base-resolution analysis of 5-hydroxymethylcytosine in the mammalian genome. Cell. 2012;149(6):1368–80.
22. Audic S, Claverie JM. The significance of digital gene expression profiles. Genome Res. 1997;7(10):986–95.
23. Li M, Wu H, Luo Z, Xia Y, Guan J, Wang T, Gu Y, Chen L, Zhang K, Ma J,

et al. An atlas of DNA methylomes in porcine adipose and muscle tissues. Nat Commun. 2012;3:850.
24. Wen L, Tang F. Genomic distribution and possible functions of DNA hydroxymethylation in the brain. Genomics. 2014;104(5):341–46.
25. Weber M, Davies JJ, Wittig D, Oakeley EJ, Haase M, Lam WL, Schubeler D. Chromosome-wide and promoter-specific analyses identify sites of differential DNA methylation in normal and transformed human cells. Nat Genet. 2005;37(8):853–62.
26. Chouliaras L, van den Hove DLA, Kenis G, Keitel S, Hof PR, van Os J, Steinbusch HWM, Schmitz C, Rutten BPF. Age-related increase in levels of 5-hydroxymethylcytosine in mouse hippocampus is prevented by caloric restriction. Curr Alzheimer Res. 2012;9(5):536–44.
27. Coppieters N, Dieriks BV, Lill C, Faull RLM, Curtis MA, Dragunow M. Global changes in DNA methylation and hydroxymethylation in Alzheimer's disease human brain. Neurobiol Aging. 2014;35(6):1334–44.
28. Bhattacharyya S, Yu YT, Suzuki M, Campbell N, Mazdo J, Vasanthakumar A, Bhagat TD, Nischal S, Christopeit M, Parekh S, et al. Genome-wide hydroxymethylation tested using the HELP-GT assay shows redistribution in cancer. Nucleic Acids Res. 2013;41(16):e157.
29. Kubiura M, Okano M, Kimura H, Kawamura F, Tada M. Chromosome-wide regulation of euchromatin-specific 5mC to 5hmC conversion in mouse ES cells and female human somatic cells. Chromosom Res. 2012;20(7):837–48.
30. Mellen M, Ayata P, Dewell S, Kriaucionis S, Heintz N. MeCP2 binds to 5hmC enriched within active genes and accessible chromatin in the nervous system. Cell. 2012;151(7):1417–30.
31. Jin SG, Wu XW, Li AX, Pfeifer GP. Genomic mapping of 5-hydroxymethylcytosine in the human brain. Nucleic Acids Res. 2011;39(12):5015–24.
32. Haffner MC, Chaux A, Meeker AK, Esopi DM, Gerber J, Pellakuru LG, Toubaji A, Argani P, Iacobuzio-Donahue C, Nelson WG, et al. Global 5-hydroxymethylcytosine content is significantly reduced in tissue stem/progenitor cell compartments and in human cancers. Oncotarget. 2011;2(8):627–37.
33. Lian CG, Xu Y, Ceol C, Wu F, Larson A, Dresser K, Xu W, Tan L, Hu Y, Zhan Q, et al. Loss of 5-hydroxymethylcytosine is an epigenetic hallmark of melanoma. Cell. 2012;150(6):1135–46.
34. Murata A, Baba Y, Ishimoto T, Miyake K, Kosumi K, Harada K, Kurashige J, Iwagami S, Sakamoto Y, Miyamoto Y, et al. TET family proteins and 5-hydroxymethylcytosine in esophageal squamous cell carcinoma. Oncotarget. 2015;6(27):23372–82.
35. Udali S, Guarini P, Moruzzi S, Ruzzenente A, Tammen SA, Guglielmi A, Conci S, Pattini P, Olivieri O, Corrocher R, et al. Global DNA methylation and hydroxymethylation differ in hepatocellular carcinoma and cholangiocarcinoma and relate to survival rate. Hepatology. 2015;62(2):496–504.
36. Gilat N, Tabachnik T, Shwartz A, Shahal T, Torchinsky D, Michaeli Y, Nifker G, Zirkin S, Ebenstein Y. Single-molecule quantification of 5-hydroxymethylcytosine for diagnosis of blood and colon cancers. Clin Epigenetics. 2017;9:70.
37. Asting AG, Caren H, Andersson M, Lonnroth C, Lagerstedt K, Lundholm K. COX-2 gene expression in colon cancer tissue related to regulating factors and promoter methylation status. BMC Cancer. 2011;11:238.
38. Yoruker EE, Mert U, Bugra D, Yamaner S, Dalay N. Promoter and histone methylation and p16(INK4A) gene expression in colon cancer. Exp Ther Med. 2012;4(5):865–70.
39. Irizarry RA, Ladd-Acosta C, Wen B, Wu ZJ, Montano C, Onyango P, Cui HM, Gabo K, Rongione M, Webster M, et al. The human colon cancer methylome shows similar hypo- and hypermethylation at conserved tissue-specific CpG island shores. Nat Genet. 2009;41(2):178–86.
40. Wen L, Li XL, Yan LY, Tan YX, Li R, Zhao YY, Wang Y, Xie JC, Zhang Y, Song CX, et al. Whole-genome analysis of 5-hydroxymethylcytosine and 5-methylcytosine at base resolution in the human brain. Genome Biol. 2014;15(3):R49.
41. Ameri K, Jahangiri A, Rajah AM, Tormos KV, Nagarajan R, Pekmezci M, Nguyen V, Wheeler ML, Murphy MP, Sanders TA, et al. HIGD1A regulates oxygen consumption, ROS production, and AMPK activity during glucose deprivation to modulate cell survival and tumor growth. Cell Rep. 2015;S2211-1247(15)00033-9.
42. Ameri K, Rajah AM, Nguyen V, Sanders TA, Jahangiri A, Delay M, Donne M, Choi HJ, Tormos KV, Yeghiazarians Y, et al. Nuclear localization of the mitochondrial factor HIGD1A during metabolic stress. PLoS One. 2013;8(4):e62758.
43. Denko N, Schindler C, Koong A, Laderoute K, Green C, Giaccia A. Epigenetic regulation of gene expression in cervical cancer cells by the tumor microenvironment. Clin Cancer Res. 2000;6(2):480–7.
44. Yamaguchi S, Ishikawa T. AHCYL2 (long-IRBIT) as a potential regulator of the electrogenic Na+-HCO3- cotransporter NBCe1-B. FEBS Lett. 2014;588(5):672–7.
45. He LH, Ma Q, Shi YH, Ge J, Zhao HM, Li SF, Tong ZS. CHL1 is involved in human breast tumorigenesis and progression. Biochem Biophys Res Commun. 2013;438(2):433–8.
46. Martin-Sanchez E, Mendaza S, Ulazia-Garmendia A, Monreal-Santesteban I, Blanco-Luquin I, Cordoba A, Vicente-Garcia F, Perez-Janices N, Escors D, Megias D, et al. CHL1 hypermethylation as a potential biomarker of poor prognosis in breast cancer. Oncotarget. 2017;8(9):15789–801.
47. Senchenko VN, Krasnov GS, Dmitriev AA, Kudryavtseva AV, Anedchenko EA, Braga EA, Pronina IV, Kondratieva TT, Ivanov SV, Zabarovsky ER *et al*: Differential expression of CHL1 gene during development of major human cancers. PLoS One 2011;6(3):e15612.
48. Calcagno DQ, Takeno SS, Gigek CO, Leal MF, Wisnieski F, Chen ES, Araujo TMT, Lima EM, Melaragno MI, Demachki S, et al. Identification of IL11RA and MELK amplification in gastric cancer by comprehensive genomic profiling of gastric cancer cell lines. World J Gastroenterol. 2016;22(43):9506–14.
49. Lu YJ, Xu Q, Chen L, Zuo YZ, Liu SC, Hu YT, Li XR, Li YH, Zhao XY. Expression of semaphorin 6D and its receptor plexin-A1 in gastric cancer and their association with tumor angiogenesis. Oncol Lett. 2016;12(5):3967–74.
50. Zhao XY, Chen L, Xu Q, Li YH. Expression of semaphorin 6D in gastric carcinoma and its significance. World J Gastroenterol. 2006;12(45):7388–90.
51. Shahrokhi M, Shafiei M, Galehdari H, Shariati G. Identification of a novel HADHB gene mutation in an Iranian patient with mitochondrial trifunctional protein deficiency. Arch Iran Med. 2017;20(1):22–7.
52. Park HD, Kim SR, Ki CS, Lee SY, Chang YS, Jin DK, Park WS. Two novel HADHB gene mutations in a Korean patient with mitochondrial trifunctional protein deficiency. Ann Clin Lab Sci. 2009;39(4):399–404.
53. Zhou Z, Zhou J, Du Y: Estrogen receptor alpha interacts with mitochondrial protein HADHB and affects beta-oxidation activity. Mol Cell Proteomics 2012, 11(7):M111 011056.
54. Revill K, Wang T, Lachenmayer A, Kojima K, Harrington A, Li J, Hoshida Y, Llovet JM, Powers S: Genome-wide methylation analysis and epigenetic unmasking identify tumor suppressor genes in hepatocellular carcinoma. Gastroenterology 2013, 145(6):1424-1435 e1421-1425.
55. Gressot LV, Doucette T, Yang YH, Fuller GN, Manyam G, Rao A, Latha K, Rao G. Analysis of the inhibitors of apoptosis identifies BIRC3 as a facilitator of malignant progression in glioma. Oncotarget. 2017;8(8):12695–704.
56. Alhourani E, Othman MAK, Melo JB, Carreira IM, Grygalewicz B, Vujic D, Zecevic Z, Joksic G, Glaser A, Pohle B, et al. BIRC3 alterations in chronic and B-cell acute lymphocytic leukemia patients. Oncol Lett. 2016;11(5):3240–6.
57. Wang DP, Berglund A, Kenchappa RS, Forsyth PA, Mule JJ, Etame AB. BIRC3 is a novel driver of therapeutic resistance in Glioblastoma. Sci Rep. 2016;6:21710.
58. Mendoza-Rodriguez M, Arevalo Romero H, Fuentes-Panana EM, Ayala-Sumuano JT, Meza I. IL-1beta induces up-regulation of BIRC3, a gene involved in chemoresistance to doxorubicin in breast cancer cells. Cancer Lett. 2017;390:39–44.

9

Metabolic and inflammatory biomarkers are associated with epigenetic aging acceleration estimates in the GOLDN study

Marguerite R. Irvin[1*], Stella Aslibekyan[1], Anh Do[1], Degui Zhi[2], Bertha Hidalgo[1], Steven A. Claas[3], Vinodh Srinivasasainagendra[4], Steve Horvath[5,6,7], Hemant K. Tiwari[4], Devin M. Absher[8] and Donna K. Arnett[3]

Abstract

Background: Recently, epigenetic age acceleration—or older epigenetic age in comparison to chronological age—has been robustly associated with mortality and various morbidities. However, accelerated epigenetic aging has not been widely investigated in relation to inflammatory or metabolic markers, including postprandial lipids.

Methods: We estimated measures of epigenetic age acceleration in 830 Caucasian participants from the Genetics Of Lipid Lowering Drugs and diet Network (GOLDN) considering two epigenetic age calculations based on differing sets of 5′-Cytosine-phosphate-guanine-3′ genomic site, derived from the Horvath and Hannum DNA methylation age calculators, respectively. GOLDN participants underwent a standardized high-fat meal challenge after fasting for at least 8 h followed by timed blood draws, the last being 6 h postmeal. We used adjusted linear mixed models to examine the association of the epigenetic age acceleration estimate with fasting and postprandial (0- and 6-h time points) low-density lipoprotein (LDL), high-density lipoprotein (HDL), and triglyceride (TG) levels as well as five fasting inflammatory markers plus adiponectin.

Results: Both DNA methylation age estimates were highly correlated with chronological age ($r > 0.90$). We found that the Horvath and Hannum measures of epigenetic age acceleration were moderately correlated ($r = 0.50$). The regression models revealed that the Horvath age acceleration measure exhibited marginal associations with increased postprandial HDL ($p = 0.05$), increased postprandial total cholesterol ($p = 0.06$), and decreased soluble interleukin 2 receptor subunit alpha (IL2sRα, $p = 0.02$). The Hannum measure of epigenetic age acceleration was inversely associated with fasting HDL ($p = 0.02$) and positively associated with postprandial TG ($p = 0.02$), interleukin-6 (IL6, $p = 0.007$), C-reactive protein (C-reactive protein, $p = 0.0001$), and tumor necrosis factor alpha (TNFα, $p = 0.0001$). Overall, the observed effect sizes were small and the association of the Hannum residual with inflammatory markers was attenuated by adjustment for estimated T cell type percentages.

Conclusions: Our study demonstrates that epigenetic age acceleration in blood relates to inflammatory biomarkers and certain lipid classes in Caucasian individuals of the GOLDN study. Future studies should consider epigenetic age acceleration in other tissues and extend the analysis to other ethnic groups.

Keywords: Epigenetics, Epigenetic age, Age acceleration, Inflammation, Inflammatory markers, Lipids, Postprandial, Cholesterol, Triglycerides, Adiponectin

* Correspondence: irvinr@uab.edu
[1]Department of Epidemiology, University of Alabama at Birmingham, 1665 University Blvd, RPHB 230J, Birmingham, AL 35294, USA
Full list of author information is available at the end of the article

Background

Increasing age is a major risk factor for chronic disease. Understanding risk factors for accelerated aging can help target strategies aimed at preventing or delaying onset of age-related disease [1, 2]. Importantly, the epigenome is an intriguing target for age-related physiological changes, as it is modifiable by the environment and is a major determinant of gene expression [3]. Recently, calculated "epigenetic age" has become a novel aging biomarker, which has been demonstrated to accurately predict chronological age across a broad spectrum of tissues and cell types [4]. Epigenetic age acceleration—or older epigenetic age in comparison to chronological age—has been robustly associated with all-cause mortality [5], obesity [6], physical fitness [7], and stress [8]. However, accelerated epigenetic aging has not been evaluated in relation to intermediate phenotypes such as postprandial blood lipid levels, inflammatory markers, or adiponectin.

Of those, postprandial blood lipid levels are especially relevant given that most people spend the majority of the day in a postprandial state [9]. Results from basic and clinical studies suggest elevated and prolonged postprandial lipemia is associated with prothrombotic and proinflammatory processes that may precipitate cardiovascular disease (CVD) and aging [10, 11]. In the current study, we evaluated the association of two measures of epigenetic age acceleration [4, 12] with fasting and postprandial lipids, five inflammatory markers, and adiponectin, using data from the Genetics of Lipid Lowering Drugs and Diet Network (GOLDN) study.

Methods

Study population

The GOLDN study determined genetic predictors of participant lipid and inflammatory response to diet and fenofibrate treatment interventions [13–15]. Participants were identified through 3-generation families previously screened in the National Heart, Lung and Blood Institute Family Heart Study (FHS) Minnesota and Utah centers. Individuals who used lipid-lowering drugs at the time of screening were required to discontinue them for 4 weeks prior to study participation. Participants fasted for at least 8 h and abstained from alcohol intake for ≥ 24 h. The postprandial lipemia intervention followed the protocol of Patsch et al. [16]. The whipping cream (83% fat) meal had 700 calories/m^2 body surface area; 3% of calories were derived from protein, and 14% from carbohydrate. Blood samples were drawn immediately before the meal with the last draw being 6 h later. During the 6-h study period, participants consumed only water and abstained from physical activity. Inflammatory markers and adiponectin were assayed only in the fasting state. The data used in this analysis were collected at the time of the postprandial lipemia challenge and, thus, except for the 6-h lipid measures, was cross-sectional.

Lipids, inflammatory markers, and adiponectin

Triglycerides (TG), high-density lipoprotein (HDL), low-density lipoprotein (LDL), and total cholesterol were measured by nuclear magnetic resonance (NMR) spectroscopy at fasting and during the postprandial intervention (Liposcience, Raleigh, NC) [17]. High-sensitivity C-reactive protein (hsCRP) was measured on the Hitachi 911 using a latex particle-enhanced immunoturbidimetric assay (Kamiya Biomedical Company, Seattle, WA). Interleukin-6 (IL6), interleukin-2 soluble receptor alpha (IL2sRα), tumor necrosis factor (TNF)-α and monocyte chemoattractant protein-1 (MCP1) were measured using quantitative sandwich enzyme immunoassays (ELISA kit assays, R&D Systems Inc., Minneapolis, MN) as described in previous publications [18, 19]. Adiponectin was measured using an ELISA kit from R&D Systems (Minneapolis, MN) [20].

DNA methylation measurements and epigenetic age calculation

DNA from a total 993 GOLDN participants was assayed using Illumina's Infinium HumanMethylation450 Beadchip as previously described by Irvin et al. [21]. Briefly, CD4+ T cells were harvested from stored buffy coats (from the fasting sample) using antibody-linked Invitrogen Dynabeads [22]. Cells were lysed and DNA was extracted using DNeasy kits (Qiagen, Venlo, Netherlands). After following standard Illumina protocols, the resulting intensity files were analyzed with Illumina's GenomeStudio to generate beta scores representing the percent of methylated sites at that location across all the cells in a sample. After previously reported QC, methylation data were available for 461,281 5′-cytosine-phosphate-guanine-3′ genomic site (CpGs) [21]. The non-normalized data were uploaded into the DNA methylation age calculator [4] using the advanced analysis in blood option. We removed 140 samples for which the predicted tissue was not blood. To err on the side of caution, we removed 23 individuals from the analysis because they were severe outliers according to the Horvath measure of epigenetic age acceleration (> 4 standard deviations away from the mean), leaving a total sample size of $n = 830$ individuals for the analysis.

In addition to the Horvath measure of epigenetic age acceleration, we considered another independent measure of age acceleration derived from the Hannum methylation age estimate [12]. Both methylation age acceleration estimates have been associated with outcomes in a side-by-side manner in previous publications [5, 23, 24]. The Horvath methylation age estimate (DNAm age) is based on 353 CpGs and has been robustly correlated with chronological age in multiple studies. DNAm age sometimes systematically underestimates chronological age [25]. To remove this systematic offset from the analysis, this study leverages epigenetic age acceleration defined by regressing DNAm age on chronological age and forming residuals. The second estimate is based on Hannum's methylation age estimate calculated from 71 CpGs. Figures 1 and 2 are the scatter plots of calculated epigenetic age versus chronological age for the Horvath and Hannum calculators, respectively, in GOLDN. The Horvath and the Hannum measures of DNAm age are related, but they capture slightly different aspects of biology (only 6 CpGs overlap) [5]. The Hannum age estimator is correlated with estimated blood cell counts, which reflects that it was constructed on the basis of whole blood DNA methylation data [5, 26]. In the current analysis, we focused on a modification of the Hannum estimate described (in previous publications) as *extrinsic* epigenetic age acceleration (EEAA) since it has been found to outperform the original Hannum measure when it comes to predicting lifespan [5]. EEAA is a residual formed from regressing the Hannum estimate weighted by the proportion of naive CD8+ T cells, exhausted CD8+ T cells, and plasmablasts on chronological age which makes the estimate more strongly reflective of immune system aging [5, 23, 27]. Chen et al. reported the Hannum estimator tracks aspects of immunosenescence exhibiting significant (albeit weak) correlations with several markers of immunosenescence, e.g., the abundance of senescent (or conversely naïve) T cells and telomere length [26, 27]. The Horvath DNAm age estimator exhibits substantially weaker correlations with estimated blood cell counts, which reflects the fact that it was constructed across a broad spectrum of tissues and cell types. Overall, the Horvath DNAm age estimator does not relate to measures of immunosenescence (including telomere length) [27]. Rather, it mostly captures cell intrinsic DNAm age changes which might reflect the actions of an innate aging process.

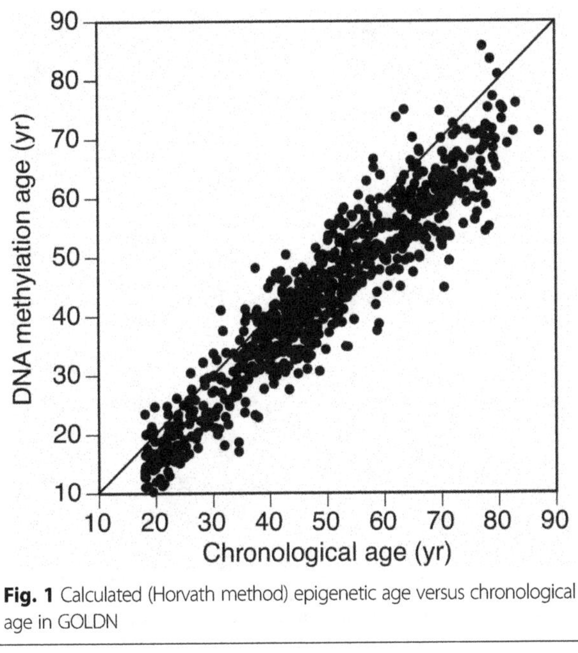

Fig. 1 Calculated (Horvath method) epigenetic age versus chronological age in GOLDN

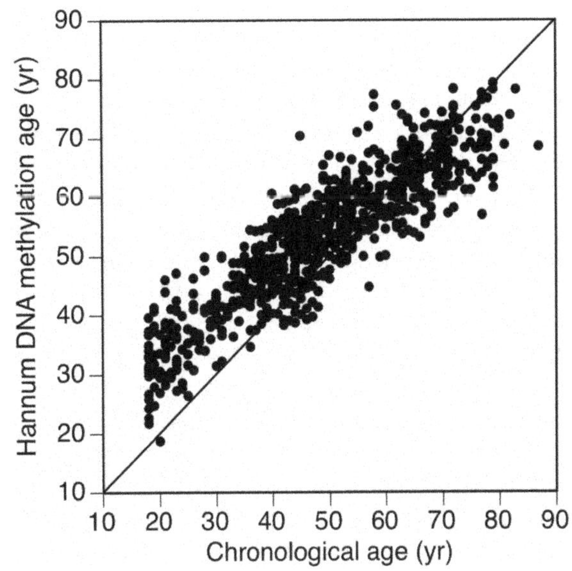

Fig. 2 Calculated (Hannum method) epigenetic age versus chronological age in GOLDN

For both methylation age acceleration estimates, a positive value indicates that the epigenetic age is higher than expected based on chronological age (i.e., accelerated epigenetic aging). We note EEAA in GOLDN is limited by the use of DNA methylation data derived from CD4+ T cells as opposed to peripheral blood mononuclear cells (PBMCs) like in previous studies. For a more direct comparison to the Horvath estimate we also report the results for the Hannum residual defined by regressing the (unweighted) Hannum methylation age estimate on chronological age in a secondary analysis.

Statistical analysis

Participant characteristics were compared by the median of each age acceleration measure using chi square tests and t-tests, as appropriate. TG, hsCRP, IL6, IL2sRα, TNFα, MCP1, and adiponectin were ln-transformed to achieve normality. Pearson correlation coefficients between lipids, inflammatory markers, adiponectin, and each measure of age acceleration were also estimated. We used linear mixed models to examine the association of the Horvath epigenetic age acceleration residual with fasting and postprandial total cholesterol, LDL, HDL, and TG as well as inflammatory markers and adiponectin (as outcomes).

The model was adjusted for age, study site, sex, corresponding fasting lipid level (if applicable), deconvolution estimated T cell type (naïve, regulatory, memory) percentages (estimated using a method developed by the GOLDN group [28]), age acceleration estimate squared (to account for a potential non-linear effect of this variable), current smoking status, current drinking status and a random effect of family relationship. Linear mixed models were implemented in the R *kinship* package (*lmekin* function) [29]. For our analysis of the EEAA estimate we used a similar model, except the model was not adjusted for estimated T cell type percentages since blood cell composition is a component of the age acceleration estimate. For both the Horvath and Hannum estimates we considered a sensitivity model adjusted for history of coronary heart disease (CHD) and diabetes status. Further, we explored a gender by age acceleration interaction term. In total we tested the association of 14 outcomes with each age acceleration estimate making the Bonferroni correction for multiple testing $p = 0.003$ (0.05/14). In secondary analysis we examined the association of each outcome with the Hannum residual, considering the model described above for EEAA both with and without adjustment for T cell percentages.

Results

The mean and standard deviation of the Horvath and Hannum (EEAA) estimates were − 3.54 (6.1) and − 1.32 (8.3), respectively. The Pearson correlation coefficient between methylation and chronological age was 0.94 ($p < 0.0001$) for the Horvath estimate and 0.91 ($p < 0.0001$) for the Hannum (EEAA) estimate. The correlation coefficient between the Horvath and Hannum (EEAA) age acceleration measures was 0.50 ($p < 0.0001$). Table 1 shows descriptive statistics of the GOLDN population, categorized by the median of each age acceleration value (− 3.33 and − 1.64 for the Horvath and Hannum (EEAA) estimates, respectively). There was a higher prevalence

Table 1 Descriptive statistics of the GOLDN study population categorized by the median of two age acceleration residuals

	Horvath age acceleration			Hannum age acceleration (EEAA)		
N (%) or mean (SD)	Below median	Above median	*p*	Below median	Above median	*p*
Center (UT)	220 (53.0)	153 (36.9)	< 0.0001	223 (46.2)	192 (43.6)	0.44
Female	226 (54.5)	193 (46.5)	0.02	222 (53.5)	197 (47.5)	0.08
Current smoker	34 (8.2)	35(8.4)	0.89	32 (7.7)	37 (8.9)	0.52
Current drinking	201 (48.4)	238 (57.4)	0.01	228(54.9)	211 (50.8)	0.23
History of CHD	16 (3.9)	27 (6.5)	0.08	15 (3.6)	28 (6.8)	0.04
Hypertension	99 (23.9)	121 (29.2)	0.08	89 (21.5)	131 (31.6)	0.001
Diabetes	22 (5.3)	41 (9.8)	0.01	23 (5.5)	40 (9.6)	0.03
Age	46.6 (16.2)	50.7 (15.5)	0.0002	46.6 (16.1)	50.7 (15.6)	0.0002
Lipids						
LDL mg/dL (0 h)	114.9 (31.8)	121.7 (32.2)	0.003	116.5 (31.8)	120.1 (32.4)	0.10
LDL mg/dL (6 h)	119.2(32.1)	125.9 (33.2)	0.003	120.8 (32.2)	124.4 (33.3)	0.12
HDL mg/dL (0 h)	46.0 (14.1)	44.5 (13.1)	0.12	47.1 (14.5)	43.4 (12.4)	< 0.0001
HDL mg/dL (6 h)	48.8 (14.6)	47.8 (14.1)	0.34	50.2 (15.2)	46.3 (133)	< 0.0001
TC mg/dL (0 h)	181.6 (38.4)	189.7 (40.0)	0.003	183.9 (38.8)	187.4(39.9)	0.20
TC mg/dL (6 h)	189.2 (39.6)	199.0 (42.9)	0.0007	191.9 (40.3)	196.3 (42.7)	0.13
TG mg/dL (0 h)	135.5 (84.8)	155.5 (108.5)	0.003	133.4 (83.0)	157.8 (109.5)	0.0003
TG mg/dL (6 h)	187.9 (130.5)	230.8 (166.8)	< 0.0001	187.0 (129.7)	231.8 (167.3)	< 0.0001
Inflammatory markers						
IL6	1.9 (2.2)	2.2 (4.4)	0.11	1.8 (26)	2.2 (4.2)	0.08
CRP	0.21 (0.3)	0.25 (0.4)	0.22	0.20 (0.4)	0.26 (0.4)	0.03
MCP1	207.8 (62.5)	211.2 (68.7)	0.45	204.3 (64.9)	214.7 (66.1)	0.02
IL2SRA	1012.3 (344.5)	1021.2 (377.1)	0.72	991.2 (330.3)	1042.3 (388.0)	0.04
Adiponectin	8498.6 (4644.7)	8047.9 (4827.6)	0.17	8568.1 (4746.8)	7978.2 (4719.4)	0.07
TNFα	3.2 (1.9)	3.9 (8.0)	0.08	3.1 (1.8)	4.0 (8.0)	0.02

EEAA extrinsic epigenetic age acceleration, *CHD* coronary heart disease, *CRP* C-reactive protein, *DNAmage* DNA methylation age, *HDL* high-density lipoprotein, *IL2SRA* interleukin-2 soluble receptor alpha, *IL6* interleukin 6, *LDL* low-density lipoprotein, *MCP1* monocyte chemotactic protein 1, *TC* total cholesterol, *TG* triglyceride, *TNFα* tumor necrosis factor alpha

of current drinking, history of CVD, hypertension, and diabetes associated with being above the median for the Horvath age acceleration measure. Similarly, being above the median of the age acceleration estimate for the Hannum method was associated with history of CVD, hypertension, and diabetes, but not with current drinking. Increasing age acceleration as measured by the Horvath method was associated with increased LDL, TC, and TG in the fasting and postprandial states. Having an age acceleration estimate above the median for the Hannum method was associated with decreased HDL and increased TG in the fasting and postprandial states. The Hannum measure of age acceleration (but not the Horvath measure) was also associated with increased C-reactive protein (CRP), IL2sRα, tumor necrosis factor alpha (TNFα), and MCP1 (Table 1). Table 2 shows the unadjusted correlation coefficients for each age acceleration estimate with lipid classes, inflammatory markers, and adiponectin. Each age acceleration measure was associated with lipid classes in the fasting and postprandial state except the Horvath measure was not associated with HDL. Each measure of age acceleration was inversely associated with adiponectin. The Hannum age acceleration estimate but not the Horvath estimate was positively associated with more than one inflammatory marker.

Regression results for the Horvath and Hannum age acceleration estimates are presented in Table 3. The Horvath epigenetic age acceleration residual was not associated with fasting lipid levels. Increasing age acceleration residual was marginally associated with higher postprandial HDL ($p = 0.05$) and postprandial total cholesterol ($p = 0.06$) after adjustment. The effect size for these associations is 0.30 mg/dL and 0.92 mg/dL for postprandial HDL and TC respectively for each 1 standard deviation change in the age acceleration estimate. The Horvath age acceleration estimate was also inversely associated (albeit marginally) with IL2sRα. The Hannum EEAA measure was inversely associated with fasting ($p = 0.02$) but not postprandial HDL levels, and was positively associated with postprandial ($p = 0.02$) but not fasting TG. The Hannum measure of epigenetic age acceleration was also strongly positively associated with IL6 ($p = 0.007$), CRP ($p = 0.0001$), and TNFα ($p = 0.0001$). The association of EEAA with CRP and TNFα were the only two associations that reached statistical significance after correction for multiple testing in Table 3. The ratio of postprandial TG, IL6, CRP, and TNFα associated with each 1 standard deviation increase in EEAA was 1.03, 1.06, 1.16, and 1.06, respectively. Additionally, adjusting for history of CHD and diabetes status in these models did not substantially change our results (data not shown). We did not find evidence of effect modification by gender of the relationship between epigenetic age acceleration and our traits except for CRP, where CRP was associated with epigenetic age acceleration (EEAA estimate) only in females ($p = 0.048$). This result does not pass significance criteria after correction for multiple testing.

In secondary analysis of the Hannum residual (Table 4), the results were consistent with those presented for EEAA in Table 3 except that the Hannum residual was not associated with IL6. After T cell type percentages were

Table 2 Marginal correlations between lipid and other biomarkers with epigenetic age acceleration in the GOLDN study

	Horvath age acceleration		Hannum age acceleration (EEAA)	
	r	*p*	*r*	*p*
Lipids				
LDL mg/dL (0 h)	0.11	0.0008	0.11	0.002
LDL mg/dL (6 h)	0.12	0.0009	0.10	0.003
HDL mg/dL (0 h)	− 0.02	0.50	− 0.13	0.0002
HDL mg/dL (6 h)	− 0.01	0.83	− 0.12	0.0004
TC mg/dL (0 h)	0.12	0.0004	0.08	0.02
TC mg/dL (6 h)	0.14	< .0001	0.09	0.007
TG mg/dL (0 h)	0.11	0.001	0.11	0.002
TG mg/dL (6 h)	0.17	< .0001	0.15	< .0001
Inflammatory markers				
IL6 (0 h)	0.05	0.18	0.09	0.02
CRP (0 h)	0.04	0.25	0.06	0.09
MCP1 (0 h)	0.01	0.81	0.07	0.05
IL2SRA (0 h)	−0.01	0.84	0.08	0.01
Adiponectin (0 h)	− 0.08	0.03	− 0.07	0.05
TNFα (0 h)	0.05	0.16	0.11	0.002

EEAA extrinsic epigenetic age acceleration, *0 h* fasting time point, *6 h* postprandial time point

Table 3 Multivariable linear regression models that relate biomarkers (rows) to epigenetic age acceleration (covariate) using the Horvath calculator and the Hannum calculator

	Horvath age acceleration			Hannum age acceleration (EEAA)		
Dependent variable	Beta*	SE	*p*	Beta#	SE	*p*
LDL mg/dL (0 h)	0.36	0.21	0.09	0.166	0.12	0.17
LDL mg/dL (6 h)	0.003	0.06	0.96	– 0.006	0.04	0.87
HDL mg/dL (0 h)	0.06	0.08	0.52	– 0.11	0.04	*0.02*
HDL mg/dL (6 h)	0.05	0.03	*0.05*	0.004	0.15	0.81
TC mg/dL (0 h)	0.44	0.25	0.08	0.091	0.14	0.52
TC mg/dL (6 h)	0.15	0.08	0.06	0.068	0.05	0.13
TG mg/dL (0 h)	0.001	0.004	0.75	0.002	0.002	0.30
TG mg/dL (6 h)	0.0005	0.002	0.84	0.004	0.001	*0.02*
IL6 (0 h)	– 0.001	0.004	0.76	0.007	0.002	*0.007*
CRP (0 h)	0.007	0.008	0.34	0.018	0.004	*0.0001*
MCP1 (0 h)	– 0.001	0.002	0.55	– 0.0003	0.001	0.76
IL2SRA(0 h)	– 0.006	0.002	*0.02*	0.002	0.001	0.09
Adiponectin (0 h)	– 0.003	0.004	0.46	– 0.003	0.002	0.24
TNFα (0 h)	– 0.0008	0.003	0.80	0.007	0.002	*0.0001*

Since the models include a quadratic term the effect of a one unit change in *x* on *y* is not constant

EEAA extrinsic epigenetic age acceleration, *0 h* fasting time point, *6 h* postprandial time point, *CRP* C-reactive protein, *HDL* high-density lipoprotein, *IL2SRA* interleukin-2 soluble receptor alpha, *IL6* interleukin-6, *LDL* low-density lipoprotein, *MCP1* monocyte chemotactic protein 1, *SE* standard error, *TC* total cholesterol, *TG* triglyceride, *TNFα* tumor necrosis factor alpha

*Model is adjusted for adjusted for age, study site, sex, fasting lipid level (if applicable), estimated T cell type percentages, epigenetic age acceleration estimate squared (i.e., a quadratic polynomial), current smoking status, current drinking status, and a random effect of family relationship

#Model is adjusted for adjusted for age, study site, sex, fasting lipid level (if applicable), epigenetic age acceleration estimate squared (i.e., a quadratic polynomial), current smoking status, current drinking status, and a random effect of family relationship

included in the model, the association with fasting HDL, CRP, and TNFα was attenuated. Postprandial TG remained marginally (0.08) associated with the Hannum residual even after adjustment for T cell type percentages.

Discussion

Measures of epigenetic age acceleration are robust biomarkers of aging independent of chronological age [4, 12]. In the current study, we tested the association of two different measures of epigenetic age acceleration with metabolic and inflammatory markers in 830 Genetics Of Lipid Lowering Drugs and Diet Network study participants. Similar to previous publications, epigenetic age acceleration was marginally associated with lipids, including postprandial lipids. We are the first to report that a measure of epigenetic age acceleration derived from the Hannum methylation age estimate (referred to as *extrinsic* epigenetic age acceleration) was strongly related to more than one inflammatory marker. However, further analysis showed this relationship was not independent of T cell type composition. Previous studies have reported each epigenetic age acceleration measure to be associated with outcomes including cancer mortality, cardiovascular disease mortality, and all-cause mortality [5, 30]. Continued research is needed to better understand if increased inflammation could be a pathway through which epigenetic aging is related to these outcomes.

A recent large meta-analysis of over 13,000 participants (including non-Hispanic whites, Hispanics, and African Americans) demonstrated that, independent of chronological age and traditional risk factors, epigenetic age acceleration assessed in blood (measured by both the Horvath and Hannum methods) predicted all-cause mortality [5]. Another study of ~ 2000 older Caucasian individuals from the ESTHER cohort (a large population-based epidemiologic study of chronic disease in Germany) reported that, for each 5 year increase of DNA methylation age (DNAmage, Horvath estimate) minus chronological age, the hazard ratio for all-cause mortality was 1.23 (95% CI 1.10–1.38), cancer mortality was 1.22 (95% CI 1.03–1.45), and cardiovascular mortality was 1.19 (95% CI 0.98–1.43) after adjustment for confounding factors [30]. Among ~ 1500 women from the Women's Health Initiative (WHI) study in a report from Horvath et al., neither measure of epigenetic age acceleration was associated with coronary heart disease (CHD) [24]. In that study, the measure of epigenetic age acceleration derived from the Horvath calculator was not robustly associated with triglyceride levels, HDL, glucose, CRP, or body mass index (BMI, $p > 0.05$) after adjustment. The extrinsic epigenetic age acceleration estimate (Hannum) was associated with fasting TG ($p = 0.04$) and CRP ($p = 0.02$), but not fasting HDL ($p = 0.80$). In our study, the direction of association of the Horvath estimate with

Table 4 Multivariable linear regression models that relate biomarkers (rows) to epigenetic age acceleration (covariate) using the Hannum residual with and without adjustment for estimated T cell type percentages

	Hannum residual					
	Model 1			Model 2		
Dependent variable	Beta	SE	*p*	Beta	SE	*p*
LDL mg/dL (0 h)	0.12	0.14	0.39	0.12	0.15	0.41
LDL mg/dL (6 h)	0.003	0.04	0.94	0.02	0.05	0.71
HDL mg/dL (0 h)	− 0.12	0.05	*0.03*	− 0.06	0.06	0.32
HDL mg/dL (6 h)	0.002	0.02	0.91	0.0008	0.02	0.97
TC mg/dL (0 h)	0.08	0.16	0.60	0.10	0.17	0.56
TC mg/dL (6 h)	0.07	0.05	0.16	0.07	0.05	0.17
TG mg/dL (0 h)	0.004	0.002	0.10	0.003	0.003	0.23
TG mg/dL (6 h)	0.003	0.002	*0.03*	0.003	0.002	0.08
IL6 (0 h)	0.002	0.003	0.53	− 0.002	0.003	0.46
CRP (0 h)	0.01	0.005	*0.005*	0.007	0.006	0.20
MCP1 (0 h)	− 0.00008	0.001	0.95	0.0006	0.001	0.62
IL2SRA (0 h)	− 0.00006	0.002	0.97	− 0.0004	0.002	0.79
Adiponectin (0 h)	− 0.003	0.002	0.20	− 0.0010	0.003	0.72
TNFα (0 h)	0.004	0.002	*0.04*	0.002	0.002	0.37

Model 1 is adjusted for adjusted for age, study site, sex, fasting lipid level (if applicable), epigenetic age acceleration estimate squared (i.e., a quadratic polynomial), current smoking status, current drinking status, and a random effect of family relationship. Model 2 adds estimated T cell type percentages to model 1. Since the models include a quadratic term, the effect of a one unit change in *x* on *y* is not constant

0 h fasting time point, *6 h* postprandial time point, *CRP* C-reactive protein, *HDL* high-density lipoprotein, *IL2SRA* interleukin-2 soluble receptor alpha, *IL6* interleukin 6, *LDL* low-density lipoprotein, *MCP1* monocyte chemotactic protein 1, *SE* standard error, *TC* total cholesterol, *TG* triglyceride, *TNFα* tumor necrosis factor alpha

fasting HDL was positive ($p = 0.52$), while the Hannum EEAA estimate was negatively associated with fasting HDL ($p = 0.02$). In the report from Horvath et al. mentioned above, the direction of association for the Horvath and Hannum estimates with HDL also conflicted. Another study reported that older epigenetic age in comparison to chronological age was associated with increased BMI in middle-aged but not in older adults, suggesting that the relationship between age acceleration and metabolic traits may change over the lifespan [6].

Since elevated postprandial lipids are predictive of aging and inflammation [9, 10], we investigated whether epigenetic age acceleration was associated with postprandial lipids. Like fasting lipids and other cardiometabolic risk factors investigated in other studies, our results demonstrate that epigenetic age acceleration is a modest predictor of postprandial lipemia. None of the results for lipids presented in Table 3 (fasting or postprandial) were significant after correction for multiple testing. Notably, after adjustment EEAA was associated with higher levels of postprandial TGs ($p = 0.02$), which is the lipid class that changes the most upon fat loading. The Horvath measure of epigenetic age acceleration was marginally associated with higher postprandial TC. With PPL and methylation measured on a single day in GOLDN, it is difficult to determine if increased metabolic parameters could lead to accelerated epigenetic age or vice versa. Longitudinal PPL and methylation data would be necessary to untangle the temporal relationship between epigenetic age acceleration and postprandial lipids. Few other studies have investigated whether diet is linked to epigenetic age acceleration. One study including > 4000 postmenopausal female participants from the WHI, as well as 402 male and female participants from the Italian cohort study, Invecchiare nel Chianti, suggested poultry intake was protective for epigenetic aging. In that same study, fish intake, alcohol, and smoking were not associated with the epigenetic age acceleration residual as measured by the Horvath age calculator.

In GOLDN, the epigenetic age acceleration measure from Horvath's calculator was associated with IL2sRα but not other inflammatory markers or adiponectin. On the other hand, EEAA was positively (but modestly) associated with three biomarkers of inflammation (IL6, CRP, and TNFα). Elevation of these three markers has been associated with a number of age-related chronic diseases [31]. Additionally, we considered the Hannum residual in a secondary analysis to help understand if the association between EEAA and inflammatory markers observed in our primary analysis could be due to a difference in probes across the two age acceleration measures or a function of the contribution of blood cell composition to the Hannum EEAA estimate. After adjustment for T cell type composition in a model considering the Hannum residual as the variable of interest, the three inflammatory markers were no longer associated with the Hannum estimate. In a previous study, EEAA was shown to be correlated with the sample estimated naïve and memory $CD8^+$ T cell populations [27]. In that same study, adjustment for T cell composition in a model correlating EEAA to leukocyte telomere length attenuated the association. In our study, the Hannum residual and Hannum EEAA estimate were strongly correlated with estimated populations of naïve CD4+ T cell percentages ($r = -0.45$, $p < 0.0001$ and -0.62, $p < 0.0001$, respectively). Overall, this lends further support to the conclusions from Chen et al. which suggested that EEAA captures information on key aspects of immunosenescence, which may help explain the stronger relationship of EEAA with mortality observed in a previous study in comparison to the Horvath estimate [5].

The current study is set in one of few observational epidemiology cohort studies with epigenetic array data and a postprandial lipemia intervention on a sizable population. Participants in the GOLDN study are, on average, middle aged, and because the study required discontinuation of lipid-lowering therapy, the study population is relatively healthy. Studies of the relationship between postprandial lipemia and epigenetic aging are still warranted in other groups (e.g., older individuals, other ethnic groups) and in other tissues.

Conclusion

Inflammatory markers associated with aging exhibit significant associations with a measure of epigenetic age acceleration. However, this association was not independent of other key aspects of immune system aging (estimated naïve T cell type percentages) in our study. The same measure of epigenetic age acceleration was weakly associated with increased postprandial triglyceride levels. Future studies should revisit these analyses by employing even larger sample sizes, different ethnic groups, and DNA methylation data from other tissues, such as saliva, which may be easier to collect.

Abbreviations

BMI: Body mass index; CHD: Coronary heart disease; CpG: 5′-Cytosine-phosphate-guanine-3′ genomic site; CRP: C-reactive protein; CVD: Cardiovascular disease; DNAm age: DNA methylation age; GOLDN: Genetics of Lipid Lowering Drugs and Diet Network (study); HDL: High-density lipoprotein; hsCRP: High-sensitivity C-reactive protein; IL2sRα: Interleukin-2 soluble receptor alpha; IL6: Interleukin-6; LDL: Low-density lipoprotein; MCP1: Monocyte chemoattractant protein-1; NMR: Nuclear magnetic resonance; PBMC: Peripheral blood mononuclear cell; TG: Triglycerides; TNFα: Tumor necrosis factor alpha; WHI: Women's Health Initiative (study)

Acknowledgements

Not applicable.

Funding

This research was funded by the US National Heart, Lung and Blood Institute grants U01 HL072524 and R01 HL104135.

Authors' contributions

MRI conceived, designed, and oversaw the analyses and drafted the manuscript. SA, DZ, BH, SAC, VS, SH, HKT, DMA, and DKA provided critical input during drafting and revision of the manuscript. AD and VS conducted the analyses. AD and SAC constructed the manuscript visuals. DMA oversaw the epigenetics laboratory. DKA conceived, designed, and oversaw the parent studies. All authors read and approved the final manusript.

Competing interests

The authors declare that they have no competing interests.

Author details

[1]Department of Epidemiology, University of Alabama at Birmingham, 1665 University Blvd, RPHB 230J, Birmingham, AL 35294, USA. [2]School of Biomedical Informatics, University of Texas Health Science Center at Houston, Houston, TX, USA. [3]College of Public Health, University of Kentucky, Lexington, KY, USA. [4]Department of Biostatistics, University of Alabama at Birmingham, Birmingham, AL, USA. [5]Human Genetics, David Geffen School of Medicine, University of California Los Angeles, Los Angeles, CA 90095, USA. [6]Biostatistics, School of Public Health, University of California Los Angeles, Los Angeles, CA 90095, USA. [7]Human Genetics, Gonda Research Center, David Geffen School of Medicine, University of California Los Angeles, Los Angeles, CA 90095-7088, USA. [8]HudsonAlpha Institute for Biotechnology, Huntsville, AL, USA.

References

1. Mather KA, Jorm AF, Parslow RA, Christensen H. Is telomere length a biomarker of aging? A review. J Gerontol A Biol Sci Med Sci. 2011;66(2):202–13. https://doi.org/10.1093/gerona/glq180.
2. Arsenis NC, You T, Ogawa EF, Tinsley GM, Zuo L. Physical activity and telomere length: impact of aging and potential mechanisms of action. Oncotarget. 2017; https://doi.org/10.18632/oncotarget.16726.
3. Pal S, Tyler JK. Epigenetics and aging. Sci Adv. 2016;2(7):e1600584. https://doi.org/10.1126/sciadv.1600584.
4. Horvath S. DNA methylation age of human tissues and cell types. Genome Biol. 2013;14(10):R115. https://doi.org/10.1186/gb-2013-14-10-r115.
5. Chen BH, Marioni RE, Colicino E, Peters MJ, Ward-Caviness CK, Tsai PC, et al. DNA methylation-based measures of biological age: meta-analysis predicting time to death. Aging (Albany NY). 2016;8(9):1844–65. https://doi.org/10.18632/aging.101020.
6. Nevalainen T, Kananen L, Marttila S, Jylhava J, Mononen N, Kahonen M, et al. Obesity accelerates epigenetic aging in middle-aged but not in elderly individuals. Clin Epigenetics. 2017;9:20. https://doi.org/10.1186/s13148-016-0301-7.
7. Marioni RE, Shah S, McRae AF, Ritchie SJ, Muniz-Terrera G, Harris SE, et al. The epigenetic clock is correlated with physical and cognitive fitness in the Lothian Birth Cohort 1936. Int J Epidemiol. 2015;44(4):1388–96. https://doi.org/10.1093/ije/dyu277.
8. Zannas AS, Arloth J, Carrillo-Roa T, Iurato S, Roh S, Ressler KJ, et al. Lifetime stress accelerates epigenetic aging in an urban, African American cohort: relevance of glucocorticoid signaling. Genome Biol. 2015;16:266. https://doi.org/10.1186/s13059-015-0828-5.
9. Pirillo A, Norata GD, Catapano AL. Postprandial lipemia as a cardiometabolic risk factor. Curr Med Res Opin. 2014;30(8):1489–503. https://doi.org/10.1185/03007995.2014.909394.
10. Munoz A, Costa M. Nutritionally mediated oxidative stress and inflammation. Oxidative Med Cell Longev. 2013;2013:610950. https://doi.org/10.1155/2013/610950.
11. Hyson D, Rutledge JC, Berglund L. Postprandial lipemia and cardiovascular disease. Curr Atheroscler Rep. 2003;5(6):437–44.
12. Hannum G, Guinney J, Zhao L, Zhang L, Hughes G, Sadda S, et al. Genome-wide methylation profiles reveal quantitative views of human aging rates. Mol Cell. 2013;49(2):359–67. https://doi.org/10.1016/j.molcel.2012.10.016.
13. Liu Y, Ordovas JM, Gao G, Province M, Straka RJ, Tsai MY, et al. Pharmacogenetic association of the APOA1/C3/A4/A5 gene cluster and lipid responses to fenofibrate: the Genetics of Lipid-Lowering Drugs and Diet Network study. Pharmacogenet Genomics. 2009;19(2):161–9. https://doi.org/10.1097/FPC.0b013e32831e030e.
14. Wojczynski MK, Parnell LD, Pollin TI, Lai CQ, Feitosa MF, O'Connell JR, et al. Genome-wide association study of triglyceride response to a high-fat meal among participants of the NHLBI Genetics of Lipid Lowering Drugs and Diet Network (GOLDN). Metabolism. 2015;64(10):1359–71. https://doi.org/10.1016/j.metabol.2015.07.001.
15. Aslibekyan S, Kabagambe EK, Irvin MR, Straka RJ, Borecki IB, Tiwari HK, et al. A genome-wide association study of inflammatory biomarker changes in response to fenofibrate treatment in the Genetics of Lipid Lowering Drug and Diet Network. Pharmacogenet Genomics. 2012;22(3):191–7. https://doi.org/10.1097/FPC.0b013e32834fdd41.
16. Patsch JR, Miesenbock G, Hopferwieser T, Muhlberger V, Knapp E, Dunn JK, et al. Relation of triglyceride metabolism and coronary artery disease. Studies in the postprandial state. Arterioscler Thromb. 1992;12(11):1336–45.
17. Kabagambe EK, Ordovas JM, Hopkins PN, Tsai MY, Arnett DK. The relation between erythrocyte trans fat and triglyceride, VLDL- and HDL-cholesterol concentrations depends on polyunsaturated fat. PLoS One. 2012;7(10):e47430. https://doi.org/10.1371/journal.pone.0047430.
18. Tsai MY, Hanson NQ, Straka RJ, Hoke TR, Ordovas JM, Peacock JM, et al. Effect of influenza vaccine on markers of inflammation and lipid profile. J Lab Clin Med. 2005;145(6):323–7. https://doi.org/10.1016/j.lab.2005.03.009.

19. Kabagambe EK, Ordovas JM, Tsai MY, Borecki IB, Hopkins PN, Glasser SP, et al. Smoking, inflammatory patterns and postprandial hypertriglyceridemia. Atherosclerosis. 2009;203(2):633–9. https://doi.org/10.1016/j.atherosclerosis.2008.08.005
20. Aslibekyan S, Do AN, Xu H, Li S, Irvin MR, Zhi D, et al. CPT1A methylation is associated with plasma adiponectin. Nutr Metab Cardiovasc Dis. 2017;27(3):225–33. https://doi.org/10.1016/j.numecd.2016.11.004.
21. Irvin MR, Zhi D, Joehanes R, Mendelson M, Aslibekyan S, Claas SA, et al. Epigenome-wide association study of fasting blood lipids in the Genetics of Lipid-lowering Drugs and Diet Network study. Circulation. 2014;130(7):565–72. https://doi.org/10.1161/circulationaha.114.009158.
22. Neurauter AA, Bonyhadi M, Lien E, Nokleby L, Ruud E, Camacho S, et al. Cell isolation and expansion using Dynabeads. Adv Biochem Eng Biotechnol. 2007;106:41–73. https://doi.org/10.1007/10_2007_072.
23. Quach A, Levine ME, Tanaka T, Lu AT, Chen BH, Ferrucci L, et al. Epigenetic clock analysis of diet, exercise, education, and lifestyle factors. Aging (Albany NY). 2017;9(2):419–46. https://doi.org/10.18632/aging.101168.
24. Horvath S, Gurven M, Levine ME, Trumble BC, Kaplan H, Allayee H, et al. An epigenetic clock analysis of race/ethnicity, sex, and coronary heart disease. Genome Biol. 2016;17(1):171. https://doi.org/10.1186/s13059-016-1030-0.
25. Gopalan S, Carja O, Fagny M, Patin E, Myrick JW, McEwen LM, et al. Trends in DNA methylation with age replicate across diverse human populations. Genetics. 2017;206(3):1659–74. https://doi.org/10.1534/genetics.116.195594.
26. Marioni RE, Shah S, McRae AF, Chen BH, Colicino E, Harris SE, et al. DNA methylation age of blood predicts all-cause mortality in later life. Genome Biol. 2015;16:25. https://doi.org/10.1186/s13059-015-0584-6.
27. Chen BH, Carty CL, Kimura M, Kark JD, Chen W, Li S, et al. Leukocyte telomere length, T cell composition and DNA methylation age. Aging (Albany NY). 2017;9(9):1983–95. https://doi.org/10.18632/aging.101293.
28. Waite LL, Weaver B, Day K, Li X, Roberts K, Gibson AW, et al. Estimation of cell-type composition including T and B cell subtypes for whole blood methylation microarray data. Front Genet. 2016;7:23. https://doi.org/10.3389/fgene.2016.00023.
29. Lourenco VM, Pires AM, Kirst M. Robust linear regression methods in association studies. Bioinformatics. 2011;27(6):815–21. https://doi.org/10.1093/bioinformatics/btr006.
30. Perna L, Zhang Y, Mons U, Holleczek B, Saum KU, Brenner H. Epigenetic age acceleration predicts cancer, cardiovascular, and all-cause mortality in a German case cohort. Clin Epigenetics. 2016;8:64. https://doi.org/10.1186/s13148-016-0228-z.
31. Singh T, Newman AB. Inflammatory markers in population studies of aging. Ageing Res Rev. 2011;10(3):319–29. https://doi.org/10.1016/j.arr.2010.11.002.

10

Promoter methylation of DNA damage repair (DDR) genes in human tumor entities: *RBBP8/CtIP* is almost exclusively methylated in bladder cancer

Jolein Mijnes[1†], Jürgen Veeck[1,2,3,4†^], Nadine T. Gaisa[1], Eduard Burghardt[1], Tim C. de Ruijter[2,3], Sonja Gostek[1], Edgar Dahl[1,4], David Pfister[5,6], Sebastian C. Schmid[7], Ruth Knüchel[1] and Michael Rose[1,4*]

Abstract

Background: Genome-wide studies identified pan-cancer genes and shared biological networks affected by epigenetic dysregulation among diverse tumor entities. Here, we systematically screened for hypermethylation of DNA damage repair (DDR) genes in a comprehensive candidate-approach and exemplarily identify and validate candidate DDR genes as targets of epigenetic inactivation unique to bladder cancer (BLCA), which may serve as non-invasive biomarkers.

Methods: Genome-wide DNA methylation datasets (2755 CpG probes of $n = 7819$ tumor and $n = 659$ normal samples) of the TCGA network covering 32 tumor entities were analyzed in silico for 177 DDR genes. Genes of interest were defined as differentially methylated between normal and cancerous tissues proximal to transcription start sites. The lead candidate gene was validated by methylation-specific PCR (MSP) and/or bisulfite-pyrosequencing in different human cell lines ($n = 36$), in primary BLCA tissues ($n = 43$), and in voided urine samples ($n = 74$) of BLCA patients. Urines from healthy donors and patients with urological benign and malignant diseases were included as controls ($n = 78$). mRNA expression was determined using qRT-PCR in vitro before ($n = 5$) and after decitabine treatment ($n = 2$). Protein expression was assessed by immunohistochemistry ($n = 42$). R 3.2.0. was used for statistical data acquisition and SPSS 21.0 for statistical analysis.

Results: Overall, 39 DDR genes were hypermethylated in human cancers. Most exclusively and frequently methylated (37%) in primary BLCA was *RBBP8*, encoding endonuclease CtIP. *RBBP8* hypermethylation predicted longer overall survival (OS) and was found in 2/4 bladder cancer cell lines but not in any of 33 cancer cell lines from entities with another origin like prostate. *RBBP8* methylation was inversely correlated with RBBP8 mRNA and nuclear protein expression while RBBP8 was re-expressed after in vitro demethylation. *RBBP8* methylation was associated with histological grade in primary BLCA and urine samples. *RBBP8* methylation was detectable in urine samples of bladder cancer patients achieving a sensitivity of 52%, at 91% specificity.

(Continued on next page)

* Correspondence: mrose@ukaachen.de
†Equal contributors
^Deceased
[1]Institute of Pathology, RWTH Aachen University, Pauwelsstr. 30, 52074 Aachen, Germany
[4]RWTH Centralized Biomaterial Bank (RWTH cBMB), Medical Faculty, RWTH Aachen University, Aachen, Germany
Full list of author information is available at the end of the article

(Continued from previous page)

Conclusions: *RBBP8* was identified as almost exclusively hypermethylated in BLCA. *RBBP8*/CtIP has a proven role in homologous recombination-mediated DNA double-strand break repair known to sensitize cancer cells for PARP1 inhibitors. Since *RBBP8* methylation was detectable in urines, it may be a complementary marker of high specificity in urine for BLCA detection.

Keywords: RBBP8/CtIP, DNA repair, Bladder cancer/BLCA, Epigenetics, Infinium HumanMethylation450 BeadChip, Urine biomarker

Background

Molecular characterization of cancer entities based on cohorts of tumor samples from all major organs created a wealth of data, allowing researchers to identify mutational landscapes across different cancer types. These studies provided novel insides into genomic signatures independent of tissue of origin [1], highlighting driver mutations potentially suitable for targeted therapies [2–4]. Next to druggable mutations, the cancer epigenome, known to regulate gene expression, holds clues to identify novel biomarkers and therapeutic approaches improving patient stratification. Genome-wide studies have recently identified pan-cancer DNA methylation (DNAm) patterns among diverse tumor entities, e.g., affected by genetic alterations in epigenetic regulators like *DNMT3* (reviewed in Witte et al. [5]). Still, the co-existence of unique DNAm patterns indicates that also entity-specific and subtype-specific targets of epigenetic deregulation could lead to the development of distinct methylation phenotypes contributing to tumorigenesis. These specific epigenetic aberrations, also referred to as epimutations, may uncover novel targets to improve disease management in many respects.

So far, DNA methylation is proposed as a molecular biomarker for cancer detection [6] but also as a biomarker for prediction and stratification of patients with risk of distinct clinical outcome and response to therapies [7]. Owing to this, methylation of DNA repair genes in general seems to be a good pool for prediction [8–12] of how patients respond to treatment with conventional chemotherapies as well as novel classes of targets such as poly (ADP-ribose) polymerase (PARP) inhibitors. Examples of predictive methylated genes are *MGMT* in glioma (temozolomide) [13, 14], *BRCA1* in breast cancer (PARP1 inhibitors, cisplatin, and chemotherapy) [15–18], and *PRKCDBP* in colon cancer (oxaliplatin) [19], among others.

In the presented study, we were, therefore, interested to reveal whether differential DNAm patterns of DNA repair genes of the DNA damage response (DDR) network were common epimutations across cancer entities, especially in those known to be impaired in DNA repair function, such as bladder cancer [20] which showed an essentially stagnant disease management since decades [21]. Since there is, to our knowledge, no systematic screen for hypermethylation of DNA repair genes, we performed a comprehensive candidate approach comprising 177 DDR genes [22] as targets of epigenetic deregulation in 32 tumor entities. Subsequently, we exemplarily aimed at the validation of the identified lead candidate gene, *RBBP8*, to assess potential biomarker performance based on a non-invasive detection approach.

Accumulating studies propose *RBBP8*, known to encode the endonuclease CtIP [23], as a novel susceptibility gene [24] whose functional loss increases sensitivity towards PARP1 inhibition [25, 26] similar to *BRCA1* inactivation as, for instance, recently demonstrated in a mice xenograft model of breast cancer [27]. Mechanistically, RBBP8, a nuclear located protein that is conserved among vertebrates, interacts with tumor suppressors such as BRCA1 and the pRb family members through binding sites that are frequently mutated in human cancers [24]. As part of the DDR network, RBBP8/CtIP has a proven role as key factor in regulating DNA-end resection and double-strand break (DSB) repair mechanisms [28, 29] by supporting homologous recombination (HR) [30], classical non-homologous end-joining (c-NHEJ) [31, 32], and alternative non-homologous end-joining (alt-NHEJ) [33]. Thus, RBBP8/CtIP is thought to be involved in the maintenance of genome integrity in a cell cycle- and DNA damage-dependent manner [34, 35]. Here, we demonstrate that *RBBP8* whose unique hypermethylation pattern in human bladder cancer was associated with its gene silencing might serve as a biomarker that can be accessed via urine tests.

Results

DNAm pattern in promoter regions of DDR genes in 32 different human cancer types

Our first aim was to identify novel DNA repair genes as targets of epigenetic inactivation unique to human cancer types, which may finally be used as a non-invasive methylation biomarker. The study design is illustrated in Additional file 1. Based on the Infinium HumanMethylation450 dataset of the publically available *The Cancer Genome Atlas* (TCGA) platform, genome-wide DNA methylation data of 7819 primary tumor samples and 659 normal samples comprising 32 tumor entities (Table 1) was assessed. Overall, we performed an integrated analysis by defining CpG probe groups including initially 2755 CpG probes (sites) located between 2000 bp downstream

Table 1 TCGA studies and sample numbers used for DNA methylation analyses in this study

Study	Study name/tumor entity	Tumors	Normals
ACC	Adrenocortical carcinoma	79	0
BLCA	Bladder urothelial carcinoma	368	17
BRCA	Breast invasive carcinoma	772	96
CESC	Cervical squamous cell carcinoma and endocervical adenocarcinoma	299	3
CHOL	Cholangiocarcinoma	35	9
COAD	Colon adenocarcinoma	265	30
DLBC	Lymphoid Neoplasm Diffuse Large B-Cell Lymphoma	47	0
ESCA	Esophageal carcinoma	182	13
GBM	Glioblastoma multiforme	129	2
HNSC	Head and neck squamous cell carcinoma	481	50
KICH	Kidney chromophobe	60	0
KIRC	Kidney renal clear cell carcinoma	271	141
KIRP	Kidney renal papillary cell carcinoma	243	34
LGG	Brain lower grade glioma	498	0
LIHC	Liver hepatocellular carcinoma	360	45
LUAD	Lung adenocarcinoma	399	22
LUSC	Lung squamous cell carcinoma	337	36
MESO	Mesothelioma	82	0
OV	Ovarian adenocarcinomas	10	0
PAAD	Pancreatic adenocarcinoma	155	7
PCPG	Pheochromocytoma and paraganglioma	152	3
PRAD	Prostate adenocarcinoma	476	40
READ	Rectum adenocarcinoma	91	7
SARC	Sarcoma	244	0
SKCM	Skin cutaneous melanoma	102	1
STAD	Stomach adenocarcinoma	300	2
TGCT	Testicular germ cell tumors	149	0
THCA	Thyroid carcinoma	484	54
THYM	Thymoma	122	2
UCEC	Uterine Corpus Endometrial Carcinoma	404	45
UCS	Uterine carcinosarcoma	56	0
UVM	Uveal melanoma	80	0

and 500 bp upstream of the reported transcription start sites (TSS) of 177 DDR genes. Subsequently, we focused on those genes whose CpG probe set with a putative regulatory impact met the following criteria: A probe set specific and (healthy-) normalized β value cutoff of ~ 0.25 (β value ~ 0.25 (90% CI 0.20–0.35)) after transformation to M values (see the "Methods" section). By that, 39 DDR genes were found to show methylation in a fraction of ≥ 5% of samples in one or more entities (see heatmap in Fig. 1). This includes known epigenetic silenced DDR genes with a therapeutic impact like *BRCA1* [17, 18], *MGMT* [13, 14], and *ERCC1* [36, 37] (Additional file 2). In addition (to these already known DDR genes), we were also able to identify novel potential targets like SLX1A which has not yet been associated with DNA methylation in tumors so far. The identified DDR genes can be classified into all essential subnetworks of DNA repair mechanisms [22], i.e., mismatch repair (MMR, e.g., *MLH1*), homologous repair (HR, e.g., *RBBP8/CtiP*), dissolution of joint DNA molecules (JMs, e.g., *TOP3A*), nucleotide excision repair (NER, e.g., *ERCC1*), and base excision repair (BER, e.g., *PARP1*).

We then reduced the selected list of candidates (i.e., CpG probe groups) by focusing on genes exhibiting hypermethylated in more than 15% of cases in at least one tumor entity with a minimum of ten analyzed normal tissue samples (Additional file 3). The list of genes with stringently tumor-specific hypermethylation includes, for instance, *ERCC1, MGMT, POLD1,* and *RBBP8/CtiP*. In all cases, hypermethylation was entity-specific as demonstrated by the conducted cluster analysis (see Fig. 1) and statistical testing applied to contingency tables of tumor samples (entity vs. relationship to the threshold, $p < 10^{-6}$).

Finally, an association between promoter methylation of defined CpG probe sets and mRNA expression of the corresponding gene across tumor types was assessed to narrow down potential candidate genes and entities for the subsequent biomarker discovery part of this study. To ensure valid statistics, only DDR genes exceeding a methylation frequency of > 5% in identified tumor entities were included. Based on that, 9 out of the identified 14 candidate genes (see Additional file 3) passed our criteria, i.e., showed a highly significant (i.e., $p < 0.001$) association with their gene expression in one or more tumor entities like *PER1* and *POLD1* (see Additional file 4). Among others (such as *ALKBH2* and *ALKBH3*), *MGMT* promoter methylation, for instance, showed a strong inverse correlation in all analyzable tumor entities (i.e., COAD, DLBC, ESCA, GBM, HNSC, LGG, READ, STAD, TGCT).

RBBP8 is almost exclusively methylated in bladder cancer correlating with lower *RBBP8* mRNA expression and a favorable prognosis

In bladder cancer, 3 out of these identified 39 DDR genes, i.e., *SLX1A*, *ERCC1*, and *RBBP8*, exhibited hypermethylation over 15%. Interestingly, *RBBP8* was almost exclusively methylated in bladder cancer (Fig. 2a–c). Overall, 137 out of 368 (37%) analyzed bladder tumors exhibited a tumor-specific *RBBP8* promoter methylation. The normal adjacent tissues showed methylation in 2 out of 17 cases. Nevertheless, the methylation was notably lower than that of the matching tumor tissues (β values 0.26 vs. 0.53 and 0.30 vs. 0.71) which might be due to an epigenetic field effect across the urothelium of bladders with cancer (e.g., [38]). Moreover, *RBBP8* promoter methylation was only

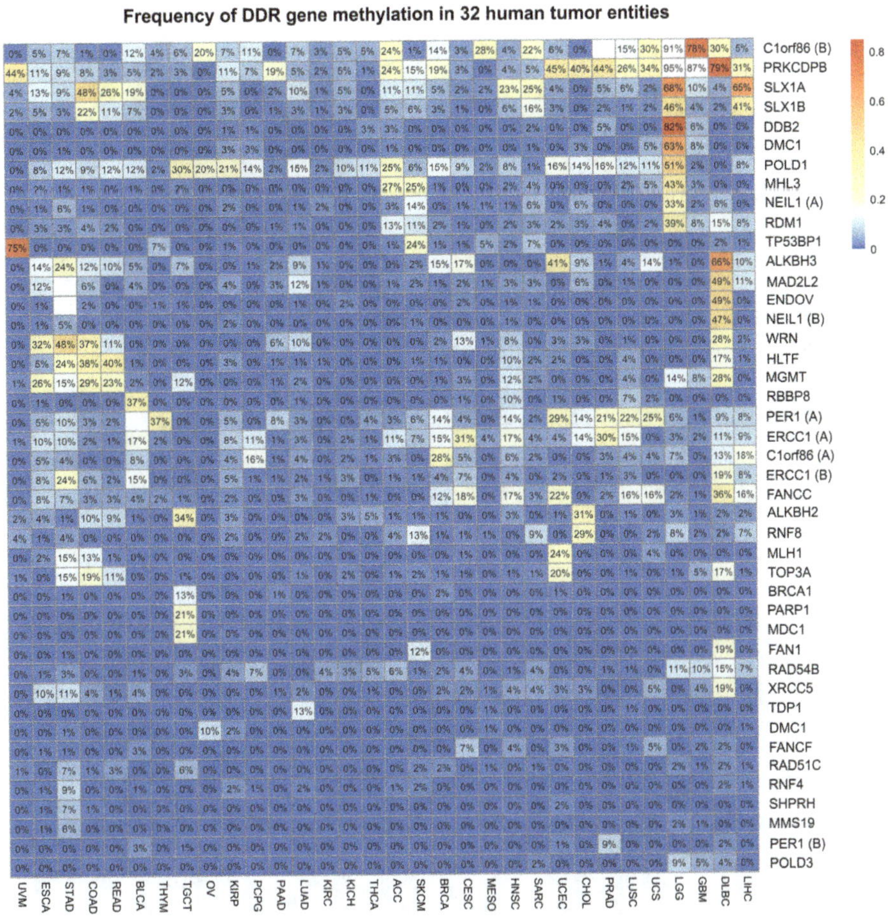

Fig. 1 Discovery analysis of DNAm pattern in promoter regions of DNA damage repair genes across tumor entities. Promoter methylation of DDR genes was present in 32 different tumor entities. The heatmap summarizes the conducted analysis of the Infinium HumanMethylation450 BeadChip data available from the TCGA project (see the "Methods" section for details). Only those genes (CpG groups near TSS (s)) for which at least one tumor entity exhibited a hypermethylation of more than 5% of cases are shown. Fields for which corresponding normal tissues were hypermethylated in more than 15% are not shown (white). Note: The tumor entities ACC, DLBC, KICH, LGG, MESO, OV, SARC, TGCT, UCS, and UVM were included despite missing corresponding normal tissue samples. Fields were clustered hierarchically in both dimensions

present at low frequency in head and neck squamous cell carcinoma (9.6%, $n = 46/481$), lung squamous carcinoma (7.1%, $n = 24/337$), uterine carcinosarcoma (1.8%, $n = 1/56$), cervical squamous cell carcinoma (1.3%, $n = 4/299$), esophageal carcinoma (1.1%, $n = 2/182$), and lung adenocarcinoma (1.0%, $n = 4/399$). In all other analyzed cancer types, *RBBP8* methylation frequency was lower than 1.0%. A multiple t tests using the Holm correction for multiple comparison analysis confirmed a significantly increased methylation frequency of *RBBP8* in bladder cancer compared to all other tested tumor entities ($p < 0.019$). In addition, a significantly inverse correlation between *RBBP8* methylation (CpG probe set as defined) and *RBBP8* mRNA expression (Spearman r −0.32; $p < 0.001$) was only demonstrated for BLCA (Fig. 2d). No association was observed for HNSC and LUSC, and *RBBP8* was thereof chosen as a lead candidate gene of this study for bladder cancer.

Given entity-specific methylation of *RBBP8* in BLCA, we aimed to provide a first insight on whether this epigenetic modification may provide a clinical impact in this entity. We divided the dataset (overall $n = 405$, for cohort characteristics see Additional file 5) into low methylated (RBBP8 β values ($\beta \leq 0.4$)) and highly methylated ($\beta > 0.4$) tumor samples and found that a prevalent loss of *RBBP8* mRNA expression was only present in tumors with high *RBBP8* promoter methylation compared to normal bladder tissue (Fig. 2e). The close association between loss of *RBBP8* mRNA expression and *RBBP8* hypermethylation was confirmed by using a Fisher's exact test (Table 2). Further associations of *RBBP8* methylation with clinicopathological characteristics were evaluated as well (Table 2), which showed a significant association of *RBBP8* methylation with higher histological tumor grade ($p = 0.041$). No further correlations between *RBBP8* methylation and clinicopathological

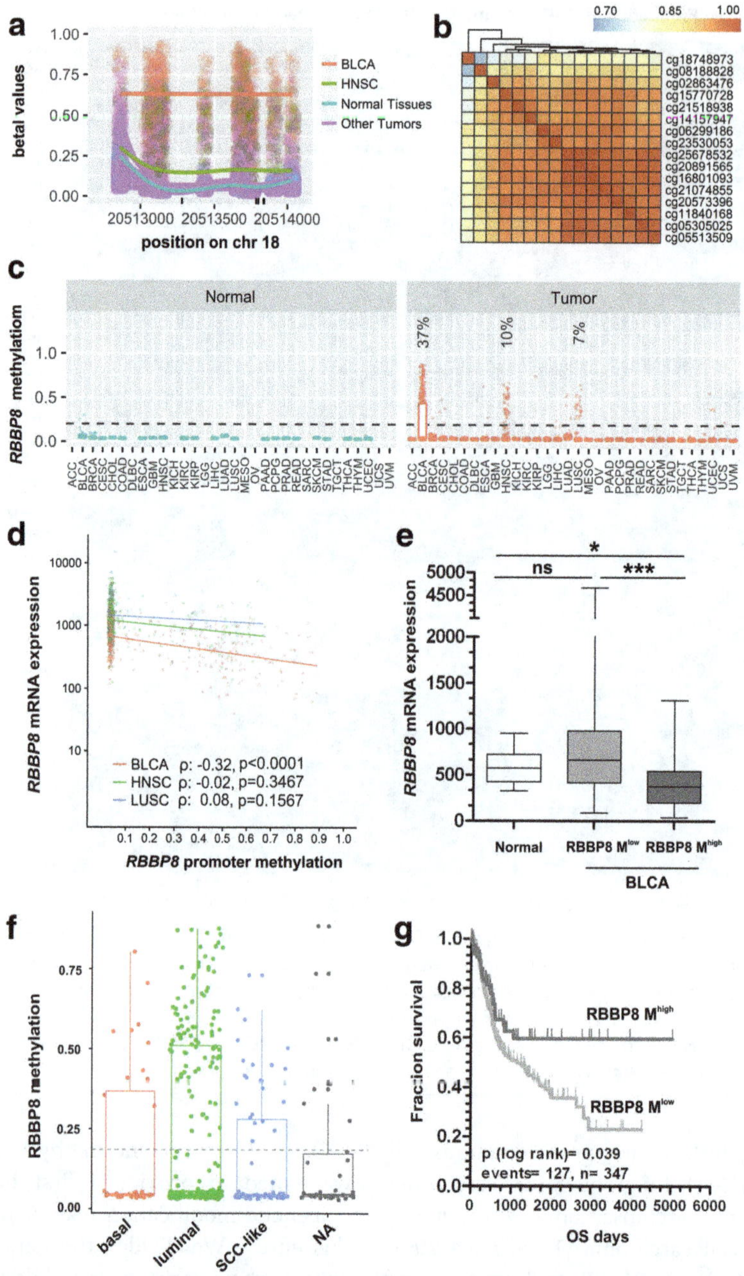

Fig. 2 *RBBP8* promoter methylation in bladder cancer of the TCGA data set. **a** Visualization of the promoter methylation of the *RBBP8* gene as a scatterplot. The β values for each sample were jittered around the probe location and plotted as points. The per sample type 90% quantiles of methylation are shown as smoothed lines. The colors represent different sample groups (BLCA, bladder cancer; HNSC, head-neck squamous cell carcinoma). **b** The Pearson correlation coefficients (ρ) for probe pairs in the core region of the promoter are shown as heatmap demonstrating a high degree of correlation between probes ($\rho > 0.7$). **c** The beta values of all probes of the promoter region were summarized by their median value, stratified by the sample as well as tissue type, and visualized as a box plot. For *RBBP8* gene loci, a frequent hypermethylation ($\beta > 0.25$ in > 5% of cases) was only observable in 37, 10, and 7% of bladder urothelial carcinoma (BLCA), head-neck squamous cell carcinoma (HNSC), and lung squamous cell carcinoma (LUSC), respectively. **d** Inverse correlation between *RBBP8* methylation (defined CpG gene set) and *RBBP8* mRNA expression in primary bladder cancer (BLCA), neck squamous cell carcinoma (HNSC), and lung squamous carcinoma (LUSC) samples of the TCGA data portal. Spearman correlation BLCA: – 0.32, $p < 0.001$; Spearman correlation HNSC: – 0.04, p = ns; Spearman correlation LUSC: 0.08, p = ns. **e** Box plot illustrates significant downregulation of RBBP8 methylation in primary tumors featuring increased *RBBP8* promoter methylation (β value > 0.4). Horizontal lines — grouped medians. Boxes — 25 to 75% quartiles. Vertical lines — range, peak, and minimum. *$p < 0.05$, **$p < 0.01$, ns: not significant. **f** Box plot shows *RBBP8* methylation in primary tumors classified by intrinsic subtypes. **g** Kaplan-Meier survival curves display overall survival (OS) of patients with high *RBBP8* methylation (β value > 0.4, dark gray curve) compared to low *RBBP8* methylation (β value ≤ 0.4, gray curve) based on TCGA datasets

Table 2 Clinicopathological parameters in relation to *RBBP8* promoter methylation of the BLCA TCGA dataset

	RBBP8 promoter methylation[b]			
	n[a]	low	high	*p* value[c]
Parameter:				
Gender				
Male	259	190	69	0.062
Female	94	78	16	
Histological tumor grade				
Low grade	20	19	1	*0.041*
High grade	330	247	83	
Tumor stage				
pT1-pT2	109	86	23	0.49
pT3-pT4	216	163	53	
pN status				
Negative	212	161	51	0.866
Positive	112	86	26	
pM status				
Negative	173	131	42	0.138
Positive	7	7	0	
RBBP8 mRNA[d]				
Low	200	124	76	*≤ 0.001*
High	200	175	25	

Significant *p* values are in italics
[a]Only patients with primary bladder cancer without any neoadjuvant therapy were included
[b]Based on TCGA 450K DNA methylation analysis
[c]Fisher's exact test
[d]RBBP8 mRNA expression was dichotomized at the median expression level

Table 3 Univariate analysis of clinicopathological parameters influencing OS

	Overall survival (OS)		
	n[a]	Events	*p* value[b]
Parameter:			
RBBP8 methylation[c]			
RBBP8 M^{low}	262	103	*0.039*
RBBP8 M^{high}	85	24	
Gender			
Male	253	91	0.920
Female	94	36	
Histological tumor grade[d]			
Low grade	15	0	0.066
High grade	329	127	
Tumor stage			
pT1-pT2	105	23	*≤ 0.001*
pT3-pT4	214	94	
pN status			
Negative	207	53	*≤ 0.001*
Nositive	111	63	
pM status			
Negative	168	52	*0.004*
Positive	7	5	

Significant *p* values are in italics
[a]Only patients with primary bladder cancer without any neoadjuvant therapy were included
[b]Log-rank test at the two-sided significance level of 0.05

characteristics were found. Classifying tumor samples by subtype, i.e., "luminal," "basal," and "SCC-like," [39] *RBBP8* promoter methylation tended to be enriched in luminal-type bladder tumors (Fig. 2f).

As dysregulation of DDR repair is known to be associated with patients' outcome, we examined overall survival (OS) as an indicator of potential clinical impact. By Kaplan-Meier analysis, we found that patients with high *RBBP8* methylation have a longer overall survival (mean OS 3197.4 days ± 310.3; 95% CI 2589.3 to 3805.5 days) compared to low *RBBP8* methylation (mean OS 1800.6 days ± 161.4; 95% CI 1484.1 to 2117.0 days) (Fig. 2g, Table 3). The multivariate hazard ratio of 0.650 (95% CI 0.312 to 1.354, $p = 0.249$) underlines a decreased risk for tumor death, although independency statistically failed in comparison to known prognostic parameters (Additional file 6).

RBBP8 methylation is exclusively present in human bladder cancer cell lines and functionally associated with *RBBP8* mRNA expression after DAC treatment

In silico analysis of the *RBBP8* gene promoter sequence using genomic DNA information (ENSEMBL contig ENS00000101773) showed a CpG-rich island between genomic positions 20512942 and 20513943 (− 353 to + 648 bp relative to the expected transcription start site (TSS: transcript variante #1: position 20513295) on chromosome 18q which met the following criteria: DNA region ≥ 200 bp; Obs/Exp ≥ 0.6; and % GC ≥ 50. The DNA region including CpG sites that are closely associated to the TSS encodes a potential regulatory core promoter and ubiquitous elements for gene regulation as determined by in silico analysis using Genomatix [40]. In order to specify the TCGA data sets, we designed both a methylation-specific PCR (MSP) and bisulfite-pyrosequencing assay close to the TSS area to screen *RBBP8* methylation status in a large set of normal and cancer cell lines from various cancer entities. The analyzed promoter region upstream of the transcription start is illustrated in Fig. 3a.

Using MSP, a methylated *RBBP8* promoter was detected in two (RT4 and RT112) out of four bladder cancer cell lines which derived from stage 2 and higher grade bladder tumors [41], while *RBBP8* was unmethylated in normal urothelial cells (UROtsa) (Fig. 3b). The analyzed *RBBP8* promoter region was also unmethylated in 33 further cancerous cell lines, i.e., cell lines from

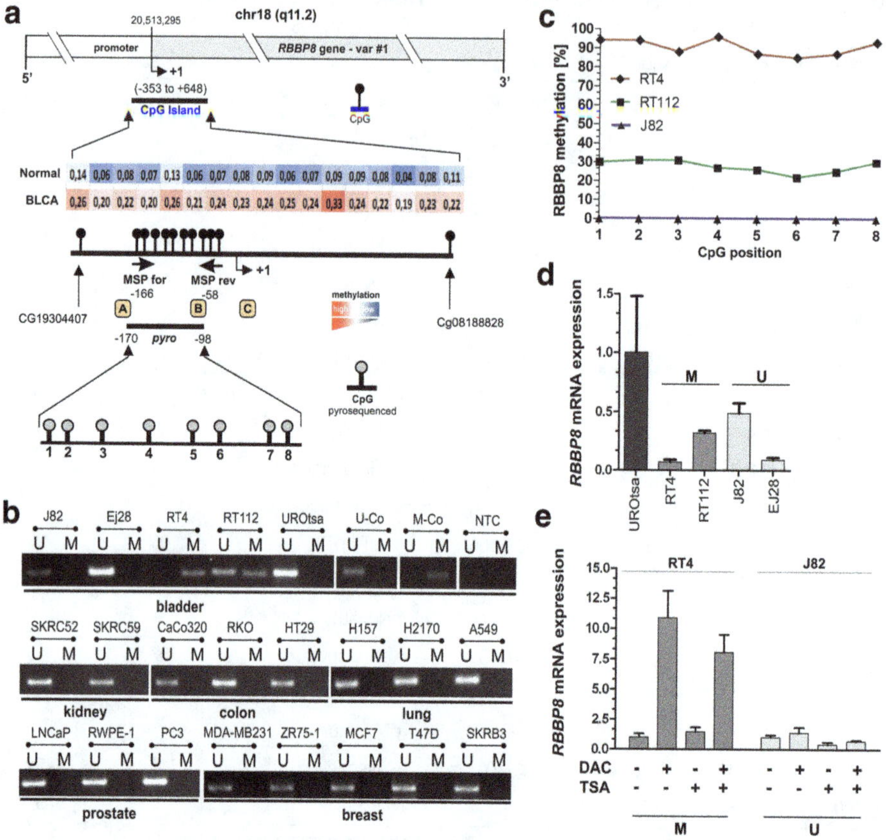

Fig. 3 *RBBP8* promoter methylation in human cancer cell lines. **a** Schematic map of the human *RBBP8* gene including the relative positions and median *β* values of 17 CpG sites based on 450K methylation array profiling in bladder cancer (TCGA dataset) within a predicted CpG island (between base − 353 and + 648). Colored boxes present methylation level (mean *ß*-values for each CpG site) of the TCGA data set. Red, high methylation; blue, low methylation. + 1, *RBBP8* transcription start site (TSS) of variant #1. The dots indicating the methylation sites closer to where they are depicted. CpG sites analyzed by MSP (black arrows) were indicated within the upstream promoter region close to the TSS. The relative position of the promoter area analyzed by bisulfite-pyrosequencing that comprises eight single CpG sites (gray dots) is shown as a black line. Orange boxes illustrate gene transcription-relevant regulatory core and ubiquitous elements statistically identified by using Genomatix [40] software (http://www.genomatix.de/). A — core promoter motif ten elements (− 200 to − 179); B — activator protein 2 (− 109 to − 94); C — activator-, mediator-, and TBP-dependent core promoter element for RNA polymerase II transcription from TATA-less promoters (+ 28 to + 39). **b** Representative MSP results of the *RBBP8* promoter methylation status in cell lines of bladder, kidney, colon, lung, prostate, and breast cancer. Bands labeled with U and M reflect unmethylated and methylated DNA, respectively. Bisulfite-converted unmethylated, genomic (U-co), and polymethylated, genomic (M-co) DNA were used as positive controls. NTC, non-template control. **c** *RBBP8* mean methylation values of analyzed CpG sites (1 to 8) using bisulfite-pyrosequencing of bladder cancer cell lines (RT4, RT112, and J82). **d** *RBBP8* mRNA expression in normal urothelial cells (UROtsa) and bladder cancer cell lines (RT4, RT112, J82, and EJ28) arranged in relation to their *RBBP8* promoter methylation status. U, unmethylated; M, methylated. Error bars: + s.e.m. **e** qPCR analysis for *RBBP8* mRNA expression after in vitro demethylation analysis demonstrating a clear *RBBP8* re-expression after treatment with both DAC (+) and TSA (+) only in RT4 with methylated *RBBP8* promoter status (M) whereas in J82 cells without any *RBBP8* methylation (U) *RBBP8* expression was not further inducible. Non-treated cells served as controls and were set to 1. Error bars: + s.e.m.

breast cancer, lung cancer, prostate cancer, colorectal cancer, and renal cancer (see the complete list in Additional file 7). Strong *RBBP8* promoter methylation in RT4 (median methylation level 90.5%) and RT112 bladder cancer cells (median methylation level: 28.5%) was confirmed by using bisulfite-pyrosequencing covering the MSP product sequence (Fig. 3c).

In all bladder cancer cell lines (RT4, RT112, J82, and EJ28), *RBBP8* mRNA was lower expressed than in normal UROtsa cells. Lowest mRNA expression was found in RT4 cells which featured the highest methylation level as well (Fig. 3d). Functionally, we confirmed this epigenetic modification as a molecular cause for *RBBP8* gene regulation by in vitro demethylation experiments. Seventy-two hours after 5-aza-2′-deoxycytidine (decitabine (DAC)) and trichostatin A (TSA) treatment upregulation of *RBBP8* mRNA expression (FC = 11) was demonstrated in RT4 tumor cells. DAC treatment without TSA supplementation already triggered an increase in *RBBP8* mRNA expression in RT4 bladder cancer cells. Treatment with both DAC and

TSA leads to a maximum of *RBBP8* mRNA re-expression. In turn, *RBBP8* mRNA was not further inducible by DAC/TSA in J82 bladder cancer cells (Fig. 3e) harboring an unmethylated *RBBP8* promoter (see Fig. 3c). These findings indicate that epigenetic alterations of the *RBBP8* gene may be caused by synergistic crosstalk between DNA methylation and histone modification.

Validation of DNAm pattern within the *RBBP8* promoter close to the TSS in primary bladder tumors

Based on MSP and bisulfite-pyrosequencing, *RBBP8* methylation was assessed in an independent cohort of primary bladder tumors. MSP analysis confirmed an unmethylated *RBBP8* promoter in healthy urothelial tissues. *RBBP8* methylation frequency was increased to 39.1% (9/23) in primary bladder tumors (Fig. 4a). None of the papillary low-grade tumors ($n = 9$) showed *RBBP8* methylation, whereas 9 out of 14 invasive BLCAs were methylated for the *RBBP8* locus. We subsequently analyzed the methylation status of eight CpG sites using pyrosequencing (Fig. 4b). The median *RBBP8* methylation for each CpG is shown in Fig. 4b for both normal urothelium and bladder tumors ($n = 20$). Nine out of 20 tumor (45%) samples showed a median *RBBP8* methylation level (including all eight CpGs) of > 5% (range 6 to 62.5%). Classifying the bladder tumors by papillary and invasive subtype, no clear differences in *RBBP8* promoter methylation were detected (Fig. 4c). However, a significant increased *RBBP8* promoter methylation was observed for high-grade bladder tumors, including pTa high-grade carcinomas, (mean methylation 20.9%; s.d. ± 4.4%) compared to low-grade BLCA (mean methylation 2.4%; s.d. ± 1.4%) (Fig. 4d). A close association between *RBBP8* and higher histological tumor grade ($p = 0.041$) was also confirmed by Fisher's exact test (Additional file 8).

RBBP8 protein expression in bladder cancer

RBBP8 protein expression was characterized in normal urothelium and in bladder tumor tissues using immunohistochemistry. We found RBBP8 protein staining in the cytoplasm and frequently in the nuclei of the normal urothelium (Fig. 5a). Advanced bladder tumors showed a similar cytoplasmatic protein level, but only sporadically a nuclear protein localization was observed (Fig. 5c–e). Interestingly, low-grade non-invasive bladder tumors retained high levels of RBBP8 protein within the nucleus (Fig. 5f).

This observation was confirmed by quantification of RBBP8 protein staining according to an adapted immunoreactive score (IRS) developed by Remmele and Stegner [42] in both the cytoplasm and the nuclei. Overall, 42 bladder carcinomas were compared evaluating the average RBBP8 protein expression in a semi-quantitative manner (for cohort characteristics, see Additional file 9). Cytoplasmatic RBBP8 protein expression remained visible in all

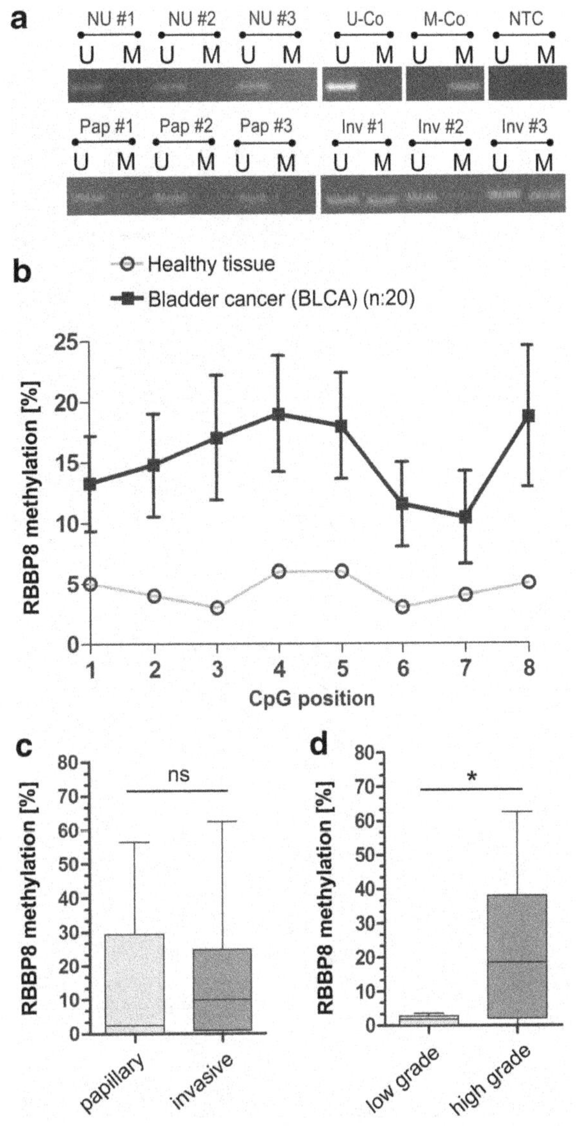

Fig. 4 Validation of *RBBP8* promoter methylation in primary bladder tumors. **a** Representative MSP analysis shows the *RBBP8* promoter methylation status of normal urothelium (NU) and both papillary (Pap) and invasive (Inv) primary bladder cancer tissues. Band labels with U and M represent an unmethylated and methylated DNA locus, respectively bisulfite-converted unmethylated, genomic (U-co) and polymethylated, genomic (M-co) DNA were used as positive controls. NTC: non-template control. **b** *RBBP8* mean methylation values of analyzed CpG sites (1 to 8) of healthy controls and bladder tumors demonstrating tumors-specific hypermethylation. **c** to **d** Box plot analysis of *RBBP8* methylation in primary bladder tumors is based on mean values of pyrosequenced CpG sites 1–8. **c** *RBBP8* methylation shows no significant differences between the two bladder cancer pathways (papillary and invasive tumors). **d** Significant enrichment of *RBBP8* methylation is demonstrated in high-grade bladder tumors. Horizontal lines—grouped medians. Boxes—25 to 75% quartiles. Vertical lines—range, peak, and minimum; $*p < 0.05$. Horizontal lines—grouped medians. Boxes—25 to 75% quartiles. Vertical lines—range, peak, and minimum; ns, not significant, $*p < 0.05$

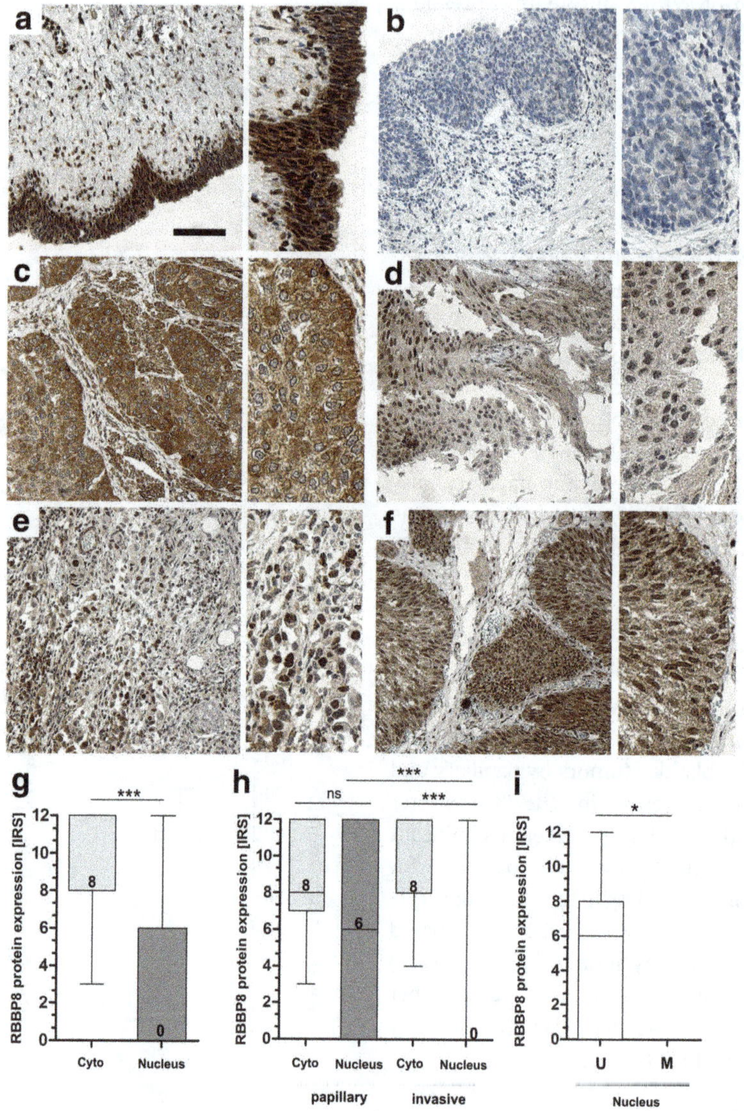

Fig. 5 RBBP8 protein loss in nuclei of bladder tumors. Immunohistochemical RBBP8 protein staining of representative tissues are shown. **a** Strong RBBP8 immunoreactivity was detected in the cytoplasm and in the nuclei of a healthy urothelium, Scale bar: 100 μm. **b** Negative control of urothelial cell layers. The application of primary antibody was omitted. **c** Strong RBBP8 immunoreactivity in the cytoplasm of high grade, invasive tumor cells which completely lack nuclear staining. **d** Moderate cytoplasmatic and heterogeneously nuclear RBBP8 protein staining in invasive tumor cells. **e** Low RBBP8 protein expression in the cytoplasm of invasive bladder cancer showing strong RBBP8 staining in the nucleus. **f** Strong nuclear and cytoplasmic RBBP8 staining in non-invasive, papillary tumor cells. **g** Box plot demonstrating overall significant loss of RBBP8 protein only in the nucleus of bladder tumors. **h** Box plot graph illustrates the loss of RBBP8 protein within the nuclei of high-grade invasive bladder tumors. **i** Box plot shows a significant RBBP8 protein loss in tumors harboring RBBP8 promoter methylation. U, unmethylated; M, methylated. Horizontal lines — grouped medians. Boxes — 25 to 75% quartiles. Vertical lines — range, peak, and minimum; ns, not significant, $*p < 0.05$, $***p < 0.001$

bladder tumors (median IRS, 8). In contrast, 71.4% ($n = 30/42$) of the analyzed bladder tumors exhibited a significant loss of RBBP8 protein expression in the nuclei with an IRS score below 3 (median IRS, 0) (Fig. 5g). Stratifying the tumor samples by substage, we revealed that the observed loss of nuclear RBBP8 protein significantly correlates with advanced invasive (pT1-pT4) bladder tumors, while pTa non-invasive tumors did not significantly differ in cytoplasmic and nuclear RBBP8 protein level (Fig. 5h).

We did not observe any association between cytoplasmatic RBBP8 staining and clinicopathological parameters. As RBBP8 is a known DNA repair protein that is functionally located in the nucleus (see for instance protein-staining pattern of breast cancer cells [43]), we further focused on nuclear RBBP8. Nuclear RBBP8 protein was significantly reduced in invasive tumors compared to papillary tumors (see Fig. 5h). A close association between loss of nuclear RBBP8 protein and both advanced tumor stages and high-grade BLCA was significantly illustrated by a Fisher's exact test (Table 4). A significant downregulation of RBBP8 protein expression in nuclei was demonstrated for bladder tumors with an increased *RBBP8* promoter methylation (> 5%) compared to those with a low *RBBP8* methylation (Fig. 5i). In line, a statistically inverse correlation between nuclear RBBP8 protein level and *RBBP8* promoter methylation was confirmed (Table 4), supporting a contribution of epigenetic *RBBP8* alterations to its protein loss in primary bladder tumors.

RBBP8 methylation is specifically detectable in urine samples derived from bladder cancer patients

As *RBBP8* is highly methylated in bladder tumor tissue, *RBBP8* methylated DNA might also be detectable in urine samples from bladder cancer patients. Therefore, urine sediments from bladder cancer patients ($n = 22$) and healthy controls ($n = 10$) were initially assessed for *RBBP8* methylation by MSP (for cohort characteristics see Additional file 10). DNA methylation of *RBBP8* was present in 11 out of 22 cancerous urine samples (50%) (Fig. 6a). In contrast, none of the control samples from healthy donors was tested positive for *RBBP8* methylation.

Table 4 Clinicopathological parameters in relation to nuclear RBBP8 protein expression

	RBBP8 IRS[b] nuclear				
	n^a	Low	High	*p* value[c]	Spearman *r*
Parameter:					
Age at diagnosis					
< 70 years	23	14	9	0.213	− 0.195
≥ 70 years	19	15	4		
Gender					
Male	33	25	8	0.075	− 0.278
Female	9	4	5		
Tumor subtype					
Non-invasive papillary	17	8	9	*0.012*	− 0.392
Invasive	25	21	4		
Histological tumor grade[d]					
Low grade	12	4	8	*0.002*	− 0.489
High grade	30	25	5		
Tumor stage[d]					
pT1-pT2	13	9	4	*0.040*	− 0.419
pT3-pT4	12	12	0		
RBBP8 methylation					
Low	11	5	6	*0.020*	− 0.564
High	7	7	0		

Significant *p* values are in italics
[a]Only patients with primary bladder cancer were included
[b]Score (IRS) according to Remmele and Stegner [42]
[c]Fisher's exact test
[d]According to WHO 2004 classification

Next, we assessed *RBBP8* methylation using bisulfite-pyrosequencing in a collective (overall $n = 103$, see Table 5) comprising 52 BLCA-derived and 51 control urine samples. Control samples included inflammatory urological diseases and malignancies of the urological tract other than bladder cancer. Please note that the used control cohort which is enriched for urological malignancies does not reflect the epidemiological composition as found in populations, but served only to evaluate entity specificity of RBBP8. Quantification of *RBBP8* methylation allows specification of cutoff levels, which are necessary for an objective assessment of biomarker performance. Summarized data of the mean *RBBP8* methylation ratio for each CpG site of BLCA-derived and control urine set #1 (including healthy, inflammatory, and benign samples) and set #2 (including set #1 samples plus testicular germ cell tumors (TGCT) and prostate adenocarcinoma (PRAD) samples) is shown in Fig. 6b. *RBBP8* methylation was clearly increased, up to 88%, in urines from bladder cancer patients. As previously observed in primary bladder cancer, *RBBP8* promoter methylation detected in urines strongly correlates with high-grade tumors (Fig. 6c). This observation was statistically confirmed using a Fisher's exact test (Table 6). Interestingly, *RBBP8* mean methylation of control urines from patients diagnosed with cystitis and benign prostatic hyperplasia (BPH) was nearly similar to healthy controls. In turn, a few urines from young patients with a testicular neoplasm (mostly seminomas) showed an increased mean *RBBP8* methylation (Fig. 6d).

In order to evaluate its diagnostic potential, we performed receiver operating characteristics (ROC) curve analysis to calculate the optimal cutoff value for *RBBP8* as single marker, with a high specificity. ROC curve statistics were performed based on the two CpG sites with the strongest discrimination impact; the methylation ratio between cancerous BLCA urines and both the benign and malignant control set revealed strongest differences for CpG number #7 and #8 (see Fig. 6b). There was no significant difference between benign and malignant control urine samples, while *RBBP8* methylation based on "best CpG sites" was highly significantly increased in BLCA-derived urines (Fig. 7a). Accordingly, *RBBP8* methylation significantly discriminates between bladder cancer patients and non-malignant patients with a sensitivity of 51.9% and a specificity of 90.9% (AUC 0.730, 95% CI 0.616–0.844) (Fig. 7b). In case of 100% specificity, *RBBP8* methylation as a single biomarker still showed a true positive rate of 25% (see Table 7). The control cohort consisted of patients with an inflammatory and benign diagnosis (benign control set). Additionally, the single *RBBP8* marker was able to distinguish bladder cancer patients from patients with neoplasms of another urological origin (malignant control set) with high specificity (90.8%, AUC 0.686, 95% CI 0.583–0.789).

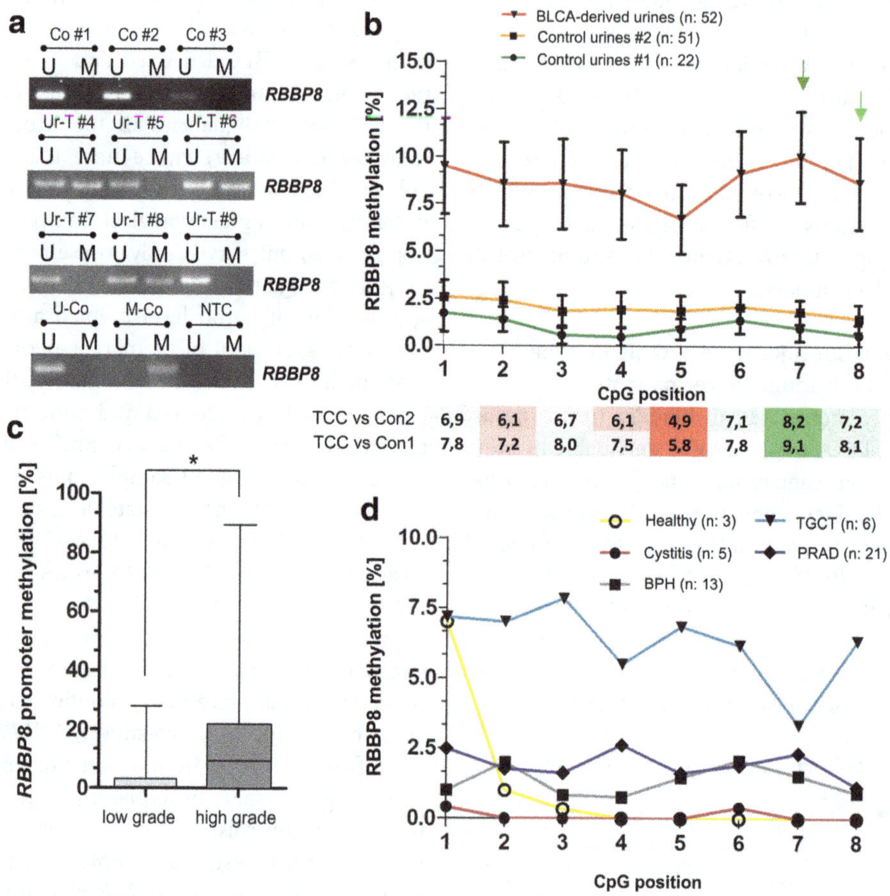

Fig. 6 *RBBP8* promoter methylation is detectable in urines from bladder cancer patients. **a** Representative MSP analysis shows the *RBBP8* promoter methylation status of human urine samples derived from healthy controls (Co) and bladder tumors (Ur-T). Band labels with U and M represent an unmethylated and methylated DNA locus. Bisulfite-converted unmethylated, genomic (U-co), and polymethylated, genomic (M-co) DNA were used as positive controls. NTC, non-template control. **b** Upper graph: *RBBP8* mean methylation values of analyzed CpG sites (1 to 8) in cancerous bladder diseases (BLCA-derived) and two control cohorts (benign: control urines #1 and malignant: control urines #2) using pyrosequencing. Lower heatmap: Differences of *RBBP8* methylation between BLCA-derived urines and both control conditions (benign and malignant) highlighting GpG sites (#7 and #8) with the strongest impact for discrimination (see green arrows). **c** Box plot demonstrating a significant increase of *RBBP8* methylation in high-grade bladder tumors. Horizontal lines — grouped medians. Boxes — 25 to 75% quartiles. Vertical lines — range, peak, and minimum; $*p < 0.05$. **d** *RBBP8* mean methylation values of analyzed CpG sites (1 to 8) of controls classified by diseases. BPH, begin prostate hyperplasia; TGCT, testicular germ cell tumors; PRAD, prostate adenocarcinoma

Sensitivity was however reduced to 40.4% (Fig. 7c). Thus, beyond a possible prognostic or predictive relevance of RBBP8 loss in human cancers, its promoter methylation may be suitable for diagnostic or monitoring applications in bladder cancer. Since a *RBBP8* methylation frequency of approximately 40% is found in bladder cancer, sensitivity is limited. Consequently, a combined application as part of a biomarker panel will be necessary to increase the true positive rate of detection.

Discussion

Dysfunction of DNA damage repair (DDR) genes in human cancer is common and, so far, mostly considered to be triggered by genetic alterations [44]. Yet, in 2015, Gao et al. proposed a notable clinical value of epigenetic alterations in distinct DDR genes in human cancer [12]. To our best knowledge, our study provides for the first time a systematic analysis of the epigenetic configuration of DNA repair genes involved in the DNA damage response across human cancer entities. As DDR genes are known to be important targets for novel therapeutic strategies [8–11] the genome-wide epigenetic configuration within promoter regions of DDR genes can be used to identify novel targets of epigenetic alterations. These targets may hold clues for non-invasive biomarker applications with predictive impact.

In the presented study, tumor-specific epigenetic deregulation of DDR genes was found to be a common event in human cancer. Statistical analysis of genome-wide 450K methylation array data identified 39 out of 177 DDR genes, whose promoter regions close to the TSS

Table 5 Clinicopathological parameters of urine samples analyzed in this study by pyrosequencing

Categorization	*n*	% analyzable
Controls:	51	
Age (median 69)		
≤ 69 years	28	54.9
> 69 years	23	45.1
Gender		
Male	48	94.1
Female	3	5.9
Diagnosis		
Disease-free	3	5.9
Cystitis	5	9.8
Benign prostatic hyperplasia	13	25.5
Prostate cancer	21	41.2
Testicular tumor	6	11.8
Other	3	5.9
BLCA asscociated[a]	52	
Age (median 71)		
≤ 71 years	27	51.9
> 71 years	25	48.1
Gender		
Male	42	80.8
Female	10	19.2
Histological tumor grade[b]		
Low grade	19	36.5
High grade	30	57.7
NA	3	5.8
Tumor stage[b]		
pTa	21	40.4
pTis	3	5.8
pT1	11	21.2
pT2	8	15.4
pT3	7	13.5
pT4	2	3.8

[a]Only urine samples of patients preoperatively diagnosed with primary bladder cancer (UC, without any other malignancy) were included
[b]According to WHO 2004 classification

Table 6 Clinicopathological parameters in relation to *RBBP8* promoter methylation in BLCA associated urine samples

	RBBP8 promoter methylation[b]			
	n[a]	Low	High	*p* value[c]
Parameter:				
Gender				
Male	42	31	11	0.687
Female	10	8	2	
Histological tumor grade				
Low grade	19	17	2	*0.046*
High grade	30	19	11	
Tumor stage				
pTa	21	19	2	*0.021*
pT1-pT4	28	17	11	
pN status				
Negative	5	3	2	0.931
Positive	8	5	3	

Significant *p* values are in italics
[a]Only patients with primary bladder cancer were included
[b]RBBP8 methylation was dichotomized at the Q75 (based on pyrosequencing)
[c]Fisher's exact test

were hypermethylated in one or several tumor entities. Most tumor entities were characterized by hypermethylation of distinct DDR genes. Among others, polymerase delta (*POLD1*) methylation was enriched in 24 out of 32 different tumor types, implying an essential role in DNA repair or tumor suppression independent of tumor entity. This includes COAD and LIHC, i.e., entities which have been associated with increased somatic mutation rates [4]. Unrepaired DNA damage is a major source of potential mutagenic lesions driving tumorigenesis, and loss of DNA repair pathways is thought to accelerate the accumulation rate of additional mutations by 100 to 1000 times [45]. The *POLD1* gene is highly conserved and encodes for the p125 subunit which provides the essential catalytic activity of polymerase δ (Polδ), mediating a key role in genome stability [46]. This raises the question whether or how methylation of the identified DDR genes may help to establish mutator phenotypes affecting the prevalence of somatic mutations in distinct tumor types. Weisenberger et al. previously revealed a close association between the CpG island methylator phenotype (CIMP), microsatellite instability, and increased BRAF mutation in COAD [47]. Moreover, sporadic cases of mismatch repair deficiency occur almost exclusively as a consequence of CIMP-associated *MLH1* methylation, a DNA repair gene involved in MMR and microsatellite instability [48], whose hypermethylation close to the TSS was confirmed for COAD in the presented study.

Beyond, our findings may provide novel implications for therapies, as DNA damage repair dysregulation sensitizes cancer cells for DNA damaging agents [12]. Novel biomarkers with a clear prognostic or predictive impact are urgently required to identify those patients likely to respond favorably to such therapy, for instance, in BLCA. There is no significant progress in systemic therapy for muscle-invasive bladder cancer (MIBC) since decades [21, 49] with the exception of immunotherapeutic approaches like PDL-1 blocking antibodies [50]. Due to the lack of biomarkers [51], disease management of BLCA and hence the selection of an adequate therapy are difficult and often insufficient [52]. Here, we show that 2%, i.e., 6 out of 368 bladder

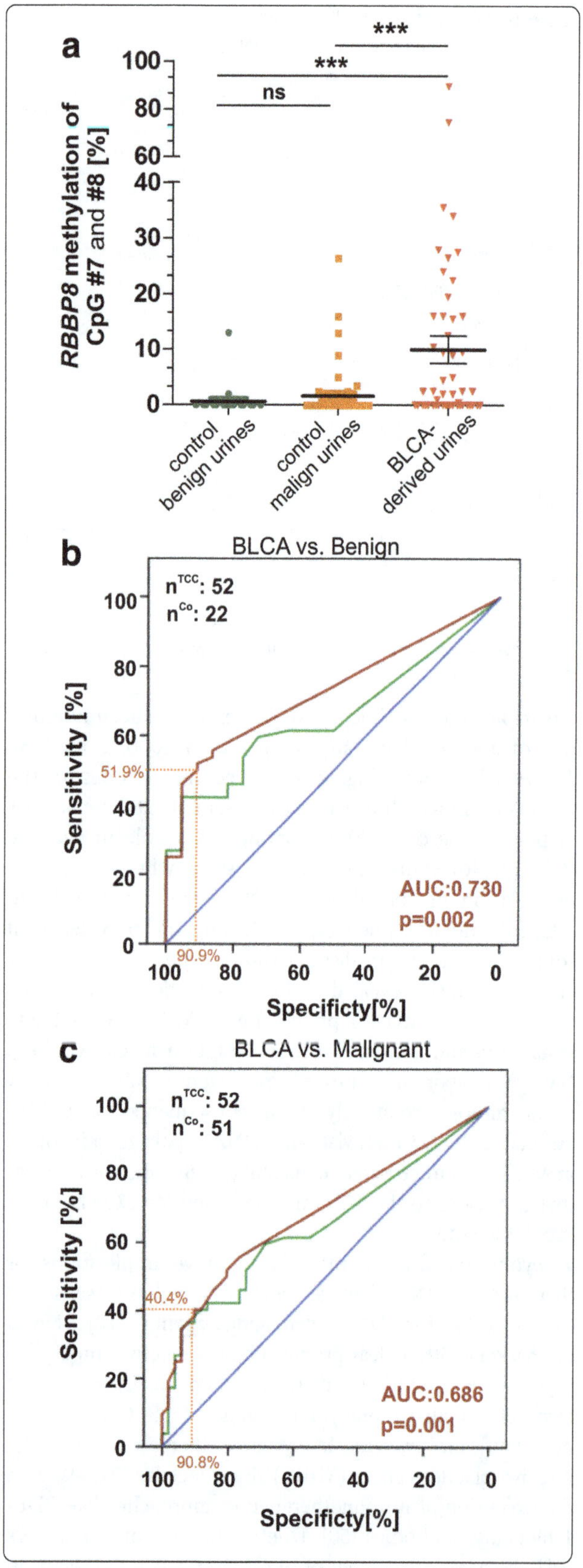

Fig. 7 Biomarker performance of *RBBP8* methylation based on a non-invasive approach. **a** *RBBP8* methylation enables significant discrimination of cancerous bladder diseases from two control conditions (benign and malignant) using urine samples. The scatterplot shows the mean methylation values of the CpG sites #7 and #8; ns, not significant; ***$p < 0.0001$. **b** to **c** ROC curve analysis illustrating RBBP8 single-biomarker performance based on all analyzed CpG sites (green curve) and CpG site #7 and #8 (red curve). **b** ROC curve in benign disease controls. Red curve (CpG #7 and #8): the cutoff value of 1.25% methylation was defined for positive detection of disease; in that case, *RBBP8* methylation achieved a specificity of 90.9% and a sensitivity of 51.9%. Area under the curve (AUC) 0.730 (95% CI, 0.616 to 0.844), $p = 0.002$. **c** ROC curve in malignant (prostate and testicular cancer) disease controls. Red curve (CpG #7 and #8): the cutoff value of 4.00% methylation was defined for positive detection of disease; in that case, *RBBP8* methylation achieved a specificity of 90.2% and a sensitivity of 40.4%. Area under the curve (AUC) 0.686 (95% CI, 0.583 to 0.789), $p = 0.001$

patients, showed O6-methylguanine-DNA methyltransferase (*MGMT*) promoter hypermethylation which is in line with previous reports [53–55]. The *MGMT* promoter status has been shown to predict response to alkylating agents in glioblastoma patients [13, 14], and in times of personalized and precision medicine even such low case numbers could be of clinical significance. Furthermore, the excision repair cross-complementing group 1 (*ERCC1)* gene, encoding for a known key enzyme of the nucleotide excision repair (NER) pathway [56], was found frequently methylated in BLCA, up to 17%. Accumulating studies propose ERCC1 protein expression as a prognostic and predictive biomarker for platinum resistance in various tumor entities [37, 57] including bladder cancer [36, 58]. In BLCA, for instance, ERCC1-negative tumors could benefit from adjuvant chemotherapy combining gemcitabine and cisplatin [36], but its predictive impact remains controversial [59]. Future studies addressing the potential clinical impact of *ERCC1* and the relation between its promoter methylation and gene silencing are important. Such a functional consequence would offer the development of predictive biomarkers based on a stable analyte (i.e., DNAm) which can be efficiently detected in bodily liquids like urine, in analogy

Table 7 RBBP8 biomarker performance

Cutoff	Specificity (%)	Sensitivity (%)	AUC	*p* value	Control group
RBBP8 CpG #7 and #8					
14.25	100	25.0	0.730	0.002	Benign
1.25	90.9	51.9			
14.25	96.1	25.0	0.686	0.001	Malignant
4.00	90.2	40.4			
RBBP8 CpG all					
11.75	100	26.9	0.660	0.030	Benign
0.69	77.3	51.9			
11.75	96.1	26.9	0.649	0.009	Malignant
3.94	90.2	38.5			

to the here exemplarily identified and validated DDR lead candidate gene *RBBP8/CtiP* in BLCA.

RBBP8/CtiP has a proven role in homologous recombination-mediated DNA double-strand break repair (HR and NHEJ pathway) [30, 32, 33], impairment of which reduces DNA repair fidelity and may promote genome instability [34, 60] also in urothelial carcinomas. Already in 2006, genomic analysis described bladder cancer as significantly impaired in DNA repair [20]. Here, we demonstrate for the first time that *RBBP8* is almost exclusively methylated in primary BLCA, suggesting the development of methylation phenotypes in a distinct molecular context. *RBBP8* methylation was confirmed to be tumor-specific in up to 45% of analyzed BLCA patients. A close association between *RBBP8* methylation and its gene expression in primary tumors as well as after demethylation treatment in vitro indicate that *RBBP8* methylation could be responsible for its gene inactivation. Hence, it seems unlikely that entity-specific *RBBP8* methylation is a silent passenger event without relevance, and we propose loss, or at least reduction, of RBBP8 mediated DNA repair function in BLCA. Interestingly, *RBBP8* methylation correlates with a favorable prognosis in the BLCA TCGA dataset. Functionally, the RBBP8 protein is known to interact with BRCA1 [61], guiding HR by recruiting Dna2 to damage sites, thus ensuring a robust DSB resection necessary for efficient homologous recombination [30]. Previously, it has been shown that BRCA1/2 deficiency results in cellular sensitivity to chemotherapy [9, 62, 63]. For example, *BRCA1* methylation has been revealed to predict significantly higher response rates to cisplatin treatment in breast and ovarian cancer patients [17], which is also traditionally used as the first-line agent in bladder cancer disease management [21]. Cisplatin-induced inter-strand adducts can lead to DNA lesions (double-strand breaks) which are regularly removed by the machinery of HR [64]. Unrepaired inter-strand cross-links as consequence of reduced RBBP8 function may thereof sensitize tumor cells to chemotherapy treatment as well. Considering that a high *RBBP8* methylation frequency correlates with increased survival of BLCA patients, *RBBP8* methylation might be a potential biomarker for better therapy response in such subsets of patients; however, further investigation is necessary to validate this hypothetical notion. Nevertheless, accumulating studies already functionally demonstrated the involvement of RBBP8 on sensitizing breast [27] and ovarian cancer cells [26] for PARP inhibitor treatment in a similar way as *BRCA1* mutations, thus unveiling novel therapeutic options for a significant subset of patients which may benefit from such approach.

The field of liquid biopsy is rapidly evolving [65] and shows that biomarkers can be detected in biological fluids like blood or urine, offering an easy and non-invasive application in diagnosis of and therapy prediction in cancer. Application of liquid biopsy tools are of importance in bladder cancer, as its clinical management remains challenging due to its high recurrence rate (up to 70%) [66] in the first 2 years after diagnosis, requiring a lifetime of surveillance, i.e., BLCA patients undergo multiple invasive procedures. One of these methods is the cystoscopy, representing the gold standard test for the detection of bladder cancer, achieving an operator-dependent sensitivity over 90%. Cystoscopy is however associated with significant discomfort, possible risk of infection, and high costs [67, 68]. Current guidelines recommend the application of non-invasive urine cytology testing complementary to cystoscopic assessment. Nevertheless, cytology is characterized by poor sensitivity, especially for low-grade and low-stage tumors like CIS [69]. In addition, previously developed non-invasive diagnostic tools, such as the "BladderCheck (point-of-care) Test" based on the protein marker NMP22, either lack sensitivity or specificity [69]. Urine-based tests assessing aberrant DNA methylation are emerging as a potential tool for cancer detection [6], and various studies described the identification of novel DNA methylation-based biomarkers. Nevertheless, although both multiple biomarker tests and single-biomarker candidates like *Vimentin* [70] were able to provide prognostic information, they did not show any predictive impact. In addition, specificity across tumor entities is disregarded in most studies. Here, we demonstrate that *RBBP8* hypermethylation was accessible through a non-invasive urine test. Using *RBBP8* as a methylation biomarker, BLCA could be detected with a 25% sensitivity (at maximal specificity of 100%) in urines from BLCA patients, i.e., enabling to distinguish early cancerous (CIS), high-grade urothelial, and even papillary subtype tumors, which are difficult to detect by urine cytology, from non-cancerous and benign ones. At 90.9% specificity, the sensitivity of *RBBP8* was even increased up to 51.9%. Importantly, in comparison to a control urine cohort including urological malignancies like prostate and testicular cancer, we were still able to detect over 40% of primary bladder tumors with high specificity. Hence, we provide a novel biomarker candidate, i.e., *RBBP8*, which has previously been shown to sensitize tumor cells for PARP1 inhibitors and which may improve entity-specificity for monitoring, early detection, and clinical management of bladder cancer in a urine biomarker panel.

Conclusions

In the current study, we systemically screened for epigenetic configuration of DNA repair genes involved in the DNA damage response (DDR) across 32 human cancer entities and identified 39 methylated DDR genes which may be important targets for novel therapeutic strategies.

This includes known epigenetic silenced repair genes like *MGMT, MLH1,* and *ERCC1* but also novel targets of epigenetic dysregulation like *RBBP8/CtiP,* which has a proven role in homologous recombination-mediated DNA double-strand break repair and is further known to sensitize cancer cells for PARP1 inhibitors. *RBBP8* was almost exclusively hypermethylated in bladder cancers and was detectable by a non-invasive approach in urines from bladder cancer patients. Hence, *RBBP8* might serve as a complementary biomarker of high specificity that can be accessed through a urine test. Further investigation of mechanisms involving RBBP8 may deliver novel therapeutic options for bladder cancer patients, finally highlighting RBBP8 as a predictive biomarker as well.

Methods

Reagents

The DNA methyltransferase (DNMT) inhibitor 5-aza-2′-deoxycytidine (decitabine (DAC); 1 mM in phosphate-buffered saline (PBS)) and the histone deacetylase inhibitor trichostatin A (TSA; 1 mM in PBS) were obtained from Sigma-Aldrich. Drugs were stored in aliquots at − 80 °C.

Cell lines

Unless stated otherwise, cell lines were obtained from the American Type Culture Collection (ATCC, Rockville, MD) and cultured as recommended by the vendor. ATCC provides molecular authentication in support of their collection through their genomics, immunology, and proteomic cores, as described, by using DNA barcoding and species identification, quantitative gene expression, and transcriptomic analyses. Cells were tested negative for mycoplasma infection before and after experiments. The 37 used cell lines were UROtsa (normal bladder urothelium), RT4, RT112, EJ28, J82 (bladder cancer), RWPE-1 (normal prostate epithelium), LNCaP, PC3, DU145 (prostate cancer), SKRC1, SKRC10, SKRC52, SKRC59 (clear cell renal cell carcinoma), HCT-116, RKO, CACO2, COLO205, HT29, SW480, CACO320 (colorectal cancer), MCF10A, MCF12A, MCF7, T-47D, ZR75-1, BT474, SKBR3, MDA-MB-231, MDA-MB-436, MDA-MB-468, UACC3199, HCC1937, BT20 (breast cancer), A549, H157, and H2170 (lung cancer).

Formalin-fixed paraffin-embedded tissue specimens

Tissues of primary bladder tumors and normal urothelium were obtained from the archives of the Institute of Pathology (RWTH Aachen University). The anonymized and retrospective study was approved by the local Ethics Committee (EK 122/04, 173/06, and 206/09). For cohort characteristics of analyzed samples, see Additional file 8. Only manually microdissected samples were used for *RBBP8* methylation analysis. RBBP8 protein expression was evaluated using whole tissue sections or tissue microarrays with representative tissue cores of 1.5 mm diameter.

Human urine samples

Voided urine samples from patients diagnosed with a primary bladder tumor ($n = 52$) were used to assess biomarker performance. Urine samples of patients with a known second malignancy such as prostate cancer were excluded from the study. Urines from healthy donors ($n = 13$) and samples derived from patients with 5 inflammatory (chronic cystitis), 13 benign (benign prostate hyperplasia), and 27 urological malignant diseases (testicular tumors and prostate cancer) served as controls. For cohort characteristics, see Table 5 and Additional file 10. All urine specimens were obtained from the RWTH centralized biomaterial bank (RWTH cBMB) and the Technical University of Munich. All patients gave written consent for retention and analysis of their samples according to local Institutional Review Board (IRB)-approved protocols of the Medical Faculty of RWTH Aachen University and the Technical University of Munich. For each sample, 20 ml of (morning) urines were centrifuged for 10 min at 2000×*g*, and sediments were stored at − 80 °C.

Genome-wide methylation analysis using TCGA data sets

Data retrieval

Infinium HumanMethylation450 BeadChip data (level 2) and RNASeqV2 data (level 3) of the tumor and normal tissue samples were obtained from the TCGA data portal [1–4]. Samples with any annotations reported via the TCGA annotation portal were excluded from the analyses. The β value of methylation was calculated according to Bibikova et al. [71] for all CpG probes with a detection p value ≤ 0.05. Probes with a detected p value above the threshold were classified as unmeasured. Multiple measurements per tumor were averaged after log-transformation of expression data and transformation of methylation data to M values [72]. In total, 7819 tumors and 659 normal samples were included in the differential CpG methylation analysis (Table 1). Five thousand one hundred ninety-one tumor samples were included in the correlation analysis of gene expression and CpG methylation. A summary of the TCGA samples that used both datasets can be found in Additional file 11.

Identification of CpG sites close to TSS of DDR genes

A list of 177 DNA damage repair genes was used for genome-wide analysis of which none was located on the sex chromosomes (Additional file 12). Information on gene location and transcription start sites (TSS) was obtained from the Ensembl database. For each gene, CpG probes (probe = CpG site) located 2000 bp downstream to 500 bp upstream of a reported TSS were determined.

Definition of probe sets near a TSS

An exploratory data analysis was performed to identify genomic regions with tumor-specific methylation, i.e., showing unmethylated CpGs in available normal tissue samples. In brief, clusters of TSS were identified (hierarchical clustering with single linkage; cut at a height of 2000 bp). Available methylation data from normal tissues were then visualized (see Additional file 13) in the regions surrounding the TSS clusters. Probes of CpGs in continuously unmethylated ($\beta < 0.25$) regions were grouped together as a set. Based on both the entity-specific patterns of methylation in tumor tissues (see Additional file 13) and the correlation coefficients between CpG sites (see Additional file 13), probe sets were further classified to define CpG (probe) sets with a putative regulatory impact within promoter regions of DDR genes. This approach led to the identification of one to four CpG (probe) sets for most candidate genes (170 out of 177). The majority (140 out of 170) of these genes showed only one CpG set, while for some genes, two (20 out of 170), three (2 out of 170) or four (1 out of 170) sets were considered. The detailed definition of used CpG probe sets for DDR genes can be found in the supplementary data (Additional file 14).

Determination of entity-specific frequency of hypermethylation

Given the definition of CpG probe sets as promoter regions potentially involved in gene regulation of the corresponding DDR gene, frequency of hypermethylation in tumor tissues from different entities was calculated for each gene. With respect to known characteristics of used tumor samples (i.e., the contamination with stromal cells (e.g., fibroblasts) in up to 40% of TCGA specimens; the copy number variations or whole genome duplications (e.g., [73]); and lastly, the prevalence of subclones) which could affect tumor-associated allele frequencies, a stepwise prioritization strategy with adjusted β value thresholds was conducted.

A CpG set specific methylation value was determined by the calculation of the median methylation level for each sample. Secondly, as the M value is more statistically valid for the differential analysis of methylation levels [72], a probe set specific ($\Delta\beta_{co}$) cutoff for the tumor samples was derived jointly from all available normal samples after transformation to M values as the arithmetic mean plus three standard deviations. To further ensure robust confirmation of these findings by alternative methods such as pyrosequencing of sodium bisulfite converted DNA (e.g., [74, 75]), we increased this cutoff by a β value of 0.1 (see Additional file 14), hence defining minimum β value differences ($\Delta\beta_{co}$) of 0.1–0.2 between normal and tumor samples which is in line with previous studies (e.g., [76]). In practice, a set specific β value above approximately 0.25 (90% CI 0.20–0.35) was considered to indicate hypermethylation of TSS regions in tumor samples. The fraction of samples with a hypermethylation event was calculated for each tumor entity separately.

In vitro genomic DNA demethylating treatment

For gene re-expression experiments, cells were seeded at 2.5×10^4 cells/cm^2 in 6-well plates. After overnight attachment, the DNMT inhibitor DAC was added and renewed every 24 h. For a combined treatment with a histone deacetylase inhibitor, TSA was added at 300 nM to cells 16 h prior to RNA extraction. After 72 h, cells were harvested, and RNA was extracted.

Nucleic acid extraction from cell lines, FFPE tissues, and urines

Sections of archival formalin-fixed paraffin-embedded (FFPE) tissue samples were microdissected, when necessary, deparaffinized in xylene, and re-hydrated in a decreasing alcohol series prior to nucleic acid extraction. Genomic DNA of bladder samples was isolated using the QIAamp® DNA Mini kit (Qiagen, Hilden, Germany). Total RNA from cell lines was extracted using the TRIzol® (Life Technologies) method according to the manufacturers' instructions.

Sediments of urine samples stored at − 80 °C were subjected to DNA extraction using the ZR Urine DNA Isolation Kit (ZR, Zymo Research, Orange, Ca, USA) following the manufacturer's instructions. The DNA yield (ng/ml urine) and purity (A_{260}/A_{280}) were determined by using the NanoDrop (Thermo Fisher Scientific, Waltham, MA, USA). Only extractions from urines with a minimal amount of 100 ng genomic DNA and a ratio of > 1.5 were finally used for MSP and pyrosequencing analyses. Note that the extracted DNA derived from FFPE tissue samples are known to be more fragmented and altered compared, for instance, to DNA from urines. Therefore, results like methylation frequencies may slightly differ between both materials.

Bisulfite conversion and methylation-specific PCR

Five hundred nanogram of the genomic DNA was bisulfite-converted for 16 h using the EZ DNA Methylation™ kit (Zymo Research, Freiburg, Germany) according to the manufacturer's instructions. Bisulfite-converted DNA was eluted in 20 μl of TRIS-EDTA buffer. MSP was performed as previously described [77]. In brief, 150 to 500 ng of converted DNA was amplified using MSP primers (designed by using MethyPrimer software [78]; for primers, see Additional file 15) that specifically met the following criteria: (1) In order to validate TCGA datasets, MSP primers recognizing either the unmethylated or methylated *RBBP8* gene sequence, covered CpG sites also used in the TCGA data analysis. (2) To reveal whether the epigenetic alteration could be responsible for *RBBP8* gene inactivation, which is a requirement for a causative impact on therapeutic responses, designed MSP primers annealed closely to the TSS (core promoter region). The EpiTect® PCR Control DNA Set (Qiagen) was used as positive controls for unmethylated and methylated DNA. Amplified products were visualized on 2% agarose gels (Biozym, Hessian Oldendorf, Germany) containing ethidium bromide (AppliChem, Darmstadt, Germany) and illuminated under UV light.

Bisulfite-pyrosequencing

In order to assess *RBBP8* methylation in detail, pyrosequencing of eight CpG sites was performed that are located in the *RBBP8* promoter area close to the transcription start site. The *RBBP8* pyrosequencing assay was designed by using the Pyromark Assay Design Software (Qiagen), and all primers are listed in Additional file 16. Initially, a 136-bp fragment of the *RBBP8* promoter region including CpG sites of both the complete MSP amplicon and the TCGA analysis was amplified by using the PyroMark PCR Kit (Qiagen). Degenerate PCR primers assured unbiased DNA amplification independently of the methylation status. A 73-pb region of the PCR amplicon, referred to as the sequence of interest, was subsequently sequenced covering eight CpG sites. Methylation ratio for each CpG of the *RBBP8* promoter was quantified based on the PyroMark96 ID device and the PyroGoldSQA reagent Kit (Qiagen) as previously specified [79].

Reverse transcription and quantitative RT-PCR

One microgram of the total RNA was reverse transcribed using the Reverse Transcription System (Promega, Mannheim, Germany). qRT-PCR was accomplished on an iQ5 Real-Time PCR Detection System (Bio-Rad, München, Germany) together with the iQ™ SYBR® Green Supermix (Bio-Rad) including 5 μM of intron-spanning oligonucleotide primers (see Additional file 17) and 20 ng of cDNA in a 20 μl reaction volume. The cycling profile was 95 °C for 10 min, followed by 40 cycles of 95 °C for 30 s and 60 °C for 60 s. All reactions were run in triplicate, and post-amplification melting curve analyses assessed the product specificity. Gene expression relative to the housekeeping gene glyceraldehyde 3-phosphate dehydrogenase (*GAPDH*) was calculated by the $\Delta\Delta C_T$ method [80].

RBBP8 immunohistochemistry

Immunohistochemical staining of RBBP8 protein was performed after heat-induced antigen retrieval (EnVision™ FLEX Target Retrieval Solution, Low pH, K8005, DAKO PT-Link, DAKO, Hamburg, Germany) according to the manufacturer's protocols. Primary anti-RBBP8 antibody (dilution 1:200) (Atlas Antibodies, HPA039890, Sigma-Aldrich, Germany) was linked with DAKO EnVision™-FLEX system and visualized with DAKO Liquid DAB Substrate Chromogen System in a DAKO Autostainer plus (K8024, K3468, DAKO). RBBP8 protein staining was quantified by a pathologist using an adapted immunoreactive scoring system (IRS) according to Remmele and Stegner [42].

Statistical analyses

Data analyses and statistical correlations of TCGA datasets were performed using R Statistical Software version 3.2.0 [81] (R Foundation for Statistical Computing, Vienna, Austria). The parameters of beta distributions were estimated by the maximum likelihood estimator implemented in the *RPMM* package [82]. Two-sided p values less than 0.05 were considered significant. In order to compare two groups, the non-parametric Mann-Whitney U test was implemented, whereas in case of more than two groups, the Dunn's multiple comparison test was used. Statistical associations between clinicopathological and molecular factors were determined by Fisher's exact test using SPSS software version 22.0 (SPSS Inc., Chicago, USA). Survival curves for overall survival (OS) were calculated using the Kaplan-Meier method with log-rank statistics. OS was measured from surgery until death and was censored for patients alive without evidence of death at the last follow-up date. Multivariate Cox regression analysis was performed to test for an independent prognostic value of *RBBP8* methylation. Receiver operating characteristics (ROC) curves were calculated to assess biomarker performance of *RBBP8* methylation in urine samples [83].

Additional files

Additional file 1: Schematic map of the underlying study design comprising the discovery and the validation step.

Additional file 2: Detailed frequency of DNAm of *BRCA1*, *MGMT*, and *ERCC1* across cancer entities and corresponding normal tissues.

Additional file 3: Heatmap of tumor-specific DNAm of DDR genes across cancer entities.

Additional file 4: Graphs illustrating the correlation between DDR gene hypermethylation and their gene expression tumor entities.

Additional file 5: This table illustrates the clinicopathological parameters of 405 bladder cancer specimens of the TCGA network analyzed in this study.

Additional file 6: This table summarizes the results from the multivariate Cox regression analysis including all factors influencing overall survival.

Additional file 7: This table lists the *RBBP8* methylation in human cell lines analyzed by MSP.

Additional file 8: This table shows the results of bivariate correlation statistics (Fisher exact test) between clinicopathological parameters and *RBBP8* methylation.

Additional file 9: A table is shown characterizing 42 bladder cancer specimens analyzed in this study by IHC.

Additional file 10: This table summarizes the clinicopathological parameters of urine samples analyzed in this study by MSP.

Additional file 11: List of 177 DDR genes analyzed in this study.

Additional file 12: This dataset illustrates a summary of the TCGA samples used in this study.

Additional file 13: Illustrating the definition of probe sets near a TSS using three different genes (*RBBP8*, *MGMT*, and *LIG4*).

Additional file 14: This dataset summarizes the beta values according to a defined cutoff of 0.1.

Additional file 15: This table shows the sequences of all primers and conditions used in this study for MSP analysis.

Additional file 16: This table lists the primer sequences for bisulfite-pyrosequencing of the *RBBP8* promoter region.

Additional file 17: Sequences of all primers and conditions for qPCR analysis are summarized in a table.

Abbreviations

ATCC: American Type Culture Collection; AUC: Area under curve; BER: Base excision repair; BLCA: Bladder cancer; BPH: Benign prostatic hyperplasia; BRCA1/2: Breast cancer 1/2, early onset; cBMB: Centralized biomaterial bank; cDNA: Copy number desoxyribonucleic acid; CIMP: CpG island methylator phenotype; CpG: 5′-deoxycytidine-phosphate-deoxyguanosine-3′; CtiP: CtBP-interacting protein; DAC: Decitabine; DDR: DNA damage repair; DNA: Deoxyribonucleic acid; DNAm: DNA methylation; DNMT: DNA methyltransferase; DSB: Double-strand break; EK: Ethics committee; ERCC1: Excision repair cross-complementing group 1; FC: Fold change; FFPE: Formalin-fixed paraffin-embedded; GAPDH: Glyeradehyde 3-phosphate dehydrogenase; HR: Homologous recombination; IHC: Immunohistochemistry; IRS: Immunoreactive score; MGMT: O6-methylguanine-DNA methyltransferase; MIBC: Muscle-invasive bladder cancer; MLH1: MutL homolog 1; MMR: Mismatch repair; mRNA: Messenger ribonucleic acid; MSP: Methylation-specific PCR; n: Number; NER: Nucleotide excision repair; NHEJ: Non-homologous end-joining; OS: Overall survival; PARP: Poly (ADP-ribose) polymerase; PBS: Phosphate-buffered saline; PCR: Polymerase chain reaction; POLD1: Polymerase delta 1; qPCR: Quantitative PCR; ROC: Receiver operating characteristic; RWTH: Rheinisch-Westfälisch Technische Hochschule; SCC: Squamous cell carcinoma; s.d.: Standard deviation; s.e.m.: Standard error of the margin; TCGA: The Cancer Genome Atlas; TSA: Trichostatin A; TSS: Transcription start site; USA: United States of America

Acknowledgements

This paper is dedicated to the memory of our unforgotten colleague and head of the working group "Translational Pathology" Dr. Jürgen Veeck who designed and initiated this study but passed away after losing his short battle with cancer. We furthermore thank Timon Heide for his great support in analyzing the statistical datasets. The excellent technical assistance of Ursula Schneider is thankfully acknowledged. Genomic 450K methylation analysis is generated by using the TCGA Research Network datasets (http://cancergenome.nih.gov), and we would like to thank them for their efforts in making this data publicly available. We finally thank the following colleagues for kindly contributing cell lines: Sven Perner (University of Bonn; LNCaP and RWPE-1 cells) and Manon van Engeland (Maastricht University; HCT116, RKO, CACO2, COLO205, HT29, SW480, CACO320, SKRC1, SKRC10, SKRC52, and SKRC59 cells).

Funding

This work was supported by a grant from the Medical Faculty of the RWTH Aachen University (START program project 113/15).

Authors' contributions

JM performed the methylation analysis and edited the manuscript. JV participated in the design of the study, drafted the manuscript, and was involved in bioinformatics. NTG, EB, TCR, and SG were involved in the experimental data acquisition and analysis. ED, DP, and SCS provided the human patients' samples. RK participated in the design of the study. MR conceived and coordinated the study, was involved in data analysis, and wrote the manuscript. All authors read, critically revised, and approved the final manuscript.

Competing interests

The authors declare that they have no competing interests.

Author details

[1]Institute of Pathology, RWTH Aachen University, Pauwelsstr. 30, 52074 Aachen, Germany. [2]Division of Medical Oncology, Maastricht University Medical Centre, Maastricht, The Netherlands. [3]GROW—School for Oncology and Developmental Biology, Maastricht University Medical Centre, Maastricht, The Netherlands. [4]RWTH Centralized Biomaterial Bank (RWTH cBMB), Medical Faculty, RWTH Aachen University, Aachen, Germany. [5]Department of Urology, RWTH Aachen University, Aachen, Germany. [6]Department of Urology, Uro-Oncology, Robot Assisted and Reconstructive Urologic Surgery, University Hospital Cologne, Cologne, Germany. [7]Department of Urology, Klinikum rechts der Isar, Technical University Munich, Munich, Germany.

References

1. Cline MS, Craft B, Swatloski T, Goldman M, Ma S, Haussler D, Zhu J. Exploring TCGA Pan-Cancer data at the UCSC Cancer Genomics Browser. Sci Rep. 2013;3:2652.
2. Cancer Genome Atlas Research Network, Weinstein JN, Collisson EA, Mills GB, Shaw KR, Ozenberger BA, Ellrott K, Shmulevich I, Sander C, Stuart JM. The Cancer Genome Atlas Pan-Cancer analysis project. Nat Genet. 2013;45:1113–20.
3. Ciriello G, Miller ML, Aksoy BA, Senbabaoglu Y, Schultz N, Sander C. Emerging landscape of oncogenic signatures across human cancers. Nat Genet. 2013;45:1127–33.
4. Alexandrov LB, Nik-Zainal S, Wedge DC, Aparicio SA, Behjati S, Biankin AV, Bignell BR, Bolli N, Borg A, Børresen-Dale AL, et al. Signatures of mutational processes in human cancer. Nature. 2013;500:415–21.
5. Witte T, Plass C, Gerhauser C. Pan-cancer patterns of DNA methylation. Genome Med. 2014;6:66.
6. Costa-Pinheiro P, Montezuma D, Henrique R, Jerónimo C. Diagnostic and prognostic epigenetic biomarkers in cancer. Epigenomics. 2015;7:1003–15.
7. Miozzo M, Vaira V, Sirchia SM. Epigenetic alterations in cancer and personalized cancer treatment. Future Oncol. 2015;11:333–48.
8. Bartkova J, Horejsí Z, Koed K, Krämer A, Tort F, Zieger K, Guldberg P, Sehested M, Nesland JM, Lukas C, et al. DNA damage response as a candidate anti-cancer barrier in early human tumorigenesis. Nature. 2005;434:864–70.
9. Asakawa H, Koizumi H, Koike A, Takahashi M, Wu W, Iwase H, Fukuda M, Ohta T. Prediction of breast cancer sensitivity to neoadjuvant chemotherapy based on status of DNA damage repair proteins. Breast Cancer Res. 2010;12:R17.
10. Kang J, D'Andrea AD, Kozono D. A DNA repair pathway-focused score for prediction of outcomes in ovarian cancer treated with platinum-based chemotherapy. J Natl Cancer Inst. 2012;104:670–81.
11. Gkotzamanidou M, Sfikakis PP, Kyrtopoulos SA, Bamia C, Dimopoulos MA, Souliotis VL. Chromatin structure, transcriptional activity and DNA repair efficiency affect the outcome of chemotherapy in multiple myeloma. Br J Cancer. 2014;111:1293–304.
12. Gao D, Herman JG, Guo M. The clinical value of aberrant epigenetic changes of DNA damage repair genes in human cancer. Oncotarget. 2016;7:37331–46.
13. Esteller M, Garcia-Foncillas J, Andion E, Goodman SN, Hidalgo OF, Vanaclocha V, Baylin SB, Herman JG. Inactivation of the DNA-repair gene MGMT and the clinical response of gliomas to alkylating agents. N Engl J Med. 2000;343:1350–4.
14. Hegi ME, Diserens AC, Gorlia T, Hamou MF, de Tribolet N, Weller M, Kros JM, Hainfellner JA, Mason W, Mariani L, et al. MGMT gene silencing and benefit from temozolomide in glioblastoma. N Engl J Med. 2005;352:997–1003.
15. Esteller M, Silva JM, Dominguez G, Bonilla F, Matias-Guiu X, Lerma E, Bussaglia E, Prat J, Harkes IC, Repasky EA, et al. Promoter hypermethylation and BRCA1 inactivation in sporadic breast and ovarian tumors. J Natl Cancer Inst. 2000;92:564 9.

16. Veeck J, Ropero S, Setien F, Gonzalez-Suarez E, Osorio A, Benitez J, Herman JG, Esteller M. BRCA1 CpG island hypermethylation predicts sensitivity to poly (adenosine diphosphate)-ribose polymerase inhibitors. J Clin Oncol. 2010;28:563–4.
17. Stefansson OA, Villanueva A, Vidal A, Martí L, Esteller M. BRCA1 epigenetic inactivation predicts sensitivity to platinum-based chemotherapy in breast and ovarian cancer. Epigenetics. 2012;7:1225–9.
18. Drew Y, Mulligan EA, Vong WT, Thomas HD, Kahn S, Kyle S, Mukhopadhyay A, Los G, Hostomsky Z, Plummer ER, et al. Therapeutic potential of poly (ADP-ribose) polymerase inhibitor AG014699 in human cancers with mutated or methylated BRCA1 or BRCA2. J Natl Cancer Inst. 2011;103:334–46.
19. Moutinho C, Martinez-Cardús A, Santos C, Navarro-Pérez V, Martínez-Balibrea E, Musulen E, Carmona FJ, Sartore-Bianchi A, Cassingena A, Siena S, et al. Epigenetic inactivation of the BRCA1 interactor SRBC and resistance to oxaliplatin in colorectal cancer. J Natl Cancer Inst. 2014;106:djt322.
20. Wu X, Gu J, Grossman HB, Amos CI, Etzel C, Huang M, Zhang Q, Millikan RE, Lerner S, Dinney CP, et al. Bladder cancer predisposition: a multigenic approach to DNA-repair and cell-cycle-control genes. Am J Hum Genet. 2006;78:464–79.
21. Knollman H, Godwin JL, Jain R, Wong YN, Plimack ER, Geynisman DM. Muscle-invasive urothelial bladder cancer: an update on systemic therapy. Ther Adv Urol. 2015;7:312–30.
22. Arcas A, Fernández-Capetillo O, Cases I, Rojas AM. Emergence and evolutionary analysis of the human DDR network: implications in comparative genomics and downstream analyses. Mol Biol Evol. 2014;31:940–61.
23. Yu X, Baer R. Nuclear localization and cell cycle-specific expression of CtIP, a protein that associates with the BRCA1 tumor suppressor. J Biol Chem. 2000;275:18541–9.
24. Chinnadurai G. CtIP, a candidate tumor susceptibility gene is a team player with luminaries. Biochim Biophys Acta. 2006;1765:67–73.
25. Gaymes TJ, Mohamedali AM, Patterson M, Matto N, Smith A, Kulasekararaj A, Chelliah R, Curtin N, Farzaneh F, Shall S, et al. Microsatellite instability induced mutations in DNA repair genes CtIP and MRE11 confer hypersensitivity to poly (ADP-ribose) polymerase inhibitors in myeloid malignancies. Haematologica. 2013;98:1397–406.
26. Lin ZP, Ratner ES, Whicker ME, Lee Y, Sartorelli AC. Triapine disrupts CtIP-mediated homologous recombination repair and sensitizes ovarian cancer cells to PARP and topoisomerase inhibitors. Mol Cancer Res. 2014;12:381–93.
27. Wang J, Ding Q, Fujimori H, Motegi A, Miki Y, Masutani M. Loss of CtIP disturbs homologous recombination repair and sensitizes breast cancer cells to PARP inhibitors. Oncotarget. 2016;7:7701–14.
28. Sartori AA, Lukas C, Coates J, Mistrik M, Fu S, Bartek J, Baer R, Lukas J, Jackson SP. Human CtIP promotes DNA end resection. Nature. 2007;450:509–14.
29. Cruz-García A, López-Saavedra A, Huertas P. BRCA1 accelerates CtIP-mediated DNA-end resection. Cell Rep. 2014;9:451–9.
30. Hoa NN, Kobayashi J, Omura M, Hirakawa M, Yang SH, Komatsu K, Paull TT, Takeda S, Sasanuma H. BRCA1 and CtIP are both required to recruit Dna2 at double-strand breaks in homologous recombination. PLoS One. 2015;10:e0124495.
31. Quennet V, Beucher A, Barton O, Takeda S, Löbrich N. CtIP and MRN promote non-homologous end-joining of etoposide-induced DNA double-strand breaks in G1. Nucleic Acids Res. 2011;39:2144–52.
32. Makharashvili N, Tubbs AT, Yang SH, Wang H, Barton O, Zhou Y, Deshpande RA, Lee JH, Lobrich M, Sleckman BP, et al. Catalytic and noncatalytic roles of the CtIP endonuclease in double-strand break end resection. Mol Cell. 2014;54:1022–33.
33. Bennardo N, Cheng A, Huang N, Stark JM. Alternative-NHEJ is a mechanistically distinct pathway of mammalian chromosome break repair. PLoS Genet. 2008;4:e1000110.
34. Gu B, Chen PL. Expression of PCNA-binding domain of CtIP, a motif required for CtIP localization at DNA replication foci, causes DNA damage and activation of DNA damage checkpoint. Cell Cycle. 2009;8:1409–20.
35. Lafranchi L, de Boer HR, de Vries EG, Ong SE, Sartori AA, van Vugt MA. APC/C (Cdh1) controls CtIP stability during the cell cycle and in response to DNA damage. EMBO J. 2014;33:2860–79.
36. Hoffmann AC, Wild P, Leicht C, Bertz S, Danenberg KG, Danenberg PV, Stöhr R, Stöckle M, Lehmann J, Schuler M, et al. MDR1 and ERCC1 expression predict outcome of patients with locally advanced bladder cancer receiving adjuvant chemotherapy. Neoplasia. 2010;12:628–36.
37. Kuhlmann JD, Wimberger P, Bankfalvi A, Keller T, Schöler S, Aktas B, Buderath P, Hauch S, Otterbach F, Kimmig R, et al. ERCC1-positive circulating tumor cells in the blood of ovarian cancer patients as a predictive biomarker for platinum resistance. Clin Chem. 2014;60:1282–9.
38. Wolff EM, Chihara Y, Pan F, Weisenberger DJ, Siegmund KD, Sugano K, Kawashima K, Laird PW, Jones PA, Liang G. Unique DNA methylation patterns distinguish noninvasive and invasive urothelial cancers and establish an epigenetic field defect in premalignant tissue. Cancer Res. 2010;70:8169–78.
39. Cancer Genome Atlas Research Network. Comprehensive molecular characterization of urothelial bladder carcinoma. Nature. 2014;507:315–22.
40. Cartharius K, Frech K, Grote K, Klocke B, Haltmeier M, Klingenhoff A, Frisch M, Bayerlein M, Werner T. MatInspector and beyond: promoter analysis based on transcription factor binding sites. Bioinformatics. 2005;21:2933–42.
41. Masters JR, Hepburn PJ, Walker L, Highman WJ, Trejdosiewicz LK, Povey S, Parkar M, Hill BT, Riddle PR, Franks LM. Tissue culture model of transitional cell carcinoma: characterization of twenty-two human urothelial cell lines. Cancer Res. 1986;46:3630–6.
42. Remmele W, Stegner HE. Recommendation for uniform definition of an immunoreactive score (IRS) for immunohistochemical estrogen receptor detection (ER-ICA) in breast cancer tissue. Pathologe. 1987;8:138–40.
43. Soria-Bretones I, Sáez C, Ruíz-Borrego M, Japón MA, Huertas P. Prognostic value of CtIP/RBBP8 expression in breast cancer. Cancer Med. 2013;2:774–83.
44. Ciccia A, Elledge SJ. The DNA damage response: making it safe to play with knives. Mol Cell. 2010;40:179–204.
45. Abbotts R, Thompson N, Madhusudan S. DNA repair in cancer: emerging targets for personalized therapy. Cancer Manag Res. 2014;6:77–92.
46. Tumini E, Barroso S, Pérez-Calero C, Aguilera A. Roles of human POLD1 and POLD3 in genome stability. Sci Rep. 2016;6:38873.
47. Weisenberger DJ, Siegmund KD, Campan M, Young D, Long TI, Faasse MA, Kang GH, Widschwendter M, Weener D, Buchanan D, et al. CpG island methylator phenotype underlies sporadic microsatellite instability and is tightly associated with BRAF mutation in colorectal cancer. Nat Genet. 2006;38:787–93.
48. Thibodeau SN, French AJ, Roche PC, Cunningham JM, Tester DJ, Lindor NM, Moslein G, Baker SM, Liskay RM, Burgart LJ, et al. Altered expression of hMSH2 and hMLH1 in tumors with microsatellite instability and genetic alterations in mismatch repair genes. Cancer Res. 1996;56:4836–40.
49. Sonpavde G, Gordetsky JB, Lockhart ME, Nix JW. Chemotherapy for muscle-invasive bladder cancer: better late than never? J Clin Oncol. 2016;34:780–5.
50. Inman BA, Longo TA, Ramalingam S, Harrison MR. Atezolizumab: a PD-L1-blocking antibody for bladder cancer. Clin Cancer Res. 2017;23:1886–90.
51. Bertz S, Otto W, Denzinger S, Wieland WF, Burger M, Stohr R, Link S, Hofstadter F, Hartmann A. Combination of CK20 and Ki-67 immunostaining analysis predicts recurrence, progression, and cancerspecific survival in pT1 urothelial bladder cancer. Eur Urol. 2014;65:218-26.
52. Otto W, Denzinger S, Fritsche HM, Burger M, Wieland WF, Hofstadter F, Hartmann A, Bertz S. The WHO classification of 1973 is more suitable than the WHO classification of 2004 for predicting survival in pT1 urothelial bladder cancer. BJU Int. 2011;107:404–8.
53. Maruyama R, Toyooka S, Toyooka KO, Harada K, Virmani AK, Zöchbauer-Müller S, Farinas AJ, Vakar-Lopez F, Minna JD, Sagalowsky A, et al. Aberrant promoter methylation profile of bladder cancer and its relationship to clinicopathological features. Cancer Res. 2001;61:8659–63.
54. Esteller M, Corn PG, Baylin SB, Herman JG. A gene hypermethylation profile of human cancer. Cancer Res. 2001;61:3225–9.
55. Christmann M, Verbeeck B, Roos WP, Kaina B. O(6)-methylguanine-DNA methyltransferase (MGMT) in normal tissues and tumors: enzyme activity, promoter methylation and immunohistochemistry. Biochim Biophys Acta. 2011;1816:179–90.
56. Westerveld A, Hoeijmakers JH, van Duin M, de Wit J, Odijk H, Pastink A, Wood RD, Bootsma D. Molecular cloning of a human DNA repair gene. Nature. 1984;310:425–9.
57. Usanova S, Piée-Staffa A, Sied U, Thomale J, Schneider A, Kaina B, Köberle B. Cisplatin sensitivity of testis tumour cells is due to deficiency in interstrand-crosslink repair and low ERCC1-XPF expression. Mol Cancer. 2010;9:248.
58. Sun JM, Sung JY, Park SH, Kwon GY, Jeong BC, Seo SI, Jeon SS, Lee HM, Jo J, Choi HY, et al. ERCC1 as a biomarker for bladder cancer patients likely to benefit from adjuvant chemotherapy. BMC Cancer. 2012;12:187.
59. Klatte T, Seitz C, Rink M, Rouprêt M, Xylinas E, Karakiewicz P, Susani M, Shariat SF. ERCC1 as a prognostic and predictive biomarker for urothelial carcinoma of the bladder following radical cystectomy. J Urol. 2015;194:1456–62.

60. Eid W, Steger M, El-Shemerly M, Ferretti LP, Peña-Diaz J, König C, Valtorta E, Sartori AA, Ferrari S. DNA end resection by CtIP and exonuclease 1 prevents genomic instability. EMBO Rep. 2010;11:962–8.
61. Yun MH, Hiom K. CtIP-BRCA1 modulates the choice of DNA double-strand-break repair pathway throughout the cell cycle. Nature. 2009;459:460–3.
62. Chaudhry P, Srinivasan R, Patel FD. Utility of gene promoter methylation in prediction of response to platinum-based chemotherapy in epithelial ovarian cancer (EOC). Cancer Investig. 2009;27:877–84.
63. Zhang S, Yuan Y, Hao D. A genomic instability score in discriminating nonequivalent outcomes of BRCA1/2 mutations and in predicting outcomes of ovarian cancer treated with platinum-based chemotherapy. PLoS One. 2014;9:e113169.
64. Galluzzi L, Senovilla L, Vitale I, Michels J, Martins I, Kepp O, Castedo M, Kroemer G. Molecular mechanisms of cisplatin resistance. Oncogene. 2012;31:1869–83.
65. Wan JC, Massie C, Garcia-Corbacho J, Mouliere F, Brenton JD, Caldas C, Pacey S, Baird R, Rosenfeld N. Liquid biopsies come of age: towards implementation of circulating tumour DNA. Nat Rev Cancer. 2017;17:223–38.
66. Kaufman DS, Shipley WU, Feldman AS. Bladder cancer. Lancet. 2009; 374:239–49.
67. van der Aa MN, Steyerberg EW, Sen EF, Zwarthoff EC, Kirkels WJ, van der Kwast TH, Essink-Bot ML. Patients' perceived burden of cystoscopic and urinary surveillance of bladder cancer: a randomized comparison. BJU Int. 2008;101:1106–10.
68. Sievert KD, Amend B, Nagele U, Schilling D, Bedke J, Horstman M, Hennenlotter J, Kruck S, Stenzl A. Economic aspects of bladder cancer: what are the benefits and costs? World J Urol. 2009;27:295–300.
69. Ye F, Wang L, Castillo-Martin M, McBride R, Galsky MD, Zhu J, Boffetta P, Zhang DY, Cordon-Cardo C. Biomarkers for bladder cancer management: present and future. Am J Clin Exp Urol. 2014;2:1–14.
70. Monteiro-Reis S, Leça L, Almeida M, Antunes S, Monteiro P, Dias P, Morais A, Oliveira J, Henrique R, Jerónimo C. Accurate detection of upper tract urothelial carcinoma in tissue and urine by means of quantitative GDF15, TMEFF2 and VIM promoter methylation. Eur J Cancer. 2014;50:226–33.
71. Bibikova M, Barnes B, Tsan C, Ho V, Klotzle B, Le JM DD, Zhang L, Schroth GB, Gunderson KL, et al. High density DNA methylation array with single CpG site resolution. Genomics. 2011;98:288–95.
72. Du P, Zhang X, Huang CC, Jafari N, Kibbe WA, Hou L, Lin SM. Comparison of Beta-value and M-value methods for quantifying methylation levels by microarray analysis. BMC Bioinf. 2010;11:587.
73. Van Loo P, Nordgard SH, Lingjærde OC, Russnes HG, Rye IH, Sun W, Weigman VJ, Marynen P, Zetterberg A, Naume B, Perou CM, Børresen-Dale AL, Kristensen VN: Allele-specific copy number analysis of tumors. Proc Natl Acad Sci U S A. 2010; 107(39):16910–5.
74. Wessely F, Emes RD. Identification of DNA methylation biomarkers from Infinium arrays. Front Genet. 2012;3 https://doi.org/10.3389/fgene.2012.0016.
75. Emes RD, Farrell WE. Make way for the 'next generation': application and prospects for genome-wide, epigenome-specific technologies in endocrine research. J Mol Endocrinol. 2012;49:19–27.
76. Shinawi T, Hill VK, Krex D, Schackert G, Gentle D, Morris MR, Wei W, Cruickshank G, Maher ER, Latif F. DNA methylation profiles of long- and short-term glioblastoma survivors. Epigenetics. 2013;8:149–56.
77. Veeck J, Niederacher D, An H, Klopocki E, Wiesmann F, Betz B, Galm O, Camara O, Durst M, Kristiansen G, et al. Aberrant methylation of the Wnt antagonist SFRP1 in breast cancer is associated with unfavourable prognosis. Oncogene. 2006;25:3479–88.
78. Li LC, Dahiya R. MethPrimer: designing primers for methylation PCRs. Bioinformatics. 2002;18:1427–31.
79. Rose M, Gaisa NT, Antony P, Fiedler D, Heidenreich A, Otto W, Denzinger S, Bertz S, Hartmann A, Karl A, et al. Epigenetic inactivation of ITIH5 promotes bladder cancer progression and predicts early relapse of pT1 high grade urothelial tumours. Carcinogenesis. 2013;35:727–36.
80. Fink L, Seeger W, Ermert L, Hanze J, Stahl U, Grimminger F, Kummer W, Bohle RM. Real-time quantitative RT-PCR after laser-assisted cell picking. Nat Med. 1998;4:1329–33.
81. R Core Team: R: a language and environment for statistical computing. R foundation for statistical computing. 2016.
82. Koestler DC, Marsit CJ, Christinsen BC, Kelsey KT, Houseman EA. A recursively partitioned mixture model for clustering time-course gene expression data. Transl Cancer Res. 2014;3:217–32.
83. Zweig MH, Campbell B. Receiver-operating characteristic (ROC) plots: a fundamental evaluation tool in clinical medicine. Clin Chem. 1993;39:561–77.

11

Exposure to NO_2, CO, and $PM_{2.5}$ is linked to regional DNA methylation differences in asthma

Mary Prunicki[1,2], Laurel Stell[3], Deendayal Dinakarpandian[2,4], Mariangels de Planell-Saguer[5], Richard W. Lucas[7], S. Katharine Hammond[8], John R. Balmes[8,9], Xiaoying Zhou[1,2], Tara Paglino[1,2], Chiara Sabatti[3,6], Rachel L. Miller[5] and Kari C. Nadeau[1,2,10*]

Abstract

Background: DNA methylation of CpG sites on genetic loci has been linked to increased risk of asthma in children exposed to elevated ambient air pollutants (AAPs). Further identification of specific CpG sites and the pollutants that are associated with methylation of these CpG sites in immune cells could impact our understanding of asthma pathophysiology. In this study, we sought to identify some CpG sites in specific genes that could be associated with asthma regulation (*Foxp3* and *IL10*) and to identify the different AAPs for which exposure prior to the blood draw is linked to methylation levels at these sites. We recruited subjects from Fresno, California, an area known for high levels of AAPs. Blood samples and responses to questionnaires were obtained ($n = 188$), and in a subset of subjects ($n = 33$), repeat samples were collected 2 years later. Average measures of AAPs were obtained for 1, 15, 30, 90, 180, and 365 days prior to each blood draw to estimate the short-term vs. long-term effects of the AAP exposures.

Results: Asthma was significantly associated with higher differentially methylated regions (DMRs) of the *Foxp3* promoter region ($p = 0.030$) and the *IL10* intronic region ($p = 0.026$). Additionally, at the 90-day time period (90 days prior to the blood draw), *Foxp3* methylation was positively associated with NO_2, CO, and $PM_{2.5}$ exposures ($p = 0.001$, $p = 0.001$, and $p = 0.012$, respectively). In the subset of subjects retested 2 years later ($n = 33$), a positive association between AAP exposure and methylation was sustained. There was also a negative correlation between the average *Foxp3* methylation of the promoter region and activated Treg levels ($p = 0.039$) and a positive correlation between the average *IL10* methylation of region 3 of intron 4 and *IL10* cytokine expression ($p = 0.030$).

Conclusions: Short-term and long-term exposures to high levels of CO, NO_2, and $PM_{2.5}$ were associated with alterations in differentially methylated regions of *Foxp3*. *IL10* methylation showed a similar trend. For any given individual, these changes tend to be sustained over time. In addition, asthma was associated with higher differentially methylated regions of *Foxp3* and *IL10*.

Keywords: Ambient air pollution, Immune system, Regulatory T cell, Epigenetics

* Correspondence: knadeau@stanford.edu
[1]Sean N. Parker Center for Allergy and Asthma Research at Stanford University, Stanford, CA 94305, USA
[2]Department of Medicine, Stanford University, Stanford, CA 94305, USA
Full list of author information is available at the end of the article

Background

Asthma is the most frequent chronic disease in children [1], and its prevalence continues to increase, raising global public health concerns [2–4]. Previous studies found that high prenatal ambient air pollutant (AAP) exposure alters epigenetic programming in utero [5] and that children are at greater risk of developing asthma when exposed to higher concentrations of AAPs [6]. This further raises concern and increases the urgency of understanding the relationship between AAP exposures and asthma and finding effective ways to prevent, treat, and/or cure asthma. Although the mechanisms by which exposures to AAPs increase asthma prevalence remain poorly understood, evidence suggests that AAPs can mediate T cell polarization and cytokine dysregulation via epigenetic modifications [7–10].

DNA methylation at least partially controls the expression of certain key genes that are known to be involved in immune tolerance [11–13]. We previously demonstrated that exposure in children to high levels of polycyclic aromatic hydrocarbons (PAHs), a component of AAPs, is associated with higher overall percent methylation of the transcriptional regulatory region of the forkhead box transcription factor 3 (*Foxp3*) locus [8]. In a subsequent study, in addition to the presence of higher *Foxp3* methylation levels, we found that exposure to higher levels of PAHs is associated with decreased expression of *IL10*, an anti-inflammatory cytokine. These associations were stronger in children with asthma, suggesting disease-linked effects [14]. Other studies have also associated air pollution with other immune parameters, such as the association of exposure to NOx with decreases in *IL10* cytokine expression and exposure to diesel exhaust with higher differentially methylated regions (DMRs) of *Foxp3* [15]. A recent review of ambient air pollutants (AAPs), epigenetic regulation, and asthma highlights the challenge that asthma is heterogeneous, responsiveness to traffic-related air pollution, and may be a distinct phenotype [16]. In addition, a study by Clifford et al. [17] found DNA methylation changes after diesel exhaust exposure in more than 500 CpG sites in the bronchial epithelial cells. Finally, AAPs and DNA methylation have been linked to other health problems, such as cardiovascular disease [18].

We sought to identify CpG sites in the *Foxp3* and *IL10* genes that have higher DMRs in children with asthma exposed to AAPs. Our primary hypothesis was that exposure to high levels of CO, O_3, NO_2, and $PM_{2.5}$ would be associated with higher DMRs within the *Foxp3* gene and the intron 4 region of the *IL10* gene. The Foxp3 gene regulates transcription of Tregs, and the Il10 gene regulates transcription of various cell types, including $CD4^+$ T cell populations, because it has been shown to act as an enhancer element [19]. In addition, our secondary hypotheses were that methylation would be sustained following continued exposure to these pollutants and that Treg levels would be negatively associated with *Foxp3* methylation at specific CpG loci in the enhancer and promoter regions.

Methods

Subjects

We recruited subjects from Fresno, California, where there is consistently high AAP. According to the 2017 American Lung Association "State of the Air" report, Fresno ranked third in the country for year-round and short-term particle pollution and O_3 exposure [20]. Fresno County also has a high childhood asthma prevalence in comparison to other counties in California (24 vs. 17%, ages 5–17) [21]. Recruiting from the Fresno Unified School district from 2010 to 2015 resulted in a convenience sample of 198 children with complete data, 188 of which were included in the analysis after quality control, with a median age of 14.7 years. In addition, we retested 33 subjects after approximately 2 years (mean 820 days, SD 243 days; again, as a convenience sample).

At each clinical visit, information on BMI, a detailed health and general history questionnaire, and blood samples were obtained. Subjects were excluded if they had taken oral immunosuppressants within 5 days of the blood draw, had a history of allergen immunotherapy within 1 year of the clinical visit, had a chronic disease other than allergies or asthma, or had an acute infection. In addition, no blood specimen was taken during an infection, sickness, or during the use of oral steroids. Subjects with asthma were defined by the participant's report of a physician's diagnosis of current asthma. Secondhand smoke exposure (SHS) was defined as exposure to cigarette smoke from other household members. Participant smoking was defined as smoking more than 100 cigarettes in their lifetime.

Collection and processing of blood specimens

Human peripheral blood mononuclear cells (PBMCs) and plasma were extracted from the blood via Ficoll procedure and stored in liquid nitrogen and at − 80 °C as per published techniques [22].

Methylation analysis

We first selected CpG sites within the upstream promoter (− 138, − 126, − 77, − 65, − 58, and − 15) and enhancer (− 4506, − 4500, − 4494, and − 4484) regions of *Foxp3* (on the X chromosome) located on the human genome (hg38) chrX at nucleotides 49264838, 49264826, 49264777, 49264765, 49264758, 49264715, and 49269206, 49,69200, 49269194, 49269184, respectively, and within the intron 4 region of *IL10* (+ 2888, + 2907, + 2921, + 3261, + 3265, and + 3281 on chromosome 1), located on the human genome (hg38) chr1 at nucleotides

206769607, 206769588, 206769574, 206769234, 206769 230, 206769214, respectively, as these sites have been shown in the literature to be key in modulating regulatory T cell (Treg) response and overall immune tolerance [11, 19, 23]. We then examined associations between exposures to CO, O_3, NO_2, and $PM_{2.5}$ and methylation levels at these CpG sites. To determine whether methylation of CpG sites is maintained with long-term exposure, we repeated measurements on a subset of samples obtained at approximately 2 years after the initial blood samples were obtained. Methylation analysis using the pyrosequencing approach was performed on the following gene loci: ten CpG sites for *Foxp3* and six CpG sites for *IL10*. Bisulfite modification and subsequent DNA amplification of specific CpG regions within the *Foxp3* and *IL10* genes were conducted by PCR using the different pairs of primers for each region enumerated in Additional file 1: Table S1. Please see Additional file 1 for further details.

CyTOF mass cytometry

We also examined Treg, *Foxp3*, and *IL10* protein expression in a subset of the subjects using mass cytometry (CyTOF). CyTOF uses antibodies tagged with heavy metal ions and allows for identifying many more cell markers in a single sample than flow cytometry and without issues of spectral overlap. Here, we performed CyTOF on a randomly selected subset of subjects ($n = 74$; 24.3% asthmatics, 75.7% non-asthmatics) for which additional blood was available from the same blood draw as that used for methylation analysis to assess for cell composition differences. Briefly, PBMCs were thawed, stimulated for 4 h with 20 ng/mL phorbol myristate acetate + 1 μg/mL ionomycin (PMA-ION), and stained for surface markers, intracellular markers, and transcription factors using CyTOF. Please see Additional file 1 for further details.

Cell composition analysis

Nine cell subtypes were measured by gating on cell surface markers obtained from the CyTOF analysis: B Cells, monocytes, CD3+ cells, CD4+, CD8+, Th17 cells, Tregs, Th1, and Th2 cells. The cell counts were converted into non-overlapping proportions, with an additional miscellaneous category (the remaining fraction of unmeasured cell types, typically < 5%) accounted for to normalize the distribution to 100%. The resulting cell distributions were compared between the asthmatic and healthy groups and used as covariates to confirm the reproducibility of differences in methylation (see Additional file 1: Table S2).

Ambient air pollution exposure estimation

Exposure to AAPs was estimated using hourly concentration data [24] of four common pollutants (CO, O_3, NO_2, and $PM_{2.5}$) measured at four air quality monitoring stations located within Fresno city limits. These data were acquired from the US Environmental Protection Agency's Air Quality System online database (https://www.epa.gov/aqs).

In order to capture both the spatial and temporal variation in the AAP exposure of each participant, we computed an index of the average outdoor residential AAP exposure for each individual using inverse distance weighting (IDW) [25, 26] of AAP measurements from the air quality monitoring stations according to their distance from each participant's residence. For each blood sample and air pollutant, exposure was defined as the mean of the IDW values over the given time period (1, 15, 30, 90, 180, or 365 days) before the sample was taken. See online Additional file 1 for further details of these data processing choices.

Statistical analysis

Statistical analysis was performed using the R statistical computing software (R 3.4.1). We used linear regression to adjust methylation values for sex, age, and BMI. Using multivariate linear regression, we evaluated associations of resulting residuals with asthma status and ambient air pollution.

Due to the presence of related subjects within our study, we also considered linear mixed-effects models fit using generalized least squares, as implemented in the "gls" function in the "nlme" R package (version 3.1.131) for non-linear mixed-effects models. Unless explicitly stated otherwise, the results from fixed-effects models are described in the main text, and the results from mixed-effects models are described in Additional file 1. Detailed descriptions of all analyses are available in Additional file 1, along with de-identified data, exposure data, and R code (see Additional files 2, 3, 4, and 5).

Multivariate linear regression was repeated on a random subset of the data for which CyTOF-derived cell counts were obtained. The proportions of different cell types were incorporated into the model to adjust for any differences. Additionally, we performed *t* tests for each cell type to look for statistically significant differences in cell distribution. Family-wise multiple testing correction was performed by using the Benjamini-Hochberg procedure [27] with a false discovery rate of 0.05.

Results

Subject characteristics

For the 188 children (50% female, 50% male) included in the study analysis, the median age (quartile 1; quartile 3) was 14.68 years (12.98; 16.87). Median body mass index (BMI) (quartile 1; quartile 3) was 21.81 kg/m^2 (18.97; 26.28). No significant differences in these variables ($p > 0.05$) were seen between the two groups (35.6% asthmatics vs. 64.4% healthy individuals, Table 1).

Table 1 Demographic characteristics of study subjects*

	Non-asthmatic	Asthmatic
Number of subjects	121	67
Total number of male	59 (48.8%)	35 (52.2%)
Median age at enrollment (years) (quartile 1; quartile 3)	14.7 (12.9; 16.9)	14.6 (13.1; 16.9)
Median BMI (kg/m^2) (quartile 1; quartile 3)	21.7 (19.1; 25.6)	22.0 (18.8; 28.0)
Total number of rhinitis	9 (7.8%)	12 (23.1%)
Total number of eczema	11 (9.8%)	8 (15.7%)
Total number of African-American	4 (3.0%21)	5 (7.5%)
Total number of Hispanic or Latino	72 (59.5%)	27 (40.3%)
Total number of Caucasian	34 (28.0%)	15 (22.4%)
Total number of mixed race	5 (4.1%)	3 (4.5%)
Total number of not reported	6 (5.0%)	17 (25.3%)
Total number of exposed to secondhand smoke	12 (10.3%)	7 (12.5%)
Total number of smokers	1 (0.9%)	0 (0%)
Total number of household income < $15,000	35 (28.9%)	15 (22.4%)
Total number of household oncome $15,000–30,000	27 (22.3%)	12 (17.9%)
Total number of household income $31,000–50,000	12 (9.9%)	3 (4.4%)
Total number of household income > $50,000	35 (28.9%)	18 (26.9%)
Total number of household income not reported	12 (9.9%)	19 (28.3%)

BMI body mass index
*Frequencies may not sum to full sample size due to missing data

Air pollution

Exposures to pollution were averaged over 1, 15, 30, 90, 180, and 365 days prior to each convenience sampling blood draw. All subjects lived within 10 km of at least one of the monitoring stations (Fig. 1a). Annual means of data recorded at each monitoring station showed limited differences between stations (Fig. 1b). Clinic visitations by subjects varied with season with the maximum number of visits occurring in April (Fig. 1c). Substantial seasonal variations were observed in the concentrations of the air pollutants over a 12-month period (Fig. 1d). A more detailed comparison of the pollution levels between air quality monitoring stations and years in Additional file 1: Figure S1 shows that there is more variability between stations than there is between yearly averages from a single station. The results of inverse weighted averaging of the pollutants on January 1, 2014, over a rectangular grid covering all participant locations are shown in Additional file 1: Figure S2, revealing that the estimate is smooth with a local extremum at each monitoring station. The distribution of pollution exposure across individuals for six different durations prior to the visit is shown in Additional file 1: Figure S3. Because subjects did not differ substantially in their average AAP exposure over the course of a year (as indicated by very short boxes for this time period in Additional file 1: Figure S3), we excluded the 365-day time period from further analyses. We defined short-term as time periods equal to or less than 90-day exposure. Long-term was defined as greater than 90-day exposure.

Normalization of methylation data

Before testing our primary hypothesis, we normalized the effects of sex, age, and BMI on *Foxp3* and *IL10* methylation. Figure 2 shows the relationship between these methylation values and sex and age from 241 visits by 198 eligible subjects, revealing a few outlier values of *Foxp3* percent methylation. Outliers were defined as values farther than three times the interquartile range (IQR) from the first quartile or third quartile; these values were excluded from the analysis presented in the main text, leaving $n = 188$ individuals. In the supplement, we report the results we would have obtained if we had not excluded these outliers, showing that the main conclusions would not have changed substantially. Figure 2a also shows that *Foxp3* DMRs in females were greater than in males and that, at the promoter sites, it decreased with age ($n = 188$, $p < 0.0001$; Additional file 1: Table S3). The relationship with sex is consistent with the presence of a hypermethylated, inactive X chromosome. The only exception was CpG-138, which had a higher DMR in males than in females (Additional file 1: Figure S4). BMI may be weakly associated with *Foxp3* methylation when adjusted for sex, age, and age-sex interaction ($p = 0.0523$). For *IL10* ($n = 179$, due to missing data for nine subjects), Fig. 3b indicates methylation generally decreases with age ($p < 0.0001$) but is not associated with sex.

For the rest of the analysis, we used the residuals from fitting methylation to a regression model with the following covariates: sex, age, BMI, and age-sex interaction. For much of the analysis, we used averages across multiple sites, so these residuals are divided by the estimated standard deviation of the error to obtain "normalized" methylation, giving equal weight to all sites in these averages.

Association between methylation and asthma status

We tested whether asthma was significantly associated with normalized methylation at each CpG site studied for *Foxp3* (Fig. 3a, Additional file 1: Table S4) using an ANOVA model. We found that asthma was significantly associated with methylation at four of the six CpG sites in the promoter region of *Foxp3* ($p < 0.05$). We also found that averaging over all six of these sites gave a stronger association than that for any individual site, so we used this average in the rest of the analysis. To aid in

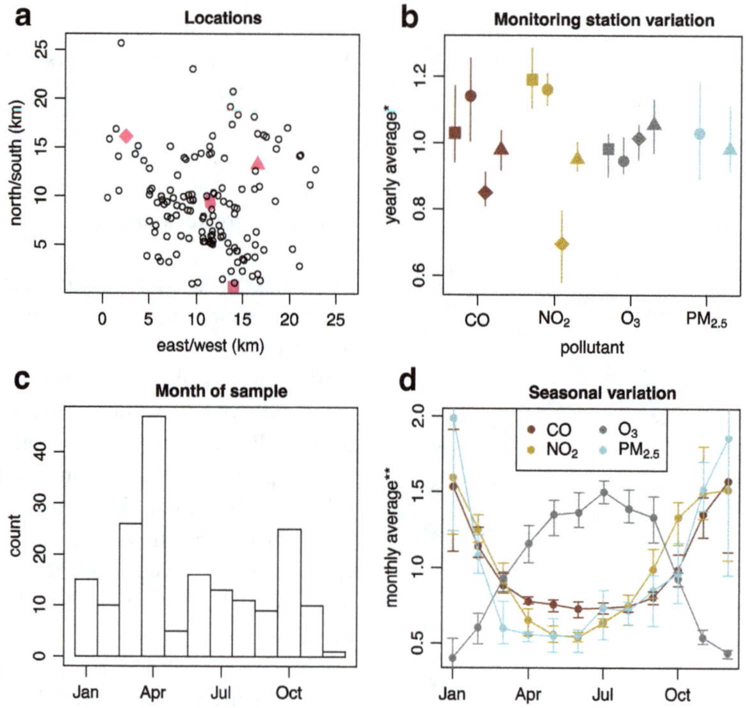

Fig. 1 Panel **a** shows the relative locations of the air quality monitoring stations (magenta symbols) and the participant home addresses (black circles). Panel **b** illustrates the variability across monitoring stations (indicated by different symbols as in the legend), which match the shapes of the magenta symbols in panel **a** for the four studied pollutants (CO, NO_2, O_3, $PM_{2.5}$), indicated with different colors as in the legend in panel **d**, using yearly averages across the study period (2010–2015); the bars show the ranges of the annual averages. Only two monitoring stations reported values for $PM_{2.5}$. Panel **c** describes the distribution of the 188 clinic visits across months of the calendar year, and panel **d** illustrates the seasonal variation in pollutants using monthly averages across monitoring stations, with the bars showing the ranges of the monthly averages across years 2010–2015. Note: In panels **b** and **d**, each value is divided by the average for the pollutant overall monitoring stations and years. Also, two stations in close proximity replaced each other, so their data are combined in panels **b** and **d**; in panel **a**, they are indicated by two magenta circles very close together in the middle of the plot

interpretation of the effect sizes in Fig. 3a, we note that the estimated standard deviation of the error for each sex at each CpG site in the *Foxp3* promoter was generally 4–6%. Hence, an effect size of 0.3 for the normalized values is roughly equivalent to 1.2–1.8 for percent methylation.

Similarly, we found that asthma was significantly associated with normalized methylation at all three CpG sites in region 3 of intron 4 of *IL10* ($p < 0.05$) (Fig. 3b, Additional file 1: Table S4). Furthermore, averaging over all three of these sites gave a stronger association than for any individual site, so we used this average in the rest of the analysis. The estimated standard deviation of the error for each sex at each CpG site in *IL10* was generally 9–11%.

Because the measured PBMC methylation is the average of all constituent cell types in a sample weighted by their proportion, an observed difference in methylation between healthy and asthmatic subjects could potentially be an artifact of differences in the underlying cell distribution. Conversely, because Treg cells constitute a small percentage of the PBMC fraction, a large difference in methylation within Treg could be masked by a small difference in cell composition. To rule out these possibilities, we performed two kinds of analyses on a random subset of the data for which cell counts of nine different cell types were obtained using CyTOF. First, we compared the proportion of each cell type. The proportion of activated Tregs was found to be statistically indistinguishable between asthmatic and healthy subjects ($p = 0.528$). After multiple testing corrections at a false discovery rate (FDR) of 0.05, Th17 cells were the only type of cell among those tested with a statistically significant difference (see Additional file 1: Table S2 for adjusted p values). We then repeated multiple linear regression to fit the average methylation in the promoter area of the *Foxp3* gene and the average methylation of region 3 of intron 4 of the *IL10* gene. The cell type composition was included as an additional covariate to adjust for any differences. For *IL10*, there was a higher DMR of *IL10* by 8.9±7.7% ($p = 0.026$) for asthmatic subjects.

Association between methylation and ambient air pollution

We investigated the association between AAP exposure (CO, O_3, NO_2, $PM_{2.5}$) and methylation of CpG sites in the *Foxp3* and *IL10* genes. The general characteristics of

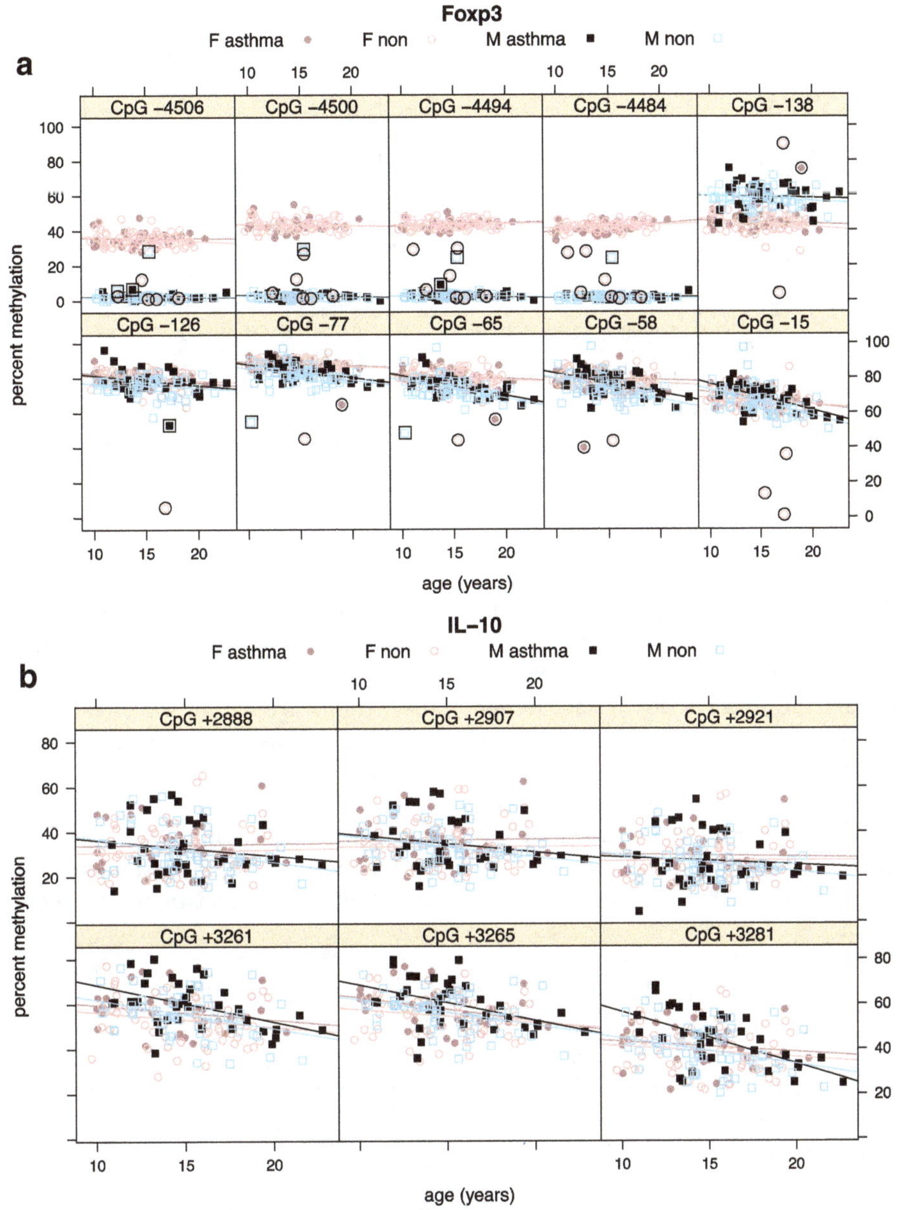

Fig. 2 Foxp3 (**a**) and IL-10 (**b**) percent methylation at measured CpG sites as a function of age, grouped by sex (M/F), and asthma status (non/asthma) as indicated. Markers of Foxp3 outliers are enclosed by black circles or squares, depending on sex. These outliers are not used in the computation of the regression lines shown for each group

our estimates of AAP exposure were described previously in this "Results" section.

To test for association with methylation, we included one pollutant at one time period along with asthma in the linear regression model. To control for other seasonal effects such as pollen (for which we do not have a direct measurement), we also considered including season in the model, which greatly increased p values for pollutants. (Additional file 1: Figures S8 and S9 show p values for all models, all pollutants, and all time periods considered.) Adding a random family effect had little effect on p values for pollutants. Therefore, we focused on the results from a model that included asthma, season, and one pollutant. The p values and effect sizes of the pollutant on averaged normalized methylation are plotted in Fig. 4. For both genes and all pollutants, the smallest p value for pollutant occurred at the 90-day exposure duration, prior to the blood draw. For *IL10*, this association was not significant for any of the four AAPs ($p > 0.1$), but all were significant ($p < 0.02$) for *Foxp3*. Table 2 shows the p values and regression coefficients for the 90-day

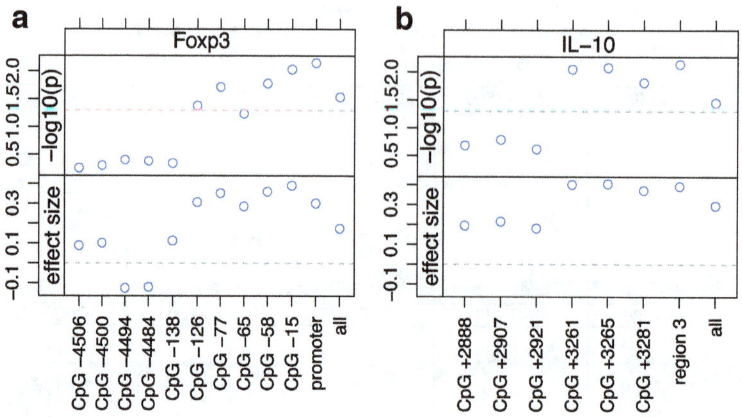

Fig. 3 The p values and effect sizes from ANOVA tests of significance of asthma status on normalized methylation for the Foxp3 (**a**) and IL-10 (**b**) genes at individual sites, and also averages over groups of sites. The horizontal dashed lines in the p value plots indicate $p = 0.05$. In the plots of effect sizes, the dashed lines indicate $y = 0$

pollution exposure prior to the blood draw and *Foxp3* promoter methylation models. The p values for the season are not significant in this model, and methylation is clearly more strongly associated with 90-day exposure. To compare the effect sizes to each other, we divided each AAP value by the 90th percentile of all monitor measurements for the pollutant, which limits the interpretability of any individual pollutant coefficient. Finally, we also considered aggregating the pollutants to increase power. We used only the first principal component (PC1) of the AAP values scaled so that each pollutant has mean zero and variance one. PC1 accounts for 93% of their total variance; the sign of the weight of O_3 was the opposite of the sign of the other three weights, and the absolute values of the weights are within 4% of each other. The last row of Table 2 shows the p values and regression coefficients for a model including PC1 along with asthma and season. The p value for PC1 is roughly the minimum of the pollutant p values in the other rows.

The p values and regression coefficients from models analyzing the associations between 90-day average

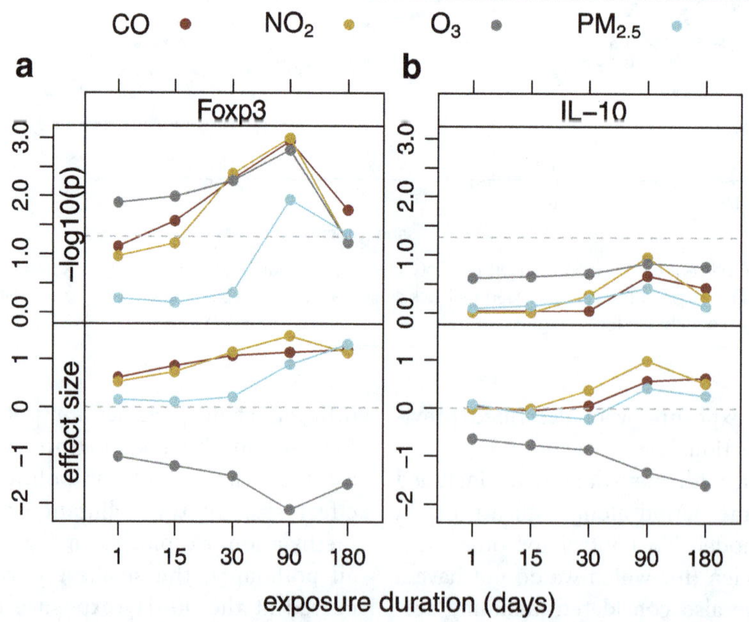

Fig. 4 The p values and effect sizes of the associations between each pollutant and normalized methylation, averaged over the sites in the promoter of Foxp3, and over the sites in region 3 of intron 4 of IL-10. Each model also includes an effect for season and one for asthma. The horizontal dashed lines in the p value plots indicate $p = 0.05$. In the plots of effect sizes, the dashed lines indicate $y = 0$. To compare effect sizes across pollutants, each AAP value is divided by the 90th percentile of all sensor measurements for the pollutant

Table 2 *p* values and regression coefficients for 90-day pollution exposure prior to blood draw and *Foxp3* promoter methylation models

	Asthma		Pollutant		Season				
Pollutant in model	*p*	Coef	*p*	Coef	*p*	Spring	Summer	Autumn	Winter
CO	0.008	0.283	0.001	1.157	0.400	− 0.828	− 0.863	− 0.858	− 1.140
NO_2	0.010	0.276	0.001	1.504	0.287	− 0.957	− 0.852	− 1.052	− 1.277
O_3	0.011	0.275	0.002	− 2.158	0.437	1.045	1.436	1.444	0.829
$PM_{2.5}$	0.016	0.261	0.012	0.903	0.145	− 0.445	− 0.608	− 0.665	− 0.770
PC1	0.011	0.273	0.001	NA	0.331	− 0.075	0.034	− 0.051	− 0.442

pollutant exposure and normalized methylation averaged over the sites in the promoter of *Foxp3*. Each row is for one model that includes 90-day exposure for the specified pollutant. Asthma and season are covariates in every model. Since season is modeled as a factor with four levels, it has a coefficient for each season. In the last row, the pollutants are aggregated by their first principal component. PC1 is scaled much differently than the exposure values used in the other rows and its sign is arbitrary, so we omit its coefficient.

Differences in percent methylation across repeated testing of methylation and estimation of ambient air pollution

In a convenience subset of the subjects, we evaluated changes in DMRs on the *Foxp3* ($n = 33$) and *IL10* ($n = 30$) genes after a period of time (mean 820 days, SD 243 days). We evaluated whether our model could explain changes in normalized methylation associated with exposure to AAPs. We predicted percent methylation for each participant at the time of repeat measure using data from 188 subjects (or 179 for *IL10*) and average normalized methylation to covariates asthma, season, and 90-day average of exposure to a single pollutant. Additional file 1: Figure S5 compares the observed values from the second time point to both the predicted values and to the original values for each gene and each pollutant for the subset of subjects with two visits. For any given individual, the actual normalized values generally change between the two time points. Furthermore, the prediction error for the second time point is generally large, but the model does correctly predict for most individuals whether an individual will have higher or lower DMRs at the second time point than at the first sample time.

Treg: *Foxp3* and *IL10* protein expression

Cell type and protein expression were measured by CyTOF. The association between both activated (a result of the PMA-ION used to stimulate *IL10* cytokine production) Tregs (CD25 high, CD127 low) in CD4+ cells and *Foxp3* protein expression vs. *Foxp3* methylation was analyzed at each CpG site for the 74 subjects for which we had performed CyTOF analysis. When analyzed using multivariate linear regression with the covariates of asthma status, age, BMI, and sex, Tregs were inversely proportional to the average *Foxp3* methylation of the CpG sites in the promoter site ($p = .039$; Additional file 1: Figure S6a). There was no significant association between *Foxp3* methylation and *Foxp3* expression (Additional file 1: Figure S6b).

The association between *IL10* cytokine expression in CD4+ T cells and average *IL10* methylation at region 3 of intron 4 was also analyzed for a subset of subjects with available cytokine data ($n = 53$). When analyzed using multivariate linear regression with the covariates of asthma status, age, BMI, and sex, *IL10* cytokine expression was positively associated with *IL10* methylation ($p = 0.030$; Additional file 1: Figure S6c).

Discussion

In this cohort study of children from Fresno, an area located in the San Joaquin Valley of California and known for high AAP exposure, we examined DMRs of *Foxp3* and *IL10*, which are genes involved in immune tolerance [28, 29]. *Foxp3* plays a key role in maintaining tolerance to common antigens in asthma and allergy [30]. *IL10* secretion by T cells can promote tolerance and suppress the production of IgE by B cells [29]. Additionally, prior studies have found an association between exposure to AAPs and *Foxp3* or *IL10* modifications [14, 31]. Overall, the results were consistent with our primary hypothesis (i.e., higher DMR with increased pollution exposure).

Our results indicate that DMRs in the *Foxp3* promoter and *IL10* intronic regions are preferentially methylated in asthmatic patients. These results are supported by other studies that have similarly found DNA methylation differences between asthmatic and control subjects at CpG loci in other genes [10, 32]. However, this DMR may be associated with asthma, regardless of the time point of pollution exposure. Furthermore, recent work indicates that heritable epigenetic alterations may mediate the increasing prevalence of atopic diseases [33, 34]. These epigenetic markers may serve as potential biomarkers to support clinical diagnosis.

Several variables measured in this study have been shown to be associated with asthma, such as age, BMI, and sex. We therefore adjusted for these factors in our analyses and found that exposure to AAPs is associated with increased DMRs in the promoter region of *Foxp3*. These results are consistent with prior studies that have demonstrated that the *Foxp3* gene is involved in overall immune tolerance [28], and more specifically that Tregs, which are suppressors of immune responses involved in asthma pathogenesis, are impaired in pediatric asthma [35]. *Foxp3* can also be present in activated CD4+ T effector cells; therefore, its presence is not a sine qua non of a Treg. We have also shown in two prior studies that increased exposure to ambient PAHs is associated with generalized higher differential DMR of the *Foxp3* locus [8, 14].

This study provides novel information by identifying specific gene regions that are sensitive to AAPs. We evaluated methylation at the enhancer and promoter regions of the *Foxp3* gene. We found methylation at the upstream promoter region of *Foxp3* to be associated with both asthma status and exposure to AAPs. However, we found no correlation between methylation and asthma status at the enhancer region. Importantly, our findings of a positive association between AAP exposure and *Foxp3* methylation in our initial cross-sectional analyses were consistent with the results of our longitudinal analyses in a subset of subjects.

We also found that individual pollutants differ in their effects on CpG methylation. Exposure to higher levels of NO_2, CO, and $PM_{2.5}$ are associated with higher DMRs of the promoter region of the *Foxp3* gene. However, O_3 exposure was inversely associated with *Foxp3* methylation. This is not surprising as O_3 is a regional pollutant with a seasonal pattern opposite to that of the other pollutants (Additional file 1: Figure S7), and we may not be observing the effect of high ozone on methylation, but, rather, the fact that the other pollutants were low.

This is the first study to our knowledge that has evaluated the association between *IL10* methylation and air pollution. We found that DMRs in the intronic region 3 are preferentially methylated in patients with asthma. However, we did not find significant associations between AAP and intron 4 methylation. In future studies, additional CpG sites, such as those in the promoter region of *IL10*, could be evaluated.

While previous investigations have suggested that exposure to higher levels of AAPs are associated with increased prevalence of asthma and allergy [36–39] and that protein expression of *IL10* decreased as PAH exposure increased from 24 h to 1 year [14], previous studies have not specified a critical time of exposure duration. Here, we determined that there was a significant positive association of *Foxp3 promoter* methylation and pollution for all subjects when there was exposure to certain AAPs (NO_2, CO, and $PM_{2.5}$) over the previous *90 days prior to the blood draw*. In addition, AAP exposure averaged over the 90 days was more strongly associated with *Foxp3* methylation than it was with season. For the *IL10* gene, there was not a significant association between pollutant exposure levels and the amount of intro region methylation, prompting our suggestion that additional *IL10 gene regions* be evaluated in future studies.

By using CyToF, we were able to link methylation and protein levels in high dimensional cell immune monitoring for these subjects. In addition, we demonstrated that methylation of the promoter region of the *Foxp3* gene is negatively associated with activated Treg levels, and *IL10* methylation at region 3 of intron 4 is positively associated with *IL10* cytokine expression. Foxp3 is produced by both Treg and activated T cells. However, *IL10* is synthesized by many immune cells and given there was a wide standard of error, it is difficult to comment on the biological significance of the *IL10* results.

We also recognize that our study is subject to a number of limitations. Blood collection occurred across all four seasons, and visits were not evenly distributed within each season. It is possible that the visit peak in April is driven by seasonal variations in airborne pollen and that the regression analyses might not remove the impact of this effect. The 90-day exposure finding could represent opposing effects (pollen/pollutant seasonal variations), which negate each other so that pollutant exposure impact can be detected. Future analyses are planned to address this. Not only do the AAP pollutants vary by season, aeroallergens such as ragweed, oak/maple, and Pinaceae pollen can affect the severity of asthma and pediatric asthma emergency department and clinic visits and have been shown to be associated with daily aeroallergen concentrations [40]. Repeat visits are limited in number and did not necessarily occur in the same season. To compensate, seasonality was included in the models used to investigate associations between methylation and AAP exposure, and 90-day exposure prior to the blood draw had a stronger effect than season, but simply using four seasons to model seasonality might not accurately reflect actual pollen levels in a given year. Furthermore, individual exposure was evaluated with the inverse distance weighting (IDW) method, rather than directly measured [25, 26]. It is also possible that other pollutants, dietary exposure, and toxins from the air, water, and other sources, not measured in this study, may contribute to DNA methylation. The generalizability of the results may be limited because the population was predominantly Hispanic and a convenience sample. And ethnicity was not adjusted in the models. Asthma was defined by self-report of physician diagnosis of asthma, rather than by clinical testing. However, in publications using the same technique, it was found that the agreement of patient self-report and physician diagnosis was correlated [41] with the questions about "physician-diagnosed asthma" having a specificity of 99% [42]; therefore, we used this method as part of our study definition of asthma. Our failure to find a significant association between *Foxp3* protein expression and *Foxp3* methylation may be related to the ongoing debate whether all Treg are *Foxp3* positive or whether all *Foxp3* positive T cells are Treg or if transcription and protein expression are directly related in Treg [43]. Given that the Treg population is a small fraction of the overall cell count, the measurement of *Foxp3* protein expression may be lost in the margin of error when measuring both it and the percentage of Tregs.

In summary, our data demonstrate that (1) CpG methylation in the promoter region of *Foxp3* and in the intronic region of *IL10* is greater in asthmatic than non-asthmatic subjects; (2) methylation levels at specific CpG sites in the *Foxp3* promoter region are associated with level of exposure to the pollutants CO, NO_2, $PM_{2.5}$, and O_3 over the previous 90 days prior to the blood draw; and (3) activated Treg levels are negatively associated with average *Foxp3* methylation in the promoter region, and *IL10* methylation at region 3 of intron 4 is positively associated with *IL10* cytokine expression. The findings from this study increase our understanding of the epigenetic effects of exposure to AAPs and may impact the development of preventative regimens and/or therapies to alter methylation of these sites and possibly prevent asthma associated with AAP exposure [44].

Conclusion

Our study suggests that asthma is significantly associated with higher DMRs within the promoter region of *Foxp3* as well as region 3 of intron 4 of *IL10*. In addition, DMRs in the promoter region of *Foxp3* are positively linked with average exposure to CO, NO_2, and $PM_{2.5}$ during the 90 days prior to the blood draw. These findings may provide important insight into understanding how pollution could exert detrimental effects relating to asthma, but need to be confirmed in future studies. Ultimately, this research may be useful in elucidating epigenetic biomarkers of asthma and in developing therapeutic targets by which to prevent or correct epigenetic damage resulting from pollution.

Acknowledgements
The authors gratefully acknowledge Dr. Robert Hamilton for his input and the assistance of Dr. Vanitha Sampath in editing the manuscript. We also thank Timothy Tyner and the clinical team at UCSF-Fresno for their help in enrolling the subjects. We also wish to thank the subjects and their families in Fresno, CA, for their involvement in this study.

Funding
Supported by: 5R01ES020926 (PI, Nadeau), Supplement 3R01ES020926 (Prunicki), Austin Family Foundation (PI, Nadeau), and some use of partial funds from Grant NIEHS/EPA Grant P20 to the University of California, Berkeley/Stanford Children's Environmental Health Center (Overall PI, Hammond; NIEHS 1P20ES018173 and EPA RD-83459601-0).

Disclaimer
This publication was developed with R01 funding awarded to Stanford University by NIEHS (PI, Nadeau), R01 Supplement (Awardee Prunicki), and in part with funds awarded to Stanford/UC Berkeley (P20; Overall PI Hammond; NIEHS 1P20ES018173 and EPA RD-83459601-0.) Its contents are solely the responsibility of the grantee and do not necessarily represent the official views of the USEPA. It has not been formally reviewed by EPA. The views expressed in this document are solely those of the authors and do not necessarily reflect those of the Agency. Further, USEPA does not endorse the purchase of any commercial any products or services mentioned in this publication.

Authors' contributions
KN conceived and designed the study and prepared and wrote the manuscript. MP coordinated the study, processed the samples, performed the CyTOF, and prepared and wrote the manuscript. RM and MdP-S designed and performed the methylation studies. LS, CS, XZ, and DD analyzed the data and created the figures. RL provided the pollution data and assisted in modeling. XZ processed the samples, performed the CyTOF, and assisted with the manuscript tables. TP assisted with the manuscript tables. JB and KH assisted in the interpretation of the data and writing of the manuscript. All authors read and approved the final manuscript.

Competing interests
The authors declare that they have no competing interests.

Author details
[1]Sean N. Parker Center for Allergy and Asthma Research at Stanford University, Stanford, CA 94305, USA. [2]Department of Medicine, Stanford University, Stanford, CA 94305, USA. [3]Department of Biomedical Data Science, Stanford University, Stanford, CA 94305, USA. [4]Center for Biomedical Informatics Research, Stanford University, Stanford, CA 94305, USA. [5]Department of Medicine, Columbia University, New York, NY 10032, USA. [6]Department of Statistics, Stanford University, Stanford, CA 94305, USA. [7]Southwest Environmental Institute, Phoenix, AZ 85087, USA. [8]School of Public Health, University of California, Berkeley, Berkeley, CA 94720, USA. [9]Department of Medicine, University of California, San Francisco, San Francisco, CA 94143, USA. [10]Division of Pulmonary and Critical Care Medicine, Department of Medicine, Stanford University, Stanford University School of Medicine, 269 Campus Drive, CCSR 3215, MC 5366, Stanford, CA 94305-5101, USA.

References
1. Fu LS, Tsai MC. Asthma exacerbation in children: a practical review. Pediatr Neonatol. 2014;55:83–91.
2. Platts-Mills TA. The allergy epidemics: 1870–2010. J Allergy Clin Immunol. 2015;136:3–13.
3. World Health Orgnization. Asthma. 2013. http://www.who.int/mediacentre/factsheets/fs307/en/. Accessed 1 June 2017.
4. Carlsten C, Rider CF. Traffic-related air pollution and allergic disease: an update in the context of global urbanization. Curr Opin Allergy Clin Immunol. 2017;17:85–9.
5. Goodrich JM, Reddy P, Naidoo RN, Asharam K, Batterman S, Dolinoy DC. Prenatal exposures and DNA methylation in newborns: a pilot study in Durban, South Africa. Environ Sci Process Impacts. 2016;18:908–17.
6. Alhanti BA, Chang HH, Winquist A, Mulholland JA, Darrow LA, Sarnat SE. Ambient air pollution and emergency department visits for asthma: a multi-city assessment of effect modification by age. J Expo Sci Environ Epidemiol. 2015;26:180–8.
7. Saunders V, Breysse P, Clark J, Sproles A, Davila M, Wills-Karp M. Particulate matter-induced airway hyperresponsiveness is lymphocyte dependent. Environ Health Perspect. 2010;118:640–6.
8. Nadeau K, McDonald-Hyman C, Noth EM, Pratt B, Hammond SK, Balmes J, et al. Ambient air pollution impairs regulatory T-cell function in asthma. J Allergy Clin Immunol. 2010;126:845–52.
9. Iwanaga K, Elliott MS, Vedal S, Debley JS. Urban particulate matter induces pro-remodeling factors by airway epithelial cells from healthy and asthmatic children. Inhal Toxicol. 2013;25:653–60.

10. Somineni HK, Zhang X, Biagini Myers JM, Kovacic MB, Ulm A, Jurcak N, et al. Ten-eleven translocation 1 (TET1) methylation is associated with childhood asthma and traffic-related air pollution. J Allergy Clin Immunol. 2015;137:797–805.
11. Brunst KJ, Leung YK, Ryan PH, Khurana Hershey GK, Levin L, Ji H, et al. Forkhead box protein 3 (FOXP3) hypermethylation is associated with diesel exhaust exposure and risk for childhood asthma. J Allergy Clin Immunol. 2013;131:592–4.
12. Prescott SL, Tulic M, Kumah AO, Richman T, Crook M, Martino D, et al. Reduced placental FOXP3 associated with subsequent infant allergic disease. J Allergy Clin Immunol. 2011;128:886–7.
13. Kohli A, Garcia MA, Miller RL, Maher C, Humblet O, Hammond SK, et al. Secondhand smoke in combination with ambient air pollution exposure is associated with increasedx CpG methylation and decreased expression of IFN-gamma in T effector cells and Foxp3 in T regulatory cells in children. Clin Epigenetics. 2012;4:17.
14. Hew KM, Walker AI, Kohli A, Garcia M, Syed A, McDonald-Hyman C, et al. Childhood exposure to ambient polycyclic aromatic hydrocarbons is linked to epigenetic modifications and impaired systemic immunity in T cells. Clin Exp Allergy. 2015;45:238–48.
15. Mostafavi N, Vlaanderen J, Chadeau-Hyam M, Beelen R, Modig L, Palli D, et al. Inflammatory markers in relation to long-term air pollution. Environ Int. 2015;81:1–7.
16. Ji H, Biagini Myers JM, Brandt EB, Brokamp C, Ryan PH, Khurana Hershey GK. Air pollution, epigenetics, and asthma. Allergy Asthma Clin Immunol. 2016;12:51.
17. Clifford RL, Jones MJ, MacIsaac JL, McEwen LM, Goodman SJ, Mostafavi S, et al. Inhalation of diesel exhaust and allergen alters human bronchial epithelium DNA methylation. J Allergy Clin Immunol. 2017;139:112–21.
18. Zhong J, Agha G, Baccarelli AA. The role of DNA methylation in cardiovascular risk and disease: methodological aspects, study design, and data analysis for epidemiological studies. Circ Res. 2016;118:119–31.
19. Tsuji-Takayama K, Suzuki M, Yamamoto M, Harashima A, Okochi A, Otani T, et al. The production of IL-10 by human regulatory T cells is enhanced by IL-2 through a STAT5-responsive intronic enhancer in the IL-10 locus. J Immunol. 2008;181:3897–905.
20. American Lung Association. Most polluted cities. 2017. http://www.lung.org/our-initiatives/healthy-air/sota/city-rankings/most-polluted-cities.html. Accessed 30 May 2017.
21. Fresno County asthma profile. 2016. https://www.cdph.ca.gov/Programs/CCDPHP/DEODC/EHIB/CPE/CDPH%20Document%20Library/County%20profiles/Fresno2016profile.pdf. Accessed 1 June 2017.
22. Fuss IJ, Kanof ME, Smith PD, Zola H. Isolation of whole mononuclear cells from peripheral blood and cord blood. Curr Protoc Immunol. 2009;Chapter 7:Unit7 1.
23. Janson PC, Winerdal ME, Marits P, Thorn M, Ohlsson R, Winqvist O. FOXP3 promoter demethylation reveals the committed Treg population in humans. PLoS One. 2008;3:e1612.
24. Environmental Protection Agency. Air data. 2016. http://www3.epa.gov/airdata/. Accessed 1 June 2017.
25. Shepard D. A two-dimensional interpolation function for irregularly-spaced data. Proceedings of the 1968 23rd ACM national conference: ACM; 1968. p. 517–24.
26. Pebesma EJ. Multivariable geostatistics in S: the gstat package. Comput Geosci. 2004;30:683–91.
27. Benjamini Y, Hochberg Y. Controlling the false discovery rate: a practical and powerful approach to multiple testing. J R Stat Soc Ser B (Methodological). 1995;57:289–300.
28. Runyon RS, Cachola LM, Rajeshuni N, Hunter T, Garcia M, Ahn R, et al. Asthma discordance in twins is linked to epigenetic modifications of T cells. PLoS One. 2012;7:e48796.
29. Akdis CA, Akdis M. Mechanisms of immune tolerance to allergens: role of IL-10 and Tregs. J Clin Invest. 2014;124:4678–80.
30. Alroqi FJ, Chatila TA. T regulatory cell biology in health and disease. Curr Allergy Asthma Rep. 2016;16:27.
31. Latzin P, Frey U, Armann J, Kieninger E, Fuchs O, Roosli M, et al. Exposure to moderate air pollution during late pregnancy and cord blood cytokine secretion in healthy neonates. PLoS One. 2011;6:e23130.
32. Acevedo N, Reinius LE, Greco D, Gref A, Orsmark-Pietras C, Persson H, et al. Risk of childhood asthma is associated with CpG-site polymorphisms, regional DNA methylation and mRNA levels at the GSDMB/ORMDL3 locus. Hum Mol Genet. 2015;24:875–90.
33. Dolinoy DC, Das R, Weidman JR, Jirtle RL. Metastable epialleles, imprinting, and the fetal origins of adult diseases. Pediatr Res. 2007;61:30R–7R.
34. Yang IV, Pedersen BS, Liu A, O'Connor GT, Teach SJ, Kattan M, et al. DNA methylation and childhood asthma in the inner city. J Allergy Clin Immunol. 2015;136:69–80.
35. Hartl D, Koller B, Mehlhorn AT, Reinhardt D, Nicolai T, Schendel DJ, et al. Quantitative and functional impairment of pulmonary CD4+CD25hi regulatory T cells in pediatric asthma. J Allergy Clin Immunol. 2007;119:1258–66.
36. Kim J, Han Y, Seo SC, Lee JY, Choi J, Kim KH, et al. Association of carbon monoxide levels with allergic diseases in children. Allergy Asthma Proc. 2016;37:1–7.
37. Kim BJ, Hong SJ. Ambient air pollution and allergic diseases in children. Korean J Pediatr. 2012;55:185–92.
38. Miller RL, Garfinkel R, Horton M, Camann D, Perera FP, Whyatt RM, et al. Polycyclic aromatic hydrocarbons, environmental tobacco smoke, and respiratory symptoms in an inner-city birth cohort. Chest. 2004;126:1071–8.
39. Jung KH, Hsu SI, Yan B, Moors K, Chillrud SN, Ross J, et al. Childhood exposure to fine particulate matter and black carbon and the development of new wheeze between ages 5 and 7 in an urban prospective cohort. Environ Int. 2012;45:44–50.
40. Zhong W, Levin L, Reponen T, Hershey GK, Adhikari A, Shukla R, et al. Analysis of short-term influences of ambient aeroallergens on pediatric asthma hospital visits. Sci Total Environ. 2006;370:330–6.
41. Baumeister H, Kriston L, Bengel J, Harter M. High agreement of self-report and physician-diagnosed somatic conditions yields limited bias in examining mental-physical comorbidity. J Clin Epidemiol. 2010;63:558–65.
42. Toren K, Brisman J, Jarvholm B. Asthma and asthma-like symptoms in adults assessed by questionnaires. A literature review. Chest. 1993;104:600–8.
43. Ziegler SF. FOXP3: of mice and men. Annu Rev Immunol. 2006;24:209–26.
44. Kawasaki H, Taira K. Induction of DNA methylation and gene silencing by short interfering RNAs in human cells. Nature. 2004;431:211–7.

12

Competing endogenous RNA expression profiling in pre-eclampsia identifies hsa_circ_0036877 as a potential novel blood biomarker for early pre-eclampsia

Xiaopeng Hu[1,2,4†], Junping Ao[3†], Xinyue Li[2], Huijuan Zhang[1], Ji Wu[1,2,4*] and Weiwei Cheng[1*]

Abstract

Background: The etiology and pathogenesis of pre-eclampsia (PE) is unclear, and there is no ideal early clinical biomarker for prediction of PE. The competing endogenous RNA (ceRNA) hypothesis is a new approach to uncover the molecular pathology of PE. The first aim of this study was to perform messenger RNA, long non-coding RNA, and circular RNA (circRNA) expression profiling of human normal and severe pre-eclampsia (SPE) placentas. circRNA, which has a stable structure, is a more suitable biomarker than other types of RNA. Therefore, the second aim of our study was to select some differentially expressed circRNAs in PE placentas as early clinical biomarkers of PE in blood circulation.

Results: Using microarray analysis, we investigated differentially expressed ceRNAs in human normal and SPE placentas. Bioinformatics, such as gene ontology, KEGG pathway, and ceRNA network analyses, were performed to evaluate the microarray data and gain further insights into the biological processes. RNAs (*Chd5*, *Furin*, lnc-ELAVL4-9:1, lnc-RAP1GAP2-5:2, hsa_circ_0036877, hsa_circ_0036878, hsa_circ_0055724, hsa_circ_0049730, and hsa_circ_0036474) were validated by quantitative real-time PCR (qRT-PCR). RNA immunoprecipitation (RIP) of AGO2 in htra-8 cells and qRT-PCR analysis of hsa_circ_0036877 expression in maternal whole peripheral blood samples of participants were then conducted to confirm that hsa_circ_0036877 is a ceRNA and potential novel blood biomarker for early PE, respectively.

Conclusion: Our study is the first systematic profiling of ceRNAs in placentas of PE patients and revealed the global ceRNA network integration in PE. Moreover, hsa_circ_0036877 can function as a ceRNA and serve as a potential novel blood biomarker for early PE.

Keywords: Pre-eclampsia, ceRNA profiling, circRNA, Biomarker

Background

At 20 weeks of gestation, pregnant women with high blood pressure and proteinuria are diagnosed with pre-eclampsia (PE) [1]. PE is one of the five kinds of gestational hypertension diseases, which can affect many organs and systems [2]. It occurs in about 2–8% of all pregnancies [3]. The etiology and pathogenesis of PE, which are unclear, may involve many factors such as trophoblast cell invasion [4], abnormal regulation of immune functions [5], endothelial cell injury [6], nutritional factors [7], and genetic factors [8, 9]. There is no single factor that can explain all causes and mechanisms of the disease. The central role of the placenta in the pathogenesis of PE is undisputed [10]. After termination of pregnancy, PE symptoms and complications are often relieved.

Many studies suggest that non-coding RNA participates in the pathogenesis of PE [11, 12]. Long non-coding RNA (lncRNA) and circular RNA (circRNA) can share micro-RNA (miRNA) response elements of linear messenger RNA (mRNA), which competitively bind to miRNAs, thus affecting the regulatory function of miRNAs and gene

* Correspondence: jiwu@sjtu.edu.cn; 18017316001@163.com
†Equal contributors
[1]International Peace Maternity and Child Health Hospital, Shanghai Jiao Tong University School of Medicine, No. 910. Hengshan Road, Xuhui District, Shanghai 200030, China
Full list of author information is available at the end of the article

expression [13, 14]. The competing endogenous RNA (ceRNA) hypothesis suggests an interaction network between miRNAs, lncRNAs, circRNAs, and mRNAs. circRNAs can function as a ceRNA to regulate gene expression. Our study focused on ceRNAs, which may facilitate uncovering the etiology and pathogenesis of PE.

In the early stage of pregnancy before the onset of PE, prediction, effective intervention, prevention, and control are of great significance for the disease [15]. At present, there is no ideal early clinical biomarker for prediction of PE [16]. Although placental growth factor (PLGF), soluble fms-like tyrosine kinase-1 (sFlt-1), and placental protein 13 (PP13) have shown potential value, these molecules need further validation [17]. Non-coding RNA studies can reveal markers to predict PE. circRNA, a kind of non-coding RNA, is structured as a closed ring and does not have a free 5′ or 3′ end compared with traditional linear RNA [18]. This structure helps circRNA to avoid the action of RNA exonuclease, which allows it to maintain stable expression and makes it a more suitable biomarker than other RNA types [19, 20]. The aim of our study was to identify a differentially expressed circRNA in PE placentas as an early clinical biomarker of PE in blood circulation.

Methods

Study design and population

This is a prospective cohort nest study. In the study, we recruited a total of 1000 "healthy" pregnant women (age from 25 to 35) followed until delivery and maternal whole peripheral blood samples were collected at 24 weeks of gestation. In all, 40 patients with PE were included in the study and 116 normal healthy women were matched based on maternal age and gestation age. This study was divided into two phases: ceRNA profiling research (discovery research) and biomarker study (prospective development research). In the first phase, we included 6 patients with severe pre-eclampsia (SPE) and 6 matched healthy pregnant women. The second phase was the prospective development study on hsa_circ_0036877 of maternal whole peripheral blood to predict PE at 24 weeks of gestation. The rest participants (34 patients with PE and 110 matched normal healthy women) were included in the phase 2 study. The study design is shown in Additional file 1: Figure S1.

Samples and setting

The study was approved by the Research Ethic Committees at the International Peace Maternity and Child Health Hospital of China Welfare Institute, SJTUM, China. A total of 110 placentas and 1000 maternal whole peripheral blood samples in the study were collected from participants (Chinese women) between December 2015 and March 2017 at the International Peace Maternity and Child Health Hospital of China Welfare Institute (Shanghai, China). Placental samples were taken from a representative block of the central portion of tissue below one third of the placenta, near maternal side. All samples were taken from the same region. This region was enriched for cytotrophoblast, syncytiotrophoblast, and villous interstitium. Samples were stored at − 80 °C until use. The demographic characteristics of participants are shown in Additional file 1: Tables S1 and S2. Forty PE patients included in the study without a history of hypertension, diabetes, or kidney disease were evaluated by an experienced obstetrician. According to the American College of Obstetricians and Gynecologists (ACOG), PE is defined as systolic blood pressure of ≥ 140 mmHg and diastolic blood pressure of ≥ 90 mmHg with proteinuria of ≥ 300 mg/day (or a protein/creatinine ratio of ≥ 0.3 mg/dl or proteinuria of ≥ 1+) or without proteinuria but with severe clinical features after 20 weeks of gestation in a woman with previously normal blood pressure [21]. Diagnosis criteria of SPE were as follows: blood pressure of ≥ 160/110 mmHg with proteinuria of ≥ 300–5000 mg/day.

RNA extraction and purification

Total RNA was extracted from placentas and whole blood using RNAiso Plus (Cat# 9109; TaKaRa) following the manufacturer's instructions and checked for a RNA integrity number (RIN) to inspect RNA integrity by an Agilent Bioanalyzer 2100 (Agilent Technologies, Santa Clara, CA, USA). RIN ≥ 7.0 and 28 s/18 s ≥ 1.9. Qualified total RNA was further purified by an RNeasy mini kit (Cat# 74106; QIAGEN, GmBH, Germany) and RNase-Free DNase Set (Cat# 79254; QIAGEN).

RNA amplification and labeling

RNA was amplified and labeled by a Low Input Quick Amp WT Labeling Kit (Cat# 5190-2943; Agilent Technologies) following the manufacturer's instructions. Labeled cRNA was purified by the RNeasy mini kit.

Quality control of the microarray

Coefficient of variation (CV) method was applied to the microarray quality control. CV, which was defined as the ratio of the standard deviation to the average, was expressed in percentage. The calculation formula is CV = Standard Deviation (SD) / Mean × 100%. The comparative analysis between the two sets of CV value data determined whether the system is stable or not. In Agilent expression profile chip experiments, the CV value of repeated probe point (repeat 10 times) signals calculated the stability of the chip and technology. According to the different chips, the probe point signals were repeated from 10 to 100 times.

Calculation method of chip detection rate: The ratio of the total number of points (flags which does not contain

A) to the total number of probes is the detection rate of the chip.

Microarray analysis

Each slide was hybridized with 1.65 μg Cy3-labeled cRNA using a Gene Expression Hybridization Kit (Cat# 5188-5242; Agilent Technologies) in a Hybridization Oven (Cat# G2545A; Agilent Technologies) according to the manufacturer's instructions. After 17 h of hybridization, the slides were washed in staining dishes (Cat# 121; Thermo Shandon, Waltham, MA, USA) with a Gene Expression Wash Buffer Kit (Cat# 5188-5327; Agilent Technologies) following the manufacturer's instructions.

Slides were scanned by an Agilent Microarray Scanner (Cat# G2565CA; Agilent Technologies) with default settings (dye channel: green; scan resolution = 3 μm; PMT: 100%, 20 bits). Data were extracted with Feature Extraction software 10.7 (Agilent Technologies). Raw data were normalized by the quantile algorithm of limma package in R. The Raw data is available and deposited in public database (GEO). The GEO accession number is GSE102897.

Bioinformatics analysis

Hierarchical clustering was performed in MeV_4_9_0 to identify and visualize patterns within the microarray dataset. Gene ontology (GO) and Kyoto Encyclopedia of Genes and Genomes (KEGG) pathway analyses were performed using GOseq and KOBAS, respectively. The p value was calculated using a right-side hypergeometric test. The Benjamini-Hochberg adjustment was used to correct for multiple tests. An adjusted p value of < 0.05 indicated a statistically significant deviation from the expected distribution. All differentially expressed RNAs were evaluated by GO and KEGG pathway analyses. The network visualization and analysis tool Cytoscape_V2_8_3 was used to identify putative target genes for the predicted miRNA sponge.

Quantitative real-time (qRT)-PCR

cDNA was synthesized from 1 μg of total RNA using HiScript reverse transcriptase (HiScript II 1st Strand cDNA synthesis kit; Vazyme, China) in a 20-μl volume containing reverse transcription primer, 25 μM oligo(dT), and 10 μM random primers. qRT-PCR was carried out with FastStart Universal SYBR Green Master (Rox) (Roche Diagnostics, Indianapolis, IN, USA) in a 10-μl reaction volume on a 7500 Real-Time PCR System using the following conditions: 95°C for 30 s, followed by 40 cycles of 95°C for 5 s and 60°C for 34 s, and then 95°C for 15 s, 60°C for 60 s, and 95°C for 15 s. 0.1 μg RNA was used for all qRT-PCR experiments. For all qRT-PCR experiments, *Gapdh* was the control gene. Data analysis was performed by the Δ cycle threshold (ΔCt) method. $\Delta Ct = CT_{RNA} - CT_{Gapdh}$, which represents the amount of RNAs normalized relative to the amount of *Gapdh*. qRT-PCR primers from Generay Biotech Co., Ltd. (Shanghai, China) are listed in Additional file 1: Table S4.

RNA immunoprecipitation (RIP)

RIP experiments were performed using a Magna RIP RNA-Binding Protein Immunoprecipitation Kit (Millipore, Bedford, MA, USA). The AGO2-RIP assay was conducted in htra-8 cells. Approximately 1×10^7 cells were pelleted and re-suspended with an equal volume of RIP lysis buffer (about 100 μl) containing protease and RNase inhibitors. Cell lysates (100 μl) were incubated with 5 μg control rabbit IgG- or anti-AGO2 antibody (Abcam)-coated beads with rotation at 4 °C overnight. After treating with proteinase K, the immunoprecipitated RNAs were extracted by an RNeasy MinElute Cleanup Kit (QIAGEN) and reverse transcribed using Prime-Script RT Master Mix (TaKaRa). The level of hsa_circ_0036877 was detected by qRT-PCR.

RNA fluorescence in situ hybridization (RNA FISH)

Oligonucleotide-modified probe sequence for hsa_circ_0036877 (GGGACTATGCAAACCAGGGGTGCGCATGCTGGAT) was applied for FISH. First, the probe of hsa_circ_0036877 was marked with BIOTIN-UTP (MEGAshortscript™ Kit, AM1354) for RNA labeling. The htra-8 cells were cultured in 24-well, and the placenta tissue was frozen in OCT and sectioned 5 μm, which were washed with PBS and fixed in 4% paraformaldehyde. After hybridization, slides were washed three times with PBS, were incubated with HRP-conjugated streptavidin to the cells or tissue, and were incubated for 60 min at room temperature (Thermo Fisher scientific, MAN0015834). After being washed for three times for 10 min at room temperature, the slides were incubated with Alexa Fluor™488 tyramide reagent (Thermo Fisher Scientific, MAN0015834) for 10 min and were sealed with tablets containing DAPI. The images were acquired using a fluorescence microscopy (Leica).

Hematoxylin and eosin (HE) assay

Placenta samples were fixed in 4% paraformaldehyde overnight. Then, the tissues were dehydrated in a graded ethanol series, cleared in a xylene solution, and embedded in paraffin. The paraffin-embedded tissues were sectioned at 5-μm thicknesses. The sections were dewaxed, hydrated, and then stained with hematoxylin and eosin. For the assessment of apoptosis in placenta, 10 high-power fields (× 100 magnifications) were selected randomly in each specimen (from the same individuals in the PE (n = 40) and non-PE groups (n = 33)), and apoptosis of trophoblastic cells was examined. The number of apoptosis cells/field was counted to represent the apoptotic index.

Statistical analyses

Statistical analyses were performed using GraphPad Prism 5.0 and Statistical Program for Social Science version 22 (SPSS 22.0). Statistically significant differences were calculated by the Student *t* test. A receiver operating characteristic (ROC) curve was established for hsa_circ_0036877 using SPSS 22.0 to determine whether it was an ideal blood biomarker for early PE.

Results

Differentially expressed mRNAs, lncRNAs, and circRNAs, and cluster analysis

Because of the central role of the placenta in PE pathogenesis, we first performed microarray analysis of six placenta samples from SPE patients and six placenta samples from matched normal controls (*N*). After applying a stringent filtering approach that compared SPE and *N* groups (adjusted *p* value, < 0.05; fold change, > 2 or < 0.5), we identified 731 upregulated and 1617 downregulated mRNAs, 5127 upregulated and 3813 downregulated lncRNAs, and 4569 upregulated and 3984 downregulated circRNAs. The top 10 upregulated and downregulated circRNAs are shown in Additional file 1: Table S3. Moreover, based on these differentially expressed mRNAs, lncRNAs, and circRNAs, a tree with a clear distinction between SPE and *N* groups was generated by MeV_4_9_0 cluster analysis (Fig. 1). The variability between controls in microarray vs variability between PE samples was shown in BOX plot (Additional file 1: Figure S2). These results suggested that ceRNA expression in the SPE group can be robustly separated from that in the *N* group.

GO enrichment of differentially expressed mRNAs, lncRNAs, and circRNAs

We identified the functional categories of these differentially expressed mRNAs, lncRNAs, and circRNAs by performing GO analysis to gain further insights into the biological processes that were potentially mediated by these differentially

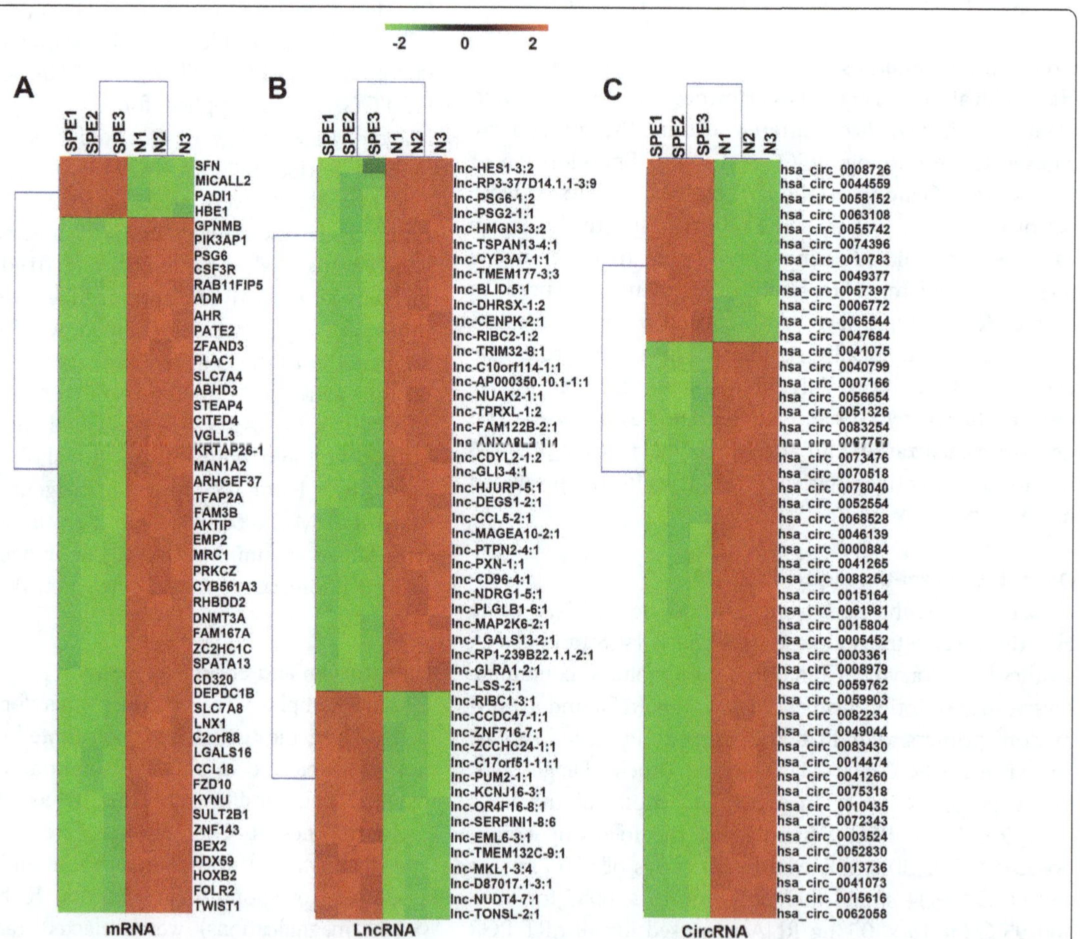

Fig. 1 Hierarchical clustering of mRNAs (**a**), lncRNAs (**b**), and circRNAs (**c**) in placenta samples between SPE and normal controls. Placenta samples were clustered based on the expression profiles of 50 twofold differentially expressed mRNAs, 50 twofold differentially expressed lncRNAs, and 50 twofold differentially expressed circRNAs. The color bar, which increases from green to red comparing SPE samples with matched normal controls, indicates mRNA, lncRNA, and circRNA expression levels

expressed molecules in PE. For differentially expressed mRNAs, 217 GO terms in the category of biological processes were significantly enriched at a false discovery rate (FDR) threshold of < 0.05. As shown in Fig. 2a, the top 10 significantly enriched biological processes were enzyme-linked receptor protein signaling pathway, tetraspanin-enriched microdomain, female pregnancy, immune system process, leukocyte migration, defense response, integral component of plasma membrane, plasma membrane, mating, and apoptotic process. Many biological processes were associated with the pathogenesis of PE, such as immune system and apoptotic processes.

There were 72 significantly enriched GO terms (FDR threshold of < 0.05) for differentially expressed lncRNAs. The top 10 significantly enriched biological processes are shown in Fig. 2b. They were CTPase activity, selenocysteine-tRNA ligase activity, vascular smooth muscle cell differentiation, response to other organism, L-aspartate transmembrane transporter activity, response to hydrostatic pressure, cellular response to osmotic stress, cell differentiation involved in embryonic placenta development, metalloendopeptidase activity, and positive regulation of apoptotic processes. Many biological processes were related to the mechanisms of PE, such as cell differentiation involved in embryonic placenta development and metalloendopeptidase activity. Four hundred and forty-four GO terms were significantly enriched (FDR threshold of < 0.05) for host genes of differentially expressed circRNAs. As shown in Fig. 2c, the top 10 significantly enriched biological processes were protein binding, cytosol, ATP binding, membrane, cytoplasm, nucleoplasm, actin binding, extracellular exosome, positive regulation of GTPase activity, and nuclear membrane. The

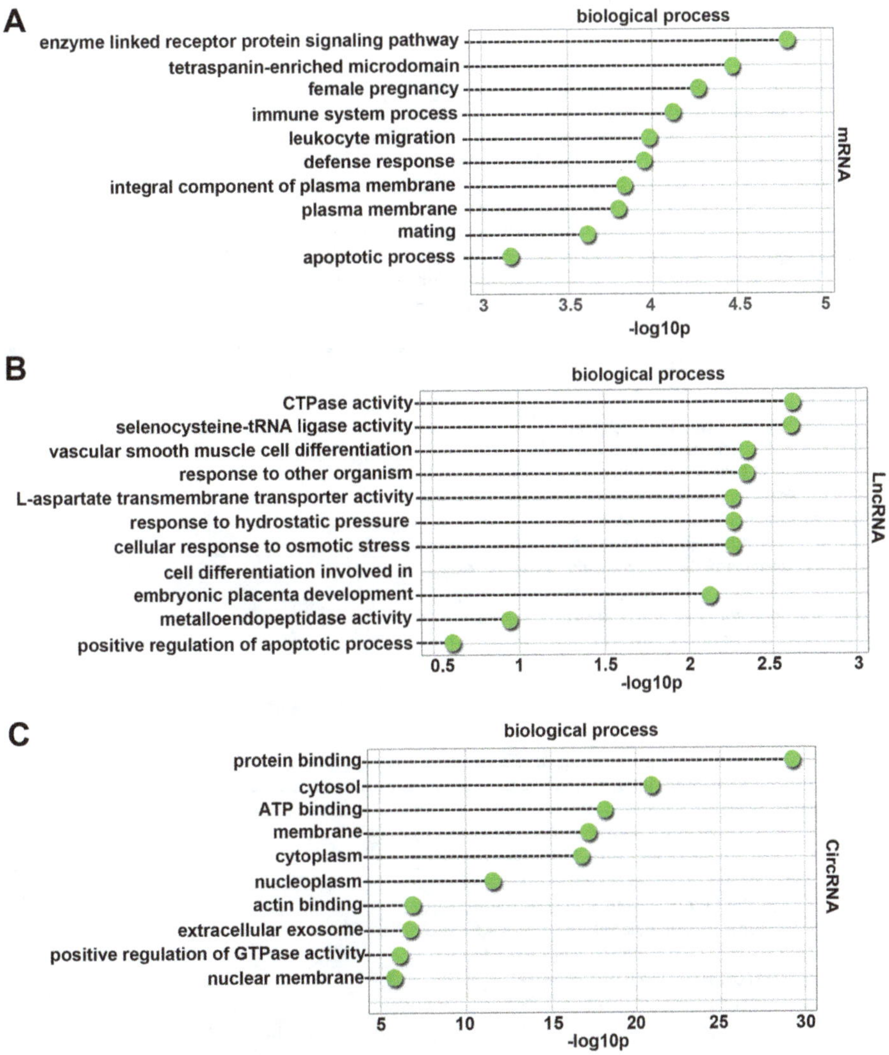

Fig. 2 Top 10 categories of GO biological processes associated with differentially expressed mRNAs (**a**), lncRNAs (**b**), and circRNAs (**c**). Dashed lines represent the *p* values of the top 10 GO biological processes. The *p* values were calculated by hypergeometric tests and corrected by the Benjamini-Hochberg adjustment. *p* values are expressed as the negative logarithm (base 10)

most abundant categories were those associated with pathological processes that may induce damage in the membrane, cytoplasm, nucleoplasm, and nuclear membrane of placental cells.

KEGG enrichment of differentially expressed mRNAs, lncRNAs, and circRNAs

Ninety-four KEGG pathways (FDR *p* value < 0.05) were associated with differentially expressed mRNAs. As shown in Fig. 3a, the top 10 enriched pathways were ECM-receptor interaction, alanine, aspartate and glutamate metabolism, sphingolipid metabolism, metabolic pathways, protein digestion and absorption, PI3K-Akt signaling pathway, proteoglycans in cancer, signaling pathways regulating pluripotency of stem cells, focal adhesion, and peroxisome. In particular, a study has shown that the phosphatidylinositide 3-kinase (PI3K)-Akt signaling pathway is associated with PE [22]. Therefore, the roles of the PI3K-Akt signaling pathway in human PE placentas were investigated further.

There were 14 KEGG pathways (FDR *p* value < 0.05) associated with differentially expressed lncRNAs. As shown in Fig. 3b, the top 10 enriched pathways were microRNAs in cancer, thiamine metabolism, terpenoid backbone biosynthesis, pentose phosphate pathway, cysteine and methionine metabolism, ether lipid metabolism, aminoacyl-tRNA biosynthesis, hepatitis B, RIG-I-like receptor signaling pathway, and protein digestion and absorption. These results indicated that differentially expressed lncRNAs in PE control gene expression on post-transcription level. One hundred and fifty-three KEGG pathways (FDR *p* value < 0.05) were associated with host genes of differentially expressed circRNAs. As shown in Fig. 3c, the top 10 enriched pathways were focal adhesion, ECM-receptor interaction, regulation of actin cytoskeleton, metabolic pathways, DNA replication,

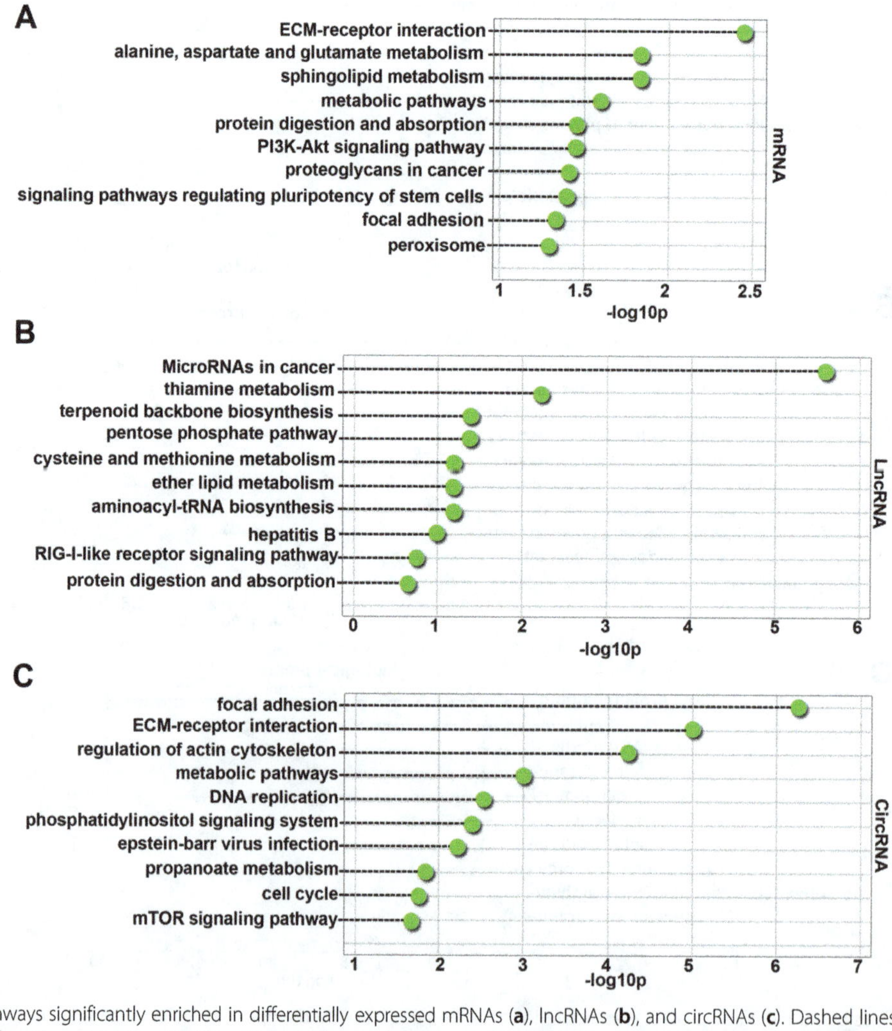

Fig. 3 Top 10 pathways significantly enriched in differentially expressed mRNAs (**a**), lncRNAs (**b**), and circRNAs (**c**). Dashed lines represent the *p* values of the significantly enriched top 10 GO pathways. The *p* values were calculated by hypergeometric tests and corrected by the Benjamini-Hochberg adjustment. *p* values are expressed as the negative logarithm (base 10)

phosphatidylinositol signaling system, Epstein-Barr virus infection, propanoate metabolism, cell cycle, and the mammalian target of rapamycin (mTOR) signaling pathway. These results indicated that host genes of differentially expressed circRNAs in PE were involved in the mTOR signaling pathway that is related to angiogenic factor expression in the placenta of rats [23].

Validation of mRNA, lncRNA, and circRNA expression

Some mRNAs (*Chd5* and *Furin*), lncRNAs (lnc-ELAVL4-9:1 and lnc-RAP1GAP2-5:2), and circRNAs (hsa_circ_0036877, hsa_circ_0036878, hsa_circ_0055724, hsa_circ_0049730, and hsa_circ_0036474) identified as differentially expressed by the microarray analysis were selected for validation (Fig. 4). qRT-PCR was performed to detect the expression of these mRNAs, lncRNAs, and circRNAs in PE ($n = 10$) and N ($n = 10$) placenta samples. As shown in Fig. 4, the qRT-PCR results were highly consistent with the microarray data. Melting curve analysis and agarose gel electrophoresis were used to check for the specificity of the qRT-PCR products.

Global ceRNA network integration in PE

Previous studies show that miRNAs (miR-210 [24], miR-181a [25], miR-126-3p and miR-126-5p [26], miR-223 [27], miR-515 [28], and miR-519d [29]) are involved in the pathogenesis of PE. Based on our microarray data and significant expression of miRNAs associated with PE in previous reports, a global ceRNA network was predicted using Cytoscape_V2_8_3. As shown in Fig. 5a, a portion of the global ceRNA network was observed and GO analysis was performed to gain further insights into the biological processes in this module. Remarkably, we observed that the target genes of this module were implicated in biological processes and molecular functions in the pathogenesis of PE, such as blood vessel maturation and angiogenesis (Fig. 5b).

Hsa_circ_0036877 can function as a ceRNA

The proprotein convertase Furin, which is required for the development of the syncytiotrophoblast structure in the labyrinth layer and normal embryonic development [30, 31], is the host gene of hsa_circ_0036877. In view of this, we explored whether has_circ_0036877 can function as a ceRNA in htra-8 cells (the htra-8 cell derived from first trimester human placenta was cell line of trophoblasts).

Firstly, we investigated the expression of hsa_circ_0036877 in placenta of patients with PE and htra-8 cells by RNA FISH. As shown in Additional file 1: Figure S3A and B, hsa_circ_0036877 was high expressed in cytoplasm of syncytial trophoblasts (arrows show) and was higher expressed in normal placenta than PE. Next, to detect the ability of hsa_circ_0036877 to sponge

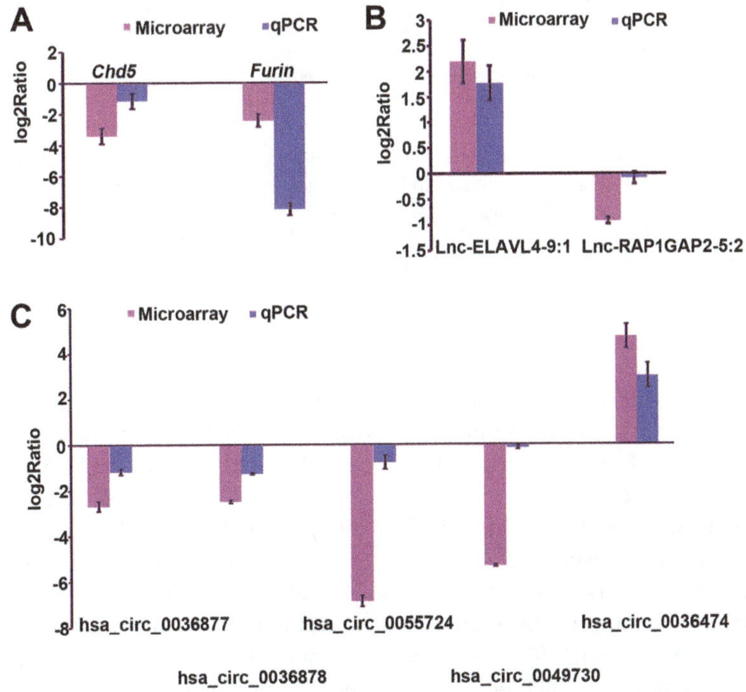

Fig. 4 mRNA (**a**), lncRNA (**b**), and circRNA (**c**) expression validated by qRT-PCR. Genes determined to be differentially expressed in all SPE patients by microarray analysis were validated by qRT-PCR. The height of the columns in the chart represents the log-transformed average fold change in expression across the two groups of patients for each of the validated genes. Bars represent standard errors

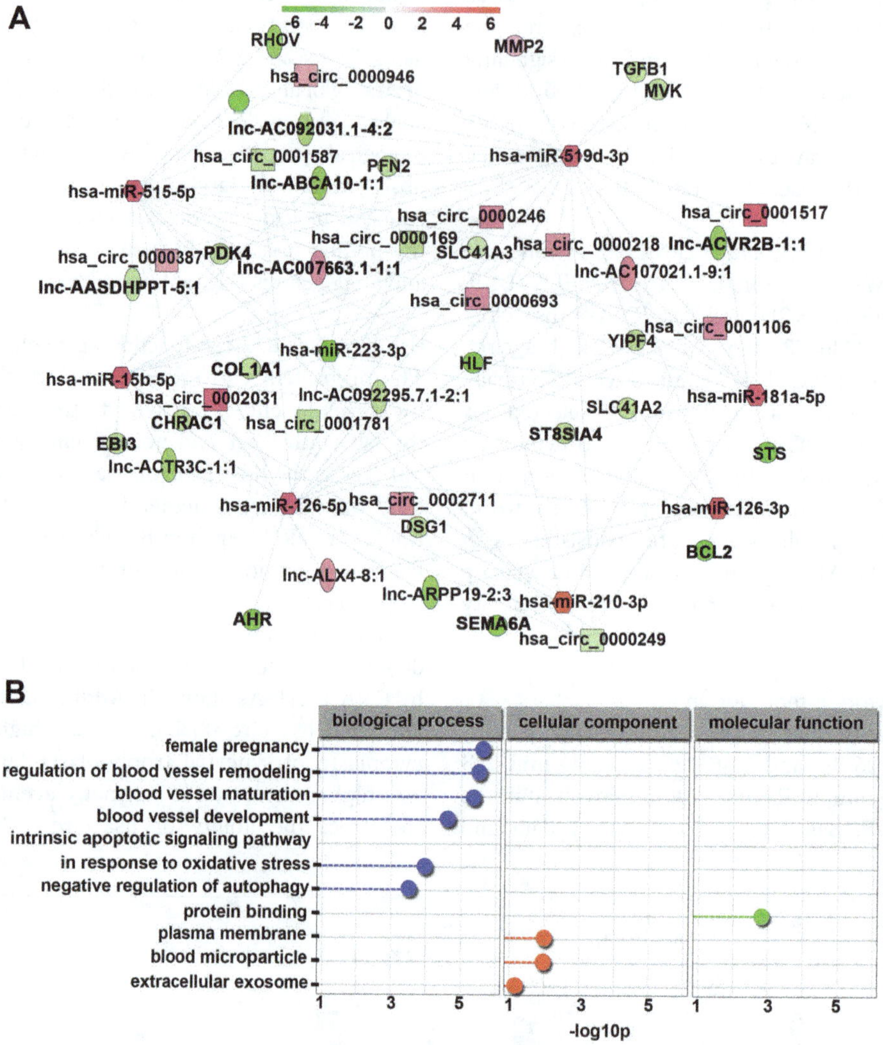

Fig. 5 Global ceRNA network integration in PE. **a** A portion of the theoretical ceRNA network in PE according to the microarray analysis and report data was predicted. The color bar, which increases from green to red comparing SPE samples with matched normal controls, indicates mRNA, lncRNA, and circRNA expression levels. **b** GO biological processes of the above module were involved in the pathogenesis of PE. Blue nodes represent biological processes, red nodes represent cellular components, and green nodes represent molecular functions. *p* values were calculated by hypergeometric tests and corrected using the Benjamini-Hochberg adjustment. *p* values are expressed as negative logarithms (base 10)

miRNAs, endogenous hsa_circ_0036877 binding of Ago2 was determined by RNA-binding protein immunoprecipitation (RIP) in htra-8 cells. RIP assay showed that the amount of endogenous hsa_circ_0036877 pulled-down using AGO2 antibody was detected by qRT-PCR and significantly higher than control using IgG antibody (Additional file 1: Figure S3C). This experiment can identify that hsa_circ_0036877 might recruit AGO2 to sponge miRNAs, because the "minimal RNA-induced silencing complex (RISC)" appears to include AGO2 bound to a short guide RNA such as a miRNA or short interfering RNA (siRNA), which direct RISC to complementary mRNAs and silence gene expression [32].

Furthermore, as predicted by Cytoscape_V2_8_3, hsa_circ_0036877 may function as a ceRNA to bind to miR-519d-3p and miR-15b-5p, thus affecting gene expression (Additional file 1: Figure S3D). GO analysis in this module was performed to gain further insights into the biological processes (Additional file 1: Figure S3E). It is worth noting that biological processes and molecular functions in the pathogenesis of PE, such as regulation of blood vessel remodeling and female pregnancy, were enriched in this module. These results suggested that hsa_circ_0036877 may function as a ceRNA and sponge miRNAs, thus implicating it in the pathogenesis of PE.

Hsa_circ_0036877 can serve as a potential novel blood biomarker for early PE

Hsa_circ_0036877 expression was lower in placenta samples of PE patients (Fig. 4c). To confirm that differentially expressed circRNAs in microarray data can serve as blood biomarkers for early PE, we selected hsa_circ_0036877 whose expression in maternal whole peripheral blood from 110 matched normal participants and 34 patients with PE at 24 weeks of gestation was detected by qRT-PCR. The qRT-PCR results showed that expression of hsa_circ_0036877 was significantly higher in blood samples of 34 patients with PE (ΔCt mean ± s.e.m., 1.779 ± 0.6888) than in those of 110 normal participants (ΔCt mean ± s.e.m., 6.651 ± 0.2192), which were diagnosed at the end of gestation based on ACOG (Fig. 6a). Higher ΔCt value indicated lower expression. Furthermore, Additional file 1: Figure S4 shows the correlation between the expression in placenta and maternal blood from the same individuals in the PE (n = 40) and non-PE groups (n = 33). These results indicated that hsa_circ_0036877 expression was lower in placenta samples of PE, but higher in whole peripheral blood samples of patients with PE than normal controls.

Leading hypotheses suggest that necrotic breaks occur in the syncytiotrophoblast as a direct consequence of an imbalance in the regulation of apoptosis, leading to increased release of trophoblast particles (TPs) into maternal circulation in PE [33]. Extracellular nucleic acids of both fetal and placental origin, packed into either trophoblast-derived apoptotic bodies or shedding syncytiotrophoblast microparticles, which are significantly increased in PE, may be detected in maternal circulation [34, 35]. In our study, hsa_circ_0036877 may be one of the extracellular nucleic acids originating from the placenta. As shown in Fig. 6b, the significantly increased apoptosis of syncytial trophoblasts (arrows) can explain the phenomenon that lower expression of hsa_circ_0036877 in PE placentas, but higher expression in blood circulation.

Furthermore, the area under the receiver operating characteristic (ROC) curve (AUC) of hsa_circ_0036877 was 0.846 [95% confidence interval (CI) 0.754–0.938]. The

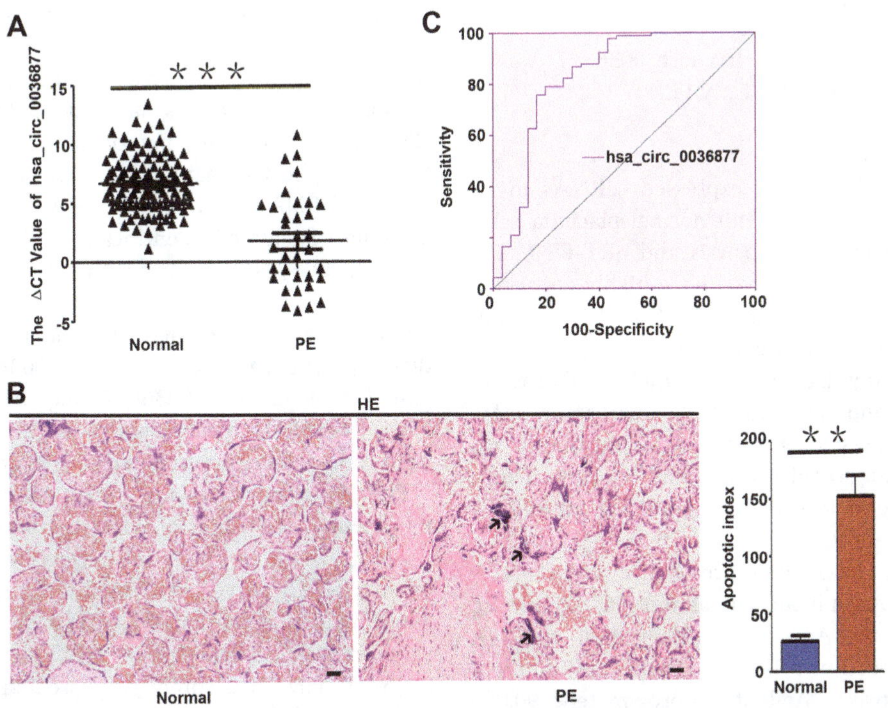

Fig. 6 Hsa_circ_0036877 can serve as a potential novel blood biomarker for early PE. **a** Expression of hsa_circ_0036877 in blood samples from 110 matched normal participants and 34 patients with PE at 24 weeks of gestation was detected by qRT-PCR. The expression of hsa_circ_0036877 in blood samples of PE (ΔCt mean ± s.e.m., 1.778 ± 0.6888) diagnosed after gestation based on ACOG was significantly higher than in normal controls (ΔCt mean ± s.e.m., 6.651 ± 0.2192). Higher ΔCt value indicated lower expression. Bars indicate means ± s.e.m. from independent experiments. ***p < 0.0001. **b** Compared with matched normal controls, significantly increased apoptosis of syncytial trophoblasts was found in the PE placenta. Right panel showed that the apoptosis index in normal and PE placenta was statisticed. Scale bar, 50 μm. **p < 0.001 **c** ROC curves showed that hsa_circ_0036877 can serve as a potential blood biomarker for prediction of PE. AUC, 0.846 (95% CI 0.754–0.938); sensitivity and specificity, 85.3 and 72.7%, respectively. The cutoff value was 5.13 (ΔCt value) (the optimal cutoff point was determined at the maximum of Youden index (YI)). The PPV of an ΔCt value of 5.13 or lower for a diagnosis of preeclampsia was 49.1%. An ΔCt value above 5.13 had a high NPV of 94.1%

cutoff value (the optimal cutoff point was determined at the maximum of Youden index (YI)) was 5.13 (ΔCt value) (Fig. 6c). The sensitivity and specificity were 85.3 and 72. 7%, respectively. The positive predictive value (PPV) of an ΔCt value of 5.13 or lower for a diagnosis of preeclampsia was 49.1%. An ΔCt value above 5.13 had a high negative predictive value (NPV) of 94.1%. These results suggested that hsa_circ_0036877 may have some predictive value for early PE.

Discussion

Main findings

In this study, we identified the ceRNA network by integrated analyses of mRNA, lncRNA, and circRNA expression profiles in human normal and SPE placentas. The global ceRNA network was predicted based on microarray data, and hsa_circ_0036877 functions as a ceRNA, thus affecting gene expression in trophoblast cells.

The second aim of our study was to identify differentially expressed circRNAs in PE placentas as early clinical biomarkers of PE in blood circulation. In prospective development study, qRT-PCR showed that the expression of hsa_circ_0036877 was significantly higher in blood samples from PE patients than normal participants. Furthermore, the ROC analyses of qRT-PCR results indicated that hsa_circ_0036877 was a potential blood biomarker for early PE.

Strength and limitations

We investigated differentially expressed ceRNAs in PE placenta samples compared with normal placenta samples by Agilent microarray analysis and qRT-PCR. The results of the microarray analysis were highly consistent with those of qRT-PCR in our study. The qRT-PCR was used to confirm the ceRNA expression profiles obtained from the microarray data. Although qRT-PCR provides higher accuracy and sensitivity than microarray, qRT-PCR data only represent one point data and microarray data can represent overall present state of participants. So microarray seems to over represent data for ceRNA compared to qRT-PCR.

Recent studies have identified some differentially expressed circRNAs in blood circulation [36, 37] and PE placentas [38] using Agilent and KangChen circRNA microarrays, respectively. Because there are different gene probes between Agilent (approximately 90,000 probes) and KangChen (301 probes) circRNA microarrays (e.g., there are no expression probes for hsa-circRNA-100782, hsa-circRNA-102682, or hsa-circRNA-104820 in the Agilent circRNA microarray) [38], our findings did not conflict with their results.

In previous studies, mRNA [39] and lncRNA [40] expression profiling of PE placentas was performed. We first systematically elucidated the CeRNA expression profiles of the placentas of PE patients and characterized the genetic pathways. Systematic comparisons demonstrated common pathological changes in the placenta of patients with PE. Molecular processes and signaling pathways controlling cell fates (e.g., the cell cycle and mTOR signaling pathway) were found to be significantly disrupted in PE based on microarray analysis. These results provide insights into the pathoetiology of PE as well as reproductive fitness at the molecular level and suggest a series of targets for therapy.

Our study has some limitations. Firstly, due to time, region, and economic problems, we investigated Chinese population, but other population was not done in this paper. Secondly, an important limitation of the study is the relatively small sample size. We will set multi-centers and recruit much more participants to investigate the hsa_circ_0036877 of biomarker research to predict PE in next project study.

Interpretation

Pre-eclampsia is the leading cause of pregnancy-associated morbidity and mortality, and the management of this complex syndrome needs to be improved [41–43]. Although the etiology and pathogenesis of PE are unclear, competing endogenous RNA (ceRNA) hypothesis is a new approach to uncover the molecular pathology of PE. Studies have revealed that non-coding RNA is involved in the pathogenesis of PE [11, 12], and further implicated that ceRNA may play role in its processes. CeRNA profiling and network analyses of SPE placentas facilitated identification of deregulated biological processes or pathways that might be regulated by ceRNAs that could serve as ideal therapeutic targets. Based on ceRNA microarray data and RIP assay, we predicted potential targets of hsa_circ_0036877, which suggested that hsa_circ_0036877 may be related to PE. Next, the ceRNA mechanism of hsa_circ_0036877 in PE need to be further investigated in vivo and in vitro.

The tissue specificity and stability of circRNA enhance its potential for use as a biomarker for the diagnosis of PE [44]. The area under the receiver operating characteristic (ROC) curve (AUC) of hsa_circ_0036877 was 0. 846 [95% confidence interval (CI) 0.754–0.938]. An ΔCt value above 5.13 had a high NPV of 94.1%. Hsa_circ_0036877 may have some early predictive value for PE and need to be further validated.

Conclusion

Our study is the first systematic profiling of ceRNAs in placentas of PE patients and revealed the global ceRNA network integration in PE. Moreover, hsa_circ_0036877 can function as a ceRNA and serve as a potential novel blood biomarker for early PE.

Additional file

Additional file 1: The demographic characteristics of the pregnant women which 12 placentas were from. The demographic characteristics of the pregnant women which blood samples were from. The top 10 differentially expressed circRNAs in placenta of PE using microarray analyses. Oligonucleotide primer sequences for qRT-PCR. Study disign. The variability between controls in microarray vs variability between PE samples was shown in BOX plot. Hsa_circ_0036877 can function as a ceRNA in the PE placenta. The correlation between the expression in placenta and maternal blood from the same individuals in the PE and non-PE grounps.

Abbreviations

ACOG: American College of Obstetricians and Gynecologists; AUC: Area under the receiver operating characteristic curve; BMI: Body mass index; CeRNA: Competing endogenous RNA; CI: Confidence interval; circRNA: Circular RNA; CV: Coefficient of variation; FDR: False discovery rate; GO: Gene ontology; HE: Hematoxylin and eosin; KEGG: Kyoto Encyclopedia of Genes and Genomes; lncRNA: Long non-coding RNA; miRNA: Micro-RNA; mRNA: Messenger RNA; NPV: Negative predictive value; PE: Pre-eclampsia; PLGF: Placental growth factor; PP13: Placental protein 13; PPV: Positive predictive value; RIN: RNA integrity number; RIP: RNA immunoprecipitation; RISC: RNA-induced silencing complex; RNA FISH: RNA fluorescence in situ hybridization; RNAi: RNA-mediated gene silencing; ROC: Receiver operating characteristic; SD: Standard deviation; sFlt-1: Soluble fms-like tyrosine kinase-1; SiRNA: Short interfering RNA; SPE: Severe pre-eclampsia; YI: Youden index; ΔCt: Δ cycle threshold

Acknowledgements

We gratefully acknowledge all the participants of the study. International Peace Maternity and Child Health Hospital of China Welfare Institute, SJTUM, China, and Ms. Huijuan Zhang are also acknowledged for their help with regard to the sample collection.

Funding

This work was supported by the National Basic Research Program of China (2017YFA0504201), National Natural Science Foundation of China (81370727 and 81720108017), Shanghai Municipal Commission of Health and Family Planning (201610361), and Shanghai Jiao Tong University Medicine-Engineering Fund (YG2017ZD11).

Microarray data accession number

Datasets are available publically at the Gene Expression Omnibus (GEO) database (http://www.ncbi.nlm.nih.gov/geo/) under accession number GSE102897.

Authors' contributions

WC and JW conceived and designed the study. XH, JA, and XL aided in the design of the study and analyzed microarray data. Validation of microarray data and biomarker were performed by XH and XL. CeRNA function was performed by XH and JA. XH and HZ wrote the manuscript. All authors edited and approved the manuscript.

Competing interests

The authors declare that they have no competing interests.

Author details

[1]International Peace Maternity and Child Health Hospital, Shanghai Jiao Tong University School of Medicine, No. 910. Hengshan Road, Xuhui District, Shanghai 200030, China. [2]Bio-X Institutes, Shanghai Jiao Tong University, No. 800. Dongchuan Road, Minhang District, Shanghai 200240, China. [3]State Key Laboratory of Oncogenes and Related Genes, Shanghai Cancer Institute, Renji Hospital, Shanghai Jiao Tong University School of Medicine, Shanghai 200032, China. [4]Key Laboratory of Fertility Preservation and Maintenance of Ministry of Education, Ningxia Medical University, Yinchuan 750004, China.

References

1. Sibai B, Dekker G, Kupferminc M. Pre-eclampsia. Lancet. 2005;365(9461):785–99.
2. Cote AM, Firoz T, Mattman A, Lam EM, von Dadelszen P, Magee LA. The 24-hour urine collection: gold standard or historical practice? Am J Obstet Gynecol. 2008;199(6):625. e621-626.
3. Steegers EA, von Dadelszen P, Duvekot JJ, Pijnenborg R. Pre-eclampsia. Lancet. 2010;376(9741):631–44.
4. Kadyrov M, Kingdom JCP, Huppertz B. Divergent trophoblast invasion and apoptosis in placental bed spiral arteries from pregnancies complicated by maternal anemia and early-onset preeclampsia/intrauterine growth restriction. Am J Obstet Gynecol. 2006;194(2):557–63.
5. Kumpel BM, Manoussaka MS. Placental immunology and maternal alloimmune responses. Vox Sang. 2012;102(1):2–12.
6. Duckitt K, Harrington D. Risk factors for pre-eclampsia at antenatal booking: systematic review of controlled studies. BMJ. 2005;330(7491):565.
7. Banerjee S, Chambers AE, Campbell S. Vitamin C and vitamin E in pregnant women at risk of pre-eclampsia. Lancet. 2006;368(9531):199. author reply 199-200.
8. Henson MC, Castracane VD. Leptin: roles and regulation in primate pregnancy. Semin Reprod Med. 2002;20(2):113–22.
9. Anderson CM, Ren J. Leptin, leptin resistance and endothelial dysfunction in pre-eclampsia. Cell Mol Biol. 2002;48 Online Pub:OL323–9.
10. Venkatesha S, Toporsian M, Lam C, Hanai J, Mammoto T, Kim YM, Bdolah Y, Lim KH, Yuan HT, Libermann TA, et al. Soluble endoglin contributes to the pathogenesis of preeclampsia. Nat Med. 2006;12(6):642–9.
11. Song X, Luo X, Gao Q, Wang Y, Gao Q, Long W. Dysregulation of LncRNAs in placenta and pathogenesis of preeclampsia. Curr Drug Targets. 2017;18:1165–70.
12. Biro O, Nagy B, Rigo J Jr. Identifying miRNA regulatory mechanisms in preeclampsia by systems biology approaches. Hypertens Pregnancy. 2017;36(1):90–9.
13. Lukiw WJ. Circular RNA (circRNA) in Alzheimer's disease (AD). Front Genet. 2013;4:307.
14. Burd CE, Jeck WR, Liu Y, Sanoff HK, Wang Z, Sharpless NE. Expression of linear and novel circular forms of an INK4/ARF-associated non-coding RNA correlates with atherosclerosis risk. PLoS Genet. 2010;6(12):e1001233.
15. Lavallee L. Clinical presentation, assessment and management of pre-eclampsia. Nurs Stand. 2015;29(45):51–9.
16. Sibai BM. First-trimester screening with combined maternal clinical factors, biophysical and biomarkers to predict preterm pre-eclampsia and hypertensive disorders: are they ready for clinical use? BJOG. 2015;122(3):282–3.
17. Robinson CJ, Johnson DD, Chang EY, Armstrong DM, Wang W. Evaluation of placenta growth factor and soluble Fms-like tyrosine kinase 1 receptor levels in mild and severe preeclampsia. Am J Obstet Gynecol. 2006;195(1):255–9.
18. Chen LL, Yang L. Regulation of circRNA biogenesis. RNA Biol. 2015; 12(4):381–8.
19. Petkovic S, Muller S. RNA circularization strategies in vivo and in vitro. Nucleic Acids Res. 2015;43(4):2454–65.
20. Lasda E, Parker R. Circular RNAs: diversity of form and function. RNA. 2014; 20(12):1829–42.
21. Hypertension in pregnancy. Report of the American College of Obstetricians and Gynecologists' Task Force on Hypertension in Pregnancy. Obstet Gynecol. 2013;122:1122–31.
22. Cudmore MJ, Ahmad S, Sissaoui S, Ramma W, Ma B, Fujisawa T, Al-Ani B, Wang K, Cai M, Crispi F, et al. Loss of Akt activity increases circulating soluble endoglin release in preeclampsia: identification of inter-dependency between Akt-1 and heme oxygenase-1. Eur Heart J. 2012;33(9):1150–8.
23. Ozmen A, Unek G, Kipmen-Korgun D, Cetinkaya B, Avcil Z, Korgun ET. Glucocorticoid exposure altered angiogenic factor expression via Akt/mTOR pathway in rat placenta. Ann Anat. 2015;198:34–40.
24. Liu C, Zhou Y, Zhang Z. MiR-210: an important player in the pathogenesis of preeclampsia? J Cell Mol Med. 2012;16(4):943–4.
25. Hu Y, Li P, Hao S, Liu L, Zhao J, Hou Y. Differential expression of microRNAs in the placentae of Chinese patients with severe pre-eclampsia. Clin Chem Lab Med. 2009;47(8):923–9.

26. Wang S, Aurora AB, Johnson BA, Qi X, McAnally J, Hill JA, Richardson JA, Bassel-Duby R, Olson EN. The endothelial-specific microRNA miR-126 governs vascular integrity and angiogenesis. Dev Cell. 2008;15(2):261–71.
27. Choi SY, Yun J, Lee OJ, Han HS, Yeo MK, Lee MA, Suh KS. MicroRNA expression profiles in placenta with severe preeclampsia using a PNA-based microarray. Placenta. 2013;34(9):799–804.
28. Zhang M, Muralimanoharan S, Wortman AC, Mendelson CR. Primate-specific miR-515 family members inhibit key genes in human trophoblast differentiation and are upregulated in preeclampsia. Proc Natl Acad Sci U S A. 2016;113(45): E7069–7076
29. Xie L, Mouillet JF, Chu T, Parks WT, Sadovsky E, Knofler M, Sadovsky Y. C19MC microRNAs regulate the migration of human trophoblasts. Endocrinology. 2014;155(12):4975–85.
30. Zhou Z, Zhang Q, Lu X, Wang R, Wang H, Wang YL, Zhu C, Lin HY, Wang H. The proprotein convertase furin is required for trophoblast syncytialization. Cell Death Dis. 2013;4:e593.
31. Vargas A, Zhou S, Ethier-Chiasson M, Flipo D, Lafond J, Gilbert C, Barbeau B. Syncytin proteins incorporated in placenta exosomes are important for cell uptake and show variation in abundance in serum exosomes from patients with preeclampsia. FASEB J. 2014;28(8):3703–19.
32. Kumar MS, Armenteros-Monterroso E, East P, Chakravorty P, Matthews N, Winslow MM, Downward J. HMGA2 functions as a competing endogenous RNA to promote lung cancer progression (retracted article. See vol. 523, 2015). Nature. 2014;505(7482):212.
33. Huppertz B, Kadyrov M, Kingdom JC. Apoptosis and its role in the trophoblast. Am J Obstet Gynecol. 2006;195(1):29–39.
34. Hromadnikova I. Extracellular nucleic acids in maternal circulation as potential biomarkers for placental insufficiency. DNA Cell Biol. 2012; 31(7):1221–32.
35. Knight M, Redman CWG, Linton EA, Sargent IL. Shedding of syncytiotrophoblast microvilli into the maternal circulation in pre-eclamptic pregnancies. Brit J Obstet Gynaec. 1998;105(6):632–40.
36. Prefumo F. Circular RNA and pre-eclampsia: on the long road from the laboratory to the bedside. BJOG. 2016;123(13):2119.
37. Zhang YG, Yang HL, Long Y, Li WL. Circular RNA in blood corpuscles combined with plasma protein factor for early prediction of pre-eclampsia. BJOG. 2016;123(13):2113–8.
38. Qian Y, Lu Y, Rui C, Qian Y, Cai M, Jia R. Potential significance of circular RNA in human placental tissue for patients with preeclampsia. Cell Physiol Biochem. 2016;39(4):1380–90.
39. Mayor-Lynn K, Toloubeydokhti T, Cruz AC, Chegini N. Expression profile of microRNAs and mRNAs in human placentas from pregnancies complicated by preeclampsia and preterm labor. Reprod Sci. 2011;18(1):46–56.
40. Long W, Rui C, Song X, Dai X, Xue X, Lu Y, Shen R, Li J, Li J, Ding H. Distinct expression profiles of lncRNAs between early-onset preeclampsia and preterm controls. Clin Chim Acta. 2016;463:193–9.
41. Staff AC, Benton SJ, von Dadelszen P, Roberts JM, Taylor RN, Powers RW, Charnock-Jones DS, Redman CW. Redefining preeclampsia using placenta-derived biomarkers. Hypertension. 2013;61(5):932–42.
42. Rana S, Powe CE, Salahuddin S, Verlohren S, Perschel FH, Levine RJ, Lim KH, Wenger JB, Thadhani R, Karumanchi SA. Angiogenic factors and the risk of adverse outcomes in women with suspected preeclampsia. Circulation. 2012;125(7):911–9.
43. Zhang J, Klebanoff MA, Roberts JM. Prediction of adverse outcomes by common definitions of hypertension in pregnancy. Obstet Gynecol. 2001;97(2):261–7.
44. Li P, Chen S, Chen H, Mo X, Li T, Shao Y, Xiao B, Guo J. Using circular RNA as a novel type of biomarker in the screening of gastric cancer. Clin Chim Acta. 2015;444:132–6.

13

Mosaicism for GNAS methylation defects associated with pseudohypoparathyroidism type 1B arose in early post-zygotic phases

Francesca Marta Elli[1*], Paolo Bordogna[2], Maura Arosio[1,2], Anna Spada[1,2] and Giovanna Mantovani[1,2]

Abstract

Background: Pseudohypoparathyroidism type 1B (PHP1B; MIM#603233) is a rare imprinting disorder (ID), associated with the GNAS locus, characterized by parathyroid hormone (PTH) resistance in the absence of other endocrine or physical abnormalities. Sporadic PHP1B cases, with no known underlying primary genetic lesions, could represent true stochastic errors in early embryonic maintenance of methylation. Previous data confirmed the existence of different degrees of methylation defects associated with PHP1B and suggested the presence of mosaicism, a phenomenon already described in the context of other IDs.

Results: With respect to mosaic conditions, the study of multiple tissues is a necessary approach; thus, we investigated somatic cell lines (peripheral blood and buccal epithelium and cells from the urine sediment) descending from different germ layers from 19 PHP patients (11 spor-PHP1B, 4 GNAS mutated PHP1A, and 4 PHP with no GNAS (epi)genetic defects) and 5 healthy controls. We identified 11 patients with epigenetic defects, further subdivided in groups with complete or partial methylation defects. The recurrence of specific patterns of partial methylation defects limited to specific CpGs was confirmed by checking methylation profiles of spor-PHP1B patients diagnosed in our lab ($n = 56$). Underlying primary genetic defects, such as uniparental disomy or deletion, potentially causative for the detected partial methylation were excluded in all samples.

Conclusions: Our data showed no differences of methylation levels between organs and tissues from the same patient, so we concluded that the epimutation occurred in early post-zygotic phases and that the partial defects were mosaics. The number of patients with no detectable (epi)genetic GNAS defects was too small to exclude epimutations occurring in later post-zygotic phases, affecting only selected tissues different from blood, thus leading to underdiagnosis during routine molecular diagnosis. Finally, we found no correlation between methylation ratios, representing the proportion of epimutated cells, and the clinical presentation, further confirming the hypothesis of a threshold effect of the GNAS loss of imprinting leading to an "all-or-none" phenotype.

Keywords: GNAS, Imprinting, Mosaicism, Pseudohypoparathyroidism, Albright hereditary osteodystrophy, PTH resistance, Epigenetics, Methylation defects

Background

Pseudohypoparathyroidism type 1B (PHP1B; MIM # 603233) is a rare imprinting disorder (ID) characterized by renal resistance to parathyroid hormone (PTH) in the absence of other endocrine or physical abnormalities. Renal resistance to PTH, the hallmark of PHP, was documented by markedly blunted or absent urinary phosphate and cAMP responses to PTH injection. More recently, resistance to the action of thyroid-stimulating hormone (TSH) has also been described in a large subset of patients, while growth hormone (GH) secretion appears to be conserved [1–3].

In 2000, the PHP1B phenotype was associated with a loss of imprinting (LOI), at one or more GNAS differentially methylated regions (DMRs), which disrupts the parental-specific expression of its transcripts (the isolated, at the A/B DMR or the broad, at the NESP DMR associated with the simultaneous LOM at AS, XL

* Correspondence: francesca.elli@unimi.it
[1]Endocrinology Unit, Department of Clinical Sciences and Community Health, University of Milan, Via Francesco Sforza, 35-20122 Milan, Italy
Full list of author information is available at the end of the article

and A/B DMRs) [2]. The autosomal dominant maternally transmitted form of the disorder (AD-PHP1B) is caused by microdeletions of long-range imprinting control elements (ICRs) that regulate GNAS imprinting [4–9]. Conversely, sporadic PHP1B cases (spor-PHP1B) present a broad GNAS LOI with no known underlying genetic lesion; thus, they could represent true stochastic errors in early embryonic maintenance of methylation [10]. In a small subset of PHP1B patients, the broad GNAS LOI resulted to be secondary to a complete or segmental uniparental disomy (UPD) of chromosome 20 [11, 12].

The DNA methylation undergoes a process of erasure, acquisition, and maintenance during gametogenesis, then it is maintained during the epigenetic reprogramming in the pre-implantation embryo, and disruptions in any of these steps may lead to IDs, resulting in the aberrant development of embryogenesis, placentation, and postnatal growth [13–15].

The examination of DNA methylation patterns in embryos and in corresponding sperm samples demonstrated no methylation errors at tested imprinted loci in sperm, suggesting that the paternal transmission of epigenetic abnormalities was unlikely [16]. The protection of imprint marks should mainly rely on maternal proteins stored in the oocyte before fertilization (i.e., *DPPA3*, *ZFP57*, *TRIM28*, and *DNMT1* gene products), because both the oocyte and the embryo are transcriptionally silent until the zygotic gene activation (ZGA), which takes place at the late four-cell stage in humans. This hypothesis was further supported by experiments in mouse embryos showing that ovarian stimulation disrupted maternal-effect gene products required for imprint maintenance [17].

The phenomenon of epigenetic mosaicism has been already described in the context of other IDs, such as Angelman syndrome (AS), Silver–Russell syndrome (SRS), Beckwith–Wiedemann syndrome (BWS), and transient neonatal diabetes (TND), and it was proposed that the absence of maternal gene products could cause complex chimeras with variable degrees of normally and aberrantly imprinted cells. Relaxation of IGF2 imprinting was previously found in BWS and in children with non-syndromic somatic overgrowth. In particular, the extent of and the location of (epi)genetic mosaicism may be responsible for the phenotype heterogeneity. Additionally, in most cases of TND, the hypomethylation was mosaic and more marked in non-leukocyte than in leukocyte samples [18–20].

The description of rare cases of monozygotic twins discordant for the methylation status of specific genes, which represent examples of post-zygotic epimutations arose after the twinning event, confirmed the existence of somatic mosaicism also for epigenetic defects [21, 22]. Single-cell DNA methylation analysis revealed the presence of epigenetic chimerism in pre-implantation embryos, emerging during the early pre-implantation phase of development, which translated into incomplete methylation patterns in whole embryos. However, further studies are needed to conclusively determine the mechanisms through which such chimerism is established [23].

Previously published data confirmed the existence of different degrees of methylation defects associated with PHP1B and suggested the presence of somatic mosaicism, with the contribution in a given tissue of both normal cells and cells with epigenetic defects [10, 24, 25]. Up to now, investigations were conducted on PHP patients' DNA samples obtained from a single tissue, mainly peripheral blood, and no specific study has been performed to confirm and characterize the mosaicism associated with partial GNAS imprinting defects.

With respect to mosaic conditions, the study of multiple tissues is a necessary approach, so we collected the genetic material of somatic cell lines descending from different germ layers (ectoderm, mesoderm, and endoderm) that eventually gives rise to tissues and organs through the process of organogenesis, and we extensively studied their genetic and epigenetic status at the GNAS locus in both PHP patients and healthy controls.

Results

We investigated genomic DNA samples obtained from different tissues of 5 healthy controls, 1 patient with PHP1A due to a large GNAS deletion, considered as a positive reference for methylation studies, and 19 PHP patients (11 spor-PHP1B, 4 GNAS-mutated PHP1A, and 4 PHP with no GNAS (epi)genetic defects).

Sanger sequencing analysis allowed to detect a point mutation in Gsα-coding exons in 4 patients (patients 12–15) and to exclude small genetic defects in the 15 other patients and 5 healthy controls. Methylation analysis identified 11 patients with broad GNAS LOI (raw methylation ratios in the Additional file 1: Table S1).

The comparison of raw methylation ratios confirmed the reproducibility and reliability of the methylation specific–multiplex ligand-dependent probe amplification (MS-MLPA) assay, allowing data validation for subsequent statistical analysis. Data obtained from the serial dilution of a sample with a GNAS maternal deletion confirmed the ability to detect different levels of methylation (Fig. 1).

After the analysis of genetic markers upstream and downstream the GNAS locus to determine whether UPD could be the primary genetic cause of the LOI, all cases resulted having at least one heterozygous VNTR in the 20q region (Additional file 1: Table S2). In patients 2 and 11, we were also able to exclude uniparental heterodisomy as parent's DNA was available. The exclusion of

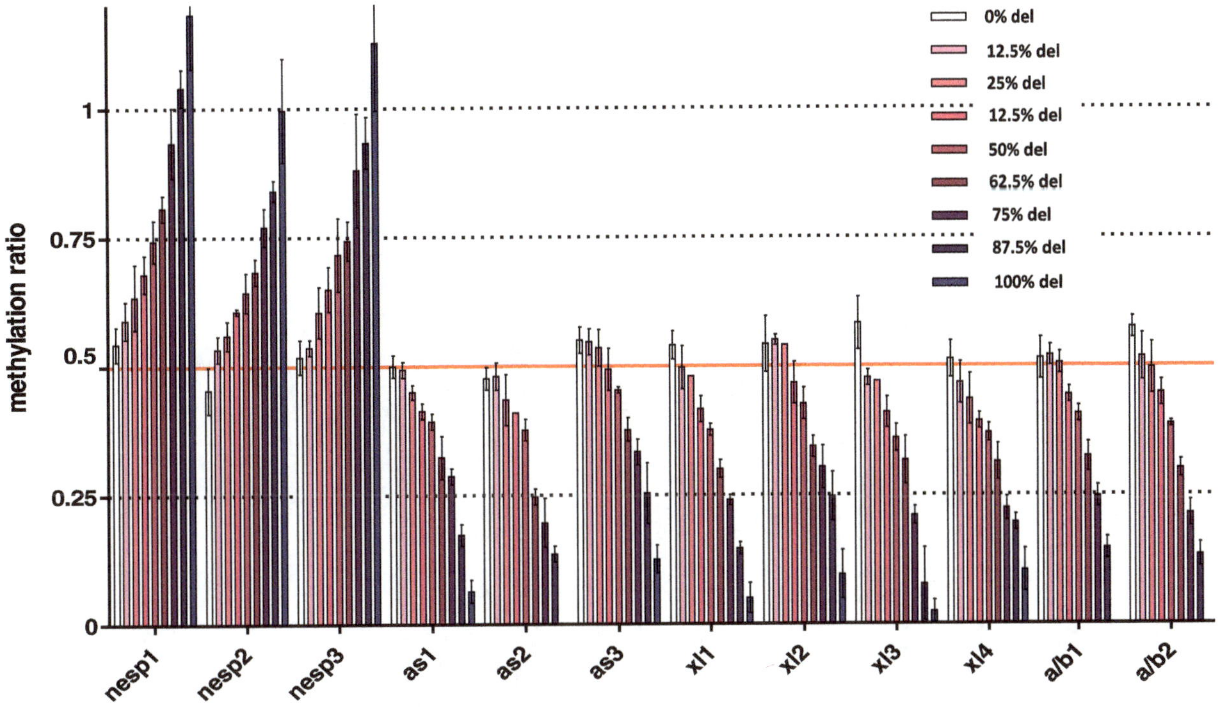

Fig. 1 Graph summarizing methylation ratio ranges detected by MS-MLPA using a 9-point serial dilution of gDNA from a PHP patient affected by a deletion of the GNAS locus on the maternal allele, from 0% (wild type, hemimethylated gDNA) to 100% (severe LOI) GNAS-deleted DNA. On the *Y* axis, mean ± SD observed methylation ratios are reported, while on the *X* axis, the 12 analyzed CpGs representative of GNAS DMRs. The red line in the *Y* axis highlights the 0.5 methylation ratio value expected in wild-type samples

uniparental isodisomy and aneuploidies as causative genetic aberration further supported that the detection of partial LOI is derived from the presence of an epigenetic mosaicism rather than a genetic mosaicism.

Single CpG methylation ratios in the three tissues (peripheral blood and buccal epithelium and cells from the urine sediment) were the same for each subject, and in the subsequent statistical analysis, we considered mean values (Table 1 and Fig. 2).

As expected, in healthy samples and in PHP patients affected by GNAS point mutations, the NESP DMR was hemimethylated on the paternal allele, while AS, XL, and A/B DMRs on the maternal allele.

The investigation of different tissues of four patients with no GNAS (epi)genetic defects failed to find an imprinting defect in cell lineages different from leucocytes, which could explain the clinical phenotype in the absence of anomalies in blood samples.

Because of the variability among different CpG methylation ratios belonging to the same DMR in spor-PHP1B with respect to negative and positive references (NESP DMR = 0.97 ± 0.17 (mean of three CpGs), AS DMR = 0.11 ± 0.11 (mean of three CpGs), XL DMR = 0.10 ± 0.11 (mean of four CpGs), and A/B DMR = 0.05 ± 0.10 (mean of two CpGs)), we considered single CpGs instead of whole DMRs in the downstream analysis. This CpG-specific analysis (raw data in the Additional file 1: Table S1) allowed subdivision of spor-PHP1B patients in two major groups, one with a "complete" methylation defect ($n = 6$) and another with a "partial" methylation defect ($n = 5$) (Fig. 3).

The "partial" cluster could be further subdivided for the presence of a partial methylation defect limited to specific CpGs. Only one patient (patient 2) showed a partial methylation defect in all CpGs, with methylation ratios significantly different (P values < 0.01 or < 0.001) from the positive deleted control. Conversely, the other four patients displayed a partial LOM limited to the AS DMR, the XL DMR, or both the AS and the XL DMRs. In particular, patient 5 had a partial LOM at the AS DMR (AS1 = 0.24 ± 0.03 and AS3 = 0.25 ± 0.04) and patient 1, a partial LOM at the XL DMR (XL1 = 0.22 ± 0.05, XL2 = 0.25 ± 0.04, XL3 = 0.18 ± 0.11, and XL4 = 0.17 ± 0.01), while patients 3 and 4 had a partial LOM at both AS and XL DMRs (AS1 = 0.21 ± 0.04/0.17 ± 0.02, AS3 = 0.21 ± 0.06/0.15 ± 0, XL1 = 0.20 ± 0.03/0.17 ± 0.01, XL2 = 0.22 ± 0.03/0.13 ± 0.01, XL3 = 0.27 ± 0.22/0.13 ± 0.02, and XL4 = 0.24 ± 0.24/0.09 ± 0, respectively) (Additional file 1: Table S1).

The methylation status of the A/B DMR of partial patients, with the exception of patient PHP2, resulted more severely affected by the LOM when compared with

Table 1 Table resuming observed by MS-MLPA methylation ratio means (± SD) at GNAS CpGs (three for NESP DMR, three for AS DMR, four for XL DMR, and two for A/B DMR)

		NESP1		NESP2		NESP3		AS1		AS2		AS3		XL1		XL2		XL3		XL4		A/B1		A/B2	
Sample	Tissue	Mean	SD	Mean	SD	Mean	SD	Mean	SD	Mean	SD	Mean	SD	Mean	SD	Mean	SD	Mean	SD	Mean	SD	Mean	SD	Mean	SD
Ctrls	B (5)	0.55	0.05	0.45	0.05	0.49	0.05	0.56	0.06	0.47	0.03	0.55	0.04	0.48	0.04	0.51	0.03	0.57	0.07	0.46	0.06	0.52	0.05	0.57	0.05
Ctrls	S (5)	0.58	0.01	0.48	0.02	0.50	0.04	0.54	0.04	0.50	0.06	0.57	0.02	0.46	0.06	0.55	0.02	0.55	0.04	0.45	0.03	0.52	0.02	0.60	0.05
Ctrls	U (5)	0.58	0.07	0.49	0.09	0.52	0.06	0.56	0.09	0.50	0.13	0.60	0.05	0.48	0.08	0.58	0.08	0.54	0.02	0.45	0.06	0.54	0.04	0.58	0.06
Mut pts	B (4)	0.56	0.02	0.51	0.05	0.54	0.03	0.57	0.04	0.46	0.03	0.59	0.03	0.54	0.06	0.54	0.06	0.56	0.04	0.50	0.05	0.56	0.04	0.55	0.03
Mut pts	S (3)	0.55	0.08	0.48	0.04	0.49	0.06	0.55	0.11	0.48	0.05	0.57	0.02	0.53	0.09	0.54	0.02	0.54	0.02	0.48	0.02	0.52	0.04	0.60	0.03
Mut pts	U (3)	0.57	0.03	0.49	0.03	0.55	0.09	0.55	0.04	0.56	0.04	0.59	0.05	0.48	0.09	0.53	0.06	0.54	0.07	0.47	0.09	0.51	0.05	0.49	0.14
No def pts	B (4)	0.56	0.06	0.48	0.06	0.52	0.04	0.54	0.08	0.48	0.06	0.57	0.03	0.54	0.05	0.53	0.07	0.56	0.03	0.48	0.03	0.54	0.04	0.56	0.01
No def pts	S (4)	0.57	0.06	0.49	0.05	0.49	0.06	0.61	0.06	0.45	0.09	0.61	0.02	0.51	0.06	0.57	0.07	0.51	0.06	0.46	0.05	0.51	0.05	0.55	0.08
No def pts	U (4)	0.58	0.05	0.47	0.04	0.46	0.09	0.60	0.08	0.55	0.1	0.61	0.03	0.56	0.04	0.54	0.06	0.55	0.04	0.50	0.07	0.51	0.06	0.59	0.08
Del pt	B (1)	1.05	0.08	0.90	0.02	1.04	0.15	0.00	0.00	0.00	0.00	0.05	0.07	0.00	0.00	0.08	0.01	0.00	0.00	0.00	0.00	0.00	0.00	0.00	0.00
PHP1B pts	B (11)	1.05	0.13	0.89	0.11	0.96	0.12	0.15	0.07	0.03	0.06	0.13	0.08	0.12	0.08	0.13	0.08	0.09	0.09	0.07	0.08	0.05	0.06	0.04	0.06
PHP1B pts	S (10)	1.08	0.16	0.92	0.13	0.90	0.12	0.15	0.07	0.02	0.05	0.14	0.09	0.08	0.09	0.12	0.09	0.06	0.08	0.05	0.08	0.04	0.07	0.02	0.06
PHP1B pts	U (11)	1.08	0.19	0.97	0.22	0.98	0.16	0.13	0.07	0.03	0.06	0.12	0.11	0.07	0.10	0.12	0.09	0.09	0.16	0.08	0.16	0.02	0.05	0.06	0.16

Data in parenthesis are the number of samples reported
B blood, *S* saliva, *U* urine

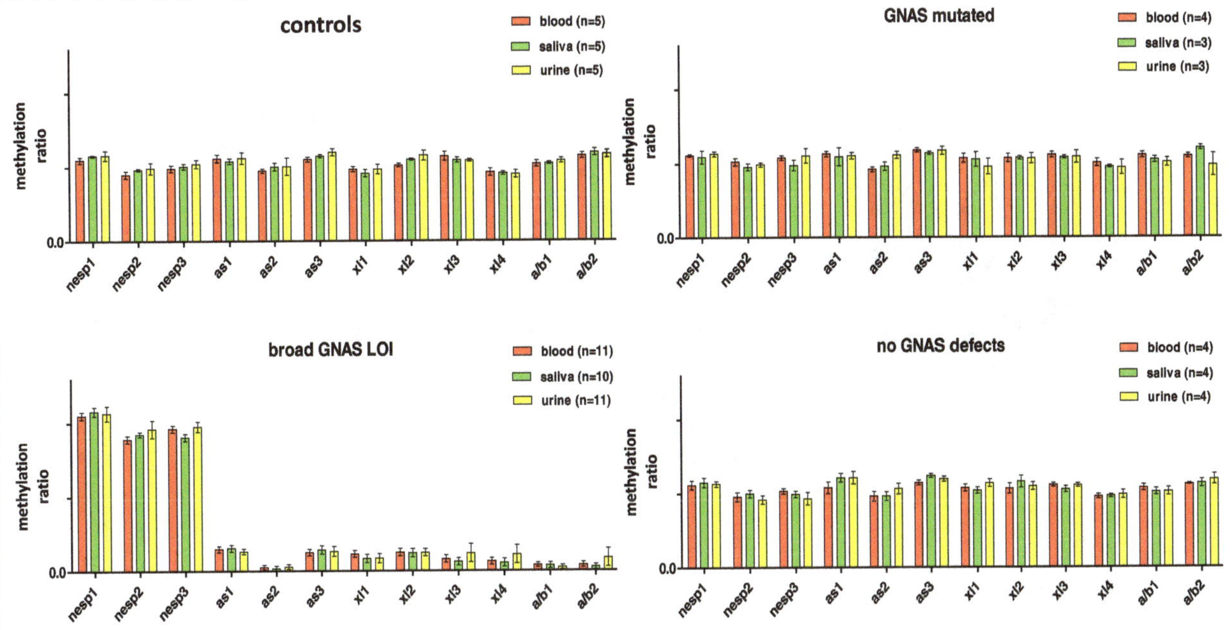

Fig. 2 Graphs showing methylation ratios (mean blood/saliva/urine replicates ± SD) at each single CpG for investigated subjects grouped as wild type controls (WT ctrls), patients bearing genetic point mutations at the *GNAS* gene (GNAS mutated), patients affected by methylation defects at all four GNAS DMRs (broad GNAS LOI), and patients with a clinical diagnosis of PHP but no detectable genetic and/or epigenetic GNAS defects (no GNAS defects)

AS and XL DMRs, with the exclusion of the AS CpG number 2 whose methylation ratio was nearly 0 in all samples. This observation further supported the hypothesis of the existence of a second independent ICR regulating their epigenetic status, independently from the A/B DMR. Moreover, the gain of methylation (GOM) at the NESP DMR was complete in all partial samples, except in patient PHP2.

To confirm our findings about "partial LOM" subclusters, we checked GNAS methylation profiles obtained from genomic DNA extracted from peripheral blood samples in our series of spor-PHP1B patients diagnosed in our lab ($n = 56$), and we observed that these patterns of partial LOM were recurrent. In particular, if we consider the whole cohort of spor-PHP1B patients ($n = 67$), we found that the prevalence of cases with partial epigenetic anomalies was about 42%: 5 patients had a partial LOM limited to the AS DMR, 12 patients had a partial LOM limited to the XL DMR, 5 patients had partial LOMs at AS and XL DMRs, and 7 patients had partial methylation defects at all 4 DMRs (Fig. 4).

Finally, we searched for an explanation of the phenotypic variability, which means the number or severity of hormonal resistances and the presence of signs of Albright hereditary osteodystrophy (AHO), according to the methylation ratio and/or the specific affected CpGs, but we failed to find any significant difference among patients with or without AHO rather than with one or more endocrine alterations.

Discussion

In the present work, we investigated GNAS imprinting in DNA samples obtained from different tissues of a small series of PHP patients, as previously published data confirmed the existence of different degrees of methylation defects associated with PHP1B and suggested the presence of epigenetic mosaicism [10, 19].

The broad GNAS LOI was previously associated with complete or segmental 20qUPD in small subsets of patients, but this hypothesis was unlikely in our case series as all patients were heterozygous for at least one genetic marker, further supporting the presence of epigenetic mosaicism in subjects with partial methylation defects [11, 12].

To study mosaic conditions, the experimental approach relies on the analysis of multiple tissues from the same subject; thus, we collected the genetic material of cell lines descending from different germ layers (ectoderm, mesoderm, and endoderm). We did not observe significant differences in methylation levels in different tissues from the same patient, so we concluded that the partial LOI was a mosaic condition due to an epimutation which occurred in early post-zygotic phases, before the germ layers' formation. In particular, in patients with partial LOI, we determined methylation ratios of 0.15–0.25, consistent with an error in methylation that occurred at the four- or eight-cell phase, i.e., the phase during which the post-zygotic genome-wide passive demethylation takes place [13–17].

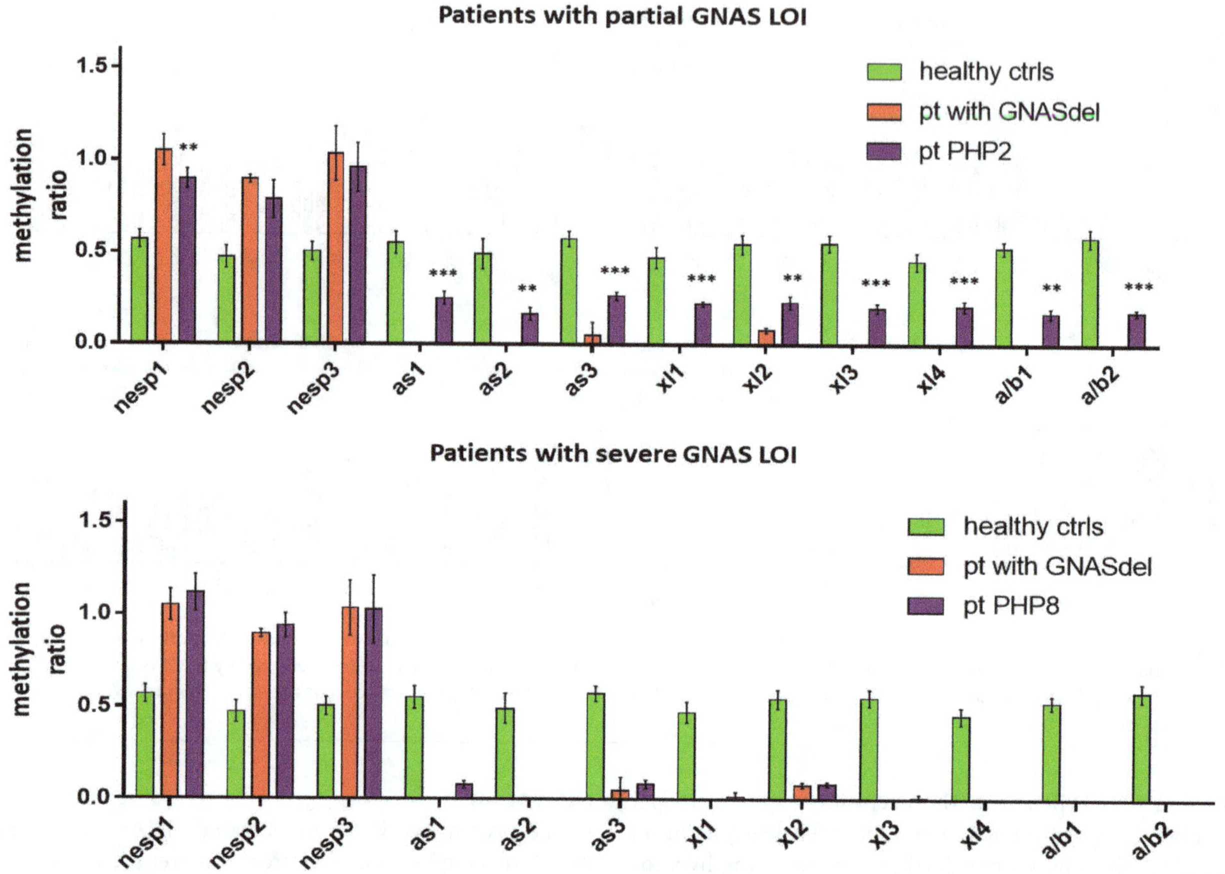

Fig. 3 Graphs showing the methylation ratio (mean blood/saliva/urine replicates ± SD) at each investigated CpG for two representative spor-PHP1B patients with partial (PHP2) and severe (PHP8) loss of imprinting (LOI) at GNAS DMRs compared to values obtained in healthy controls (negative ctrls) and the patient with the GNAS locus deletion (positive ctrl). All methylation ratios observed in spor-PHP1B patients were significantly different from those in wild type ($P < 0.001$). Methylation ratios determined in spor-PHP1B patients could be not significantly different (no symbol above the column) or significantly different (*$P < 0.05$; **$P < 0.01$; ***$P < 0.001$) from those due to ablation of the maternal allele

Following fertilization, parental genomes undergo a global demethylation to facilitate the remodeling from two distinct differentiated gamete-specific states to a pluripotent embryonic state, with the exception of imprinted loci whose differential methylation is preserved by maternal zygotic effect genes accumulated during the oocyte growth. Maternal-effect proteins that protect imprinted methylation sites during pre-implantation development identified up to now include developmental pluripotency-associated 3 (DPPA3; also called STELLA/PGC7), zinc finger protein 57 (ZFP57), tripartite motif-containing 28 protein (TRIM28; also called KAP1/TIF1b) and DNA methyltransferase 1 (DNMT1) [16, 17]. Mutations in ZFP57 were associated with TND, the first heritable global ID compatible with life described in humans, and perhaps additional methylation anomalies of imprinted loci are not yet described [26].

Although the underlying molecular cause of spor-PHP1B is not clear, the mosaicism in cases with partial GNAS methylation defects is consistent with a failure of methylation maintenance in the early zygote, and a maternal-effect mutation might be postulated. On the other hand, in patients affected by complete broad methylation defects, an imprinting defect originating in gametes, resulting in unstable methylation of the ICRs afterwards, could be considered, but further studies to detect factors associated with the GNAS imprinting maintenance are needed. Conversely, defects affecting cells from a specific tissue would derive from molecular errors during later phases of the embryo development, but unfortunately, the number of investigated patients with no detectable GNAS (epi)genetic defects was too small to fully exclude epimutations occurring in later post-zygotic phases.

Studies in the mouse model performed to investigate structure and regulation of the GNAS-imprinted cluster identified 2 candidate ICRs with a different mode of action, one at exon A/B, acting as an insulator model, and one covering AS and XL promoters, acting through a mechanism involving antisense RNAs [27]. The detection

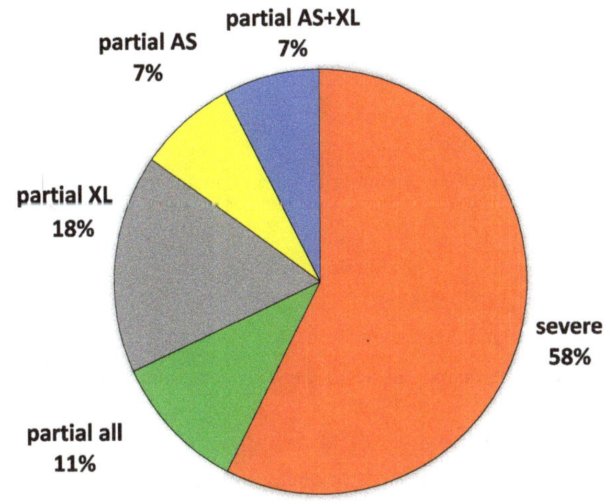

Fig. 4 Pie chart showing the prevalence of different sub-clusters of methylation defects detected in our cohort of PHP1B patients with broad GNAS imprinting defects. In particular, patients were firstly divided into two main groups, the severe and the partial methylation defect (58 and 42%, respectively), and then the partial group was further subdivided into partial LOM limited to the XL DMR (18%, 12 of 67 pts), partial LOM limited to the AS DMR (7%, 5 of 67 pts), partial LOM limited to AS and XL DMRs (7%, 5 of 67 pts), and partial LOI at all 4 DMRs (10%, 7 of 67 pts)

of different patterns of mild epigenetic anomalies in our patients, in particular, partial LOMs limited to the AS DMR, the XL DMR, or both AS and XL DMRs associated with a complete LOM at the A/B DMR, uphold the assumption that two independent and interacting ICRs regulate GNAS methylation and highlighted the hypothesis that different molecular mechanisms might be involved in the epigenetic dysregulation associated to PHP1B. Additionally, a recent work published by Court and colleagues showed that the ICR in the AS-XL region is not a single regulatory unit and that its two DMRs are partitioned by an interval of about 200-bp [28]. These data were in accordance with our finding of patients with partial LOM limited to the AS DMR or to the XL DMR.

Some DMRs, defined as germline or primary DMRs, acquire their allelic methylation during gametogenesis and are stably maintained throughout the post-zygotic development. Conversely, somatic or secondary DMRs acquire methylation during development and are regulated by nearby germline DMRs [28]. Previous studies found that AS, XL, and A/B DMRs are germline DMRs and that the AS DMR affects the somatic NESP DMR methylation status, as its antisense transcript could act in a similar manner to Air [29]. As a matter of fact, the isolated LOM at the A/B DMR, both in sporadic and inherited patients, does not affect the imprinting of the NESP DMR [30]. Our observations further supported this hypothesis because the GOM at the NESP DMR was complete also in partial patients, except for patient 2, who displayed a complete LOM at the CpG AS2, raising the possibility that this region contains a *cis*-acting sequence involved in the NESP DMR methylation establishment.

Finally, in our previous work, conducted in 63 patients with PHP type 1 and GNAS imprinting defects, we found no correlation between the degree of methylation defects and the severity of clinical parameters [25]. The absence of correlation between methylation ratios and the phenotype observed in the present study further confirms our previous findings and can be explained by a threshold effect leading to an "all-or-none" phenotype.

Conclusions

To conclude, further studies to unravel the mechanisms underlying GNAS LOI are needed and, in particular, it will be crucial to determine whether GNAS LOI in spor-PHP1B patients is associated with a primary or secondary epigenetic defect, with the final aim to correctly evaluate the recurrence risk of this imprinting syndrome.

Methods

The present study included 5 healthy controls, 1 subject affected by a whole GNAS locus deletion (g.56′657′752_59′228′953del, previously described in reference 34), used as positive reference for methylation defects at GNAS DMRs, and 19 PHP patients (11 with methylation defects at the GNAS locus, 4 with point mutations in GNAS Gsα-coding exons, and 4 with no GNAS/PDE4D/PRKAR1A (epi)genetic defects and no deletions of the long arm of chromosome 2). Some of these PHP patients (1–6, 9–10, 12–14, and 16–17) were presented in our previous works [25, 28, 29, 31]. The clinical diagnosis was based upon the presence or absence of specific clinical and biochemical signs, i.e., hypocalcemia, hyperphosphatemia, and raised serum PTH levels in the absence of vitamin D deficiency and/or typical AHO manifestations, considered major and minor criteria for the diagnosis of PHP [32–35]. Clinical details, including some additional patient-specific features, and molecular diagnosis are summarized in Table 2. Informed consent for genetic and epigenetic studies was obtained from all subjects involved in the study.

Genomic DNA was extracted from samples of the peripheral blood (Nucleon BACC2 genomic DNA purification kit, cod.RPN8502, GE Healthcare), saliva, and urine (Puregene Core kit, cod. 158622, Qiagen), in order to obtain the genetic material from somatic cell lines descending from different germ layers. Buccal epithelial cells are of ectodermal derivation and urine sediment cells are derived from the mesoderm, while leukocytes are from the endoderm. Mutation analysis was performed by direct sequencing (BigDye™Terminator v3.1 Cycle Sequencing Kit, cod.4337456, Applied

Table 2 Clinical characteristics and molecular analysis of patients included in the present study

pt ID	GNAS point mut	GNAS meth def	Sex	PTH	TSH	SS	Ob	RF	Br	MR/BD	OS	Additional features
1	No	Yes	F	183	2.7							
2	No	Yes	M	899	2.6		Yes					Long QT syndrome
3	No	Yes	M	258	4.1							Hypertension, Fahr syndrome, and renal damage
4	No	Yes	F	215	2.5							
5	No	Yes	M	454	4.9							
6	No	Yes	M	114	5.4							Subclinic hypothyroidism
7	No	Yes	M	X					Yes			Long QT syndrome
8	No	Yes	F	152	0.29					Yes		Leukopenia, normocytic microcromica anemia, autoimmune primary hypothyroidism, and osteopenia
9	No	Yes	M	288	7							Asperger syndrome
10	No	Yes	F	615	1.8							Asthenia associated with lipothymia, genu valgo, andhypertension
11	No	Yes	M	338	2.1		Yes					LGA at birth
12	Yes	No	F	373	8.34						Yes	Popliteal cyst, aortic stenosis, rGHRH, and genu valgo
13	Yes	No	F	83.6	1.49	Yes			Yes		Yes	Irregular menses and hypertension
14	Yes	No	F	X	4.48							
15	Yes	No	F	138	34					Yes		Oligohydramnios,congenital hyperthyroidism, rickets, spastic diplegia, and amenorrhea
16	No	No	F	10.6	7.9		Yes	Yes	Yes	Yes		Cholelithiasis, hypoadrenalism
17	No	No	M	77	X				Yes			Congenital adrenal hyperplasia
18	No	No	F	77.3	1.65							Hashimoto thyroiditis, favism, and multiple fractures
19	No	No	F	37	X		Yes					Oligomenorrhoea

Age (years at diagnosis)

PTH PTH serum levels, normal range 10–65 pg/mL, *TSH* TSH serum levels, normal range 0.4–3.9 mU/L, *X* elevated, but value not available, *Ob* obesity, *RF* round face, *MR/BD* mental retardation and/or behavioral defects, *Br* brachydactyly, *OS* ectopic ossifications, *SS* short stature, *LGA* large for gestational age

Biosystems) of GNAS 1–13 exons and flanking intronic sequences (ENSEMBL ID: ENSG00000087460). Informative genetic markers in the 20q region were evaluated to exclude a possible misdiagnosis of spor-PHP1B in the presence of aneuploidies (monosomy or trisomy) or uniparental disomy (UPD). According to sample availability, the analysis was performed in blood, saliva, and urine samples. For variable number tandem repeat (VNTR) genotyping, we set up a cost-effective three-primer approach based on the simultaneous use of a couple of sequence-specific primers, the reverse one containing a poliA tail at the 5′ end to allow easier allele scoring, associated with a fluorescently labeled universal forward M13-tailed FAM oligonucleotide. All primers and experimental conditions are available upon request. Copy number variant (CNV) analysis of STX16 and GNAS loci and methylation analysis of GNAS DMRs were performed by MS-MLPA (cod. ME031-100R+ EK1-FAM, MRC-Holland) (methylation-specific probe location, GR37/hg19, summarized in Additional file 1: Figure S1). MS-MLPA data analysis was performed using the Coffalyser.Net (MRC-Holland). The detection of expected MS-MLPA methylation ratios of about 0.5 reflected a normal hemimethylated status in healthy controls (considered as a negative reference), while finding of MS-MLPA methylation ratios of about 1 and 0 reflected the apparent LOI in the GNAS-locus-deleted subject (considered as positive reference). At least two technical replicates were performed for each biological sample. A serial dilution, in triplicate, of GNAS-deleted DNA (0, 12.5, 25, 37.5, 50, 62.5, 75, 87.5, and 100%) in wild type DNA was created to define the MS-MLPA detection range of different percentages of epigenetic mosaics. Statistical analysis was performed using GraphPad Prism version 5 for Windows (www.graphpad.com). The exploratory data analysis included means ± SD, median, and interquartile ranges for values measured in the blood, saliva, and urine. Based on data distribution, means ± SD were used for further comparisons. One-way ANOVA with Bonferroni's Multiple Comparison test was used to evaluate the intercluster variability at single CpGs. After Bonferroni correction, a P value < 0.05 was deemed to indicate statistical significance. Continuous variables, i.e., hormonal and biochemical parameters, were reported as means ± SD, whereas dichotomous variables, i.e., the presence of AHO signs, were expressed as proportions. Differences between means and proportions were checked by

Student's *t* and chi-squared tests, respectively. In particular, for the epigenotype–phenotype correlation investigation, we considered the following clinical parameters: the precocity of the disease (defined as the age at diagnosis), the severity of hormonal resistances (defined as PTH, calcium, phosphorus, and TSH levels at diagnosis), and the severity of AHO, defined as the number of AHO signs.

Abbreviations

AHO: Albright hereditary osteodystrophy; AS: Angelman syndrome; BWS: Beckwith–Wiedemann syndrome; cAMP: Cyclic adenosine monophosphate; DMRs: Differentially methylated regions; GH: Growth hormone; GOM: Gain of methylation; Gsα: Alpha subunit of the stimulatory G protein; ICRs: Imprinting control elements; ID: Imprinting disorder; LOI: Loss of imprinting; LOM: Loss of methylation; MS-MLPA: Methylation-specific–multiplex ligand-dependent probe amplification;
PHP: Pseudohypoparathyroidism; PTH: Parathyroid hormone; SD: Standard deviation; SRS: Silver–Russell syndrome; TND: Transient neonatal diabetes; TSH: Thyroid-stimulating hormone; UPD: Uniparental disomy; VNTR: Variable number tandem repeat; ZGA: Zygotic gene activation

Acknowledgements

The authors are members of and acknowledge the Euro-Pseudohypoparathyroidism network (EuroPHP) and the EUCID.net (COST action BM1208 on imprinting disorders; www.imprinting-disorders.eu).

Funding

This work was supported by the Italian Ministry of Health under Grant GR-2009-1608394, Fondazione IRCCS Ca' Granda Policlinico Ospedale Maggiore under Grant Ricerca Corrente Funds.

Authors' contributions

FMC conceived and designed the project, analyzed and interpreted the data, and was a major contributor in writing the manuscript. PB acquired and analyzed the data. GM conceived and designed the project, followed patients, interpreted the data, and was a major contributor in writing the manuscript. AS and MA conceived the project, followed patients, and were minor contributors in writing the manuscript. All authors read and approved the final manuscript.

Competing interests

The authors declare that they have no competing interests.

Author details

[1]Endocrinology Unit, Department of Clinical Sciences and Community Health, University of Milan, Via Francesco Sforza, 35-20122 Milan, Italy. [2]Endocrinology and Metabolic Diseases Unit, Fondazione IRCCS Ca' Granda Ospedale Maggiore Policlinico, Milan, Italy.

References

1. Barret D, Breslau NA, Wax MB, Molinoff PB, Downs RW Jr. New form of pseudohypoparathyroidism with abnormal catalytic adenylate cyclase. Am J Phys. 1989;257(2 Pt 1):E277–83.
2. Liu J, Litman D, Rosenberg MJ, Yu S, Biesecker LG, Weinstein LS. A GNAS1 imprinting defect in pseudohypoparathyroidism type IB. J Clin Invest. 2000; 106(9):1167–74.
3. Mantovani G, Bondioni S, Linglart A, Maghnie M, Cisternino M, Corbetta S, Lania AG, Beck-Peccoz P, Spada A. Genetic analysis and evaluation of resistance to thyrotropin and growth hormone-releasing hormone in pseudohypoparathyroidism type Ib. J Clin Endocrinol Metab. 2007;92: 3738–42.
4. Bastepe M, Frohlich LF, Hendy GN, Indridason OS, Josse RG, Koshiyama H, Korkko J, Nakamoto JM, Rosenbloom AL, Slyper AH, et al. Autosomal dominant pseudohypoparathyroidism type Ib is associated with a heterozygous microdeletion that likely disrupts a putative imprinting control element of GNAS. J Clin Invest. 2003;112(8):1255–63.
5. Bastepe M, Frohlich LF, Linglart A, Abu-Zara HS, Tojo K, Ward LM, Juppner H. Deletion of the NESP55 differentially methylated region causes loss of maternal GNAS imprints and pseudohypoparathyroidism type Ib. Nat Genet. 2005;37(1):25–7.
6. Linglart A, Gensure RC, Olney RC, Juppner H, Bastepe M. A novel STX16 deletion in autosomal dominant pseudohypoparathyroidism type Ib redefines the boundaries of a cis-acting imprinting control element of GNAS. Am J Hum Genet. 2005;76(5):804–14.
7. Chillambhi S, Turan S, Hwang D, Chen H, Juppner H, Bastepe M. Deletion of the noncoding GNAS antisense transcript causes pseudohypoparathyroidism type Ib and biparental defects of GNAS methylation in cis. J Clin Endocrinol Metab. 2010;95(8):3993–4002. https://doi.org/10.1210/jc.2009-2205.
8. Richard N, Abeguilè G, Coudray N, Mittre H, Gruchy N, Andrieux J, Cathebras P, Kottler M. A new deletion ablating NESP55 causes loss of maternal imprint of A/B GNAS and autosomal dominant pseudohypoparathyroidism type Ib. J Clin Endocrinol Metab. 2012;97(5):E863–7. https://doi.org/10.1210/jc.2011-2804.
9. Elli FM, de Sanctis L, Peverelli E, Bordogna P, Pivetta B, Miolo G, Beck-Peccoz P, Spada A, Mantovani G. Autosomal dominant pseudohypoparathyroidism type Ib: a novel inherited deletion ablating STX16 causes loss of imprinting at the A/B DMR. J Clin Endocrinol Metab. 2014;99(4):E724–8. https://doi.org/10.1210/jc.2013-3704.
10. Garin I, Mantovani G, Aguirre U, Barlier A, Brix B, Elli FM, Freson K, Grybek V, Izzi B, Linglart A, de Nanclares GP, Silve C, Thiele S, Werner R. European guidance for the molecular diagnosis of pseudohypoparathyroidism not caused by point genetic variants at GNAS : an EQA study. Eur J Hum Genet. 2015;23(4):560. https://doi.org/10.1038/ejhg.2015.40.
11. Bastepe M, Lane AH, Jüppner H. Paternal uniparental isodisomy of chromosome 20q—and the resulting changes in GNAS1 methylation—as a plausible cause of pseudohypoparathyroidism. Am J Hum Genet. 2001;68(5):1283–9.
12. Dixit A, Chandler KE, Lever M, Poole RL, Bullman H, Mughal MZ, Steggall M, Suri M. Pseudohypoparathyroidism type 1b due to paternal uniparental disomy of chromosome 20q. J Clin Endocrinol Metab. 2013;98(1):E103–8. https://doi.org/10.1210/jc.2012-2639.
13. Reik W, Dean W, Walter J. Epigenetic reprogramming in mammalian development. Science. 2001;293(5532):1089–93.
14. Morgan HD, Santos F, Green K, Dean W, Reik W. Epigenetic reprogramming in mammals. Hum Mol Genet. 2005;14:R47–58.
15. Shi L, Wu J. Epigenetic regulation in mammalian preimplantation embryo development. Reprod Biol Endocrinol. 2009;7:59. https://doi.org/10.1186/1477-7827-7-59.
16. Shi X, Chen S, Zheng H, Wang L, Wu Y. Abnormal DNA methylation of imprinted loci in human preimplantation embryos. Reprod Sci. 2014; 21(8):978–83.
17. Denomme MM, Mann MR. Maternal control of genomic imprint maintenance. Reprod BioMed Online. 2013;27(6):629–36. https://doi.org/10.1016/j.rbmo.2013.06.004.
18. Okamoto K, Morison IM, Taniguchi T, Reeve AE. Epigenetic changes at the insulin-like growth factor II/H19 locus in developing kidney is an early event in Wilms tumorigenesis. Proc Natl Acad Sci U S A. 1997; 94(10):5367–71.
19. Itoh N, Becroft DM, Reeve AE, Morison IM. Proportion of cells with paternal 11p15 uniparental disomy correlates with organ enlargement in Wiedemann-Beckwith syndrome. Am J Med Genet. 2000;92(2):111–6.
20. Mackay DJ, Boonen SE, Clayton-Smith J, Goodship J, Hahnemann JM, Kant SG, Njølstad PR, Robin NH, Robinson DO, Siebert R, et al. A maternal hypomethylation syndrome presenting as transient neonatal diabetes mellitus. Hum Genet. 2006;120(2):262–9.
21. Galetzka D, Hansmann T, El Hajj N, Weis E, Irmscher B, Ludwig M, Schneider-Rätzke B, Kohlschmidt N, Beyer V, Bartsch O, et al. Monozygotic twins discordant for constitutive BRCA1 promoter methylation, childhood cancer and secondary cancer. Epigenetics. 2012;7(1):47–54. https://doi.org/10.4161/epi.7.1.18814.

22. Bliek J, Alders M, Maas SM, Oostra RJ, Mackay DM, van der Lip K, Callaway JL, Brooks A, van 't Padje S, Westerveld A, et al. Lessons from BWS twins: complex maternal and paternal hypomethylation and a common source of haematopoietic stem cells. Eur J Hum Genet. 2009;17(12):1625–34. https://doi.org/10.1038/ejhg.2009.77.
23. Lorthongpanich C, Cheow LF, Balu S, Quake SR, Knowles BB, Burkholder WF, Solter D, Messerschmidt DM. Single-cell DNA-methylation analysis reveals epigenetic chimerism in preimplantation embryos. Science. 2013;341(6150): 1110–2. https://doi.org/10.1126/science.1240617.
24. Maupetit-Mehouas S, Mariot V, Reynes C, Bertrand G, Feillet F, Carel JC, Simon D, Bihan H, Gajdos V, Devouge E, et al. Quantification of the methylation at the GNAS locus identifies subtypes of sporadic pseudohypoparathyroidism type Ib. J Med Genet. 2011;48(1):55–63. https://doi.org/10.1136/jmg.2010.081356.
25. Elli FM, de Sanctis L, Bollati V, Tarantini L, Filopanti M, Barbieri AM, Peverelli E, Beck-Peccoz P, Spada A, Mantovani G. Quantitative analysis of methylation defects and correlation with clinical characteristics in patients with pseudohypoparathyroidism type I and GNAS epigenetic alterations. J Clin Endocrinol Metab. 2014;99(3):E508–17. https://doi.org/10.1210/jc.2013-3086.
26. Mackay DJ, Callaway JL, Marks SM, White HE, Acerini CL, Boonen SE, Dayanikli P, Firth HV, Goodship JA, Haemers AP, et al. Hypomethylation of multiple imprinted loci in individuals with transient neonatal diabetes is associated with mutations in ZFP57. Nat Genet. 2008;40(8):949–51. https://doi.org/10.1038/ng.187.
27. Williamson CM, Ball ST, Nottingham WT, Skinner JA, Plagge A, Turner MD, Powles N, Hough T, Papworth D, Fraser WD, et al. A cis-acting control region is required exclusively for the tissue-specific imprinting of Gnas. Nat Genet. 2004;36(8):894–9.
28. Court F, Tayama C, Romanelli V, Martin-Trujillo A, Iglesias-Platas I, Okamura K, Sugahara N, Simón C, Moore H, Harness JV, et al. Genome-wide parent-of-origin DNA methylation analysis reveals the intricacies of human imprinting and suggests a germline methylation-independent mechanism of establishment. Genome Res. 2014;24(4):554–69. https://doi.org/10.1101/gr.164913.113.
29. Hayward BE, Bonthron DT. An imprinted antisense transcript at the human GNAS1 locus. Hum Mol Genet. 2000;9(5):835–41.
30. Elli FM, Linglart A, Garin I, de Sanctis L, Bordogna P, Grybek V, Pereda A, Giachero F, Verrua E, Hanna P, Mantovani G, Perez de Nanclares G. The prevalence of GNAS deficiency-related diseases in a large cohort of patients characterized by the EuroPHP Network. J Clin Endocrinol Metab. 2016; 101(10):3657–68.
31. Garin I, Elli FM, Linglart A, Silve C, de Sanctis L, Bordogna P, Pereda A, Clarke JT, Kannengiesser C, Coutant R, Tenebaum-Rakover Y, Admoni O, de Nanclares GP, Mantovani G. Novel microdeletions affecting the GNAS locus in pseudohypoparathyroidism: characterization of the underlying mechanisms. J Clin Endocrinol Metab. 2015;100(4):E681–7. https://doi.org/10.1210/jc.2014-3098.
32. Elli FM, deSanctis L, Ceoloni B, Barbieri AM, Bordogna P, Beck-Peccoz P, Spada A, Mantovani G. Pseudohypoparathyroidism type Ia and pseudo-pseudohypoparathyroidism: the growing spectrum of GNAS inactivating mutations. Hum Mutat. 2013;34(3):411–6.
33. Elli FM, Bordogna P, de Sanctis L, Giachero F, Verrua E, Segni M, Mazzanti L, Boldrin V, Toromanovic A, Spada A, et al. Screening of PRKAR1A and PDE4D in a large Italian series of patients clinically diagnosed with Albright hereditary osteodystrophy and/or pseudohypoparathyroidism. J Bone Miner Res. 2016;31(6):1215–24. https://doi.org/10.1002/jbmr.2785.
34. Mantovani G, Spada A, Elli FM. Pseudohypoparathyroidism and Gsα-cAMP-linked disorders: current view and open issues. Nat Rev Endocrinol. 2016; 12(6):347–56. https://doi.org/10.1038/nrendo.2016.52.
35. Thiele S, Mantovani G, Barlier A, Boldrin V, Bordogna P, De Sanctis L, Elli FM, Freson K, Garin I, Grybek V, et al. From pseudohypoparathyroidism to inactivating PTH/PTHrP signalling disorder (iPPSD), a novel classification proposed by the EuroPHP network. Eur J Endocrinol. 2016;175(6):P1–P17.

14

An epigenome-wide study of obesity in African American youth and young adults: novel findings, replication in neutrophils, and relationship with gene expression

Xiaoling Wang[1*], Yue Pan[1], Haidong Zhu[1], Guang Hao[1], Yisong Huang[1], Vernon Barnes[1], Huidong Shi[2], Harold Snieder[3], James Pankow[4], Kari North[5], Megan Grove[6], Weihua Guan[4], Ellen Demerath[4], Yanbin Dong[1] and Shaoyong Su[1]

Abstract

Background: We conducted an epigenome-wide association study (EWAS) on obesity in healthy youth and young adults and further examined to what extent identified signals influenced gene expression and were independent of cell type composition and obesity-related cardio-metabolic risk factors. Genome-wide DNA methylation data from leukocytes were obtained from 700 African Americans aged 14–36. We also measured genome-wide DNA methylation data from neutrophils as well as genome-wide gene expression data from leukocytes in a subset of samples ($n = 188$).

Results: The EWAS identified 76 obesity-related CpG sites in leukocytes with $p < 1 \times 10^{-7}$. In silico replication in the ARIC study of 2097 African Americans aged 47–70 validated 54 CpG sites. Out of the 54 CpG sites, 29 associations with obesity were novel and 37 were replicated in neutrophils. Fifty one CpG sites were associated with at least one cardio-metabolic risk factor; however, the number reduced to 9 after adjustment for obesity. Sixteen CpG sites were associated with expression of 17 genes in *cis*, of which 5 genes displayed differential expression between obese cases and lean controls. We also replicated 71.5% of obesity-related CpG sites previously reported.

Conclusion: In this study of youth and young adults, we identified 29 novel CpG sites associated with obesity and replicated the majority of the CpG sites previously identified. We further demonstrated that the majority of the obesity-related CpG sites in leukocytes were not driven by cell composition or obesity-related cardio-metabolic risk factors. We also provided the direct link between DNA methylation-gene expression-obesity for 5 genes.

Keywords: DNA methylation, Youth, African Americans, Obesity, Leukocytes, Neutrophils

Background

Obesity is a complex disease resulting from interactions between genes and environmental factors that can be modified and/or mediated by epigenetic changes. DNA methylation is a pivotal and stable epigenetic mechanism, and DNA methylation levels at particular loci have been associated with obesity and its related cardio-metabolic traits [1]. Recently, four large-scale epigenome-wide association studies (EWAS) [2–5] in middle-aged and older adults identified multiple DNA methylation loci in blood leukocytes that were associated with body mass index (BMI). However, the high prevalence of obesity comorbidities and use of medications in middle-aged or older populations may hide or bias obesity-related DNA methylation changes. For this reason, we investigated 700 healthy African American youth and young adults. With genome-wide DNA methylation data from leukocytes in the full data set and genome-wide DNA methylation data from purified neutrophils and genome-wide gene expression data from leukocytes in a subset of 188 subjects, the present study has three objectives. First, we conducted an EWAS of obesity in youth and young adults to identify

* Correspondence: xwang@augusta.edu
[1]Department of Pediatrics, Georgia Prevention Institute, Medical College of Georgia, Augusta University, HS-1640, Augusta, GA 30912, USA
Full list of author information is available at the end of the article

new signals and further validate the findings with replication in an independent cohort of 2097 middle-aged African Americans from the Atherosclerosis Risk in Communities (ARIC) study [2]. Second, for these obesity-related DNA methylation loci, we checked whether the associations can be replicated in one purified cell type (neutrophils), whether the associations were driven by obesity-related cardio-metabolic traits, and whether the DNA methylation status of these loci was associated with gene expressions. Third, we examined to what extent we can replicate the findings previously reported in middle-aged and older adults. The identification of obesity-related DNA methylation changes in youth and young adult may provide new insights into the mechanisms linking obesity to associated clinical conditions at the early stages of the disease process and may provide new targets for early prevention.

Methods

Subjects

A total of 700 African American youths and young adults aged 14–36 were included in the current study. These subjects were participants from 3 existing cohorts (for details, see Additional file 1): the Epigenetic Basis of Obesity-Induced Cardiovascular Disease and Type 2 Diabetes (EpiGO) study [6] (96 obese [BMI percentile ≥ 95%] vs. 92 lean controls [BMI percentile ≤ 50%] aged 14–20), the LACHY study [7] (284 participants from the general population aged 14–18), and the BP stress study [8] (228 participants from the general population aged 18–36). All of these participants were free of chronic or acute disease and not on daily prescription medication for treatment of diseases. All participants were recruited from the southeastern USA. Height and weight were measured by standard methods using a wall-mounted stadiometer and a scale, respectively. BMI was calculated as weight/height^2, and BMI percentile was calculated according to their age, sex, height, and weight. These studies were approved by the Institutional Review Board of Augusta University and performed following the guidelines of the Declaration of Helsinki. Written informed consent was provided by all participants or by their parents if they were less than 18 years.

DNA extraction and genome-wide DNA methylation

For the participants from the EpiGO study, DNA was extracted from both peripheral leukocytes and neutrophils using the QIAamp DNA Mini Kit (QIAGEN). Peripheral neutrophils were obtained using the approach previously described [9]. For the other participants, DNA was extracted from stored buffy coats using the same kit.

Genome-wide DNA methylation levels of all these samples were analyzed by the Illumina Infinium Human Methylation 450K Beadchip (Illumina Inc.). The Minfi package [10] and CPACOR (incorporating Control Probe Adjustment and reduction of global CORrelation) package [11] were used for initial quantification, data preprocessing, and quality control (QC). The key QC steps included the following: (1) Detectable probes were defined as the probes with detection p value $< 1 \times 10^{-16}$ in more than 95% samples; (2) Detectable samples were defined as the samples with more than 95% CpG sites having a detection p value $< 1 \times 10^{-16}$ and correct classification of gender based on the genome-wide DNA methylation data; (3) Probes on the X and Y chromosomes and the 65 SNP markers were excluded; (4) Illumina background correction and quantile normalization were applied to all intensity values, and beta value was further calculated and used as the index of CpG methylation levels; (5) A principal component analysis (PCA) of the control probe intensities (excluding negative control probes) was performed and the resulting PCs 1 to 30 were stored; (6) White blood cell sub-populations were estimated using the approach described by Houseman et al. [12]; and (7) A linear regression model was conducted for each CpG site with DNA methylation level as the dependent variable and the 30 PCs from the control probe intensities as well as the estimated cell compositions as the independent variables. The residuals were calculated and used as indices of DNA methylation levels in further analysis. The above steps were conducted for each cohort separately.

RNA extraction and genome-wide gene expression assays

For the participants of the EpiGO study, RNA samples were extracted from the peripheral leukocytes stored in the RNA cell protection reagents (QIAGEN Inc.) using the QIAamp RNA mini Kit (QIAGEN Inc.). RNA concentration and purity were evaluated on a NanoDrop spectrophotometer 2000 (Thermo Scientific Inc.). RNA integrity (RIN) was evaluated on a Bioanalyzer 2100 (Agilent Inc.). The RIN scores of all these samples were greater than 8, indicating the high quality of RNA.

Genome-wide gene expression data were obtained using the Illumina HumanHT-12 v4 Expression BeadChip (Illumina Inc). This chip targets more than 48,000 probes that provide genome-wide coverage of well-characterized genes, gene candidates, and splice variants. The GenomeStudio Gene Expression Module (Illumina Inc.) was used for initial quantification, and the lumi package [13] was used for data preprocessing and QC. The key QC steps included the following: (1) Probes with detection p value $<$ 0.05 in more than 50% of the samples were defined as "present"; (2) Log transformation and quartile normalization were applied to the gene expression data; and (3) A linear regression model was conducted for each probe with gene expression level as the dependent variable and batches (16 batches with 12 samples in each batch) as the independent variables. The residuals were calculated and used as the indices of gene expression levels in further analysis.

Statistical analysis

The R package Limma [14] was used for the identification of differentially methylated CpG sites and differentially expressed genes related to the obesity phenotypes.

For DNA methylation analysis on peripheral leukocytes, the residual derived from the regression of each single CpG site methylation level (beta) on cell compositions and PCs from the control probes was used as dependent variable with age and sex as covariates. The test of interest was group (obese vs. lean) in the EpiGO study and BMI in the LACHY and BP stress cohort. Meta-analysis across the three cohorts was conducted using METAL [15] by converting the direction of effect and p value observed in each study into a signed Z score. This approach is very flexible and allows results to be combined when the β-coefficients and standard errors from individual studies are in different units. To account for multiple testing, a standard Bonferroni correction for the 473,788 CpG sites gives $p < 1 \times 10^{-07}$ as the significance threshold.

For DNA methylation analysis on peripheral neutrophils, the residual derived from the regression of each single CpG site methylation level on PCs from the control probes was used as dependent variable with age and sex as covariates. The test of interest was group (obese vs. lean).

For gene expression analysis on peripheral leukocytes, the residual derived from the regression of each probe gene expression level on batches was used as dependent variable with age and sex as covariates. The test of interest was group (obese vs. lean).

The differentially methylated CpG sites identified for obesity and BMI in peripheral leukocytes with a p value< 1×10^{-07} were carried forward for replication in the African American participants of the ARIC study [2] ($n = 2097$, 64% females, age range from 47 to 70). Leukocyte DNA and the same Illumina 450K platform for methylation analysis were used in ARIC study. Replication was defined as consistent direction of the β-coefficient and FDR < 0.05 in the BMI-related CpG sites from the ARIC study. The replicated CpG sites were taken forward in the following analyses: First, they were checked in obesity-related CpGs identified from neutrophils. Replication was defined as consistent direction of the β-coefficient and FDR< 0.05 in neutrophils. Second, their associations with seven cardio-metabolic traits including SBP, fasting glucose, fasting insulin, fasting triglycerides (TG), fasting total cholesterol (TC), fasting HDL-cholesterol (HDLC), and fasting LDL-cholesterol (LDLC) were tested in EpiGO and LACHY cohorts with and without the adjustment of obesity status/BMI. A p value < 0.05 was defined as significant. Third, *cis*-regulation of these CpG sites of gene expression (within ± 250 kb of the CpG sites) was explored. Partial correlation of gene expression and DNA methylation was conducted with age, gender, and group (obese vs. lean) as covariates. A Bonferroni corrected p value < 0.05 according to the number of genes tested for each CpG site (range from 0 to 28) was defined as significant correlation. Obesity-related differentially expressed genes were defined as genes with their expression levels showing significant difference between obese cases and lean controls at p value < 0.05.

Pathway enrichment analysis was conducted for the genome-wide DNA methylation obtained from leukocytes using gene set enrichment analysis (GSEA) [16]. GSEA was performed on an unfiltered, ranked list of genes (ranked by the p values without consideration of directions), and a running-sum statistic was used to determine the enrichment of an a priori defined gene sets (pathways) based on the gene ranks. Statistical significance of pathway enrichment scores were ascertained by permutation testing over size-matched random gene sets and multiple testing was controlled by the false discovery rate (FDR). A FDR of 5% was used. Kyoto Encyclopedia of Genes and Genomes (KEGG) gene sets were used as the reference gene sets. The CpG site showing the most significant p value within a gene was used to represent the DNA methylation level of the gene.

We also checked whether we could replicate previously identified obesity-related CpG sites ($n = 277$) in our current study of youth and young adult [2–5]. Replication was defined as a consistent direction of the β-coefficient and FDR < 0.05.

Results

Discovery meta-analysis in the youth and young adult

Table 1 lists the general characteristics of the subjects. We identified 76 CpG sites significantly associated ($p < 1 \times 10^{-07}$) with obesity in the meta-analysis of the three cohorts (Manhattan and QQ-plot, Fig. 1; Additional file 2: Table S1). Obesity was positively associated with the methylation of 65 CpG sites and negatively associated with the methylation of 11 CpG sites. The top CpG site (cg12170787, $p = 1.13 \times 10^{-16}$) locates in the intron 5 of the *SBNO2* gene (Strawberry Notch Homolog 2). Two more CpG sites (cg18608055, $p = 3.69 \times 10^{-16}$; cg07573872, $p = 1.12 \times 10^{-09}$) locating in the same region also passed the threshold for genome-wide significance. CpG site cg07573872 is located in a CpG island shore region and has been reported to be associated with BMI previously [2]. CpG sites cg18608055 and cg12170787 are 4524 bp and 4623 bp away from cg07573872 (Additional file 3: Figure S1). The *SBNO2* gene is expressed in peripheral leukocytes and is a key player in the IL-10-regulated anti-inflammatory signaling pathway [17].

Table 1 General characteristics of the subjects

General characteristics	EpiGO		LACHY	BP stress cohort
	Lean	Obese		
N	92	96	284	228
Female (%)	50.0	51.0	50.0	57.5
Age (years)	17.7 ± 1.7	17.7 ± 1.8	16.2 ± 1.3	27.8 ± 3.3
Age range (years)	14.0–20.9	14.1–21.0	13.8–19.0	18.9–35.6
BMI (kg/m^2)	18.8 ± 1.3	39.8 ± 6.8	24.1 ± 5.6	31.4 ± 8.6
BMI range (kg/m^2)	15.0–21.7	28.1–70.1	16.4–45.9	17.6–59.6
BMI percentile (%)	18.7 ± 11.0	98.8 ± 1.1	65.7 ± 28.3	–
BMI percentile range (%)	0.8–41.7	95.0–99.9	2.3–99.7	–

In silico replication with ARIC study

Of the 76 CpG sites significantly associated with obesity in our discovery meta-analysis, 54 replicated (FDR < 0.05) in the ARIC study (Table 2), of which 33 survived Bonferroni correction ($p < 6.58 \times 10^{-4}$). These 54 CpG sites annotated to 45 genes. In addition to *SBNO2* which exhibits 3 significant CpG sites, *SOCS3* (suppressor of cytokine signaling 3: cg18181703, cg04610187, and cg10508317), *CISH* (Cytoking-Inducible Src-Homology 2 –containing protein: cg21585138 and cg23005227), and *VMP1* (Vacuole Membrane Protein: cg16936953, cg12054453, cg24174557, cg18942579, and cg010409343) also have 2 or more significant CpG sites. The locations of these CpG sites within each gene and their correlations were provided in Additional file 3: Figure S1. Out of the 54 CpG sites associated with obesity, 29 CpG sites (annotated to 25 genes) were novel signals (highlighted in gray in Table 2).

Replication of obesity-related CpG sites identified from mixed cells in purified neutrophils

The 54 CpG sites were taken forward to check whether the associations with obesity could be validated in one purified cell type: neutrophils. The results were listed in Additional file 2: Table S2. Thirty-seven CpG sites were found to be associated with obesity in neutrophils (FDR < 0.05 and consistent directions of effect), confirming that for the majority of the CpG sites (68.5%), the significant associations with obesity are not driven by potential cell compositions in leukocytes. For the 17 CpG sites that were not validated in neutrophils, it is difficult to determine whether these signals are driven by cell compositions or that neutrophils are not the biologically relevant cell type to target. The fact that 6 of the 17 CpG sites were hypermethylated (i.e., beta > 0.8) in neutrophils compared with 0 in the 37 replicated CpG sites ($p = 1.2E\text{-}4$) indicated that at least for some of the obesity-related CpG sites which could not be validated in neutrophils, neutrophils might not be the relevant cell type to target.

Association with cardio-metabolic phenotypes

We examined the associations between the 54 replicated CpG sites and 7 cardiometabolic traits (SBP, fasting insulin, fasting glucose, fasting lipid panel including TG, TC, HDLC, and LDLC). Without the adjustment of obesity or BMI, we observed 148 significant associations ($p < 0.05$, Additional file 2: Table S3) with 39 for SBP, 45 for insulin, 1 for glucose, 14 for TG, 5 for TC, 25 for HDLC, and 19 for LDLC. CpGs that were significantly associated with higher SBP, insulin, glucose, TG, TC, and LDLC were also associated with higher BMI levels. For HDLC, CpGs were associated with lower BMI levels (Fig. 2). After the adjustment of obesity or BMI, only 11 associations remained significant (Additional file 2: Table S4). The results indicate that the majority of the associations of these CpG sites with cardiometabolic phenotypes are driven by obesity.

Gene expression analyses

Of the 54 CpG sites, 16 were significantly associated with expression of 17 unique genes in cis (Bonferroni corrected *p* value < 0.05) (Additional file 2: Table S5).

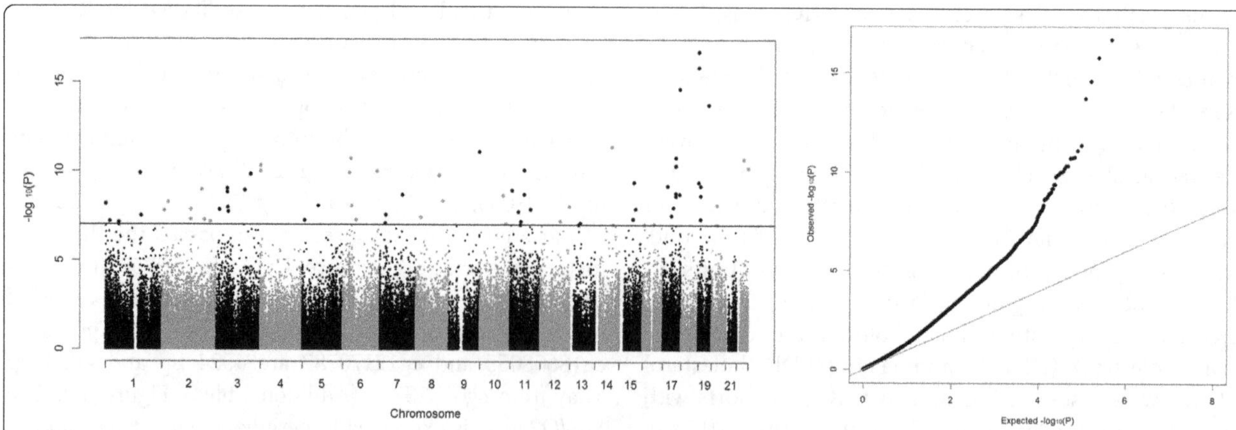

Fig. 1 Left panel: Manhattan plot of the genome-wide DNA methylation analysis in youths and young adults. The dotted line indicates the Bonferroni threshold of 1E–07 for significance. Right panel: QQ plot of the genome-wide DNA methylation analysis in youth and young adults

Table 2 Validated CpG sites in the ARIC study

TargetID	Closest gene	Chr.	Position	The youth and young adult discovery panel		ARIC		
				Directions*	P value	Beta**	P value	FDR
cg12170787	SBNO2	19	1130965	---	1.13E-16	-0.00347	1.30E-05	7.60E-05
cg18181703	SOCS3	17	76354621	---	1.94E-16	-0.00679	3.80E-07	4.13E-06
cg18608055	SBNO2	19	1130866	---	3.69E-16	-0.00460	5.80E-04	1.34E-03
cg26470501	BCL3	19	45252955	---	4.87E-14	-0.00247	1.84E-02	2.65E-02
cg09349128	CRELD2	22	50327986		1.15E-13	-0.00590	1.40E-08	2.66E-07
cg16611584	AKAP10	17	19809078	+++	7.37E-12	0.00810	2.08E-04	5.27E-04
cg03940776	SYNJ2	6	158490013	---	8.82E-12	-0.00306	1.40E-04	4.09E-04
cg04610187	SOCS3	17	76360794	---	8.95E-12	-0.00510	1.89E-03	3.34E-03
cg10919522	ELMSAN1	14	74227441	---	1.18E-11	-0.00548	4.00E-06	3.04E-05
cg08548559	PIK3IP1	22	31686097	---	1.49E-11	-0.00743	1.40E-07	1.77E-06
cg12593793	LMNA	1	156074135	---	1.79E-11	-0.00385	1.59E-04	4.32E-04
cg06178669	HRASLS2	11	63334608	---	3.50E-11	-0.00507	3.12E-03	5.15E-03
cg21585138	CISH	3	50645106	---	4.52E-11	-0.00572	1.10E-06	9.29E-06
cg07136133	PRR5L	11	36422377	---	6.77E-11	-0.00484	6.70E-09	2.10E-07
cg01671681	PLCH1	3	155421735	---	2.02E-10	-0.00440	1.48E-04	4.17E-04
cg03957124	COX6A1P2	6	37016869	---	2.91E-10	-0.00268	2.77E-03	4.67E-03
cg16936953	VMP1	17	57915665	---	3.17E-10	-0.00777	2.40E-05	1.22E-04
cg10601624	PLEKHG6	12	6404377	---	3.34E-10	-0.00454	6.90E-05	2.91E-04
cg07037944	DAPK2	15	64290807	---	5.48E-10	-0.00349	2.47E-04	6.06E-04
cg17178175	NFE2L2	2	178109973	---	5.56E-10	-0.00397	1.38E-03	2.69E-03
cg06568880	SMG6	17	2166583	+++	6.00E-10	0.00258	1.63E-03	3.10E-03
cg10508317	SOCS3	17	76355146	---	7.45E-10	-0.00197	1.31E-03	2.62E-03
cg09152259	MAP3K2	2	128156114	---	8.03E-10	-0.00429	7.10E-04	1.54E-03
cg21163717	DOK2	8	21769903	---	8.41E-10	-0.00339	1.27E-04	3.86E-04
cg07573872	SBNO2	19	1126342	---	1.12E-09	-0.00689	2.80E-08	4.26E-07
cg23005227	CISH	3	50645426	---	1.26E-09	-0.00416	1.73E-03	3.20E-03
cg22866430	SNORA59A	1	12566378	+++	2.68E-09	0.00179	1.30E-02	1.90E-02
cg12054453	VMP1	17	57915717	---	2.71E-09	-0.00745	8.10E-05	3.08E-04
cg07094298	TNIP2	4	2748026	---	3.08E-09	-0.00534	8.10E-05	3.08E-04
cg24174557	VMP1	17	57903544	---	3.35E-09	-0.00556	1.91E-04	5.01E-04
cg19750657	UFM1	13	38935967	+++	5.50E-09	0.00805	5.50E-06	3.80E-05
cg23076949	FBRSL1	12	133016265	+++	5.58E-09	0.00316	1.01E-03	2.13E-03
cg06647068	CHST11	12	104853274	---	6.48E-09	-0.00367	1.20E-02	1.78E-02
cg17061862	WEE1	11	9590431	---	6.70E-09	-0.00458	1.26E-03	2.59E-03
cg03183540	LOC101927822	8	134931756	---	6.97E-09	-0.00282	2.50E-03	4.31E-03
cg05845030	DCN	12	91573247	---	9.27E-09	-0.00260	2.51E-02	3.54E-02
cg24531955	LOXL2	8	23154691	---	1.20E-08	-0.00416	3.80E-05	1.70E-04
cg03257930	RNU6-996P	9	110399293	---	1.50E-08	-0.00251	6.11E-03	9.67E-03
cg00760203	PLXDC1	17	37254921	+++	1.64E-08	0.00458	9.20E-05	3.18E-04
cg20849150	LINC01358	1	59522993	---	2.34E-08	-0.00401	3.40E-05	1.62E-04
cg18942579	VMP1	17	57915773	---	2.52E-08	-0.00658	8.90E-05	3.18E-04
cg02734358	GPRIN3	4	90227074	---	4.22E-08	-0.00525	3.29E-04	7.81E-04
cg22143698	ANKRD33B	5	10608058	+++	4.46E-08	0.00628	1.50E-05	8.14E-05
cg08857797	VPS25	17	40927699	+++	4.98E-08	0.00634	3.40E-09	2.10E-07
cg07960624	SAMD12	8	119208486	---	6.13E-08	-0.00578	6.98E-04	1.54E-03
cg03929796	ALAS1	3	52231840	---	6.94E-08	-0.00317	8.36E-03	1.30E-02
cg08239103	SOX6	11	16623818	---	7.32E-08	-0.00342	4.74E-03	7.66E-03
cg06946797	RIM2	16	11422409	---	7.38E-08	-0.00702	8.30E-09	2.10E-07
cg04163119	PRICKLE4	6	41754006	---	7.77E-08	-0.00153	9.49E-03	1.44E-02
cg13134297	CRHR2	7	30737556	---	8.47E-08	-0.00374	1.10E-04	3.48E-04
cg01409343	VMP1	17	57915740	---	8.53E-08	-0.00546	1.03E-04	3.40E-04
cg14531564	SDF4	1	1154853	---	8.54E-08	-0.00410	1.10E-05	6.97E-05
cg06164260	BCL6	3	187454439	---	9.42E-08	-0.00410	5.30E-07	5.04E-06
cg23018755	MAFG	17	79881529	+++	9.85E-08	0.00339	1.86E-03	3.34E-03

Newly discovered associations are highlighted in gray

*"+" indicates that DNA methylation levels increase with obesity status or BMI. The order is Epigo, LACHY, and BP stress cohort

**DNA methylation changes with 1 unit increase in BMI

Furthermore, of these 17 genes, the expression levels of 5 genes were significantly associated with obesity ($p < 0.05$) (Additional file 2: Table S5). Figure 3 shows the corresponding relationships between DNA methylation and gene expression for these 5 genes. With the exception of the correlation between cg06178669 and *HRASLS2* (HRAS-like suppressor 2), increased methylation was associated with decreased gene expressions. For

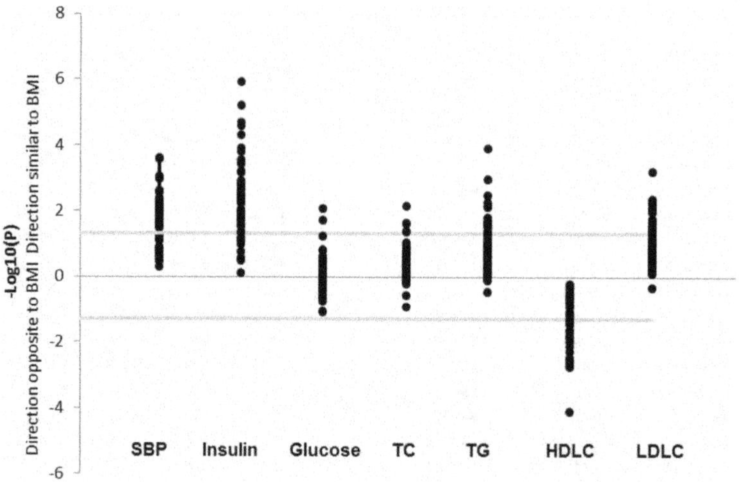

Fig. 2 Manhattan plot depicting the $-\log_{10}(p$ values) and effect direction (respectively to obesity) of the associations between the 55 replicated CpG sites and each cardiometabolic phenotype. The lines indicate the threshold of 0.05 for significance

SOCS3, *CISH*, *PIM3* (Pim-3 proto-oncogene, serine/threonine kinase), and *KLF4* (Kruppel-like factor 4), obesity was associated with decreased methylation and increased gene expression, while for *HRASLS2*, obesity was associated with decreased methylation and decreased gene expression (Additional file 2: Table S5).

Pathway analyses

The pathway analyses yielded significant (FDR < 0.05) enrichment of 33 KEGG pathways for obesity-related DNA methylation changes in peripheral leukocytes (Additional file 2: Table S6). These pathways represent processes involved in inflammatory pathways (e.g., cell adhesion molecules, JAK-STAT signaling pathway, intestinal immune network for IGA production), autoimmune response (e.g., type 1 diabetes, allograft rejection, graft versus host disease), and obesity-related comorbidities (e.g. type 2 diabetes, vascular smooth muscle contraction, cancer, and asthma).

Replication of previously reported CpG sites for obesity in middle-aged and elderly adults

We attempted to replicate the previously reported CpG sites for obesity. At the time this study was conducted, 4 large EWASs (with replication cohorts) for obesity were available: the ARIC study by Demerath E et al. [2] (reported 37 CpG sites), the Cardiogenics Consortium study by Dick K et al. [4] (reported 3 CpG sites), the GOLDN study by Aslibekyan S et al. [5] (reported 8 CpG sites), and the study reported by Wahl S et al. [3] (reported 254 CpG sites). These 4 studies resulted in 277 unique CpG sites associated with obesity. Out of these 277 CpG sites, 198 (71.5%) could be replicated with consistent direction of effect and a FDR < 0.05 in our study (Additional file 2: Table S7), indicating that majority of the obesity-related CpG sites identified in middle-aged and elderly adults already show changes in youth and young adulthood.

Discussion

In this epigenome-wide association study of African American youth and young adults, we identified 29 novel CpG sites associated with obesity and the replicated majority of the CpG sites previously identified in middle-aged and older adults. We further demonstrated that majority of the obesity-related CpG sites identified from leukocytes are not driven by cell compositions or obesity-related cardio-metabolic risk factors. We also provided direct links between DNA methylation, gene expression, and obesity status for 7 CpG sites in 5 genes.

Unlike genetic markers that are the same in all cells and unlikely to change over a lifetime, epigenetic regulation is tissue specific and plastic (i.e., findings may reflect the consequence rather than the cause of the disease) [18]. In addition to availability, the choice of leukocytes in this study as well as in the previous epigenome-wide association studies of obesity in middle-aged and elder people is based on the fact that obesity is characterized by a state of chronic, low-grade inflammation [19]. With the established role of epigenetic regulation in shaping the immune and inflammatory response [20], identification of the epigenetic markers specifically involved in obesity-induced inflammation has the potential to provide novel insight into the pathogenesis of obesity-related disorders. The choice of leukocytes also assumes that the observed epigenetic changes will reflect consequences rather than causes of obesity. Although the cross-sectional design of the current and previous studies [2–5] does not provide information on the direction of causality, the Mendelian randomization model

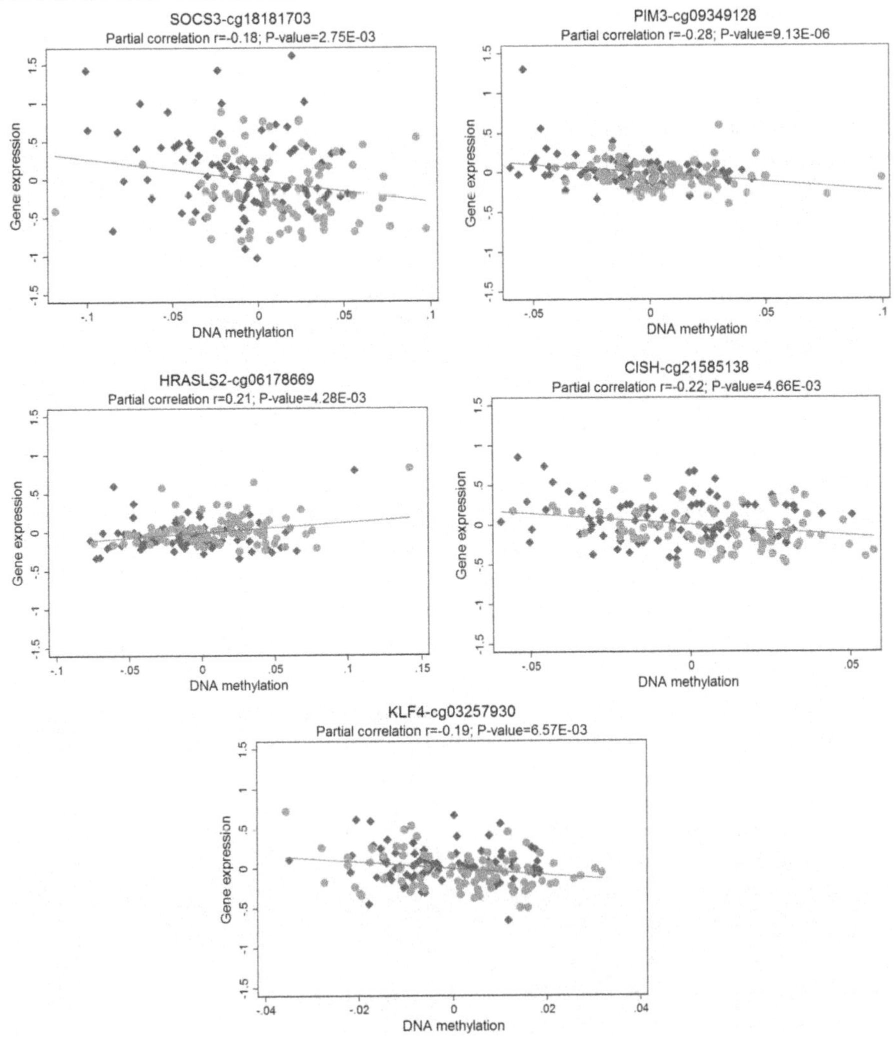

Fig. 3 Partial correlations between DNA methylation and gene expression. Covariates included age, sex, and obesity status. Gray dots represent the lean group and black diamonds represent the obese group. For the SOCS3 gene, similar correlation was observed for cg04610187 ($r = -0.20$, $p = 1.77E{-}03$); for the CISH gene, similar correlation was observed for cg23005227 ($r = -0.21$, $p = 7.14E{-}03$)

used in one [3] of the previous adult studies strongly suggested that obesity-related DNA methylation changes identified in peripheral leukocytes are predominately the consequence rather than the cause of obesity. One concern in analyzing epigenetic changes in peripheral leukocytes in obese individuals is that the effect of obesity itself on the immune system can be hidden or biased by the coexistence of obesity-related diseases and the use of medication, which is very common in middle-aged and elderly individuals. To avoid this problem, in this study, we focused on youth and young adults. This is a population having shown obesity-related metabolic risk that has not developed into clinical disease yet. We did observe that many obesity-related CpG sites were associated with cardiometabolic traits. However, after the adjustment of obesity, this number decreased dramatically, indicating that a large majority of the associations of these CpG sites with cardiometabolic phenotypes is driven by obesity.

In comparing with the previous studies in middle-aged adults and elderly [2–5], we identified 29 novel CpG sites (annotated to 25 genes). We were also able to present triangular relationships between DNA methylation, gene expression, and obesity at 5 genes including *SOCS3, CISH, PIM3, KLF4*, and *HRASLS2*. With the exception of *HARSLS2*, obesity was associated with decreased DNA methylation level and increased gene expressions. Interestingly, both *SOCS3* and *CISH* are involved in the JAK-STAT signaling pathway and are the key negative regulators of the activation of this pathway [21]. The JAK-STAT signaling pathway is activated during inflammation and used by a variety of cytokines. The JAK-STAT signaling pathway activates its own suppressors: suppressors of cytokine signaling (SOCS) molecules including SOCS1-7 and CISH. This negative feedback control is essential for the effective dissipation of cytokine signaling to prevent excessive inflammation and detrimental effect on other signaling pathways. However, the increased levels of SOCS proteins can induce insulin resistance in peripheral organs [22] and leptin resistance in the central nervous system [23]. There are very limited studies on *PIM3*, *KLF4*, and *HARSLS2*. However, PIM1, a protein from the same family and structurally and functionally similar to PIM3, is also primarily involved in the JAK/STAT signaling pathway. PIM-1 transcription is initiated by STAT factors and can also bind to regulators of the JAK/STAT pathway, resulting in a negative feedback loop [24]. Taken together, the activation of the JAK/STAT signaling pathway in obesity transcriptionally upregulates its own suppressors through DNA methylation mechanisms. On the one hand, the increased production of negative regulators can prevent excessive inflammation, while on the other hand, these increased negative feedback products may increase the risk of obesity-related disorders, a compensatory mechanism that has been observed in the development of many diseases.

Our study in healthy youth and young adults also replicated 71.5% of obesity-related CpG sites previously reported in middle-aged and elderly adults, indicating that the majority of the obesity-related CpG sites already show changes in adolescence. It will be interesting to find out the age of onset of these changes. In a recent study exploring this question on the first EWAS-identified gene (*HIF3A*), Pan et al. [25] observed that DNA methylation levels at the three previously described *HIF3A* CpG sites were already associated with greater weight and adiposity at birth. On the other hand, the strong consistency of obesity-related DNA methylation signals across ethnic groups (African Americans in this study comparing with Caucasians, Asians, and African Americans in previous studies) and age emphasizes the importance of conducting large-scale epigenome-wide meta-analysis similar to what has been done in the GWAS. This action will discover more obesity-related epigenome-wide changes and enable the recognition of the overall picture of the role of DNA methylation in obesity and its related disorders.

One possible concern in these EWAS studies on obesity using peripheral blood is the heterogeneity of leukocytes since different cell populations have distinct epigenetic signatures [26]. This concern was dramatically reduced with the development of algorithms estimating the cell subset compositions based on genome-wide DNA methylation data [12]. Our study further confirms this through successfully replication of 68.5% of the obesity-related CpG sites from leukocytes in one purified cell type: neutrophils. The reason that neutrophils were selected is that previous studies including ours [9, 27] have observed that obesity is consistently associated with neutrophilia, manifesting not only by elevated neutrophil count but also increased percentage. However, we believe that replication of the findings from leukocytes in a variety of other single cell types remains important to guide further functional in vitro studies.

Several limitations to the present study need to be recognized. First, although the study by Wahl S et al. [3] in adults have shown that obesity-related DNA methylation changes identified in peripheral leukocytes are predominately the consequence rather than the cause of obesity, we cannot test the direction of the causality of these newly identified obesity-related CpG sites in youth and young adults due to the cross-sectional design and the lack of genotype data. Second, although 71% of the signals from the discovery cohort were validated in the replication cohort, the lack of replication of other signals might be due to the age difference between the discovery cohort and the replication cohort. Third, due to the lack of genotype data, we cannot adjust the potential bias resulted from ancestry compositions.

Conclusion

In summary, this EWAS study in healthy youth and young adult confirmed the majority of previously identified obesity-related DNA methylation loci in middle-aged and elderly adults and identified 29 novel CpG sites associated with obesity. The findings from the current study have the potential to enable development of new strategies for early prevention and treatment.

Additional files

Additional file 1: Detailed description of the participants for each study.

Additional file 2: Table S1. CpG sites with $p < 1E-7$ in this youth and young adult study. **Table S2.** Performance of the 55 CpG sites in neutrophils. **Table S3.** Association of the 55 CpG sites with cardiometabolic traits without adjustment of obesity/BMI. **Table S4.** The significant associations between CpG sites and metabolic traits after the adjustment of obesity/BMI. **Table S5.** DNA methylation, gene expression, and obesity. **Table S6.** Significantly enriched pathways (FDR < 0.05). **Table S7.** Replication of previous reported CpG sites identified in middle-aged and elderly population.

Additional file 3: Figure S1. Positions and correlations of the multiple CpG sites in SBNO2, SOCS3, VMP1, and CISH genes.

Abbreviations

ARIC: Atherosclerosis Risk in Communities; BMI: Body mass index; BP: Blood pressure; CISH: Cytoking-Inducible Src-Homology 2–containing protein; CPACOR: Incorporating Control Probe Adjustment and reduction of global CORrelation; CpG: 5'—C—phosphate—G—3'; DNA: Deoxyribonucleic acid; EpiGO: Epigenetic Basis of Obesity-Induced Cardiovascular Disease and Type 2 Diabetes; EWAS: Epigenome-wide association study; FDR: False discovery rate; GOLDN: Genetics of Lipid Lowering Drugs and Diet Network; GSEA: Gene set enrichment analysis; GWAS: Genome-wide association study; HDLC: Fasting HDL-cholesterol; HIF3A: Hypoxia-inducible factor 3 alpha subunit; HRASLS2: HRAS-like suppressor 2; IL-10: Interleukin-10; JAK-STAT: Janus kinase/signal transducers and activators of transcription; KEGG: Kyoto Encyclopedia of Genes and Genomes; KLF4: Kruppel-like factor

4; LACHY: Lifestyle, Adiposity, and Cardiovascular Health in Youth; LDLC: Fasting LDL-cholesterol; PCA: Principal component analysis; PIM1: Pim-1 proto-oncogene, serine/threonine kinase; PIM3: Pim-3 proto-oncogene, serine/threonine kinase; QC: Quality control; RIN: RNA integrity; SBNO2: Strawberry notch homolog 2; SBP: Systolic blood pressure; SNP: Single-nucleotide polymorphism; SOCS: Suppressors of cytokine signaling; SOCS3: Suppressor of cytokine signaling 3; TC: Fasting total cholesterol; TG: Fasting triglycerides; VMP1: Vacuole membrane protein

Acknowledgements
Not applicable.

Funding
This study was supported by grant HL105689 and HL125577 from the National Institute of Health (NIH) and GRNT20480211 from AHA.

Authors' contributions
XW and SS designed the study and drafted the manuscript; YP, GH, YH, and WG conducted the data analysis; HZ, XW, VB, HS, and YD participated in the data collection; HS made critical changes to the manuscript; JP, KN, MC, and ED conducted the in silico replication of the study. All authors read and approved the final manuscript.

Competing interests
The authors declare that they have no competing interests.

Author details
[1]Department of Pediatrics, Georgia Prevention Institute, Medical College of Georgia, Augusta University, HS-1640, Augusta, GA 30912, USA. [2]Cancer Center, Augusta University, Augusta, GA, USA. [3]Department of Epidemiology, University of Groningen, University Medical Center Groningen, Groningen, the Netherlands. [4]Division of Epidemiology and Community Health, School of Public Health, University of Minnesota, Minneapolis, MN 55454, USA. [5]Department of Epidemiology, University of North Carolina at Chapel Hill, Chapel Hill, NC 27514, USA. [6]Human Genetics Center, School of Public Health, University of Texas Health Sciences Center at Houston, Houston, TX 77030, USA.

References

1. van Dijk SJ, Tellam RL, Morrison JL, Muhlhausler BS, Molloy PL. Recent developments on the role of epigenetics in obesity and metabolic disease. Clin Epigenetics. 2015;7:66.
2. Demerath EW, Guan W, Grove ML, Aslibekyan S, Mendelson M, Zhou YH, Hedman AK, Sandling JK, Li LA, Irvin MR, et al. Epigenome-wide association study (EWAS) of BMI, BMI change and waist circumference in African American adults identifies multiple replicated loci. Hum Mol Genet. 2015; 24(15):4464–79.
3. Wahl S, Drong A, Lehne B, Loh M, Scott WR, Kunze S, Tsai PC, Ried JS, Zhang W, Yang Y, et al. Epigenome-wide association study of body mass index, and the adverse outcomes of adiposity. Nature. 2017;541(7635):81–6.
4. Dick KJ, Nelson CP, Tsaprouni L, Sandling JK, Aissi D, Wahl S, Meduri E, Morange PE, Gagnon F, Grallert H, et al. DNA methylation and body-mass index: a genome-wide analysis. Lancet. 2014;383(9933):1990–8.
5. Aslibekyan S, Demerath EW, Mendelson M, Zhi D, Guan W, Liang L, Sha J, Pankow JS, Liu C, Irvin MR, et al. Epigenome-wide study identifies novel methylation loci associated with body mass index and waist circumference. Obesity (Silver Spring). 2015;23(7):1493–501.
6. Xu X, Su S, Barnes VA, De Miguel C, Pollock J, Ownby D, Shi H, Zhu H, Snieder H, Wang X. A genome-wide methylation study on obesity: differential variability and differential methylation. Epigenetics. 2013;8(5):522–33.
7. Gutin B, Johnson MH, Humphries MC, Hatfield-Laube JL, Kapuku GK, Allison JD, Gower BA, Daniels SR, Barbeau P. Relationship of visceral adiposity to cardiovascular disease risk factors in black and white teens. Obesity (Silver Spring). 2007;15(4):1029–35.
8. Wang X, Poole JC, Treiber FA, Harshfield GA, Hanevold CD, Snieder H. Ethnic and gender differences in ambulatory blood pressure trajectories: results from a 15-year longitudinal study in youth and young adults. Circulation. 2006;114(25):2780–7.
9. Xu X, Su S, Wang X, Barnes V, De Miguel C, Ownby D, Pollock J, Snieder H, Chen W. Obesity is associated with more activated neutrophils in African American male youth. Int J Obes. 2015;39(1):26–32.
10. Aryee MJ, Jaffe AE, Corrada-Bravo H, Ladd-Acosta C, Feinberg AP, Hansen KD, Irizarry RA. Minfi: a flexible and comprehensive bioconductor package for the analysis of Infinium DNA methylation microarrays. Bioinformatics. 2014;30(10):1363 9.
11. Lehne B, Drong AW, Loh M, Zhang W, Scott WR, Tan ST, Afzal U, Scott J, Jarvelin MR, Elliott P, et al. A coherent approach for analysis of the Illumina HumanMethylation450 BeadChip improves data quality and performance in epigenome-wide association studies. Genome Biol. 2015;16:37.
12. Houseman EA, Accomando WP, Koestler DC, Christensen BC, Marsit CJ, Nelson HH, Wiencke JK, Kelsey KT. DNA methylation arrays as surrogate measures of cell mixture distribution. BMC Bioinformatics. 2012;13:86.
13. Du P, Kibbe WA, Lin SM. lumi: a pipeline for processing Illumina microarray. Bioinformatics. 2008;24(13):1547–8.
14. Smyth GK, Michaud J, Scott HS. Use of within-array replicate spots for assessing differential expression in microarray experiments. Bioinformatics. 2005;21(9):2067–75.
15. Willer CJ, Li Y, Abecasis GR. METAL: fast and efficient meta-analysis of genomewide association scans. Bioinformatics. 2010;26(17):2190–1.
16. Subramanian A, Tamayo P, Mootha VK, Mukherjee S, Ebert BL, Gillette MA, Paulovich A, Pomeroy SL, Golub TR, Lander ES, et al. Gene set enrichment analysis: a knowledge-based approach for interpreting genome-wide expression profiles. Proc Natl Acad Sci U S A. 2005;102(43):15545–50.
17. El Kasmi KC, Smith AM, Williams L, Neale G, Panopoulos AD, Watowich SS, Hacker H, Foxwell BM, Murray PJ. Cutting edge: a transcriptional repressor and corepressor induced by the STAT3-regulated anti-inflammatory signaling pathway. J Immunol. 2007;179(11):7215–9.
18. Egger G, Liang G, Aparicio A, Jones PA. Epigenetics in human disease and prospects for epigenetic therapy. Nature. 2004;429(6990):457–63.
19. Karalis KP, Giannogonas P, Kodela E, Koutmani Y, Zoumakis M, Teli T. Mechanisms of obesity and related pathology: linking immune responses to metabolic stress. FEBS J. 2009;276(20):5747–54.
20. Wilson AG. Epigenetic regulation of gene expression in the inflammatory response and relevance to common diseases. J Periodontol. 2008;79(8 Suppl):1514–9.
21. Wunderlich CM, Hovelmeyer N, Wunderlich FT. Mechanisms of chronic JAK-STAT3-SOCS3 signaling in obesity. JAKSTAT. 2013;2(2):e23878.
22. Galic S, Sachithanandan N, Kay TW, Steinberg GR. Suppressor of cytokine signalling (SOCS) proteins as guardians of inflammatory responses critical for regulating insulin sensitivity. Biochem J. 2014;461(2):177–88.
23. Lubis AR, Widia F, Soegondo S, Setiawati A. The role of SOCS-3 protein in leptin resistance and obesity. Acta Med Indones. 2008;40(2):89–95.
24. Bachmann M, Moroy T. The serine/threonine kinase Pim-1. Int J Biochem Cell Biol. 2005;37(4):726–30.
25. Pan H, Lin X, Wu Y, Chen L, Teh AL, Soh SE, Lee YS, Tint MT, MacIsaac JL, Morin AM, et al. HIF3A association with adiposity: the story begins before birth. Epigenomics. 2015;7(6):937–50.
26. Reinius LE, Acevedo N, Joerink M, Pershagen G, Dahlen SE, Greco D, Soderhall C, Scheynius A, Kere J. Differential DNA methylation in purified human blood cells: implications for cell lineage and studies on disease susceptibility. PLoS One. 2012;7(7):e41361.
27. Pecht T, Gutman-Tirosh A, Bashan N, Rudich A. Peripheral blood leucocyte subclasses as potential biomarkers of adipose tissue inflammation and obesity subphenotypes in humans. Obes Rev. 2014;15(4):322–37.

15

Pharmacological inhibition of EZH2 disrupts the female germline epigenome

Lexie Prokopuk[1,2], Kirsten Hogg[1,2] and Patrick S. Western[1,2*]

Abstract

Background: Recently discovered drugs that target epigenetic modifying complexes are providing new treatment options for a range of cancers that affect patients of reproductive age. Although these drugs provide new therapies, it is likely that they will also affect epigenetic programming in sperm and oocytes. A promising target is Enhancer of Zeste 2 (EZH2), which establishes the essential epigenetic modification, H3K27me3, during development.

Results: In this study, we demonstrate that inhibition of EZH1/2 with the clinically relevant drug, tazemetostat, severely depletes H3K27me3 in growing oocytes of adult female mice. Moreover, EZH2 inhibition depleted H3K27me3 in primary oocytes and in fetal oocytes undergoing epigenetic reprogramming. Surprisingly, once depleted, H3K27me3 failed to recover in growing oocytes or in fetal oocytes.

Conclusion: Together, these data demonstrate that drugs targeting EZH2 significantly affect the germline epigenome and, based on genetic models with oocyte-specific loss of EZH2 function, are likely to affect outcomes in offspring.

Keywords: Germline, Oocyte, Pharmacology, Epigenetic, PRC2, H3K27me3, Inheritance

Background

Although many studies indicate that epigenetic changes in gametes can influence development and health in offspring, the mechanisms are poorly understood (reviewed in [1, 2]). Despite this, new pharmaceuticals that specifically target epigenetic modifying enzymes are currently being developed for the treatment of cancer and other diseases, and these drugs are being administered to patients of reproductive age. While these therapies are likely to offer significant improvements in cancer treatment, their potential impacts on the germline epigenome, and on offspring, remain unknown.

Altered epigenetic states can result in disease, and more than 50% of cancers harbour mutations in chromatin-associated proteins. This has driven recent interest in the development of drugs that specifically target epigenetic modifying complexes with the aim of providing new cancer treatments [3]. A prominent target is Enhancer of Zeste 2 (EZH2), which is commonly subject to gain of function mutations or overexpression in a range of tumours [3–6]. EZH2 catalyses methylation of lysine 27 on histone 3 (H3K27me3), an epigenetic modification that is critical for repressing developmental genes during embryogenesis. EZH2 is the catalytic component of polycomb repressive complex 2 (PRC2), which also contains embryonic ectoderm development (EED) and Suppressor of Zeste 12 (SUZ12). Inactivation of any one of these three protein subunits severely compromises the enzymatic activity of PRC2 and results in the loss of H3K27me3 [7–10].

Recently developed pharmaceuticals that inhibit EZH2 include EPZ-6438, also known as the proprietary product, tazemetostat [11]. Tazemetostat is currently in stage I/II clinical trials in patients for the treatment of multiple cancers, including lymphomas, mesothelioma, myelomas, solid tumours, and malignant rhabdoid tumours of the kidney and ovary. Patient cohorts include children and adults of reproductive age (12 current NIH Clinical Trials 02860286, 02875548, 03028103, 03010982, 02601937, 01897571, 02601950, 03009344, 03213665, 02220842, 03217253, 03155620). Three studies include the recruitment of children, aged 6 months to 21 years (NIH Clinical Trials 02601937, 03213665, 03155620).

* Correspondence: patrick.western@hudson.org.au
[1]Centre for Reproductive Health, Hudson Institute of Medical Research, Clayton, Victoria 3168, Australia
[2]Department of Molecular and Translational Science, Monash University, Clayton, Victoria 3168, Australia

As H3K27me3 is enriched in developing germ cells during epigenetic reprogramming and in mature oocytes [12–16], it is likely that drugs targeting EZH2 will disrupt the sperm and oocyte epigenome. Current guidelines for tazemetostat typically recommend avoiding pregnancy for 30 days post-treatment (NIH Clinical Trials Register), significantly less time than the ~ 350 days required for human oocyte growth and maturation [17]. Other studies do not stipulate any form of contraception after treatment with tazemetostat. As these drugs are systemic and the germline will be exposed in patients undergoing treatment, determining whether current treatments affect the germline epigenome is of significant importance for developing informed therapeutic guidelines and providing advice to patients with regard to post-treatment reproductive management. Moreover, although the use of these drugs during pregnancy is contra-indicated, there is little empirical data to support this advice. This is important, as recent studies have provided examples of drugs taken during pregnancy that have disrupted fetal or ovarian development [18, 19]. Of particular note, the epigenetic modifying drug valproic acid (Epilim) has been extensively used for the treatment of epilepsy, bipolar mania and migraine prophylaxis, but recent evidence of affects in children of women who took the drug during pregnancy have raised concerns over its clinical management [19]. While the effects of these, and other drugs, on the fetus have been of central concern, their potential impacts on the germline epigenome have been largely overlooked. These examples underline the need to understand the germline effects of epigenetic modifying drugs to allow appropriate development of informed clinical guidelines.

The developing germline plays a central role in regulating epigenetic information transmitted by gametes to offspring. To ensure transmission of appropriate epigenetic information to offspring, epigenetic information is reset during germline development [14, 20–24]. During this period of germline epigenetic reprogramming, H3K27me3 is highly enriched in primordial germ cells and in both male and female germ cells compared to somatic cells of the developing gonad [13, 14, 21, 25]. Moreover, H3K27me3 undergoes EZH2-dependent reorganisation while DNA methylation levels are at their lowest, indicating important roles for EZH2 and H3K27me3 for setting the germline epigenome [14]. Consistent with this, genome-wide mapping demonstrated H3K27me3 enrichment at developmental genes during epigenetic programming in the mouse fetal germline and in mature sperm [15, 26–29]. Given that many of these genes are not expressed during germline development, it has been speculated that these epigenetic modifications are established to regulate outcomes in offspring [15]. This concept is consistent with observations that deletion of *Ezh2* in growing oocytes affects preimplantation development and birth weight in offspring [16].

Females are born with a finite pool of primordial follicles, which provide the lifelong oocyte reserve that supports fertility. Primordial follicles are continually activated during reproductive life, resulting in the formation of primary follicles and oocyte growth [30–32]. As activated follicles grow from primary to pre-ovulatory stages, epigenetic modifications and maternal factors are established in the oocyte that are important for offspring development [33]. These maternal factors are produced through co-ordinate regulation of gene expression in the growing oocyte, a process that is considered to depend on appropriate epigenetic regulation throughout this period. An important example is provided by EZH2, which performs an essential role in the oocyte that profoundly affects offspring development and growth [16].

Here, we show that the EZH1/2-specific inhibitor, tazemetostat, substantially alters H3K27me3 in the developing female germline and maturing oocytes. Tazemetostat severely reduced H3K27me3 in growing oocytes in vivo, and H3K27me3 was not recovered after treatment withdrawal for half of the mouse oocyte growth period. Moreover, tazemetostat significantly reduced H3K27me3 in developing germ cells and in primary oocytes. Together, these data demonstrate that systemic pharmacological inhibition of EZH2 affects H3K27me3 at all stages of oocyte development and growth. While tazemetostat and similar drugs that target epigenetic pathways offer important therapeutic options to patients, our findings highlight an urgent need for a greater understanding of their impacts on the germline and the reassessment of clinical guidelines to ensure safe management in patients who may wish to conceive after treatment.

Results

PRC2 and H3K27me3 are enriched in growing oocytes of adult female mice

To determine the potential for PRC2 to catalyse H3K27me3 in growing oocytes of adult females, we assessed EZH2, EED, SUZ12 and H3K27me3 enrichment in postnatal day (PND) 24 ovaries using immunofluorescent staining. EED, EZH2 and SUZ12 were all detected in the nucleus of growing oocytes in PND24 ovaries (Fig. 1a–c), coinciding with H3K27me3 enrichment (Fig. 1d).

EZH2 inhibition potently depletes H3K27me3 in growing oocytes

As tazemetostat and other similar drugs are systemic, treatment of females of reproductive age is expected to

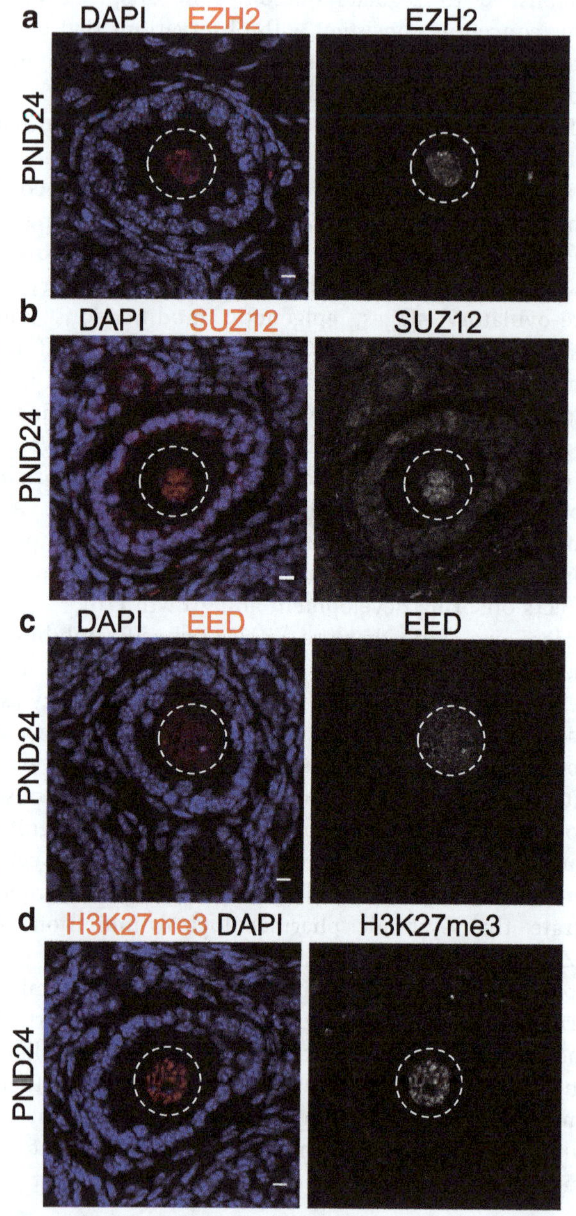

Fig. 1 PRC2 and H3K27me3 are enriched in growing oocytes. Confocal images of EZH2, SUZ12 and EED immunofluorescence in sections of ovary at postnatal day 24. Left panels show merged images. **a** EZH2 (red) and DAPI (DNA; blue). **b** SUZ12 (red) and DAPI (DNA; blue). **c** EED (red) and DAPI (DNA; blue). **d** H3K27me3 (red) and DAPI (DNA; blue). Right panels show single channel images of EED/EZH2/SUZ12/H3K27me3 (greyscale). Oocyte nuclei are shown within the white dashed line. Images are representative of three biological replicates. 10 μm scale bars

result in oocyte exposure to these EZH2-inhibiting drugs. To determine whether pharmacological inhibition of EZH1/2 affected H3K27me3 enrichment in the adult female germline, we treated adult females with tazemetostat. This is an especially important question as females are born with a finite supply of oocytes and disruption of oocyte epigenetic state may affect offspring outcomes. Previous in vivo preclinical studies of tazemetostat have shown that 220 mg/kg administered twice daily is required to induce effective tumour regression in mouse models carrying grafted malignant rhabdoid cells [4]. To investigate whether this dose caused depletion of H3K27me3 in growing oocytes in vivo, 7-week-old adult female mice were injected subcutaneously with either 220 mg/kg tazemetostat ($n = 3$) or sham control (0.5% NaCMC, 0.1% Tween80; $n = 3$) for 10 days. Notably, we injected mice once a day, thereby delivering less drug than in the preclinical cancer model, in which the drug was administered twice daily at 220 mg/kg by oral gavage [4]. Immunofluorescent analysis of H3K27me3 enrichment in secondary follicles revealed that H3K27me3 was depleted by 84% in the oocytes of females injected with tazemetostat compared to sham injected controls ($P < 0.0001$, Student's t test; Fig. 2). This demonstrated potent disruption of EZH1/2 function in growing oocytes of adult females.

Adult oocytes failed to recover H2K27me3 after withdrawal of EZH2 inhibition

To assess whether growing oocytes could recover after the extensive loss of H3K27me3 resulting from tazemetostat treatment, we carried out an in vivo recovery experiment. One cohort of 7-week-old adult female mice were injected subcutaneously with either 220 mg/kg tazemetostat ($n = 3$) or sham control ($n = 3$) once a day for 10 days and collected. An additional cohort was injected with either 220 mg/kg tazemetostat ($n = 3$) or sham control ($n = 3$) once a day for 10 days and then allowed to recover for a further 10 days with no treatment. After treatment or treatment/recovery regimes, immunofluorescence was performed on ovaries and secondary follicles to assess H3K27me3 enrichment in oocytes. Consistent with the initial in vivo depletion experiment in growing oocytes, H3K27me3 was robustly depleted in growing oocytes after 10 days of EZH2 inhibition compared to sham injected controls (Fig. 3). However, remarkably, we did not observe any H3K27me3 rescue in oocytes allowed to recover for 10 days ($P < 0.0001$, one-way ANOVA with post hoc Tukey's multiple comparisons test; Fig. 3). Instead, after the 10-day recovery period, H3K27me3 was depleted by a further 50% in oocytes.

Together, these data demonstrate that systemic tazemetostat treatment at the minimal preclinical dose that effectively controls tumour growth in mice also results in severe depletion of H3K27me3 in maturing oocytes. Moreover, our data indicate that once depleted, H3K27me3 does not recover in a window corresponding to half the growth period for mouse oocytes.

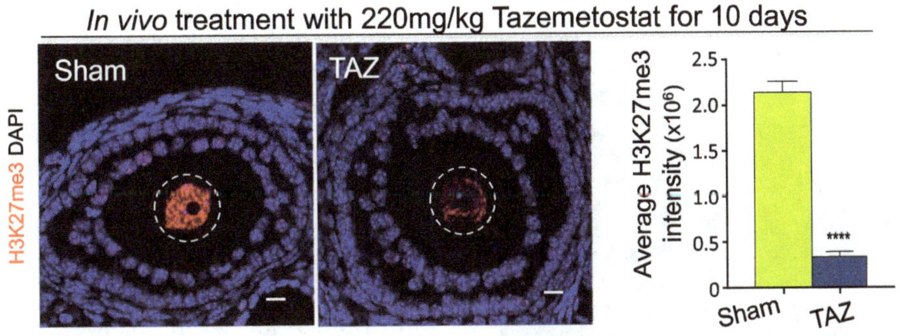

Fig. 2 Tazemetostat treatment of adult female mice substantially reduced H3K27me3 in growing oocytes. Confocal images of immunofluorescence in ovary sections from adult mice treated for 10 days with vehicle control (sham; 0.5% NaCMC, 0.1% Tween 80) or 220 mg/kg tazemetostat injected daily. Each panel shows merged colour images with H3K27me3 shown in red and DAPI (DNA) in blue. Oocyte nuclei are shown within the white dashed line. Images are representative of three biological replicates. 10 μm scale bars. Mean fluorescence intensity for H3K27me3 is shown in the graph to the right analysed by ROI manager, ImageJ. ****$P < 0.0001$ one-way ANOVA plus post hoc Tukey's multiple comparisons test; $n = 4$ biological replicates per treatment, 5–7 oocytes measured per replicate. Error bars ± SEM

EZH2 inhibition depletes H3K27me3 in female fetal germ cells undergoing epigenetic reprogramming

Although use of tazemetostat during pregnancy is contra-indicated, empirical evidence for this position is lacking. Previous studies provide examples where similar drugs have been used in pregnancy [19], raising the possibility that drugs targeting epigenetic modifying enzymes may be similarly used in the future. Since exposure of the fetus would also expose the germline of future offspring to the drug, we determined the ability of EZH2 inhibitors to alter H3K27me3 in developing oocytes. To achieve this, we performed a series of experiments on germ cells using ex vivo cultured fetal gonads treated with tazemetostat. Germ cells undergo significant epigenetic reprogramming during fetal life that results in removal of existing epigenetic modifications and the establishment of new sex-specific germline epigenomes. This developmental period in germ cells is therefore considered susceptible to modification by agents that disrupt epigenetic programming and may alter the germline epigenome in mature gametes. As H3K27me3 is significantly reorganised in germ cells undergoing epigenetic reprogramming [14], we initially determined the potential for EZH2 inhibition to affect H3K27me3 enrichment in fetal germ cells during this period.

Female Swiss mice were time-mated to *Oct4GFP* transgenic males (129T2svJ) to allow stage-specific collection of embryonic gonads with *Oct4GFP* expressed in germ cells but not in somatic cells [14, 34, 35]. We treated E12.5 XX (female) fetal gonads grown in ex vivo organ culture with tazemetostat or vehicle control (DMSO) for 24–72 h. At the end of the culture period, the gonads were dissociated and H3K27me3 levels measured in individual germ and somatic cells using flow cytometry ([14, 36]; Additional file 1: Figure S1). Robust depletion of H3K27me3 was observed in germ cells of XX E12.5 gonads treated for 72 h with 100 nM–5 μM tazemetostat (Fig. 4a, b; Additional file 1: Figure S1C). Treatment with 100 nM tazemetostat resulted in significant depletion of H3K27me3, although slightly less efficiently than that at higher doses. Tazemetostat was very well tolerated in culture, with even the highest doses having no noticeable effect on gonad growth or the proportions of germ cells at the end of the culture period (Fig. 4c, Additional file 1: Figures. S1C, S2A-B). This is consistent with our previous observations that cell viability was unaffected by a similar EZH2-inhibiting drug, GSK126, in this culture system [14].

A major milestone for female germ cell development is their entry into meiosis, which occurs between E13.5 and E15.5 [37, 38]. To assess the impact of EZH2 inhibitors on female germ cell development, E12.5 gonads were treated for 72 h allowing sufficient time for germ cells to enter meiosis. Cell cycle state was assessed by incorporation of EdU during the final 2 h of gonad culture and staining germ cells with propidium iodide to determine individual cell DNA content using flow cytometry ([38–40]; Additional file 1: Figure S2). XX germ cells arrested in meiosis with normal timing and in normal numbers in E12.5 gonads treated for 72 h with tazemetostat, indicating that EZH2 inhibition and loss of H3K27me3 did not prevent E12.5 germ cells from reaching this key developmental milestone (Fig. 4c). Similarly, somatic cells proliferated at a normal rate in XX gonads indicating that EZH2 inhibition did not impact gonad growth during the treatment period, despite loss of H3K27me3 (Additional file 1: Figure S2B).

H3K27me3 failed to recover in female fetal germ cells following EZH2 inhibition

Collectively, these data demonstrate that tazemetostat potently depletes H3K27me3 in XX fetal germ cells as

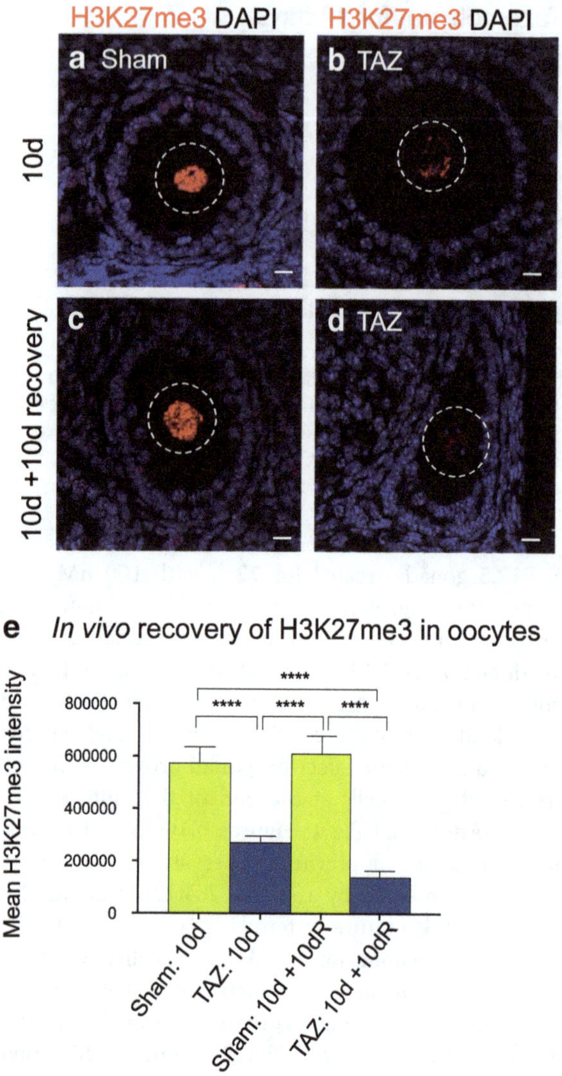

Fig. 3 H3K27me3 was not recovered in oocytes of adult mice after tazemetostat treatment. Confocal images of immunofluorescence in ovary sections from adult mice treated. **a** Treatment for 10 days with vehicle control (sham; 0.5% NaCMC, 0.1% Tween 80). **b** Treatment for 10 days with 220 mg/kg tazemetostat injected daily. **c.** Treatment for 10 days with vehicle control (sham; 0.5% NaCMC, 0.1% Tween 80) followed by a 10-day no treatment recovery period. **d.** Treatment for 10 days with 220 mg/kg tazemetostat followed by a 10-day no treatment recovery period. Each panel shows merged colour images with H3K27me3 shown in red and DAPI (DNA) in blue. Oocyte nuclei are shown within the white dashed line. Images are representative of three biological replicates. 10 μm scale bars. **e.** Mean fluorescence intensity for H3K27me3 for each treatment, analysed by ROI manager, ImageJ. ****$P < 0.0001$ one-way ANOVA plus post hoc Tukey's multiple comparisons test; $n = 4$ biological replicates, 7–12 oocytes measured per replicate. Error bars ± SEM

they undergo epigenetic reprogramming and entry into meiosis. However, all PRC2 components have been detected in fetal XX germ cells at E11.5 and E12.5 [14] indicating that germ cells may be able to recover H3K27me3 after drug exposure. To determine whether H3K27me3 could be re-established after depletion in fetal germ cells undergoing epigenetic reprogramming, we cultured E11.5 gonads for 24 h with DMSO, 100 nM tazemetostat or 1 μM tazemetostat; removed the drug by washing three times with drug-free culture media; and continued culture for an additional 48 h in the presence of 100 nM, 1 μM tazemetostat or DMSO (Fig. 5a). To ensure collection of control and experimental data at the end of the initial drug depletion period and after the recovery period, treatments were carried out on four treatment groups: (1) treatment with DMSO for 24 h followed by treatment with DMSO for 48 h, which provided a negative control to determine the H3K27me3 levels after 72 h culture without the drug; (2) treatment with tazemetostat for 24 h only, which determined the reduction of H3K27me3 after 24 h of treatment as a pre-recovery control; (3) treatment with tazemetostat for 24 h, followed by treatment with DMSO for 48 h, which determined the extent to which H3K27me3 recovered after tazemetostat exposure; and (4) treatment with tazemetostat for 24 h followed by treatment with tazemetostat for 48 h, providing a positive control to determine the H3K27me3 depletion after 72 h of drug treatment (Fig. 5a). Flow cytometry was used to determine the levels of H3K27me3 in the germ cells after each treatment. Germ cell H3K27me3 levels were depleted to a lesser extent at 100 nM, compared to 1 μM tazemetostat at 24 h, and these levels were maintained without restoration across the 48-h recovery period (Fig. 5b). At the higher dose (1 μM), germ cell H3K27me3 levels were depleted by 54% after 24 h and continued to decline over the 48-h recovery period (DMSO; $P < 0.01$, one-way ANOVA post hoc Tukey's multiple comparisons test; Fig. 5b). Together, these data demonstrate that EZH2 inhibition rapidly, and potently, depleted germ cells of H3K27me3 and that recovery of H3K27me3 in fetal germ cells was dependent on tazemetostat dose.

EZH2 inhibition potently depletes H3K27me3 in primary oocytes

As tazemetostat is currently in clinical trials for treatment of cancer in patients aged 6 months to 18 years, it is possible that oocytes in the primordial follicle reserve will be affected by the drug in these patients. This is of particular relevance as the primordial follicle reserve provides all oocytes for the female reproductive life. To assess whether H3K27me3 was depleted in primary oocytes after birth, we cultured E18.5 mouse ovaries for 7 days with either vehicle control (DMSO) or 5 μM TAZ (Fig. 6). Primordial oocytes of E18.5 ovaries treated with 5 μM TAZ were significantly less enriched for H3K27me3 compared to controls (Fig. 6).

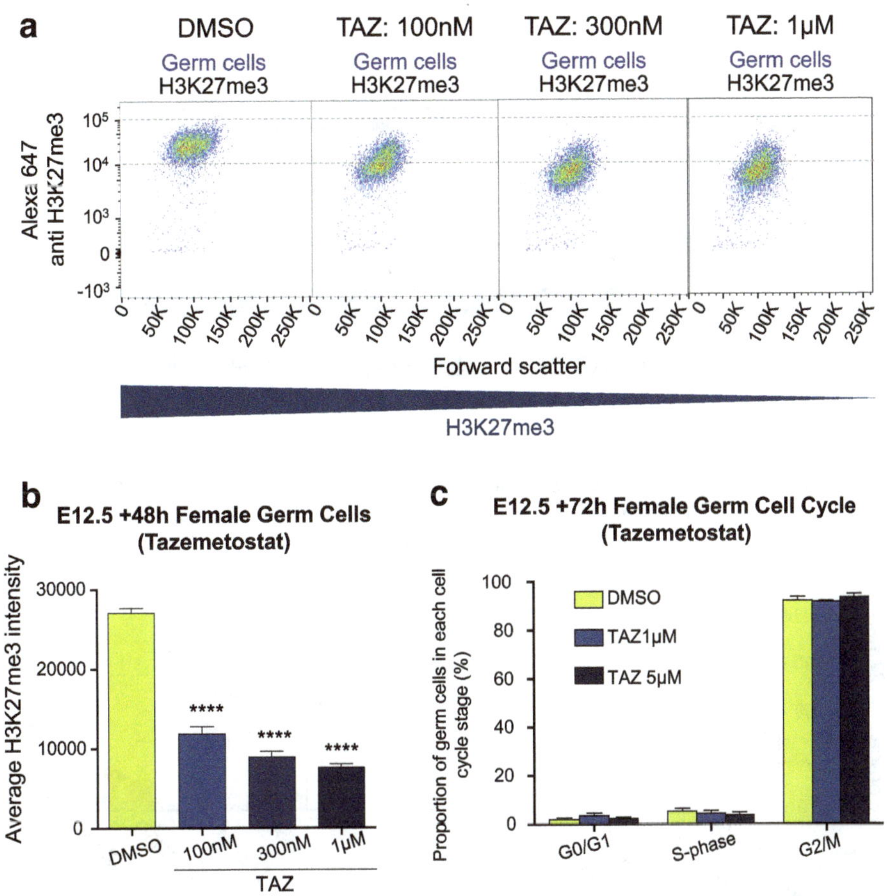

Fig. 4 EZH2 inhibition potently reduced H3K27me3 levels in fetal oocytes undergoing epigenetic reprogramming. **a.** Flow scatter plots showing H3K27me3 mean intensity of germ cells measured by flow cytometry of XX E12.5 gonads cultured for 48 h with DMSO, 100 nM, 300 nM or 1 μM tazemetostat. Examples of flow cytometric gating are shown in Additional file 1: Figure S1. **b** Average H3K27me3 staining intensity in germ cells from XX female E12.5 gonads cultured for 48 h with DMSO, 100 nM, 300 nM, 1 μM tazemetostat. ****$P < 0.0001$, one-way ANOVA plus post hoc Tukey's multiple comparisons test; $n = 3–5$ biological replicates. Error bars ± SEM. **c** Cell cycle state in germ cells from XX female E12.5 gonads cultured for 72 h with DMSO, 1 μM and 5 μM tazemetostat. No significant differences between DMSO control and treatments. One-way ANOVA plus post hoc Tukey's multiple comparisons test; $n = 3–5$ biological replicates. Error bars ± SEM

Discussion

Drugs that target epigenetic modifying complexes hold great promise in oncology and potentially for treatment of a range of other diseases and disorders. These drugs are therefore likely to make a significant contribution to the treatment of human disease and provide substantial improvements in health outcomes. From this point of view, drugs targeting epigenetic modifiers are highly desirable and may be of significant benefit. However, these drugs also have the potential to affect epigenetic programming in the germline, with significant implications for health and developmental outcomes in offspring. There is therefore a need to assess the germline impacts of drugs that inhibit epigenetic modifying proteins to enable the informed clinical management of these drugs in patients of reproductive age.

In this study, we investigated the potential for drugs that inhibit EZH2 to alter H3K27me3 in growing oocytes, primary oocytes and the developing female germline. Significantly, tazemetostat prevented H3K27me3 enrichment in growing oocytes of adult females in vivo, and this effect was relatively stable as H3K27me3 did not recover after 10 days of drug withdrawal. In addition, EZH2 inhibition reduced H3K27me3 in the primary oocyte pool, indicating that the lifelong primordial follicle reserve is affected by these drugs. Finally, tazemetostat severely depleted H3K27me3 in developing oocytes undergoing epigenetic reprogramming and established that once depleted, H3K27me3 did not recover in these cells within the window analysed. Combined, these findings demonstrate that EZH2 inhibitors potently reduce H3K27me3 at all stages of female germline development.

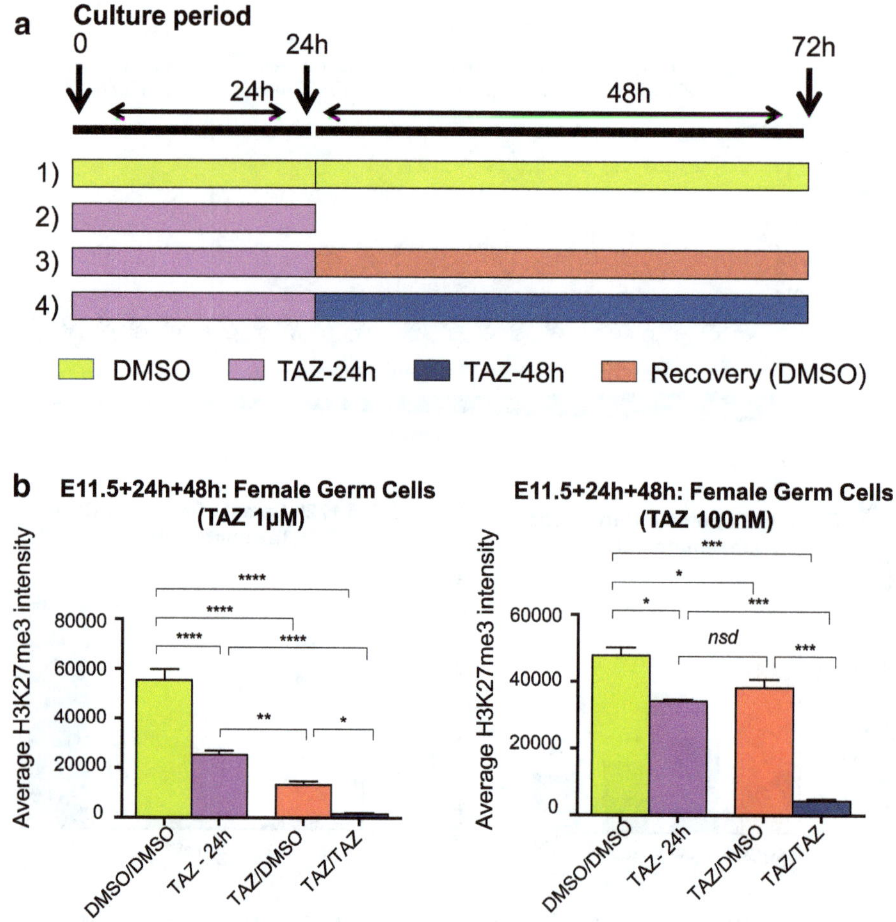

Fig. 5 H3K27me3 was not recovered in oocytes after treatment of fetal ovaries with tazemetostat. Data summary from flow cytometric analyses of E11.5 XX gonads cultured for 24 h with DMSO (green), 100 nM or 1 μM tazemetostat (Blue), followed by drug removal and additional culture for 48 h in the presence of DMSO (green), 100 nM or 1 μM tazemetostat. Drugs were removed by washes with culture media after the initial 24 h of culture. Four treatment groups were used to collect control and experimental data. Treatment 1: DMSO/DMSO—24 h DMSO followed by 48 h DMSO (negative control). Treatment 2: TAZ—24 h tazemetostat (H3K27me3 depletion after 24 h drug treatment). Treatment 3: TAZ/DMSO—24 h tazemetostat followed by 48 h DMSO (H3K27me3 recovery after 48 h drug withdrawal). Treatment 4: TAZ/TAZ—24 h tazemetostat followed by 48 h tazemetostat (H3K27me3 depletion after 72 h drug treatment). **a** Summary of experimental pipeline for assessing H3K27me3 recovery after drug depletion in germ cells undergoing epigenetic reprogramming. **b** Average H3K27me3 staining intensity in germ cells for treatments 1–4 DMSO/DMSO, TAZ, TAZ/DMSO and TAZ/TAZ using 1 μM (left) and 100 nM (right) tazemetostat from cultured E11.5 XX female gonads (1 μM, $n = 5$ biological replicates, 100 nM $n = 4$ biological replicates). $^{*}P < 0.05$, $^{**}P < 0.01$, $^{***}P < 0.001$, $^{****}P < 0.0001$; one-way ANOVA plus post hoc Tukey's multiple comparisons test. Error bars ± SEM

Previous work, and our own experiments, using a mouse genetic model in which EZH2 was specifically deleted in growing oocytes demonstrated that maternal H3K27me3 was lost in the oocyte. Moreover, offspring had abnormal preimplantation development and were born with substantial growth restriction ([16], Prokopuk et al. unpublished data). Growth restriction is a risk factor for lifelong health impacts including metabolic disease [41–43]. Moreover, de novo germline mutations in human EZH2 result in Weaver syndrome, characterised by growth and skeletal defects and intellectual disability [44–46]. As these combined studies indicate that altered H3K27me3 in growing oocytes affects outcomes in offspring, it is likely that maternal exposure to EZH2 inhibitors and similar epigenetic modifying drugs will have the potential to impact on offspring growth and development. Although the specific impacts of EZH2 inhibitors on oocytes and offspring are yet to be determined, it is clear that much greater understanding of the potential germline impacts of these drugs in patients of reproductive age is required.

Understanding the impacts of drugs on both the parental germline epigenome and on offspring is of significant importance as a range of studies have shown that environmental impacts in the parent can affect outcomes in offspring through epigenetic mechanisms that are, by and large, poorly understood [47–59]. Moreover, although studies of other epigenetic modifying

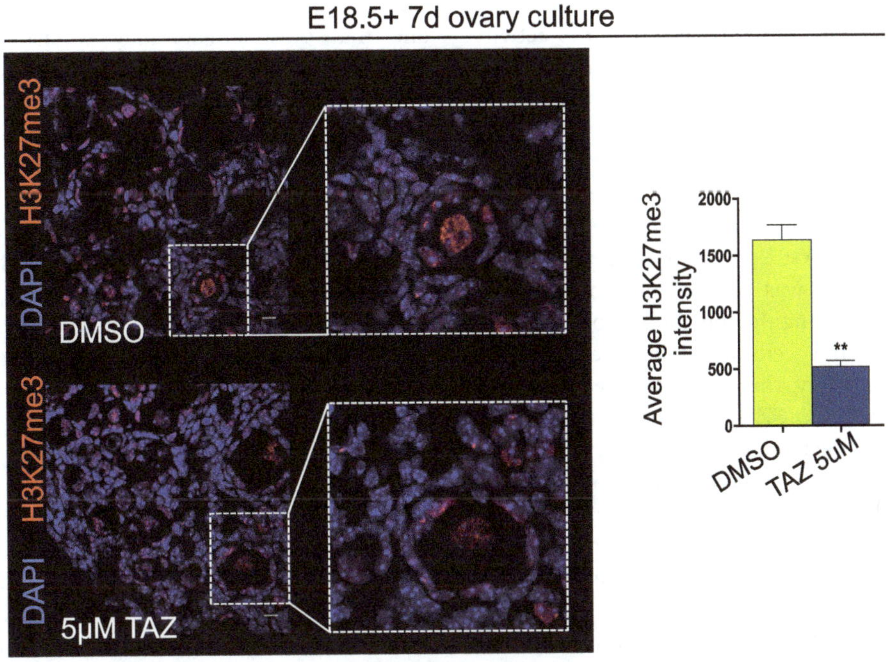

Fig. 6 Tazemetostat depleted H3K27me3 in primary oocytes. Confocal images of H3K27me3 (red) and DAPI (blue) immunofluorescence in sections of E18.5 mouse ovaries cultured for 7 days with either DMSO (top panel) or 5 μM tazemetostat (bottom panel; 10 μm scale bars). Graphical representation of mean H3K27me3 staining intensity in DMSO treatment in green and tazemetostat treatment in blue, analysed by ROI manager, ImageJ. $P < 0.005$, Student's t test; DMSO $n = 4$ and tazemetostat $n = 3$ biological replicates, three primary oocytes analysed per replicate. Error bars ± SEM

compounds, such as valproic acid, have demonstrated direct effects on the unborn fetus and on children of mothers treated during pregnancy [19], these studies have not addressed the potential intergenerational or transgenerational effects of drugs that target other epigenetic mechanisms in the germline.

In this study, tazemetostat caused severe depletion of H3K27me3 from growing oocytes after only 10 days of treatment and H3K27me3 had not recovered 10 days after treatment of the females had been terminated. This recovery period is equivalent to approximately half of the period required for a mouse oocyte to reach maturity from the primordial follicle stage [17]. The human oocyte takes approximately 350 days to grow and mature after recruitment from the primordial follicle pool [60, 61]. However, the current clinical guidelines recommend not to become pregnant for at least 30 days after treatment has been terminated. Consequently, after the termination of treatment, growing oocytes that were exposed to tazemetostat will remain for almost 11 months, and offspring conceived during this period may be also affected. Our findings in mice indicate that even after drug withdrawal there is a risk that H3K27me3 levels in oocytes will be affected for a significant period of oocyte growth and maturation. Based on oocyte growth and maturation periods of 21 days for mouse [17] and 350 days for human [60], we estimate that a similar withdrawal period in humans would require at least a full cycle of oocyte growth to allow the clearance of potentially affected oocytes. This is significantly longer than the current 30-day period recommended in most current tazemetostat clinical trials before patients should consider becoming pregnant. Therefore, it is possible that even after tazemetostat treatment has ceased in human patients, there will be a protracted period during which the oocyte epigenome will be affected and may have consequences for offspring.

Our data demonstrate that in growing oocytes, tazemetostat potently depleted H3K27me3 and H3K27me3 levels continued to decline until at least 10 days after treatment was withdrawn from the mice. Despite this, all core components of PRC2 were detected in growing oocytes, and H3K27me3 was enriched during oocyte growth demonstrating that PRC2 is normally active in growing oocytes. Similarly, H3K27me3 was not recovered in female fetal germ cells after tazemetostat treatment of fetal ovaries. We have previously shown that *Ezh2* is transcribed, EZH2 protein is present and EZH2 is required for redistributing H3K27me3 in XX germ cells during epigenetic reprogramming, demonstrating a functional role for EZH2 during this developmental period [14]. A possible explanation for the lack of H3K27me3 recovery after drug withdrawal is that once inhibited, EZH2 activity cannot recover, possibly because the drug irreversibly blocks and inhibits activity. This observation also implies that new EZH2 was either not synthesised in oocytes or the drug continued to block its activity throughout the withdrawal period. Retention of drug activity is unlikely as a previous study demonstrated an in vivo half-life for tazemetostat of only 4 h in mice [4], indicating that greater than 90% drug clearance in the first 24 h after drug withdrawal. Similarly, tazemetostat was washed out of the fetal ovarian cultures by changing the media for drug-free media and washing the wells multiple times. It therefore appears more likely that once blocked in either growing or fetal oocytes, EZH2 activity cannot readily recover. This may affect all stages of oocyte development and growth as EZH2 inhibition also compromised H3K27me3 in primary oocytes. It is therefore possible that tazemetostat and similar drugs may have persistent effects on all oocytes, including those in the primordial follicle pool. This is an important consideration when female children or patients of reproductive age are treated with the drug and is of direct relevance in current clinical trials involving patients aged 6 months to 18 years.

The current clinical guidelines clearly state that use of EZH2-inhibiting drugs is contra-indicated in patients during pregnancy. This position is presumably based on the direct impacts of EZH2 on somatic development in the fetus, but empirical evidence for this position is currently lacking. Recent reports of adverse impacts of the anti-epilepsy drug Epilim (valproic acid) [19] have highlighted the importance of a direct evidence-based position in developing stringent guidelines for these drugs in pregnancy. In addition to teratogenic impacts on somatic development in the fetus, in utero exposure to valproic acid has been associated with long-term effects on children, including decreased learning ability, autism and behavioural anomalies [19]. Similar outcomes in the fetus are likely for other drugs that inhibit epigenetic modifying complexes. However, it is also possible that drugs targeting epigenetic modifiers will cause intergenerational or transgenerational epigenetic effects in the patients' children or grandchildren. Using gonad culture and in vivo treatments, respectively, we have clearly demonstrated that germline exposure to EZH2 inhibiting drugs severely affects epigenetic programming in the fetal and adult oocytes, highlighting the potent ability of these drugs to disrupt epigenetic programming in the germline and a need to further understand the impacts of these drugs on the germline.

Although new drugs that target epigenetic modifying enzymes offer important new therapeutic options for patients, it is clear that these drugs also have the capacity to significantly alter the germline epigenome and that these effects may persist for a significant period of time. One obvious way to avoid such effects in patients of reproductive age undergoing treatment with drugs that target epigenetic modifiers would be to employ germline preservation methods, such as sperm and oocyte freezing. However, as gamete preservation techniques are imperfect and not available to all patients, it is also clear that significantly more work is required to determine the molecular and phenotypic effects of EZH2 inhibitors in the germline and their potential to adversely affect subsequent children of female patients.

Conclusions

Significantly, the potential impacts on the germline of drugs that target epigenetic modifying enzymes appear to be largely "off the radar" when the clinical safety of these drugs is being considered—most attention is reserved for the potential teratogenicity of the drugs rather than the potential germline impacts and subsequent effects on offspring. This study highlights an urgent need to determine risks of these and similar treatments for oogenesis and offspring outcomes.

Methods

Mouse strains, animal housing, breeding and ethics

Mice were housed at Monash Medical Centre Animal Facility using a 12-h light-dark cycle. Food and water were available ad libitum and room temperature was 21–23 °C with controlled humidity. Embryos were collected from *Oct4* [*Pou5f1*]-eGFP on 129T2svJ background males crossed with Swiss females. Females were checked for vaginal plugs daily and detection of a plug was noted as E0.5. Embryos E12.5 or older were sexed by the presence (male) or absence (female) of testis cords in gonads. E11.5 embryos were genetically sexed using PCR as described [62].

Gonad collection and organ culture

All culture reagents were purchased from Life Technologies unless otherwise stated. Embryos were collected from Swiss females mated to 129T2svJ *Oct4*-eGFP transgenic males. Gonad plus mesonephros was cultured on 30 mm organotypic cell culture inserts (Merck Millipore; PICM03050) in 1200 μL culture media (250 μM sodium pyruvate, 15 mM Hepes, 1× non-essential amino acids) (Life Technologies, 11140), 1 mg/ml N-acetylcysteine (Sigma, A9165), 55 μM β-mercaptoethanol (Life Technologies, 21985) and 10% FCS in DMEM/F12 with Glutamax (Life Technologies, 10565) containing either DMSO (vehicle control) or tazemetostat (EPZ6438; SelleckChem, S7128). Culture media also contained 1× penicillin/streptomycin (Life

Technologies, 15070). Gonads were randomly allocated to each culture treatment condition and cultured for 48 h in 37 °C/5% CO_2 conditions. Culture media was refreshed daily. Gonads were processed for flow cytometry, FACS and immunofluorescence (IF).

Flow cytometry

Gonad collection, dissociation, fixation, antibody staining and flow cytometry were performed as described [14, 40]. Gonad samples stained with rabbit IgG control antibody were used as negative controls to set flow cytometry gates for H3K27me3 intensity and mesonephros or limb samples were used as a germ cell negative control to gate for eGFP. Cell proliferation was assessed by dosing cultured gonads with 20 μM 5-ethynyl-2 deoxyuridine (EdU) for the final 2 hours of culture prior to tissue collection, dissociation and fixation. Cell cycle analysis was carried out as described [40, 63] with germ cells identified by their expression of mouse vasa homologue (MVH). Cells were stained with 20 μg/ml propidium iodide, allowing quantitation of cellular DNA content. Proliferation was measured by gating EdU-positive cells against propidium iodide to identify cells actively in S-phase. Cells in G1 and G2/M were identified by their DNA content and the absence of S-phase activity. All flow cytometry was performed on a FACS Canto instrument and data were analysed in FlowJo and Graphpad Prism. For all analyses, at least three biological replicates were analysed and statistical significance was determined using one-way ANOVA with Tukey's multiple comparison or t test as appropriate. P values < 0.05 were considered significant.

Tissue fixation and embedding

Gonads were fixed in 4% paraformaldehyde (PFA) in PBS for immunofluorescence (IF) overnight at 4 °C. Samples were washed twice in PBS and left in 30% sucrose in PBS overnight at 4 °C. Samples were then placed in disposable cryostat moulds (Sakura Finetek, 4565) filled with OCT (Sakura Finetek, 4583) and frozen in dry ice and stored at − 80 °C.

Immunofluorescence

Immunofluorescence was carried out as previously described [14]. Eight micron sections were cut from OCT-embedded gonads fixed in 4% PFA, mounted on Superfrost Plus slides and dried for 5 min before immersing in 1× PBS. Sections were then permeabilized by incubation in 1% Triton X 100 (Sigma, T8787) in PBS for 10 min at room temperature (RT). Slides were washed three times for 5 min each in PBS. Sections were blocked in PBS containing 5% BSA (Sigma, A9647) and 10% donkey serum (Sigma, D9663) and incubated for 45 min at RT. Blocking solution was replaced by PBS containing 1% BSA and appropriately diluted primary antibodies (rabbit anti-H3K27me3 1:400, Cell Signaling Technology #C36B11; sheep anti-EED 1:100, R&D #AF5827; rabbit anti-EZH2 1:400, Cell Signaling Technology #D2C9; rabbit anti-SUZ12 1:100, Cell Signaling Technology #D39F6) and incubated for 1 h at RT. Slides were washed three times for 5 min in PBS and secondary antibodies diluted at 1:300 in 1% BSA in 1× PBS (Alexa Fluor, Life Technologies, Donkey anti Sheep 647 #A21447; Donkey anti Rabbit 594 #A21207). Secondary antibody incubation was carried out in a dark humidity chamber for 1 h at RT. Slides were washed three times in PBS (5 min each wash) and mounted in ProLong Gold® containing DAPI (Life Technologies, #P36931) and left in a dark box overnight to dry. For control slides, only a secondary antibody was applied. Confocal images were taken as single optical sections using a Nikon® C1 inverted confocal microscope. All pictures were taken at ×80, using a ×40 oil immersion lens. H3K27me3 mean intensity was measured in at least three biological replicates using ImageJ ROI manager to calculate the mean intensity for H3K27me3, and unpaired t tests were used to statistically analyse groups, with $P \leq 0.05$ considered significant.

In vivo injection of tazemetostat

Seven-week old C57Bl/6J females were subcutaneously injected with 220 mg/kg/day tazemetostat. Mice were weighed daily to ensure correct dosage. Dosage regime involved injecting mice once a day for 9 consecutive days and collecting females on the 10th day. Females were culled via cervical dislocation and ovaries were collected and processed for IF.

Additional file

Additional file 1: Figure S1. Representative flow cytometric scatter plots demonstrating separation, gating and analysis of germ and somatic cells derived from gonads cultured with DMSO or tazemetostat. A. Representative flow cytometric plots of cells analysed from female cultured gonads. Oct4GFP-positive germ cells and Oct4GFP-negative somatic cells were separated and gated based on their respective positive or negative expression of Oct4GFP (left plot). Mean H3K27me3 staining intensity of individual germ (middle plot) and somatic cells (right plot) was quantified using FlowJo. B. Representative flow cytometric plots of cells analysed from limb control cells, which do not express Oct4GFP. This and similar controls facilitated the gating of Oct4GFP-positive and Oct4GFP-negative populations shown in A and B. C. Average H3K27me3 staining intensity in germ cells of E12.5 XX gonads cultured with DMSO, 1 μM and 5 μM tazemetostat for 72 h. **Figure S2.** Representative flow cytometric scatter plots demonstrating separation, gating and cell cycle analysis of germ and somatic cells derived from female E12.5 gonads cultured with DMSO or tazemetostat for 72 h. A. Oct4GFP positive germ cells and Oct4GFP negative somatic cells were separated and gated based on their respective positive or negative expression of Oct4GFP (left plots). The middle and right-hand plots represent cell cycle analyses based on incorporation of EdU and propidium iodide (PI) staining quantified using FlowJo (germ cell cycle-middle plots; somatic cell cycle-right plots). B. Average H3K27me3 staining intensity (left) and cell cycle state (right) in somatic cells from female E12.5 gonads cultured with DMSO or tazemetostat. $^{****}P < 0.0001$, one-way ANOVA plus post hoc Tukey's multiple comparisons test; $n = 3–5$ biological replicates.

Abbreviations

E: Embryonic day; EED: Embryonic ectoderm development; eGFP: Enhanced GFP; EPZ: EZH1/2 inhibitor, TAZ, tazemetostat/EPZ-6438; EZH1: Enhancer of Zeste 1; EZH2: Enhancer of Zeste 2; FACS: Fluorescence-activated cell sorting; GSK126: EZH1/2 inhibitor, GSK; H3K27me3: Trimethylated lysine 27 on histone 3; MVH: Mouse vasa homologue (also known as DDX4); *Nsd*: No significant difference; PRC2: Polycomb repressive complex 2; SUZ12: Suppressor of Zeste 12

Acknowledgements

We thank Monash Animal Research Platform staff for assistance with mouse care. We thank Jessica Stringer and Karla Hutt for manuscript review and Ellen Jarred for technical assistance with ovary culture experiments.

Funding

This work was supported by National Health and Medical Research Grants GNT1043939 and GNT1051223 awarded to PSW, funding from the Monash University Faculty of Medicine, Nursing and Health Sciences funding granted to PSW and the Victorian Government's Operational Infrastructure Support Program. LP is supported by an Australian Postgraduate Award.

Authors' contributions

PSW conceived and designed the study, obtained financial support, collected and analysed the data and drafted the manuscript. LP collected and processed the samples, optimised and performed experiments, analysed the data and drafted the manuscript. KH optimised and performed experiments, analysed data and drafted the manuscript. All authors read and approved the final manuscript.

Authors' information

K.H and L.P are now located at the Stem Cells and Cancer Division of the Walter and Eliza Hall Institute of Medical Research, Parkville, Victoria, Australia.

Competing interests

The authors declare that they have no competing interests.

References

1. Stringer J, Barrand S, Western P. Fine-tuning evolution: germ-line epigenetics and inheritance. Reproduction. 2013;146:R37–48.
2. Hogg K, Western PS. Refurbishing the germline epigenome: out with the old, in with the new. Semin Cell Dev Biol. 2015;45:104–13.
3. Jones PA, Issa JPJ, Baylin S. Targeting the cancer epigenome for therapy. Nat Rev Genet. 2016;17(10):630–41.
4. Knutson SK, Kawano S, Minoshima Y, Warholic NM, Huang KC, Xiao YH, Kadowaki T, Uesugi M, Kuznetsov G, Kumar N, et al. Selective inhibition of EZH2 by EPZ-6438 leads to potent antitumor activity in EZH2-mutant non-Hodgkin lymphoma. Mol Cancer Ther. 2014;13(4):842–54.
5. McCabe MT, Ott HM, Ganji G, Korenchuk S, Thompson C, Van Aller GS, Liu Y, Graves AP, Della Pietra A, Diaz E, et al. EZH2 inhibition as a therapeutic strategy for lymphoma with EZH2-activating mutations. Nature. 2012; 492(7427):108.
6. Huang Y, Zhang J, Yu ZT, Zhang HL, Wang YZ, Lingel A, Qi W, Gu J, Zhao KH, Shultz MD, et al. Discovery of first-in-class, potent, and orally bioavailable embryonic ectoderm development (EED) inhibitor with robust anticancer efficacy. J Med Chem. 2017;60(6):2215–26.
7. Pasini D, Bracken AP, Jensen MR, Denchi EL, Helin K. Suz12 is essential for mouse development and for EZH2 histone methyltransferase activity. EMBO J. 2004;23(20):4061–71.
8. Faust C, Schumacher A, Holdener B, Magnuson T. The Eed mutation disrupts anterior mesoderm production in mice. Development. 1995;121(2):273–85.
9. O'Carroll D, Erhardt S, Pagani M, Barton SC, Surani MA, Jenuwein T. The polycomb-group gene Ezh2 is required for early mouse development. Mol Cell Biol. 2001;21(13):4330–6.
10. Shen X, Liu Y, Hsu YJ, Fujiwara Y, Kim J, Mao X, Yuan GC, Orkin SH. EZH1 mediates methylation on histone H3 lysine 27 and complements EZH2 in maintaining stem cell identity and executing pluripotency. Mol Cell. 2008;32(4):491–502.
11. Knutson SK, Warholic NM, Wigle TJ, Klaus CR, Allain CJ, Raimondi A, Scott MP, Chesworth R, Moyer MP, Copeland RA, et al. Durable tumor regression in genetically altered malignant rhabdoid tumors by inhibition of methyltransferase EZH2. Proc Natl Acad Sci U S A. 2013;110(19):7922–7.
12. Hajkova P, Jeffries SJ, Lee C, Miller N, Jackson SP, Surani MA. Genome-wide reprogramming in the mouse germ line entails the base excision repair pathway. Science. 2010;329(5987):78–82.
13. Saitou M, Kagiwada S, Kurimoto K. Epigenetic reprogramming in mouse pre-implantation development and primordial germ cells. Development. 2012;139(1):15–31.
14. Prokopuk L, Stringer JM, Hogg K, Elgass KD, Western PS. PRC2 is required for extensive reorganization of H3K27me3 during epigenetic reprogramming in mouse fetal germ cells. Epigenet Chromatin. 2017;10:1–20.
15. Lesch BJ, Dokshin GA, Young RA, McCarrey JR, Page DC. A set of genes critical to development is epigenetically poised in mouse germ cells from fetal stages through completion of meiosis. Proc Natl Acad Sci U S A. 2013; 110(40):16061–6.
16. Erhardt S, Su IH, Schneider R, Barton S, Bannister AJ, Perez-Burgos L, Jenuwein T, Kouzarides T, Tarakhovsky A, Surani MA. Consequences of the depletion of zygotic and embryonic enhancer of zeste 2 during preimplantation mouse development. Development. 2003;130(18):4235–48.
17. Peters H. The development of the mouse ovary from birth to maturity. Acta Endocrinol. 1969;62(1):98–116.
18. Stefansdottir A, Johnston ZC, Powles-Glover N, Anderson RA, Adams IR, Spears N. Etoposide damages female germ cells in the developing ovary. BMC Cancer. 2016;16(1):482.
19. Gotlib D, Ramaswamy R, Kurlander JE, DeRiggi A, Riba M: Valproic acid in women and girls of childbearing age. Curr Psychiat Rep 2017, **19**(9).
20. Hajkova P, Erhardt S, Lane N, Haaf T, El-Maarri O, Reik W, Walter J, Surani MA. Epigenetic reprogramming in mouse primordial germ cells. Mech Dev. 2002;117(1-2):15–23.
21. Hajkova P, Ancelin K, Waldmann T, Lacoste N, Lange UC, Cesari F, Lee C, Almouzni G, Schneider R, Surani MA. Chromatin dynamics during epigenetic reprogramming in the mouse germ line. Nature. 2008;452(7189):877–81.
22. Li Y, Cang M, Lee AS, Zhang K, Liu D. Reprogramming of sheep fibroblasts into pluripotency under a drug-inducible expression of mouse-derived defined factors. PLoS One. 2011;6(1):e15947.
23. Seki Y, Yamaji M, Yabuta Y, Sano M, Shigeta M, Matsui Y, Saga Y, Tachibana M, Shinkai Y, Saitou M. Cellular dynamics associated with the genome-wide epigenetic reprogramming in migrating primordial germ cells in mice. Development. 2007;134(14):2627–38.
24. Seisenberger S, Andrews S, Krueger F, Arand J, Walter J, Santos F, Popp C, Thienpont B, Dean W, Reik W. The dynamics of genome-wide DNA methylation reprogramming in mouse primordial germ cells. Mol Cell. 2012;48(6):849–62.
25. Gkountela S, Li Z, Vincent JJ, Zhang KX, Chen A, Pellegrini M, Clark AT. The ontogeny of cKIT+ human primordial germ cells proves to be a resource for human germ line reprogramming, imprint erasure and in vitro differentiation. Nat Cell Biol. 2013;15(1):113–22.
26. Sachs M, Onodera C, Blaschke K, Ebata KT, Song JS, Ramalho-Santos M. Bivalent chromatin marks developmental regulatory genes in the mouse embryonic germline in vivo. Cell Rep. 2013;3(6):1777–84.
27. Ng JH, Kumar V, Muratani M, Kraus P, Yeo JC, Yaw LP, Xue K, Lufkin T, Prabhakar S, Ng HH. In vivo epigenomic profiling of germ cells reveals germ cell molecular signatures. Dev Cell. 2013;24(3):324–33.

28. Hammoud SS, Nix DA, Zhang H, Purwar J, Carrell DT, Cairns BR. Distinctive chromatin in human sperm packages genes for embryo development. Nature. 2009;460(7254):473–8.
29. Brykczynska U, Hisano M, Erkek S, Ramos L, Oakeley EJ, Roloff TC, Beisel C, Schubeler D, Stadler MB, Peters AH. Repressive and active histone methylation mark distinct promoters in human and mouse spermatozoa. Nat Struct Mol Biol. 2010;17(6):679–87.
30. Oktem O, Urman B. Understanding follicle growth in vivo. Hum Reprod. 2010;25(12):2944–54.
31. Tingen C, Kim A, Woodruff TK. The primordial pool of follicles and nest breakdown in mammalian ovaries. Mol Hum Reprod. 2009;15(12):795–803.
32. Kerr JB, Myers M, Anderson RA. The dynamics of the primordial follicle reserve. Reproduction. 2013;146(6):R205–15.
33. Li R, Albertini DF. The road to maturation: somatic cell interaction and self-organization of the mammalian oocyte. Nat Rev Mol Cell Biol. 2013;14(3):141–52.
34. Szabo PE, Hubner K, Scholer H, Mann JR. Allele-specific expression of imprinted genes in mouse migratory primordial germ cells. Mech Dev. 2002;115(1-2):157–60.
35. van den Bergen JA, Miles DC, Sinclair AH, Western PS. Normalizing gene expression levels in mouse fetal germ cells. Biol Reprod. 2009;81:362–70.
36. Gustin SE, Hogg K, Stringer JM, Rastetter RH, Pelosi E, Miles DC, Sinclair AH, Wilhelm D, Western PS. WNT/beta-catenin and p27/FOXL2 differentially regulate supporting cell proliferation in the developing ovary. Dev Biol. 2016;412(2):250–60.
37. Bullejos M, Koopman P. Germ cells enter meiosis in a rostro-caudal wave during development of the mouse ovary. Mol Reprod Dev. 2004;68(4):422–8.
38. Miles DC, van den Bergen JA, Sinclair AH, Western PS. Regulation of the female mouse germ cell cycle during entry into meiosis. Cell Cycle. 2010; 9(2):408–18.
39. Western PS, Miles DC, van den Bergen JA, Burton M, Sinclair AH. Dynamic regulation of mitotic arrest in fetal male germ cells. Stem Cells. 2008;26(2):339–47.
40. Wakeling SI, Miles DC, Western PS. Identifying disruptors of male germ cell development by small molecule screening in ex vivo gonad cultures. BMC Res Notes. 2013;6(1):168.
41. Thornburg KL, O'Tierney PF, Louey S. The placenta is a programming agent for cardiovascular disease. Placenta. 2010;31:S54–9.
42. Gatford KL, Simmons RA, De Blasio MJ, Robinson JS, Owens JA. Placental programming of postnatal diabetes and impaired insulin action after IUGR. Placenta. 2010;31:S60–5.
43. Maltepe E, Bakardjiev AI, Fisher SJ. The placenta: transcriptional, epigenetic, and physiological integration during development. J Clin Inv. 2010;120(4): 1016–25.
44. Cooney E, Bi WM, Schlesinger AE, Vinson S, Potocki L. Novel EED mutation in patient with Weaver syndrome. Am J Med Genet A. 2017;173(2):541–5.
45. Gibson WT, Hood RL, Zhan SH, Bulman DE, Fejes AP, Moore R, Mungall AJ, Eydoux P, Babul-Hirji R, An JH, et al. Mutations in EZH2 cause Weaver syndrome. Am J Hum Genet. 2012;90(1):110–8.
46. Tatton-Brown K, Hanks S, Ruark E, Zachariou A, Duarte SD, Ramsay E, Snape K, Murray A, Perdeaux ER, Seal S, et al. Germline mutations in the oncogene EZH2 cause Weaver syndrome and increased human height. Oncotarget. 2011;2(12):1127–33.
47. Francis D, Diorio J, Liu D, Meaney MJ. Nongenomic transmission across generations of maternal behavior and stress responses in the rat. Science. 1999;286(5442):1155–8.
48. Wolff GL, Kodell RL, Moore SR, Cooney CA. Maternal epigenetics and methyl supplements affect agouti gene expression in Avy/a mice. FASEB J. 1998; 12(11):949–57.
49. Waterland RA, Jirtle RL. Transposable elements: targets for early nutritional effects on epigenetic gene regulation. Mol Cell Biol. 2003;23(15):5293–300.
50. Cropley JE, Suter CM, Beckman KB, Martin DI. Germ-line epigenetic modification of the murine Avy allele by nutritional supplementation. Proc Natl Acad Sci U S A. 2006;103(46):17308–12.
51. Waterland RA, Travisano M, Tahiliani KG. Diet-induced hypermethylation at agouti viable yellow is not inherited transgenerationally through the female. FASEB J. 2007;21(12):3380–5.
52. Morgan HD, Sutherland HG, Martin DI, Whitelaw E. Epigenetic inheritance at the agouti locus in the mouse. Nat Genet. 1999;23(3):314–8.
53. Padmanabhan N, Jia D, Geary-Joo C, Wu X, Ferguson-Smith AC, Fung E, Bieda MC, Snyder FF, Gravel RA, Cross JC, et al. Mutation in folate metabolism causes epigenetic instability and transgenerational effects on development. Cell. 2013; 155(1):81–93.
54. Gapp K, Jawaid A, Sarkies P, Bohacek J, Pelczar P, Prados J, Farinelli L, Miska E, Mansuy IM. Implication of sperm RNAs in transgenerational inheritance of the effects of early trauma in mice. Nat Neurosci. 2014;17(5):667–9.
55. Ng SF, Lin RC, Laybutt DR, Barres R, Owens JA, Morris MJ. Chronic high-fat diet in fathers programs beta-cell dysfunction in female rat offspring. Nature. 2010;467(7318):963–6.
56. Jimenez-Chillaron JC, Isganaitis E, Charalambous M, Gesta S, Pentinat-Pelegrin T, Faucette RR, Otis JP, Chow A, Diaz R, Ferguson-Smith A. Intergenerational transmission of glucose intolerance and obesity by in utero undernutrition in mice. Diabetes. 2009;58(2):460–8.
57. Radford EJ, Ito M, Shi H, Corish JA, Yamazawa K, Isganaitis E, Seisenberger S, Hore TA, Reik W, Erkek S, et al. In utero effects. In utero undernourishment perturbs the adult sperm methylome and intergenerational metabolism. Science. 2014;345(6198):1255903.
58. Guerrero-Bosagna C, Settles M, Lucker B, Skinner MK. Epigenetic transgenerational actions of vinclozolin on promoter regions of the sperm epigenome. PLoS One. 2010;5(9):e13100.
59. Lambrot R, Xu C, Saint-Phar S, Chountalos G, Cohen T, Paquet M, Suderman M, Hallett M, Kimmins S. Low paternal dietary folate alters the mouse sperm epigenome and is associated with negative pregnancy outcomes. Nat Commun. 2013;4
60. Gougeon A, Testart J. Germinal vesicle breakdown in oocytes of human atretic follicles during the menstrual cycle. J Reprod Fertil. 1986;78(2):389–401.
61. McGee EA, Hsueh AJW. Initial and cyclic recruitment of ovarian follicles. Endocr Rev. 2000;21(2):200–14.
62. McFarlane L, Truong V, Palmer JS, Wilhelm D. Novel PCR assay for determining the genetic sex of mice. Sex Dev. 2013;7(4):207–11.
63. Hogg K, Western PS. Differentiation of fetal male germline and gonadal progenitor cells is disrupted in organ cultures containing knockout serum replacement. Stem Cells Dev. 2015;24(24):2899–911.

16

Profile of epigenetic mechanisms in lung tumors of patients with underlying chronic respiratory conditions

Mercè Mateu-Jimenez[1,2], Víctor Curull[1,2], Alberto Rodríguez-Fuster[3], Rafael Aguiló[3], Albert Sánchez-Font[1,2], Lara Pijuan[4], Joaquim Gea[1,2] and Esther Barreiro[1,2*]

Abstract

Background: Chronic lung diseases such as chronic obstructive pulmonary disease (COPD) and epigenetic events underlie lung cancer (LC) development. The study objective was that lung tumor expression levels of specific microRNAs and their downstream biomarkers may be differentially regulated in patients with and without COPD.

Methods: In lung specimens (tumor and non-tumor), microRNAs known to be involved in lung tumorigenesis (miR-21, miR-200b, miR-126, miR-451, miR-210, miR-let7c, miR-30a-30p, miR-155 and miR-let7a, qRT-PCR), DNA methylation, and downstream biomarkers were determined (qRT-PCR and immunoblotting) in 40 patients with LC (prospective study, subdivided into LC-COPD and LC, $N = 20$/group).

Results: Expression of miR-21, miR-200b, miR-210, and miR-let7c and DNA methylation were greater in lung tumor specimens of LC-COPD than of LC patients. Expression of downstream markers *PTEN*, *MARCKs*, *TPM-1*, *PDCD4*, *SPRY-2*, *ETS-1*, *ZEB-2*, *FGFRL-1*, *EFNA-3*, and *k-RAS* together with *P53* were selectively downregulated in tumor samples of LC-COPD patients. In these patients, tumor expression of miR-126 and miR-451 and that of the biomarkers *PTEN*, *MARCKs*, *FGFRL-1*, *SNAIL-1*, *P63*, and *k-RAS* were reduced.

Conclusions: Biomarkers of mechanisms involved in tumor growth, angiogenesis, migration, and apoptosis were differentially expressed in tumors of patients with underlying respiratory disease. These findings shed light into the underlying biology of the reported greater risk to develop LC seen in patients with chronic respiratory conditions. The presence of an underlying respiratory disease should be identified in all patients with LC as the differential biological profile may help determine tumor progression and the therapeutic response. Additionally, epigenetic events offer a niche for pharmacological therapeutic targets.

Keywords: Increased susceptibility to lung cancer, Underlying chronic respiratory disease, Tumor microRNAs, DNA methylation, Lung tumorigenesis biomarkers

Background

Lung cancer (LC) continues to be the most common cause of cancer-related mortality worldwide, rising up to one third of all-cause mortality in certain regions [1]. Major respiratory conditions such as chronic obstructive pulmonary disease (COPD) have been consistently proposed as risk factors of LC development in patients [2–7]. Specifically, the presence of emphysema was demonstrated to be the most important risk factor in LC pathogenesis [2–7]. Despite the relevance of this problem, identification of the underlying biology that predisposes patients with airway obstruction and emphysema to LC remains at its infancy.

Several mechanisms such as greater levels of oxidative stress [8–11] and inflammatory markers [8, 12, 13], along with a relative predominance of Th1 cytokines and M1 macrophages, were demonstrated in the tumors

* Correspondence: ebarreiro@imim.es
[1]Pulmonology Department, Lung Cancer and Muscle Research Group, Hospital del Mar-IMIM, Parc de Salut Mar, Health and Experimental Sciences Department (CEXS), Universitat Pompeu Fabra (UPF), Parc de Recerca Biomèdica de Barcelona (PRBB), C/ Dr. Aiguader, 88, E-08003 Barcelona, Spain
[2]Centro de Investigación en Red de Enfermedades Respiratorias (CIBERES), Instituto de Salud Carlos III (ISCIII), Barcelona, Spain
Full list of author information is available at the end of the article

and blood of patients with LC and COPD [14]. In patients with underlying chronic respiratory conditions, these biological mechanisms are likely to participate in the neoplastic transformation as they may interfere with important cell processes such as repair, angiogenesis, and apoptosis [8, 12, 13].

Epigenetic events, defined as the process whereby gene expression is regulated by heritable mechanisms that do not alter DNA sequence, significantly contribute to adaptation to environmental factors. In this regard, cigarette smoking-mediated effects were shown to induce epigenetic modifications in the airways and lungs of patients [15–17]. Alterations in several epigenetic mechanisms such as chromatin remodeling, DNA methylation, and either histone acetylation or methylation were shown to occur in the airways of COPD patients and in lung tumors of patients irrespective of COPD [18, 19]. Interestingly, in patients with COPD and LC, methylation of immune-related genes was demonstrated in their tumor samples [20]. In keeping with, several specific immune-related genes were shown to be hypermethylated in tumor samples of patients with underlying COPD, suggesting that methylation of those specific genes may contribute to the epithelial cell transformation to cancer in patients with chronic respiratory conditions [21, 22]. On the other hand, non-coding single-stranded RNA molecules (microRNAs) which regulate cellular processes, namely proliferation, cell invasion and migration, adaptation to hypoxia, apoptosis, and angiogenesis have also been proposed to underlie lung tumorigenesis in patients with chronic respiratory conditions [23–27]. Additionally, specific microRNA expression patterns may also help predict mortality and response to treatment in LC patients [25, 28]. Whether these mechanisms may take place in the actual tumor lesions of LC patients with underlying respiratory conditions remains to be fully explored.

On this basis, we hypothesized that expression levels of specific microRNAs and DNA methylation may be differentially expressed in the lung tumors of patients with underlying respiratory diseases versus those without the presence of chronic respiratory conditions. Moreover, we also hypothesized that expression of a selected panel of biomarkers known to be specifically regulated by the target microRNAs may also differ in the tumors and non-tumor lungs of patients with LC with and without COPD. These downstream biomarkers were carefully chosen on the basis of currently available literature on the biological processes that are regulated by the target LC-associated microRNAs. Hence, the specific study objectives were to assess prospectively in tumor and non-tumor lung specimens of patients with non-small cell LC (NSCLC), with and without underlying COPD: (1) expression levels of microRNAs known to underlie lung tumorigenesis and total DNA methylation and (2) levels of their downstream pathways known to promote cellular processes involved in lung tumorigenesis and progression.

Methods

Study patients

This was a prospective, controlled study in which a group of 40 Caucasian patients (33 males, Table 1) with LC, undergoing thoracotomy for their lung neoplasm, were recruited consecutively from the Lung Cancer Clinic of the Respiratory Medicine Department at *Hospital del Mar* (Barcelona, Spain). The patients were always recruited before having received any treatment for their lung neoplasm including chemotherapy and/or radiotherapy. Tumor and non-tumor lung specimens were obtained ($n = 40$), and patients were subdivided into two groups depending on the presence of underlying COPD [26, 27, 29]: (1) 20 patients with LC who also had COPD (LC-COPD group) and (2) 20 patients with LC without COPD (LC group). As part of the prospective ongoing cohort "Lung Cancer-COPD" in our center, both LC and LC-COPD patients simultaneously participated in a previous study aimed to assess Th1 and Th2 inflammatory profiles and their implications in lung tumors of patients with chronic respiratory conditions (14).

Approval was obtained from the institutional Ethics Committee on Human Investigation (*Hospital del Mar–IMIM*, Barcelona, project number 2014/5776/1) in accordance with the World Medical Association guidelines (Helsinki Declaration of 2008) for research on human beings. Informed written consent was obtained from all patients at study entry and prior to initiation of therapies.

Anthropometrical and functional assessment

Lung function and anthropometry were evaluated in all patients as previously described [8, 14, 30–32].

Sample collection

During the surgical intervention (minimal resection or lobectomy), in patients that underwent thoracotomy ($n = 40$), lung samples were obtained (tumor and non-tumor specimens) by the expert lung pathologist. Non-tumor samples were collected from the distant surrounding parenchyma with respect to where the tumor was localized (7-cm minimum distance from the tumor site in all the samples), which enabled us to study non-tumor lung specimens. Briefly, non-tumor samples were carefully selected as a result of visual and manual detection (palpation) of any potential nodules that might modify disease staging. The presence of ground-glass opacities in the non-tumor specimens was always ruled

Table 1 Clinical and functional characteristics of the study patients

Anthropometric variables	Lung cancer $N = 20$	Lung cancer-COPD $N = 20$
Age, years	64 (12)	65 (9)
Male, *N*/female, *N*	13/7	20/0
BMI, kg/m^2	26 (5)	26 (5)
Smoking history		
Current: *N*, %	12, 60	14, 70
Ex-smoker: *N*, %	5, 25	6, 30
Never smoker: *N*,%	3, 15	0, 0¶
Pack-years	53 (25)	57 (20)
Lung function testing		
vFEV$_1$, % pred	92 (8)	61 (14)¶¶¶
FEV$_1$/FVC, % pred	77 (6)	60 (8)¶¶¶
DLCO, % pred	88 (12)	72 (21)¶¶¶
KCO, % pred	88 (11)	73 (17)¶¶¶
TNM staging		
Stage IA: *N*, %	5, 25	5, 25
Stage IB: *N*, %	0, 0	4, 20
Stage IIA: *N*, %	1, 5	6, 30
Stage IIB: *N*, %	4, 20	2, 10
Stage IIIA: *N*, %	3, 15	3, 15
Stage IIIB: *N*, %	4, 20	0, 0
Stage IV: *N*, %	3, 15	0, 0
Histological diagnosis		
Squamous cell carcinoma: *N*, %	6, 30	5, 25
Adenocarcinoma: *N*, %	11, 55	14, 70
Others: *N*, %	3, 15	1, 5
Blood parameters		
Total leucocytes/μL	8.3 10^3 (1.9 10^3)	9.2 10^3 (2.1 10^3)
Total neutrophils/μL	5.7 10^3 (2.1 10^3)	6.3 10^3 (1.7 10^3)
Total lymphocytes/μL	1.7 103 (650)	2.1·10^3 (617)
Albumin (g/dL)	4.1 (0.4)	4.0 (0.5)¶¶
Total proteins (g/dL)	7.4 (0.5)	7.1 (0.6)
Fibrinogen (mg/dL)	485 (99)	409 (77)¶¶
CRP (mg/dL)	1.1 (1.1)	1.7 (1.2)
GSV (mm/h)	20 (7.4)	30 (16.8)¶
Ceruloplasmin (g/dL)	26.2 (4.8)	26.5 (4.8)
Body weight loss, kg		
0, *N*, %	18, 90	17, 85
1–4, *N*, %	2, 10	1, 5
5–8, *N*, %	0, 0	2, 10
9–12, *N*, %	0, 0	0, 0

Continuous variables are presented as mean (standard deviation), while categorical variables are presented as the number of patients in each group and percentage of the total population

Abbreviations: *N* number, *kg* kilograms, *m* meters, *BMI* body mass index, *FEV$_1$* forced expiratory volume in the first second, *pred* predicted, *FVC* forced vital capacity, *DLco*, carbon monoxide transfer, *K$_{CO}$* Krogh transfer factor, *TNM* tumor, nodes, metastasis, *CRP* C-reactive protein, *GSV* globular sedimentation velocity, *L* liter

$^{¶}p < 0.05$, $^{¶¶}p < 0.01$, $^{¶¶¶}p < 0.001$ between LC-COPD and LC patients. Comparisons of the clinical and physiological variables between LC-COPD and LC patients were assessed using the Student's *t* test. Differences between the study groups in the qualitative variables were assessed using the chi-square test

out by previously analyzing the CT scan sections in all the study patients. Additionally, hematoxylin-eosin staining was performed in all non-tumor lung specimens to further confirm the absence of cancer cells. For ethical reasons, this was the only approach approved to study non-tumor lungs in COPD and non-COPD patients in our institution. In all cases, the expert lung pathologist selected a fragment of lung tumor and non-tumor specimens of approximately 10×10 mm^2 size from the fresh samples after a careful collection of the specimens required for diagnosis purposes. On the day of thoracotomy, blood samples were obtained for conventional routine blood tests (hemogram and nutritional parameters). Importantly, a minimum amount of 50% of cancer cells was similarly identified in all tumor types from all the study patients. The remaining cell components were inflammatory and stromal cells in all the analyzed tumors. On the day of thoracotomy, blood samples were obtained for conventional routine blood tests (hemogram and nutritional parameters).

Sample preservation

Lung specimens (tumor and non-tumor) were snap-frozen in liquid nitrogen and stored at − 80 °C for further use.

Molecular biology analyses

The biology analyses were all conducted blind in our molecular biology laboratory (IMIM).

MicroRNAs and target genes

RNA and DNA isolations and quantitative real time-PCR amplification (qRT-PCR) were used to quantify in the lung specimens, the target microRNAs and downstream biomarkers (genes involved in key cellular processes related to tumorigenesis and cancer progression; Additional file 1: Tables S1 and S2, Tables 2, 3, and 4) of the microRNAs analyzed in the current study [30, 32–34].

Methylated DNA

Global 5-methylcytosine was quantified using the Methyl-Flash Methylated Kit and previous studies [30, 34].

Immunoblotting of 1D electrophoresis

Protein levels of the different molecular markers in lung specimens were explored using methodologies previously published [11, 31–33, 35].

Immunohistochemistry

Levels of ki-67 (marker of cell proliferation) were identified in the lung specimens as previously described [11, 31, 32, 35].

Table 2 Downstream targets of the microRNAs analyzed in tumor and non-tumor lungs of the study patients

MicroRNAs	Downstream targets	LC patients		LC-COPD patients	
		Non-tumor	Tumor	Non-tumor	Tumor
miR-21					
	PTEN, gene expression	78.5 (59.3)	115.6 (89.7)	82.4 (70.2)	0.26 (0.60)$^{*, \S\S\S}$
	MARCKs, gene expression	0.4 (0.2)	0.5 (0.2)	0.5 (0.5)	0.2 (0.1)$^{*, \S}$
	TPM-1, gene expression	2.8 (2.1)	11.0 (10.4)**	5.8 (4.9)	1.8 (1.5)§§
	PDCD4, gene expression	5.4 (3.4)	5.2 (4.4)	4.0 (2.5)	1.4 (1.0)§
	SPRY-2, gene expression	6.0 (3.3)	8.4 (7.1)	3.4 (1.9)	1.2 (1.0)§§§
miR-200b					
	ETS-1, gene expression	4.6 (3.7)	3.3 (2.5)	2.8 (2.5)	0.6 (0.3)§
	ZEB-2, gene expression	2.3 (1.3)	3.5 (2.7)	0.7 (0.2)$^{\#}$	0.4 (0.3)§§§
miR-126					
	EGFL-7, gene expression	4.0 (2.0)	5.0 (3.0)	5.0 (5.0)	1 (0.7)
	TOM-1, gene expression	0.6 (0.3)	2.2 (1.1)***	1.3 (1.0)	0.8 (0.6)§§§
	CRK, gene expression	8.6 (7.1)	21.3 (19.7)*	6.6 (5.8)	3.7 (3.5)§§§
	Ang-2, protein content	0.3 (0.1)	0.3 (0.2)	0.3 (0.07)	0.5 (0.2)$^{*, \S}$
	Fibulin-3, protein content	0.6 (0.2)	0.6 (0.3)	0.5 (0.2)	0.4 (0.2)
	Fibulin-2, protein content	0.04 (0.03)	0.1 (0.04)*	0.04 (0.02)	0.04 (0.03)
	Fibulin-5, protein content	0.3 (0.1)	0.4 (0.1)	0.5 (0.1)$^{\#}$	0.5 (0.1)
miR-451					
	MIF, gene expression	0.6 (0.8)	2.5 (2.1) **	1.3 (1.1)	0.3 (0.2) §§§
	RAB-14, gene expression	6.3 (5.1)	4.1 (1.9)	1.5 (1.3) $^{\#\#}$	2.4 (2.1)
miR-210					
	FGFRL-1, gene expression	2.5 (1.8)	3.2 (2.0)	4.1 (2.3)	1.3 (1.0)$^{***, \S}$
	EFNA-3, gene expression	0.3 (0.2)	1.0 (0.9)*	0.2 (0.1)	0.1 (0.08)§§
	P-62, protein content	0.1 (0.04)	0.3 (0.1)*	0.1 (0.02)	0.3 (0.1)*
	LC3II/LC3II, protein content	0.1 (0.05)	0.4 (0.1)***	0.2 (0.1)	0.4 (0.1)*
	Beclin-1, protein content	0.3 (0.09)	0.3 (0.05)	0.2 (0.1)	0.3 (0.1)
	BAX, protein content	0.2 (0.06)	0.3 (0.2)	0.2 (0.1)	0.3 (0.2)
	BCL-2, protein content	0.04 (0.02)	0.2 (0.1)***	0.1 (0.04)	0.2 (0.05)**
miR-30a-30p					
	SNAIL-1, gene expression	2.3 (1.4)	3.4 (2.8)	2.8 (1.7)	0.6 (0.4)$^{*, \S\S\S}$
	P53, gene expression	0.4 (0.3)	0.7 (0.5)	0.5 (0.3)	0.3 (0.2)§
	CDKN2A, gene expression	4.7 (3.9)	1.9 (1.8)*	9.8 (7.8)$^{\#}$	19.4 (16.5)§§§
	P63, gene expression	0.1 (0.08)	0.1 (0.05)	0.8 (0.5)$^{\#\#\#}$	0.4 (0.3)*
	CDKN1A, gene expression	11.8 (10.4)	5.7 (3.5)*	13.5 (7.7)	6.4 (4.8)**
	Ki-67 positive cells, %	42.6 (19.0)	96.5 (3.0)***	42.6 (19.0)	96.2 (4.7)***
miR-let7c					
	k-RAS, gene expression	3.0 (2.0)	2.2 (1.0)	2.7 (2.1)	1.1 (0.5)$^{*, \S}$

Variables are represented as mean (standard deviation)

Abbreviations: *miR* microRNA, *rel.expresion* relative expression, *prot.content* protein content, *PTEN* phosphatase and tensin homolog 10, *MARCKS* myristoylated alanine-rich protein kinase C substrate, *TPM1* tropomyosin 1 (alpha), *PDCD4* programmed cell death 4, *SPRY2* sprouty homolog 2, *ETS1* v-ets avian erythroblastosis virus E26 oncogene homolog 1, *ZEB2* zinc finger E-box binding homeobox 2, *EGFL7* EGF-like-domain, multiple 7, *TOM1* target of myb1, *CRK* v-crk avian sarcoma virus CT10 oncogene homolog 17, *Ang-2* angiopoietin-2, *MIF* macrophage migration inhibitory factor, *RAB14* member RAS oncogene family 14, *FGFRL-1* fibroblast growth factor receptor-like 1, *EFNA3* ephrin-A3, *LC3* light chain 3, *BAX* bcl-2 associated X protein, *BCL-2* B cell lymphoma-2, *SNAIL-1* snail family zinc finger 1, *P53* tumor protein p53, *CDKN2A* cyclin-dependent kinase inhibitor 2A, *P63* protein p63, *CDKN1A* cyclin-dependent kinase inhibitor 1A, and *k-RAS* Kirsten rat sarcoma viral oncogene homolog 11

$^{\S}p < 0.05$, $^{\S\S}p < 0.01$, $^{\S\S\S}p < 0.001$ between tumor lungs of LC-COPD and tumor specimens of LC patients; $^{*}p < 0.05$, $^{**}p < 0.01$, $^{***}p < 0.001$ between tumor and non-tumor lungs in either LC or LC-COPD patients; $^{\#}p < 0.05$, $^{\#\#}p < 0.01$, $^{\#\#\#}p < 0.001$ between non-tumor specimens of LC-COPD and non-tumor lungs of LC patients. Absence of any statistical symbol means no differences between the study groups

Table 3 Summary of epigenetic events in the tumor specimens of LC patients with and without the chronic respiratory condition

Epigenetic events	LC patients	
	Non-COPD	COPD
Lung tumors		
MicroRNAs		
miR-21, miR-200b, miR-210, miR-let7c	↓	↑
miR-126, miR451, miR30a-30p, miR-155, miR-let7a	=	=
Histone modifications		
HDAC2, *Sirtuin-1*	=	=
DNA methylation	↓	↑

Abbreviations: *miR* microRNA, *HDAC2* histone deacetylase-2, = there were no significant differences for the specific tumor markers between LC-COPD and LC patients without COPD

Statistical analyses

Data are expressed as mean (standard deviation). Normality of the variables was explored using the Shapiro-Wilk test. For the quantitative variables in the lungs, differences between study groups were assessed using one-way analysis of variance (ANOVA) and Tukey's post hoc analysis to adjust for multiple comparisons of all the study variables. Chi-square test was used to assess potential differences between the study groups for the qualitative variables. Statistical significance was established at $P \leq 0.05$.

Table 4 Summary of biological processes represented by the downstream markers of the epigenetic events explored in the study in the tumor specimens of LC patients with and without COPD

Downstream markers	LC patients	
	Non-COPD	COPD
Tumor suppressor genes		
P53, PTEN, PDCD4, TPM-1, k-RAS	↑	↓
CDKN2A	↓	↑
Sirtuin-1	=	=
Cell proliferation and invasion (through ↓ *SPRY-2, MIF* and *TOM-1*)	↓	↑
Apoptosis (through ↓ *ETS-1*)	↑	↓
Cell differentiation (through ↓ *ETS-1* and *FGFRL-1*)	↑	↓
Epithelial mesenchymal transition (through ↓ *ZEB2* and *SNAIL-1*)	↑	↓
Cell- mediated immunity (through ↓ *MIF*)	↓	↑
Angiogenesis (through ↑ angiopoietin-2 and ↓ EFNA-3)	↓	↑
Cell adhesion and migration (through ↓ *CRK, TOM-1* and *MARCKs*)	↑	↓

= there were no significant differences for the specific tumor markers between LC-COPD and LC patients without COPD

Results

Clinical characteristics

Clinical and functional characteristics of LC-COPD and LC patients recruited in the study are shown in Table 1. Age, gender, and BMI did not significantly differ between LC-COPD and LC patients (Table 1). Interestingly, smoking history was similar in both study groups (Table 1). The functional parameters forced expiratory volume in 1 s (FEV_1), FEV_1/forced vital capacity (FVC), and diffusion lung capacity for carbon monoxide (DL_{CO}) were significantly lower in LC-COPD than LC patients (Table 1). Furthermore, no significant differences were found in either TNM or histological subtypes between LC-COPD and LC groups (Table 1). In LC-COPD compared to LC patients, levels of albumin and fibrinogen were significantly decreased, whereas those of globular sedimentation (GSV) were increased and C-reactive protein (CRP) levels did not differ between groups (Table 1).

Differential microRNA profile and downstream targets in lung tumors in patients with underlying respiratory disease

In LC-COPD compared to LC patients, miR-21 expression was significantly increased in the tumors, whereas that of its downstream targets *PTEN, MARCKs, TPM-1, PDCD4,* and *SPRY-2* was significantly reduced (Fig. 1a and Table 2). However, non-tumor lung expression of miR-21, *PTEN, MARCKs, TPM-1, PDCD4,* and *SPRY-2* did not significantly differ between LC-COPD and LC patients (Fig. 1a and Table 2). Tumor miR-200b expression was significantly greater in LC-COPD than in LC patients, while that of its downstream markers *ETS-1* and *ZEB-2* was significantly reduced (Fig. 1b and Table 2). Non-tumor lung expression of miR-200b also significantly increased in LC-COPD compared to LC patients, and only the expression of *ZEB-2* significantly decreased (Fig. 1b and Table 2). Tumor expression levels of miR-126 did not significantly differ between LC-COPD and LC patients, whereas in the former patients, an almost significant decrease in *EGFL-7* expression was observed ($p = 0.073$, Fig. 1c and Table 2), together with a decrease in *TOM-1* and *CRK* expression and a rise in angiopoietin-2 content (Table 2). Tumor protein levels of fibulin-3, fibulin-2, and fibulin-5 did not differ between LC-COPD and LC patients (Table 2 and Additional file 1: Figure S1).

Tumor and non-tumor expression of miR-451 did not differ between LC-COPD and LC patients (Fig. 1d), while *MIF* tumor expression was significantly lower in LC-COPD than LC patients, and RAB-14 expression was also significantly reduced in the non-tumors of the former patients (Table 2). Tumor expression of miR-210 significantly increased in LC-COPD compared to LC patients, while that of its downstream targets *FGFRL-1* and *EFNA-3*

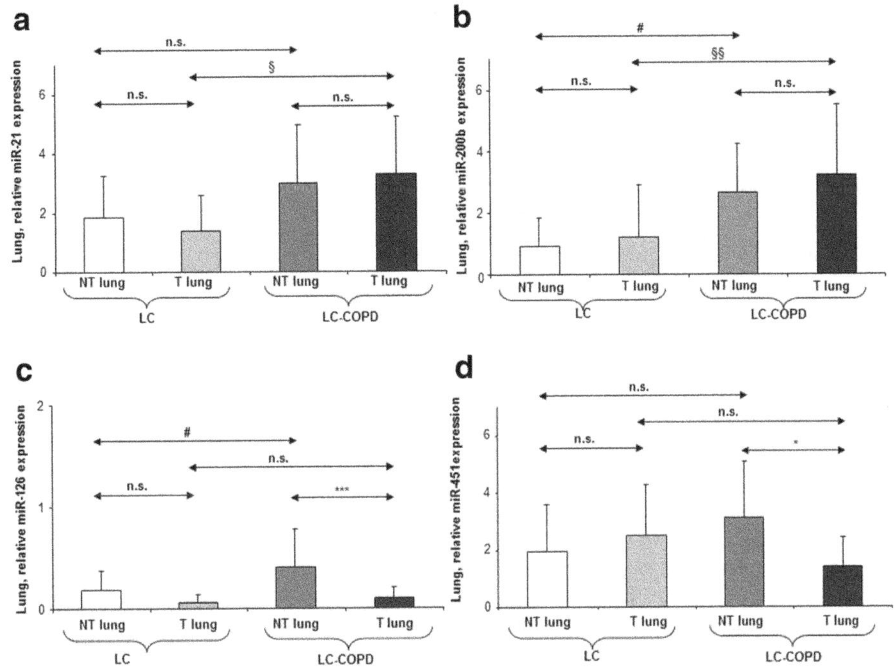

Fig. 1 Mean values and standard deviation (relative expression) of miR-21 (**a**), miR-200b (**b**), miR-126 (**c**), and miR-451 (**d**). Definition of abbreviations: miR, microRNA. Statistical significance: $^{*}p < 0.05$, $^{***}p < 0.001$ between tumor and non-tumor lungs in either LC or LC-COPD patients; $^{\#}p < 0.05$ between non-tumor specimens of LC-COPD and non-tumor lungs of LC patients; $^{\S}p < 0.05$, $^{\S\S}p < 0.01$ between tumor lungs of LC-COPD and tumor specimens of LC patients; and n.s., non-significant differences between the study groups

was reduced in the former patients (Fig. 2a and Table 2). Tumor protein levels of autophagy and apoptosis markers P62, LC3II/LC3I, beclin-1, BAX, and BCL-2 did not differ between LC-COPD and LC patients (Table 2 and Additional file 1: Figure S2). In LC-COPD, tumor expression of miR30a-30p was similar to that seen in LC patients (Fig. 2b). However, tumor expression of its downstream markers *SNAIL*-1 and *P53* was significantly lower in LC-COPD than LC patients, while that of *CDKN2A* was greater and that of *P63*, *CDKN1A*, and ki-67 did not differ in tumors between patient groups (Table 2 and Additional file 1: Figure S3). Furthermore, non-tumor lung expression levels of miR-210 and miR30a-30p and their downstream markers *FGFRL-1*, *EFNA-3*, P62, LC3II/LC3I, beclin-1, BAX, BCL-2, *SNAIL-1*, *P53*, *CDKN1A*, and ki-67 did not significantly differ between LC-COPD and LC patients (Fig. 2a, b, Additional file 1: Figures S2, S3 and Table 2). Nonetheless, non-tumor lung expression of *CDKN2A* and *P63* was significantly higher in LC-COPD than LC patients (Table 2). Tumor expression of miR-let7c was significantly greater in LC-COPD than LC patients (Fig. 2c), while that of its downstream marker *k-RAS* significantly decreased in the former patients (Table 2). Tumor expression of miR-155 and miR-let7a did not significantly differ between LC-COPD and LC patients (Figs. 2d and 3, respectively). Additionally, non-tumor lung expression levels of miR-let7c, *k-RAS*, miR-155, and miR-let7a markers did not significantly differ between LC-COPD and LC patients (Figs 2c, d and 3 and Table 2).

Differential profile of histone deacetylases and DNA methylation in lung tumors of patients with underlying chronic respiratory disease

Tumor expression levels of the markers *SIRT-1* and histone deacetylase-2 (HDAC2) did not differ between the two study groups (Fig. 3a, b and Additional file 1: Figure S4). Nevertheless, in LC-COPD compared to LC patients, non-tumor *SIRT-1* expression was greater, whereas HDAC2 non-tumor protein levels did not differ between the study groups (Fig. 4a, b and Additional file 1: Figure S4). Total DNA methylation levels were significantly greater in both tumor and non-tumor lungs of LC-COPD than in LC patients (Fig. 4c).

Discussion

In the current study, the study hypothesis has been confirmed. Importantly, the most relevant findings encountered in the investigation were that expression levels of miR-21, miR-200b, miR-210, miR-let7c, and DNA methylation were significantly greater in lung tumors of patients with underlying COPD than in those

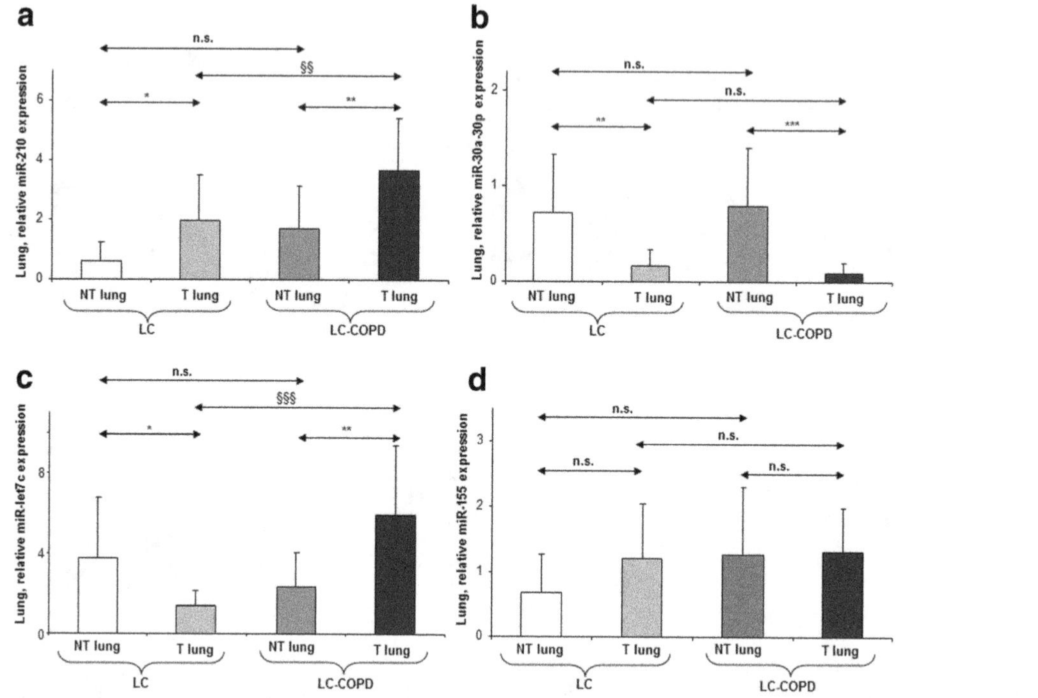

Fig. 2 Mean values and standard deviation (relative expression) of miR-210 (**a**), miR-30a-30ap (**b**), miR-let7c (**c**), miR-155 (**d**), and miR-let7a (**e**) in tumor (T) and non-tumor (NT) lungs of LC and LC-COPD patients. Definition of abbreviations: miR, microRNA. Statistical significance: $^{*}p < 0.05$, $^{**}p < 0.01$, $^{***}p < 0.001$ between tumor and non-tumor lungs in either LC or LC-COPD patients; $^{\S\S}p < 0.01$, $^{\S\S\S}p < 0.001$ between tumor lungs of LC-COPD and tumor specimens of LC patients; and n.s., non-significant differences between the study groups

without this chronic condition (Table 3). Furthermore, expression levels of the downstream markers of the corresponding microRNAs, namely *PTEN, MARCKs, TPM-1, PDCD4, SPRY-2, ETS-1, ZEB-2, FGFRL-1, EFNA-3,* and *k-RAS* were downregulated in the lung tumor lesions of patients with the underlying condition compared to non-COPD patients (Table 4). Importantly, levels of the tumor suppressor gene *P53* were also downregulated in the tumors of patients with COPD. These are biological markers of the underlying processes that are involved in tumorigenesis and tumor progression. Remarkably, these are novel findings that may partly explain the underlying biology of the reported greater risk of patients with COPD to develop lung tumors.

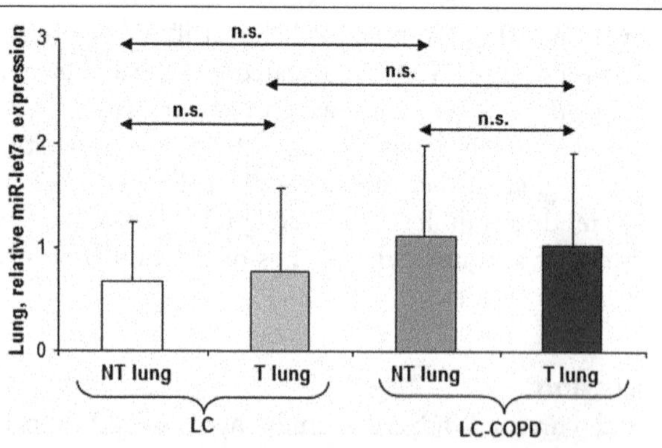

Fig. 3 Mean values and standard deviation (relative expression) of miR-let7a in tumor (T) and non-tumor (NT) lungs of LC and LC-COPD patients. Definition of abbreviations: miR, microRNA. Statistical significance: n.s. non-significant differences between the study groups

Downregulation of the study genes may entail alterations in the target pathways such as increased cell proliferation, migration, adhesion, invasion and angiogenesis, potential development of metastatic tumors, and adaptation of the cancer cells to hypoxia [25]. Clearly, all these biological processes promote tumor growth and favor disease progression in the patients. Previous investigations have demonstrated that levels of miR-21, miR-200b, miR-210, and miR-let7c were also upregulated in the tumor lesions of lung cancer cells in several experimental models and in patients [25, 36–42]. Interestingly, in other investigations, cancer cells were also shown to be more resistant to radiation or chemotherapy when those markers were elevated [43, 44]. In the present investigation, these results suggest that upregulation of miR-21, miR-200b, miR-210, and miR-let7c expression and that of DNA methylation may partly underlie the increased susceptibility of COPD patients to develop lung tumors. In keeping with, aberrant methylation status of tumor suppressor (*CDKN2A*) and DNA repair genes has already been identified in tumors of patients with LC and COPD [45, 46]. Furthermore, it has also been proposed that cancer cells express specific

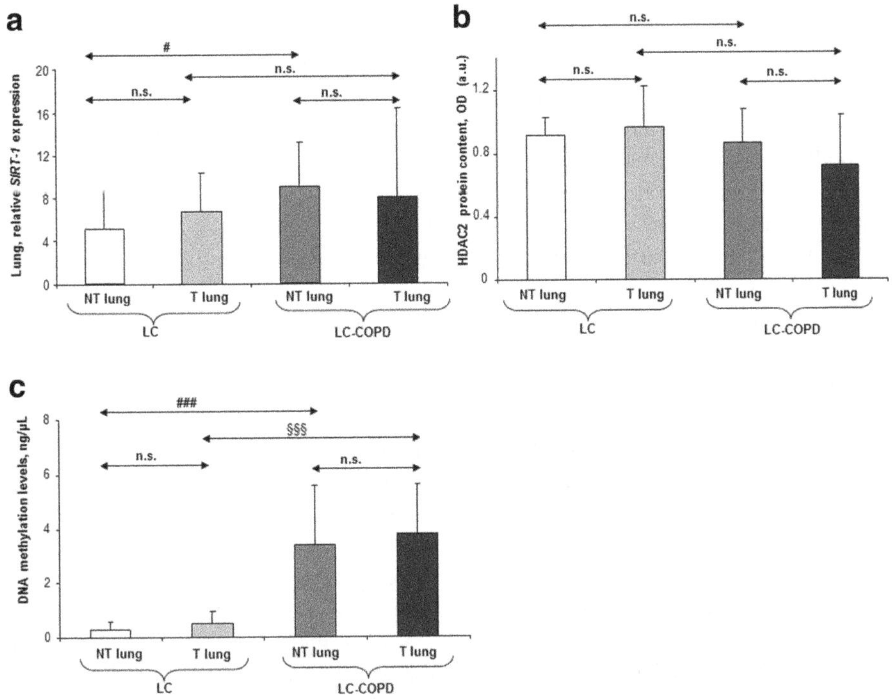

Fig. 4 Mean values and standard deviation (relative expression) of *SIRT-1* (**a**), HDAC2 (**b**), and DNA methylation levels (**c**) in tumor (T) and non-tumor (NT) lungs of LC and LC-COPD patients. Definition of abbreviations: miR, microRNA; *SIRT-1*, sirtuin-1; and HDAC2, histone deacetylase 2. Statistical significance: $^{\#}p < 0.05$, $^{\#\#\#}p < 0.001$ between non-tumor specimens of LC-COPD and non-tumor lungs of LC patients; $^{\S\S\S}p < 0.001$ between tumor lungs of LC-COPD and tumor specimens of LC patients; and n.s., non-significant differences between the study groups

patterns of microRNA profiles that may contribute to the process of tumorigenesis [46]. Whether these epigenetic events may also confer a greater resistance to cancer treatment in patients with COPD will remain a matter of future research.

As the approach used in the study enabled us to analyze the target markers also in the surrounding non-tumor parenchyma in both groups of patients with LC, it is worth mentioning that levels of expression of miR-200b, miR-126, and DNA methylation were significantly greater in non-tumor specimens of patients with COPD than in those without this chronic condition. Additionally, expression levels of the downstream markers *ZEB-2* and *RAB-14* were downregulated, while those of the tumor suppressors *CDKN2A*, *P63*, and *SIRT-1* were upregulated in the non-tumor specimens of LC patients with underlying respiratory disease compared to non-COPD patients. These are relevant findings that reveal the underlying biology of the lung parenchyma in patients with COPD. These results also imply that in COPD, a differential epigenetic regulation of cell cycle and proliferation also takes place in the lung parenchyma regardless of the presence of cancer cells. In fact, it has been clearly demonstrated that transition of cancer cells at the invasive site to a mesenchyme-like phenotype, commonly known as epithelial-to-mesenchymal transition, is crucial for invasion and distant metastasis in cancer progression [47]. In the current investigation, expression levels of the epithelial-to-mesenchymal transition inducers *SNAIL*-1 and *ZEB*-2 were significantly downregulated in tumors of patients with LC-COPD compared to those without underlying COPD. Thus, these results may imply that epithelial-to-mesenchymal transition may not play a major role in lung tumorigenesis in those patients, probably as result of areas of lung destruction. Clearly, future avenues of research should specifically address this question.

A third group of novel findings observed in this investigation were that within each study group of patients, in the lung tumors compared to non-tumor specimens, expression levels of miR-126 and miR-451 decreased in LC-COPD patients, while those of miR-30a-30p were reduced in both groups of patients. Compared to non-tumor specimens, levels of miR-let7c were also lower in lung tumors of patients without COPD, while a rise was seen in those with underlying COPD. The last findings are somehow counter to those previously reported in patients with COPD, who exhibited a decrease in miR-let7c expression in the sputum macrophages and bronchial airway epithelial cells [24]. As miR-let7c acts a tumor suppressor in tumor cells, it is likely that COPD induces a positive feedback on its expression in order to offset the deleterious effects of cancer biology. Levels of miR-let7c, which negatively correlated with metastasis, vascular invasion, and poor survival, were also downregulated in patients with NSCLC in another investigation [42]. However, whether patients also had underlying chronic respiratory disease was not explored in that study [42].

Posttranslational modifications of histones regulate gene transcription in normal and disease-related cellular processes. Levels of markers regulated by histone acetylation such as *PTEN*, *MARCKs*, EGFL-7 (almost significant decrease), *FGFRL-1*, *SNAIL-1*, *P63*, and *k-RAS* were significantly reduced in the lung tumors compared to non-tumors only in patients with LC-COPD. Indeed, proliferation markers and *k-RAS* mutations were reduced in lung tumors among COPD patients [48]. However, expression levels of downstream markers *TPM-1*, *TOM-1*, *CRK*, fibulin-2, *MIF*, and *EFNA-3* were greater in the lung tumors than in non-tumor specimens only in patients without COPD. Interestingly, in the tumors of both groups of patients, the autophagy markers P62 and LC3, the anti-apoptotic BCL-2, and the proliferation marker ki-67 were increased compared to non-tumor specimens, while those of the inhibitor of cell proliferation *CDKN1A* were reduced. These findings also confirm that epigenetics play a significant role in the regulation of cellular mechanisms such as apoptosis, angiogenesis, and cell migration and adhesion that underlie tumorigenesis itself in both groups of patients, with a specific pattern of expression in patients with COPD.

Study critique

Since epigenetic events may be influenced by cigarette smoking, results might differ between smokers and nonsmokers. Nonetheless, as no differences in smoking history or pack-years were observed between the two study groups, the results encountered in the investigation are likely to be attributed to the presence of the lung tumor and COPD in the patients with the underlying condition. Another factor that might have affected the study results is aging. Nevertheless, as age did not significantly differ between the two patient groups, the encountered findings can also be mostly recognized to the presence of the neoplasm and to COPD in the patients with this disease. Another limitation in the study refers to the relatively small number of lung specimens analyzed from both patient groups. Nevertheless, for ethical reasons, tumor and non-tumor lung specimens could only be obtained from patients undergoing thoracotomy for the treatment of their lung neoplasm (approximately 25% of all patients with LC). It should also be acknowledged that in three patients of the LC group, the lung neoplasms were in stage IV. These patients underwent surgery, chemotherapy, and/or radiotherapy for the treatment of the single metastasis always following thoracotomy for their primary lung neoplasm. It should also be mentioned that the approach used in the investigation enabled us to assess the effects of COPD itself without the cancer lesions on the epigenetic targets as distant non-tumor samples were also obtained from both groups of study patients. This is a unique approach commonly used in our group and the only acceptable from an ethical standpoint as also previously reported [11, 14]. Finally, future studies may be conducted in which the markers analyzed in this study will be validated in large-scale cohorts of patients. Nonetheless, it should also be emphasized that the results reported in the present investigation have been obtained within the frame of a hypothesis-driven prospective study.

Clinical impact of the study findings and future perspectives

Epigenetic regulation of cellular processes may explain disease pathogenesis. In the study, LC patients with an underlying respiratory condition exhibited a differential expression profile of several epigenetic markers, namely DNA methylation and microRNA expression along with that of downstream markers that are involved in tumorigenesis and tumor suppression. The clinical relevance of these findings is based on the following principles: (1) the target biological processes analyzed in the study may be eventually used as potential biomarker panels for the early diagnosis of LC in patients with COPD (the vast majority of patients with LC); (2) the epigenetic mechanisms could be used as potential biomarkers of disease progression (clinical staging) and prognosis, especially in patients with chronic respiratory diseases; (3) microRNAs such as miR-21 and miR-let7c may be targeted pharmacologically [49, 50], and thus, they may act as suitable biomarkers for the treatment of LC, which in turn may also help to gauge the response to therapy in these patients; and (4) the presence of an underlying respiratory disease should be identified in all patients with LC as the differential biological profile may help determine tumor progression and the therapeutic response. Future investigations should focus on the elucidation of whether microRNAs may serve as biomarkers of tumor progression, clinical staging, and recurrence in patients with underlying respiratory diseases.

Conclusions

A differential epigenetic regulation characterized by increased expression of several microRNAs and DNA methylation that control cellular processes involved in lung tumorigenesis exists in patients with LC and underlying respiratory disease. Fingerprint biomarkers of mechanisms involved in tumor growth, angiogenesis, migration, and apoptosis were also differentially expressed in tumors of patients with COPD. These findings shed light into the underlying biology of the reported greater risk to develop

LC in patients with chronic respiratory conditions. Furthermore, they also have potential therapeutic implications as epigenetic events may be specifically targeted pharmacologically.

Abbreviations

ANG-2: Angiopoietin-2; ANOVA: One-way analysis of variance; BAX: Bcl-2-associated X protein; BCL-2: B cell lymphoma-2; BMI: Body mass index; *CDKN1A*: Cyclin-dependent kinase inhibitor 1A; *CDKN2A*: Cyclin-dependent kinase inhibitor 2A; COPD: Chronic obstructive pulmonary disease; *CRK*: v-crk avian sarcoma virus CT10 oncogene homolog 17; CRP: C-reactive protein; DLco: Carbon monoxide transfer; *EFNA3*: Ephrin-A3; *EGFL7*: EGF-like-domain, multiple 7; *ETS1*: v-ets avian erythroblastosis virus E26 oncogene homolog 1; FEV_1: Forced expiratory volume in the first second; *FGFRL-1*: Fibroblast growth factor receptor-like 1; FVC: Forced vital capacity; GAPDH: Glyceraldehyde-3-phosphate dehydrogenase; GSV: Globular sedimentation velocity; HDAC2: Histone deacetylase-2; K_{CO}: Krogh transfer factor; *k-RAS*: Kirsten rat sarcoma viral oncogene homolog 11; L: Liter; LC: Lung cancer; LC3: Light chain 3; *MARCKS*: Myristoylated alanine-rich protein kinase C substrate; *MIF*: Macrophage migration inhibitory factor; miR: MicroRNA; *N*: Number; NSCLC: Non-small cell lung cancer; *P53*: Tumor protein p53; *P63*: Protein p63; *PDCD4*: Programmed cell death 4; *PTEN*: Phosphatase and tensin homolog 10; qRT-PCR: Quantitative real time polymerase chain reaction; *RAB14*: Member RAS oncogene family 14; SD: Standard deviation; *SIRT-1*: Sirtuin-1; *SNAIL-1*: Snail family zinc finger 1; *SPRY2*: Sprouty homolog 2; TNM: Tumor, nodes, metastasis; *TOM1*: Target of myb1; *TPM1*: Tropomyosin 1 (alpha); *ZEB2*: Zinc finger E-box binding homeobox 2

Acknowledgements

The authors are thankful to Ms. Arianne Bercowsky for her help with the ki-67 counting, to Ms. Mireia Admetlló for her help with the patient clinical assessment, and Mr. Sergi Mojal for his help with the comprehensive statistical analyses.

Funding

This study has been supported by Instituto de Salud Carlos III (Ministry of Economy and Competitiveness (Spain): FIS 11/02029 (FEDER), FIS 14/00713 (FEDER), PT13/0010/0005 (FEDER), and CIBERES (Lung Cancer Program, which is a member of the International Association for the Study of Lung Cancer, *Instituto de Salud Carlos III*), SEPAR 2016, FUCAP 2016, unrestricted grant from Menarini SA 2014 (Laboratorios Menarini S.A.), and the *Xarxa de Bancs de tumors sponsored by Pla Director d'Oncologia de Catalunya* (XBTC), Catalan Government.

Authors' contributions

EB, VC, and LP contributed to the study conception and design. VC, MMJ, ARF, RA, ASF, and LP contributed to the patient assessment and recruitment and sample collection. LP contributed to the pathological diagnosis. MMJ and EB contributed to the molecular biology analyses. EB, MMJ, and VC contributed to the statistical analyses and data interpretation. EB, MMJ, VC, ARF, RA, and JG contributed to the manuscript drafting and intellectual input. EB contributed to the manuscript writing of the final version. All authors read and approved the final manuscript.

Consent for publication

Not applicable

Competing interests

The authors declare that they have no competing interests.

Author details

[1]Pulmonology Department, Lung Cancer and Muscle Research Group, Hospital del Mar-IMIM, Parc de Salut Mar, Health and Experimental Sciences Department (CEXS), Universitat Pompeu Fabra (UPF), Parc de Recerca Biomèdica de Barcelona (PRBB), C/ Dr. Aiguader, 88, E-08003 Barcelona, Spain. [2]Centro de Investigación en Red de Enfermedades Respiratorias (CIBERES), Instituto de Salud Carlos III (ISCIII), Barcelona, Spain. [3]Thoracic Surgery Department, Hospital del Mar-IMIM, Parc de Salut Mar, Barcelona, Spain. [4]Pathology Department, Hospital del Mar-IMIM, Parc de Salut Mar, Barcelona, Spain.

References

1. Siegel RL, Miller KD, Jemal A. Cancer statistics, 2015. CA Cancer J Clin. 2015; 65(1):5–29. https://doi.org/10.3322/caac.21254.
2. Portillo K, Perez-Rodas N, Garcia-Olive I, Guasch-Arriaga I, Centeno C, Serra P, et al. Lung cancer in patients with combined pulmonary fibrosis and emphysema and idiopathic pulmonary fibrosis. A descriptive study in a Spanish series. Arch Bronconeumol. 2016; https://doi.org/10.1016/j.arbres.2016.10.004.
3. Alvarez FV, Trueba IM, Sanchis JB, Lopez-Rodo LM, Rodriguez Suarez PM, de Cos Escuin JS, et al. Recommendations of the Spanish Society of Pneumology and Thoracic Surgery on the diagnosis and treatment of non-small-cell lung cancer. Arch Bronconeumol. 2016;52(Suppl 1):2–62. https://doi.org/10.1016/S0300-2896(16)30198-3.
4. Gonzalez J, de Torres JP. Lung cancer and emphysema. Arch Bronconeumol. 2016; https://doi.org/10.1016/j.arbres.2016.07.010.
5. Sanchez-Salcedo P, Berto J, de Torres JP, Campo A, Alcaide AB, Bastarrika G, et al. Lung cancer screening: fourteen year experience of the Pamplona early detection program (P-IELCAP). Arch Bronconeumol. 2015;51(4):169–76. https://doi.org/10.1016/j.arbres.2014.09.019.
6. Sanchez-Salcedo P, Wilson DO, de Torres JP, Weissfeld JL, Berto J, Campo A, et al. Improving selection criteria for lung cancer screening. The potential role of emphysema. Am J Respir Crit Care Med. 2015;191(8):924–31. https://doi.org/10.1164/rccm.201410-1848OC.
7. de CJ S, Hernandez JH, Lopez MF, Sanchez SP, Gratacos AR, Porta RR. SEPAR guidelines for lung cancer staging. Arch Bronconeumol. 2011;47(9):454–65. https://doi.org/10.1016/j.arbres.2011.06.013.
8. Barreiro E, Fermoselle C, Mateu-Jimenez M, Sanchez-Font A, Pijuan L, Gea J, et al. Oxidative stress and inflammation in the normal airways and blood of patients with lung cancer and COPD. Free Radic Biol Med. 2013;65:859–71. https://doi.org/10.1016/j.freeradbiomed.2013.08.006.
9. Gupta A, Srivastava S, Prasad R, Natu SM, Mittal B, Negi MP, et al. Oxidative stress in non-small cell lung cancer patients after chemotherapy: association with treatment response. Respirology. 2010;15(2):349–56. https://doi.org/10.1111/j.1440-1843.2009.01703.x.
10. Masri FA, Comhair SA, Koeck T, Xu W, Janocha A, Ghosh S, et al. Abnormalities in nitric oxide and its derivatives in lung cancer. Am J Respir Crit Care Med. 2005;172(5):597–605. https://doi.org/10.1164/rccm.200411-1523OC. Pubmed PMID: PMC2718532
11. Mateu-Jimenez M, Sanchez-Font A, Rodriguez-Fuster A, Aguilo R, Pijuan L, Fermoselle C, et al. Redox imbalance in lung cancer of patients with underlying chronic respiratory conditions. Mol Med. 2016; https://doi.org/10.2119/molmed.2015.00199. Pubmed PMID: PMC5004710
12. Cho WC, Kwan CK, Yau S, So PP, Poon PC, Au JS. The role of inflammation in the pathogenesis of lung cancer. Expert Opin Ther Targets. 2011 Sep; 15(9):1127–37.
13. O'Byrne KJ, Dalgleish AG. Chronic immune activation and inflammation as the cause of malignancy. Br J Cancer. 2001 Aug 17;85(4):473–83.
14. Mateu-Jimenez M, Curull V, Pijuan L, Sanchez-Font A, Rivera-Ramos H, Rodriguez-Fuster A, et al. Systemic and tumor Th1 and Th2 inflammatory profile and macrophages in lung cancer: influence of underlying chronic respiratory disease. J Thorac Oncol. 2017;12(2):235–48. https://doi.org/10.1016/j.jtho.2016.09.137.
15. Breitling LP, Yang R, Korn B, Burwinkel B, Brenner H. Tobacco-smoking-related differential DNA methylation: 27K discovery and replication. Am J Hum Genet. 2011;88(4):450–7. https://doi.org/10.1016/j.ajhg.2011.03.003. Pubmed PMID: PMC3071918
16. Gao X, Jia M, Zhang Y, Breitling LP, Brenner H. DNA methylation changes of whole blood cells in response to active smoking exposure in adults: a systematic review of DNA methylation studies. Clin Epigenetics. 2015;7:113. https://doi.org/10.1186/s13148-015-0148-3. Pubmed PMID: PMC4609112
17. Zhang Y, Elgizouli M, Schottker B, Holleczek B, Nieters A, Brenner H. Smoking-associated DNA methylation markers predict lung cancer incidence. Clin Epigenetics. 2016;8:127. https://doi.org/10.1186/s13148-016-0292-4. Pubmed PMID: PMC5123284

18. Sundar IK, Mullapudi N, Yao H, Spivack SD, Rahman I. Lung cancer and its association with chronic obstructive pulmonary disease: update on nexus of epigenetics. Curr Opin Pulm Med. 2011;17(4):279–85. https://doi.org/10.1097/MCP.0b013e3283477533. Pubmed PMID: PMC3730439
19. Wang S, Wang Z. Epigenetic aberrant methylation of tumor suppressor genes in small cell lung cancer. J Thorac Dis. 2013;5(4):532–7. https://doi.org/10.3978/j.issn.2072-1439.2013.08.21. Pubmed PMID: PMC3755684
20. Chen C, Hua H, Han C, Cheng Y, Cheng Y, Wang Z, et al. Prognosis value of MGMT promoter methylation for patients with lung cancer: a meta-analysis. Int J Clin Exp Pathol. 2015;8(9):11560–4. Pubmed PMID: PMC4637707
21. Suzuki M, Wada H, Yoshino M, Tian L, Shigematsu H, Suzuki H, et al. Molecular characterization of chronic obstructive pulmonary disease-related non-small cell lung cancer through aberrant methylation and alterations of EGFR signaling. Ann Surg Oncol. 2010;17(3):878–88. https://doi.org/10.1245/s10434-009-0739-3.
22. Wauters E, Janssens W, Vansteenkiste J, Decaluwe H, Heulens N, Thienpont B, et al. DNA methylation profiling of non-small cell lung cancer reveals a COPD-driven immune-related signature. Thorax. 2015;70(12):1113–22. https://doi.org/10.1136/thoraxjnl-2015-207288.
23. Houghton AM. Mechanistic links between COPD and lung cancer. Nat Rev Cancer. 2013;13(4):233–45. https://doi.org/10.1038/nrc3477.
24. Van Pottelberge GR, Mestdagh P, Bracke KR, Thas O, van Durme YM, Joos GF, et al. MicroRNA expression in induced sputum of smokers and patients with chronic obstructive pulmonary disease. Am J Respir Crit Care Med. 2011;183(7):898–906. https://doi.org/10.1164/rccm.201002-0304OC.
25. Liloglou T, Bediaga NG, Brown BR, Field JK, Davies MP. Epigenetic biomarkers in lung cancer. Cancer Lett. 2014;342(2):200–12. https://doi.org/10.1016/j.canlet.2012.04.018.
26. Miravitlles M, Soler-Cataluna JJ, Calle M, Molina J, Almagro P, Quintano JA, et al. Spanish guidelines for management of chronic obstructive pulmonary disease (GesEPOC) 2017. Pharmacological treatment of stable phase. Arch Bronconeumol. 2017;53(6):324–35. https://doi.org/10.1016/j.arbres.2017.03.018.
27. Vogelmeier CF, Criner GJ, Martinez FJ, Anzueto A, Barnes PJ, Bourbeau J, et al. Global strategy for the diagnosis, management, and prevention of chronic obstructive lung disease 2017 report: GOLD executive summary. Arch Bronconeumol. 2017;53(3):128–49. https://doi.org/10.1016/j.arbres.2017.02.001.
28. Blandino G, Fazi F, Donzelli S, Kedmi M, Sas-Chen A, Muti P, et al. Tumor suppressor microRNAs: a novel non-coding alliance against cancer. FEBS Lett. 2014;588(16):2639–52. https://doi.org/10.1016/j.febslet.2014.03.033.
29. Miravitlles M. What was the impact of the Spanish COPD guidelines (GesEPOC) and how can they be improved? Arch Bronconeumol. 2016;52(1):1–2. https://doi.org/10.1016/j.arbres.2015.04.001.
30. Puig-Vilanova E, Ausin P, Martinez-Llorens J, Gea J, Barreiro E. Do epigenetic events take place in the vastus lateralis of patients with mild chronic obstructive pulmonary disease? PLoS One. 2014;9(7):e102296. https://doi.org/10.1371/journal.pone.0102296.
31. Puig-Vilanova E, Rodriguez DA, Lloreta J, Ausin P, Pascual-Guardia S, Broquetas J, et al. Oxidative stress, redox signaling pathways, and autophagy in cachectic muscles of male patients with advanced COPD and lung cancer. Free Radic Biol Med. 2015;79:91–108. https://doi.org/10.1016/j.freeradbiomed.2014.11.006.
32. Puig-Vilanova E, Martinez-Llorens J, Ausin P, Roca J, Gea J, Barreiro E. Quadriceps muscle weakness and atrophy are associated with a differential epigenetic profile in advanced COPD. Clin Sci (Lond). 2015;128(12):905–21. https://doi.org/10.1042/CS20140428.
33. Chacon-Cabrera A, Gea J, Barreiro E. Short- and long-term hindlimb immobilization and reloading: profile of epigenetic events in gastrocnemius. J Cell Physiol. 2016; https://doi.org/10.1002/jcp.25635.
34. Puig-Vilanova E, Aguilo R, Rodriguez-Fuster A, Martinez-Llorens J, Gea J, Barreiro E. Epigenetic mechanisms in respiratory muscle dysfunction of patients with chronic obstructive pulmonary disease. PLoS One. 2014;9(11):e111514. https://doi.org/10.1371/journal.pone.0111514. Pubmed PMID: PMC4219759
35. Mateu-Jimenez M, Fermoselle C, Rojo F, Mateu J, Pena R, Urtreger AJ, et al. Pharmacological approaches in an experimental model of non-small cell lung cancer: effects on tumor biology. Curr Pharm Des. 2016;22(34):5300–10.
36. Fasanaro P, D'Alessandra Y, Di SV, Melchionna R, Romani S, Pompilio G, et al. MicroRNA-210 modulates endothelial cell response to hypoxia and inhibits the receptor tyrosine kinase ligand Ephrin-A3. J Biol Chem. 2008;283(23):15878–83. https://doi.org/10.1074/jbc.M800731200. Pubmed PMID: PMC3259646
37. Schliekelman MJ, Gibbons DL, Faca VM, Creighton CJ, Rizvi ZH, Zhang Q, et al. Targets of the tumor suppressor miR-200 in regulation of the epithelial-mesenchymal transition in cancer. Cancer Res. 2011;71(24):7670–82. https://doi.org/10.1158/0008-5472.CAN-11-0964. Pubmed PMID: PMC3419137
38. Zhang JG, Wang JJ, Zhao F, Liu Q, Jiang K, Yang GH. MicroRNA-21 (miR-21) represses tumor suppressor PTEN and promotes growth and invasion in non-small cell lung cancer (NSCLC). Clin Chim Acta. 2010;411(11–12):846–52. https://doi.org/10.1016/j.cca.2010.02.074.
39. Zhu S, Si ML, Wu H, Mo YY. MicroRNA-21 targets the tumor suppressor gene tropomyosin 1 (TPM1). J Biol Chem. 2007;282(19):14328–36. https://doi.org/10.1074/jbc.M611393200.
40. Trang P, Medina PP, Wiggins JF, Ruffino L, Kelnar K, Omotola M, et al. Regression of murine lung tumors by the let-7 microRNA. Oncogene. 2010;29(11):1580–7. https://doi.org/10.1038/onc.2009.445. Pubmed PMID: PMC2841713
41. Wang PY, Sun YX, Zhang S, Pang M, Zhang HH, Gao SY, et al. Let-7c inhibits A549 cell proliferation through oncogenic TRIB2 related factors. FEBS Lett. 2013;587(16):2675–81. https://doi.org/10.1016/j.febslet.2013.07.004.
42. Zhao B, Han H, Chen J, Zhang Z, Li S, Fang F, et al. MicroRNA let-7c inhibits migration and invasion of human non-small cell lung cancer by targeting ITGB3 and MAP4K3. Cancer Lett. 2014;342(1):43–51. https://doi.org/10.1016/j.canlet.2013.08.030.
43. Oh JS, Kim JJ, Byun JY, Kim IA. Lin28-let7 modulates radiosensitivity of human cancer cells with activation of K-Ras. Int J Radiat Oncol Biol Phys. 2010;76(1):5–8. https://doi.org/10.1016/j.ijrobp.2009.08.028.
44. Zhong M, Ma X, Sun C, Chen L. MicroRNAs reduce tumor growth and contribute to enhance cytotoxicity induced by gefitinib in non-small cell lung cancer. Chem Biol Interact. 2010;184(3):431–8. https://doi.org/10.1016/j.cbi.2010.01.025.
45. Guzman L, Depix MS, Salinas AM, Roldan R, Aguayo F, Silva A, et al. Analysis of aberrant methylation on promoter sequences of tumor suppressor genes and total DNA in sputum samples: a promising tool for early detection of COPD and lung cancer in smokers. Diagn Pathol. 2012;7(87) https://doi.org/10.1186/1746-1596-7-87. Pubmed PMID: PMC3424112
46. Wang DC, Shi L, Zhu Z, Gao D, Zhang Y. Genomic mechanisms of transformation from chronic obstructive pulmonary disease to lung cancer. Semin Cancer Biol. 2017;42:52–9. https://doi.org/10.1016/j.semcancer.2016.11.001.
47. Courtney JM, Spafford PL. The role of epithelial-mesenchymal transition in chronic obstructive pulmonary disease. Cells Tissues Organs. 2017;203(2):99–104. https://doi.org/10.1159/000450919.
48. Saber A, van der Wekken AJ, Kerner GS, van den Berge M, Timens W, Schuuring E, et al. Chronic obstructive pulmonary disease is not associated with KRAS mutations in non-small cell lung cancer. PLoS One. 2016;11(3):e0152317. https://doi.org/10.1371/journal.pone.0152317. Pubmed PMID: PMC4805285
49. Tufman A, Tian F, Huber RM. Can microRNAs improve the management of lung cancer patients? A clinician's perspective. Theranostics. 2013;3(12):953–63. https://doi.org/10.7150/thno.6615. Pubmed PMID: PMC3881097
50. Markou A, Zavridou M, Lianidou ES. miRNA-21 as a novel therapeutic target in lung cancer. Lung Cancer (Auckl). 2016;7:19–27. https://doi.org/10.2147/LCTT.S60341. Pubmed PMID: PMC5310696

Epigenetic gestational age acceleration: a prospective cohort study investigating associations with familial, sociodemographic and birth characteristics

Jasmine N. Khouja[1,2,3*], Andrew J. Simpkin[1,2], Linda M. O'Keeffe[1,2], Kaitlin H. Wade[1,2], Lotte C. Houtepen[1,2], Caroline L. Relton[1,2], Matthew Suderman[1,2] and Laura D. Howe[1,2]

Abstract

Background: Gestational age at delivery is associated with health and social outcomes. Recently, cord blood DNA methylation data has been used to predict gestational age. The discrepancy between gestational age predicted from DNA methylation and determined by ultrasound or last menstrual period is known as gestational age acceleration. This study investigated associations of sex, socioeconomic status, parental behaviours and characteristics and birth outcomes with gestational age acceleration.

Results: Using data from the Avon Longitudinal Study of Parents and Children ($n = 863$), we found that pre-pregnancy maternal overweight and obesity were associated with greater gestational age acceleration (mean difference = 1.6 days, 95% CI 0.7 to 2.6, and 2.9 days, 95% CI 1.3 to 4.4, respectively, compared with a body mass index < 25 kg/m^2, $p < .001$). There was evidence of an association between male sex and greater gestational age acceleration. Greater gestational age acceleration was associated with higher birthweight, birth length and head circumference of the child (mean differences per week higher gestational age acceleration: birthweight 0.1 kg, 95% CI 0.1 to 0.2, $p < .001$; birth length 0.4 cm, 95% CI 0.2 to 0.7, $p < .001$; head circumference 0.2 cm, 95% CI 0.1 to − 0.4, $p < .001$). There was evidence of an association between gestational age acceleration and mode of delivery (assisted versus unassisted delivery, odds ratio = 0.9 per week higher gestational age acceleration, 95% CI 0.7, 1.3 ($p = .05$); caesarean section versus unassisted delivery, odds ratio = 0.6, 95% CI 0.4 to 0.9 per week higher gestational age acceleration ($p = .05$)). There was no evidence of association for other parental and perinatal characteristics.

Conclusions: The associations of higher maternal body mass index and larger birth size with greater gestational age acceleration may imply that maternal overweight and obesity is associated with more rapid development of the fetus in utero. The implications of gestational age acceleration for postnatal health warrant further investigation.

Keywords: DNA methylation, Epigenetics, Gestational, Age acceleration, ALSPAC, ARIES

* Correspondence: jasmine.khouja@bristol.ac.uk
[1]MRC Integrative Epidemiology Unit at the University of Bristol, Bristol, England
[2]Population Health Sciences, Bristol Medical School, University of Bristol, Bristol, England
Full list of author information is available at the end of the article

Background

Preterm birth (≤ 37 weeks gestation) is associated with numerous health consequences such as increased mortality [1], hypertension [2, 3], insulin resistance [4] and respiratory problems in later life [5, 6]. Indeed, each additional gestational day at birth is associated with improved medical and neuropsychological outcomes in childhood [7]. Gestational age (GA) at delivery is typically determined via early obstetric ultrasound or last menstrual period (LMP), with ultrasound methods considered the more reliable [8], 'gold standard' procedure.

Recently, DNA methylation (DNAm) has been used to predict GA at delivery [9, 10]. This method builds on work that used DNAm to predict chronological age [11] and subsequent work, showing that the differences between predicted and chronological age are associated with disease outcomes. Those with DNAm-predicted ages that exceeded their chronological ages (age acceleration, AA) have a higher risk of cancer incidence [12–14], Alzheimer's disease [15] and mortality [15–20]. Of note, the term AA is commonly used in the literature to describe both positive and negative differences (i.e. predicted ages above or below chronological ages), which could be misleading, but we use the term to be consistent with previous literature.

In a similar way, the gestational epigenetic clocks developed by Bohlin et al. [10] and Knight et al. [9] can be compared with actual GA to determine gestational age acceleration (GAA). There is little existing research on the association of potential predictors of GAA or the potential outcomes of GAA.

The aim of this study was to apply a previously published model for predicting GA from DNAm [10] and use this model to estimate GAA in order to (i) explore potential predictors of GAA by assessing the association of a broad range of socioeconomic variables and parental characteristics with GAA and (ii) explore potential outcomes of GAA by assessing associations of GAA with delivery and postnatal factors, using data from the Accessible Resource for Integrated Epigenomic Studies (ARIES) project, a subsample of child-mother pairs from the Avon Longitudinal Study of Parents and Children (ALSPAC).

Results

Study sample characteristics

The characteristics of the 863 participants from the ARIES cohort included in our analysis are displayed in Tables 1 and 2, and Additional file 1: Table S1 describes the differences between these participants and the full ALSPAC cohort from which ARIES is a subsample. Additional file 1: Table S2 shows the full range of GAs of the 863 participants included in the analysis.

Modelling of GA estimates

GA was estimated from ARIES cord blood DNAm using the model of Bohlin et al. [10]. Correlation between estimated and reported GA was high (correlation coefficient $r = 0.65$) though not as high as that reported in the original publication ($r = 0.81$). Some reduction, however, was expected because the Bohlin et al. [10] model was trained and tested in distinct subsets of the same Norwegian cohort. We elected not to use the model of Knight et al. [9] because we were less confident that it would produce meaningful GAA estimates given its low correlation with GA in ARIES ($r = 0.37$) [21].

Associations of gender, socioeconomic and parental factors with GAA

Females had lower GAA than males by 0.8 days after adjusting for sex and cell type proportion (mean difference [MD] = – 0.8 days; 95% CI – 1.4, – 0.1, $p = .024$; Table 3).

Maternal pre-pregnancy overweight and obese status was associated with higher GAA compared with maternal pre-pregnancy body mass index (BMI) of < 25 kg/m^2 (MD = 1.6 days, 95% CI 0.7, 2.6 for overweight; MD = 2.9 days, 95% CI 1.3, 4.4 for obese, $p < .001$, see Table 4) after adjusting for sex, cell type proportion and parental socioeconomic factors. As GAA calculated using Bohlin et al. methods [10] is correlated with birthweight [21], we further adjusted these models including birthweight as a covariate to assess whether birthweight may be driving this effect. The results were not substantially different when additionally adjusting for birthweight (Additional file 1: Table S3).

No clear associations were found for parental education, relationship status, smoking, alcohol consumption, depression or age, nor with housing tenure, financial difficulties, parity or pregnancy complications with GAA (Tables 3 and 4).

Associations of GAA with delivery and birth outcomes

There were strong positive associations of GAA with birthweight (MD = 0.1 kg of birthweight per week higher GAA, 95% CI 0.1, 0.2, $p < .001$), birth length (MD = 0.4 cm of birth length per week higher GAA, 95% CI 0.2, 0.7, $p < .001$) and head circumference (MD = 0.2 cm of head circumference per week higher GAA, 95% CI 0.1, 0.4, $p < .001$) (see Table 5).

No association was observed between GAA and Appearance, Pulse, Grimace, Activity, and Respiration (APGAR) score at 5 min. GAA was inversely associated with assisted delivery (excluding caesarean section) (odds ratio [OR] = 0.9 per week higher GAA, 95% CI 0.7, 1.3, see Table 5) and caesarean section (OR = 0.6 per week higher GAA, 95% CI 0.4, 0.9, $p = .05$).

There were no substantial differences between the imputed and observed data sets (Additional file 1: Table S4).

Table 1 Characteristics of the study population (count and percent of the total sample). $N = 863$

	Count (*n*)	Percentage
Female	442	51.22
Maternal smoking during pregnancy		
Never smoker	513	60.64
Former smoker	238	28.13
Current smoker	95	11.23
Paternal smoking		
Never smoker	479	70.34
Former smoker	28	4.11
Current smoker	174	25.55
Maternal alcohol consumption during pregnancy		
Heavy/binge drinker	113	13.40
Light/moderate drinker	380	45.08
Pregnancy abstainer	308	36.54
Never drinker	42	4.98
Paternal alcohol consumption during pregnancy		
Heavy/binge drinker	583	83.05
Light/moderate drinker	97	13.82
Never drinker	22	3.13
Maternal depression (EPDS)—likely to be depressed	231	27.83
Paternal depression (EPDS)—likely to be depressed	61	9.36
Maternal pre-pregnancy BMI		
Under/normal weight	651	81.07
Overweight	114	14.20
Obese	38	4.73
Paternal BMI		
Under/normal weight	357	54.42
Overweight	250	38.11
Obese	49	7.47
Parental relationship status during pregnancy		
Married	709	83.22
Cohabiting	114	13.38
Single	29	3.40
Parity		
0	702	83.87
1	102	12.19
2+	33	3.94
Maternal age (years)		
35+	115	13.33
25–34	640	74.16
15–24	108	12.51
Paternal age (years)		
35+	219	27.17
25–34	542	67.25
15–24	45	5.58

Percentages reflect the proportion of the total sample
EPDS Edinburgh Postnatal Depression Scale, *BMI* body mass index

Table 2 Socioeconomic and perinatal characteristics of the study population (count, percent of total sample, mean and SD). $N = 863$

	Count (*n*)	%/mean (SD)
Non-manual parental social class	713	85.59
Maternal education		
Degree	172	20.28
A level	253	29.83
O level	279	32.90
Less than O level	144	16.98
Paternal education		
Degree	214	25.60
A level	252	30.14
O level	181	21.65
Less than O level	189	22.61
Housing tenure		
Owned/mortgaged	737	89.77
Rented (private)	28	3.41
Rented (council/HA)	56	6.82
Financial difficulties		
No financial difficulties	352	42.16
Some financial difficulties	347	41.56
Many financial difficulties	136	16.29
Delivery method		
Unassisted	320	60.72
Assisted	126	23.91
Caesarean section	81	15.37
Delivery complications	142	16.53
Term/post-term GA at delivery	839	97.22
APGAR score at 5 min		9.52 (0.69)
Birthweight (kg)	850	3.49 (0.49)
Birth length (cm)	735	50.77 (2.12)
Head circumference (cm)	737	34.92 (1.41)

Percentages reflect the proportion of the total sample
HA owned by the housing association, *APGAR* scores are based on Appearance, Pulse, Grimace, Activity, and Respiration at birth

Table 3 Associations of gender and parental socioeconomic factors with gestational age acceleration. $N = 863$

Exposure	Mean difference in gestational age acceleration (days)		
	Mean difference	95% CI	p
Female	− 0.8	− 1.4, − 0.1	0.024
High/non-manual parental social class	0.1	− 0.9, 1.0	0.91
Maternal education			
Degree	(Ref)		0.72
A level	0.8	− 0.1, 1.8	
O level	− 0.1	− 1.0, 0.8	
Less than O level	− 0.3	− 1.4, 0.8	
Paternal education			
Degree	(Ref)		0.51
A level	− 0.8	− 1.6, 0.1	
O level	− 0.2	− 1.2, 0.7	
Less than O level	0.3	− 0.7, 1.2	
Housing tenure			
Owned/mortgaged	(Ref)		0.42
Rented (private)	0.7	− 1.1, 2.5	
Rented (council/HA)	0.2	− 1.1, 1.5	
Financial difficulties			
None	(Ref)		0.55
Some	− 0.1	− 0.8, 0.6	
Many	− 0.4	− 1.3, 0.6	

Results are from multiply imputed data; coefficients are mean differences adjusted for sex (except for when sex is the exposure) and cell type proportion

Adjusting for cell type proportion did not substantially alter our results (see Additional file 1: Tables S5 to S7 for unadjusted results) and neither did adjustment for socioeconomic status (SES) and other potential confounders.

Discussion

Our analyses indicated that male sex, higher maternal pre-pregnancy BMI and vaginal delivery are associated with higher GAA. Our results also indicated that higher GAA was associated with birth size (birthweight, birth length and head circumference). There was no clear evidence of any associations of GAA with parental education, relationship status, smoking, alcohol consumption, depression or age, nor with housing tenure, financial difficulties, parity, pregnancy complications or APGAR scores.

Unlike in AA research, where AA has been associated with negative outcomes such as all-cause mortality and Alzheimer's disease [15–20], it is currently unclear whether accelerated GA at birth is beneficial or detrimental to a fetus or newborn. From previous research using ARIES data, we know sex, birthweight, caesarean section and maternal BMI have also been associated with AA [22]. A recent study has also shown associations of GAA with birth size and sex [23]. However, in their main analysis, associations with birth size were in the opposite direction to our analysis when the raw GAA-GA difference was used as the outcome, i.e. higher GAA was associated with smaller size at birth. When calculating GAA using the residuals from a regression of DNAm-predicted GA on reported GA, as GAA was calculated in this study, there was no clear association between GAA and size at birth. In further contrast, we did not replicate their associations with maternal age, APGAR scores (at 1 min) and pregnancy complications (pre-eclampsia). The discrepancies in the results could be related to the focus on raw differences rather than residuals in the main analysis of Girchenko et al. [23]. We did not estimate GAA as the difference between DNAm-predicted GA and reported GA because the confounding effect of GA is not accounted for in this approach, whereas the residual-based approach ensures GAA is uncorrelated with GA.

Another explanation for the discrepancies between our findings and the findings of Girchenko et al. [23] is their use of the Knight et al. [9] GA prediction model rather than the Bohlin et al. [10] model applied in this study. We have previously noted several key methodological differences in the derivation of the Knight et al. [9] and the Bohlin et al. [10] models that influence the accuracy of the GA prediction in this cohort [21], such as the inclusion of preterm infants in the test set of the Knight et al. model [9] which is inappropriate for a data set with few pre-term births (as in this study). Additionally, the number of CpGs (148) included in the Knight et al. [9] training model was close to the sample size of the training set (207) and the model was then tested with a much larger sample size which may have resulted in an overfitting of the model. In contrast, the number of CpGs (96) in the Bohlin et al. [10] training model was much lower than the sample size of the training set (1068). Thus, the Bohlin et al. [10] model provided us with the best estimate of GAA for this cohort [21], which was reflected in the stronger correlation found between reported GA in the ARIES cohort and the model predictions of GA compared to the Knight et al. [9] model. The Bohlin et al. [10] model for prediction of GA from DNAm performed well in our data, adding support to the notion that DNAm could potentially be used as a marker of GA in data sets where GA has not been measured.

In this study, we were able to apply the epigenetic clock created by Bohlin et al. [10] in ARIES data. Despite the original model being trained only on a Norwegian cohort, the methods of Bohlin et al. [10] transferred to a UK cohort with considerable accuracy ($r = 0.65$). Additionally, the use of ARIES and ALSPAC data (a large and rich

Table 4 Associations between parental factors and gestational age acceleration. $N = 863$

Exposure	Mean difference in gestational age acceleration (days)					
	Model 1			Model 2		
	MD	95% CI	*p*	MD	95% CI	*p*
Maternal smoking						
Never smoker	(Ref)		0.49	(Ref)		0.50
Former smoker	0.01	− 0.8, 0.7		0.03	− 0.7, 0.8	
Current smoker	0.5	− 0.5, 1.6		0.5	− 0.7, 1.6	
Paternal smoking						
Never smoker	(Ref)		0.41	(Ref)		0.40
Former smoker	− 0.9	− 2.7, 0.9		− 0.9	− 2.7, 0.9	
Current smoker	0.1	− 0.8, 0.9		0.1	− 0.8, 0.9	
Maternal alcohol consumption						
Heavy/binge drinker	(Ref)		0.26	(Ref)		0.25
Light/moderate drinker	− 0.2	− 1.2, 0.8		− 0.3	− 1.3, 0.8	
Pregnancy abstainer	− 0.4	− 1.4, 0.7		− 0.4	− 1.4, 0.6	
Never drinker	− 1.2	− 2.9, 0.5		− 1.2	− 2.9, 0.5	
Paternal alcohol consumption						
Never drinker	(Ref)		0.54	(Ref)		0.67
Light/moderate drinker	− 0.9	− 1.9, 0.1		− 0.8	− 1.9, 0.2	
Heavy/binge drinker	0.2	− 1.8, 2.2		0.4	− 1.7, 2.4	
Maternal depression depressed	0.4	− 0.4, 1.1	0.32	0.4	− 0.3, 1.2	0.28
Paternal depression depressed	−0.5	− 1.8, 0.8	0.42	− 0.6	− 1.8, 0.8	0.49
Maternal pre-pregnancy BMI						
Under/normal weight	(Ref)		< 0.001	(Ref)		< 0.001
Overweight	1.5	0.6, 2.5		1.6	0.7, 2.6	
Obese	2.7	1.2, 4.3		2.9	1.3, 4.4	
Paternal BMI						
Under/normal weight	(Ref)		0.53	(Ref)		0.58
Overweight	0.1	− 0.7, 0.9		0.1	− 0.7, 0.9	
Obese	0.4	− 0.9, 1.8		0.4	− 1.0, 1.8	
Parental relationship status						
Married	(Ref)		0.37	(Ref)		0.47
Cohabiting	0.1	− 0.8, 1.1		0.1	− 0.9, 1.1	
Single	0.8	− 1.0, 2.5		0.7	− 1.1, 2.6	
Parity						
0	(Ref)		0.88	(Ref)		0.83
1	− 0.3	− 1.3, 0.7		− 0.4	− 1.3, 0.7	
2+	0.1	− 1.6, 1.8		0.1	− 1.6, 1.8	
Maternal age						
35+	(Ref)		0.60	(Ref)		0.69
25–34	− 0.5	− 1.5, 0.5		− 0.5	− 1.4, 0.5	
15–24	− 0.1	− 1.3, 1.2		0.03	− 1.3, 1.4	
Paternal age						
35+	(Ref)		0.27	(Ref)		0.32
25–34	− 0.4	− 1.2, 0.3		− 0.4	− 1.1, 0.4	

Table 4 Associations between parental factors and gestational age acceleration. $N = 863$ *(Continued)*

Exposure	Mean difference in gestational age acceleration (days)					
	Model 1			Model 2		
	MD	95% CI	*p*	MD	95% CI	*p*
15–24	− 0.7	− 2.2, 0.8		− 0.6	− 2.2, 0.9	
Pregnancy complications	− 0.4	− 1.2, 0.5	0.42	− 0.6	− 1.5, 0.3	0.16

Results are from multiply imputed data; coefficients are mean differences (MD) adjusted for sex and cell type proportion (model 1) and additionally for parental social class, education, housing tenure and financial difficulties (model 2). Parental depression was measured using the Edinburgh Postnatal Depression Scale. The pregnancy complication analysis additionally adjusted for all other parental behaviour covariates
BMI body mass index

source of longitudinal data for children and their families) allowed us to assess the associations of GAA with a wide range of socioeconomic, parental and perinatal factors. The longitudinal nature of ARIES also enabled comparisons between GAA and AA at multiple ages.

Although the ARIES sub-sample is a more affluent sample of the full ALSPAC cohort, our results were robust to adjustment for SES. This is in line with some evidence that such differences are unlikely to severely bias association studies [24–27]. To account for missing data, we used multiple imputation, which maximised our statistical power. The results were consistent when using complete-case observed data.

Following Gervin et al.'s [28] methods, the regression analyses were adjusted for cell type proportions, even though GA is associated with variation in cell type proportions and this adjustment could therefore potentially bias the results. However, comparing the data before and after adjustment, there were no substantial differences in the results. Additionally, only weak associations were found between GA and cell type composition in this study (Additional file 1: Figure S1). Another potential issue with adjusting for cell type composition arises from deriving cord blood references from full-term births only; cord blood cell counts may be inaccurate for cord blood methylation profiles of preterm infants. However, a small proportion of the participants in our study were pre-term (3%) so it is unlikely that this will have substantially impacted the results.

Interestingly, there is little overlap between probes used in the Bohlin et al. [10] model of GA predication and the Horvath [11] model of age prediction, with only one CpG site (cg08965235 in the latent-transforming growth factor beta-binding protein 3 gene) overlapping between the models. In contrast to the Horvath [11] model, which compares accurate measures of chronological age and epigenetic predictions, the Bohlin et al. [10] model compares potentially inaccurate LMP/ultrasound estimates to epigenetic predictions. Consequently, inaccurate GA estimates may have impacted upon the GAA estimates in this research, especially as the majority of the GA estimates in ALSPAC are derived from LMP, since ultrasound estimation of GA was not common at the time of recruitment. Additionally, the GA predictions using the Bohlin et al. [10] model were more accurate using ultrasound methods rather than LMP. This may mean that our estimates may not be as accurate as if ultrasound GAs had been used and this could explain the discrepancy in accuracy between the Bohlin et al. [10] test data and the ARIES data, as detailed by Simpkin and colleagues [21].

Table 5 Associations between gestational age acceleration and perinatal factors. $N = 863$

Outcome	Mean difference in perinatal outcome per 1 week higher gestational age acceleration					
	Model 1			Model 2		
	MD	CI	*p*	MD	CI	*p*
Birthweight (kg)	0.1	0.1, 0.2	< 0.001	0.1	0.1, 0.2	< 0.001
Birth length (cm)	0.5	0.3, 0.7	< 0.001	0.4	0.2, 0.7	< 0.001
Head circumference (cm)	0.3	0.1, 0.4	< 0.001	0.2	0.1, 0.4	< 0.001
APGAR scores (0–10)	− 0.01	− 0.1, 0.1	0.79	− 0.02	− 0.1, 0.1	0.73
	OR	CI	*p*	OR	CI	*p*
Delivery method						
Unassisted	–	(Ref)		–	(Ref)	
Assisted	0.9	0.7, 1.2		0.9	0.7, 1.3	
Caesarean section	0.7	0.5, 1.0	0.05	0.6	0.4, 0.9	0.05

Results are from multiply imputed data; coefficients are mean differences (MD) or odds ratios (OR) adjusted for sex and cell type proportion in model 1 and additionally adjusted for parental social class, education, smoking, alcohol use, depression, body mass index, age and relationship status as well as housing tenure, financial difficulties and parity in model 2. APGAR scores are based on Appearance, Pulse, Grimace, Activity, and Respiration at birth

Conclusions

Our results suggest that higher maternal BMI is strongly associated with higher GAA and that higher GAA is strongly associated with larger size at birth (birthweight, birth length and head circumference). In addition, we found weaker associations of sex and delivery method with GAA. Our results may indicate that having a BMI over 25 kg/m^2 is associated with more rapid development of the fetus in utero. The implications of GAA for postnatal growth, development and health warrant further investigation.

Methods

Study population

This study used DNAm data generated under the auspices of the ALSPAC [29, 30]. ALSPAC recruited 14,541 pregnant women with expected delivery dates between April 1991 and December 1992. Of these initial pregnancies, there were 14,062 live births and 13,988 children who were alive at 1 year of age. The study website contains details of all the data that are available through a fully searchable data dictionary (http://www.bris.ac.uk/alspac/researchers/data-access/data-dictionary).

As part of the ARIES [31] project (http://www.ariesepigenomics.org.uk), a sub-sample of 1018 ALSPAC child-mother pairs had DNAm measured using the Infinium HumanMethylation450 BeadChip (Illumina, Inc.) [32]. The ARIES sub-sample was selected based on availability of DNA samples at three time points (birth, mean 7.5 years and mean 15.5 years). DNAm was measured three times in ALSPAC offspring, from cord blood at birth and from peripheral blood at approximately ages 7 and 17.

Laboratory methods, quality control and pre-processing

All DNAm wet-lab and pre-processing analyses were performed at the University of Bristol as part of the ARIES project. Following extraction, DNA was bisulphite converted using the Zymo EZ DNA MethylationTM kit (Zymo, Irvine, CA). Infinium HumanMethylation450 BeadChips were used to measure genome-wide DNAm levels at over 485,000 CpG sites. The arrays were scanned using an Illumina iScan, with initial quality review using GenomeStudio. The level of DNAm is expressed as a 'beta' value (β value), ranging from 0 (no cytosine methylation) to 1 (complete cytosine methylation). β values are reported as percentages. Several quality control steps were included in the laboratory pipeline which are described in detail elsewhere [33].

Epigenetic GA prediction

Using a recently published model [10], we derived epigenetic gestational age (EGA) from cord blood DNAm. The Bohlin et al. [10] model was chosen over the Knight et al. [9] model due to its much stronger correlation with GA in ARIES ($r = 0.65$ compared to $r = 0.37$). This epigenetic clock for GA at delivery uses 96 CpG sites to predict GA from cord blood methylation. We obtained GAA as the residuals from a regression of EGA on observed GA. GA was gathered from clinical records and determined by LMP for the majority; however, on some occasions, this measure was updated following a dating ultrasound. It is not known for which individual GA was based on LMP or ultrasound but as updating GA based on ultrasound was not common practice at the time of the measurement, the numbers are likely to be low. To be consistent with previous literature, we have used the terms 'AA' and 'GAA' to describe both positive and negative differences (i.e. predicted ages above or below chronological/gestational ages). A positive GAA corresponds to an EGA that was higher than actual GA and vice versa.

Socioeconomic, parental and perinatal characteristics

Socioeconomic factors included housing tenure, social class, parental education and financial difficulties. Parental factors included parental smoking, alcohol use, mental health, relationship status, BMI and age. Finally, perinatal variables considered were child's sex, birthweight, birth length, head circumference and APGAR score at 5 min as well as the occurrence of any pregnancy complications and the delivery type. All variables were measured through questionnaires at different times during pregnancy (socioeconomic and parental variables), by trained ALSPAC staff shortly after birth (anthropometry at birth) or from obstetric records (pregnancy complications, child's sex and APGAR score). Full details of measurement of these factors are in Additional file 1.

Statistical analysis

Sex, SES, parental behaviours and pregnancy complications were analysed as potential determinants of GAA. Associations between these factors and GAA were assessed in linear regression models with GAA as the outcome. Models with parental behaviours as the exposure were adjusted for SES variables as confounders. Birth size, delivery method and APGAR score were considered as potential outcomes of GAA. Associations of GAA with these factors were assessed using linear or multinomial logistic regression as appropriate, with GAA as an exposure and parental behaviour and SES variables included as potential confounders. We performed the analysis in this way due to the temporal ordering of the variables, although we do not necessarily hypothesise a direct causal effect of GAA on these outcome variables. The associations were analysed in two models: (1) adjusted for sex and cell type proportion and (2) with additional adjustment for potential confounders, as appropriate for the specific model. The Gervin et al. [28] methods were used for cell-type proportion estimations. Due to missingness in the observed data set, analyses were completed using 100 multiply imputed data sets (see Additional file 1: Table S8 for further information). There were no substantial differences between the analysis of the observed data and the multiply imputed data sets.

Abbreviations

AA: Age acceleration; ALSPAC: Avon Longitudinal Study of Parents and Children; APGAR: Appearance, Pulse, Grimace, Activity, and Respiration; ARIES: Accessible Resource for Integrated Epigenomic Studies; BMI: Body mass index; DNAm: DNA methylation; EGA: Epigenetic gestational age; EPDS: Edinburgh Postnatal Depression Scale; GA: Gestational age; GAA: Gestational age acceleration; HA: Owned by the housing association; LMP: Last menstrual period; MD: Mean differences; OR: Odds ratio; SD: Standard deviation; SES: Socio-economic status

Acknowledgements

We are extremely grateful to all the families who took part in this study, the midwives for their help in recruiting them and the whole ALSPAC team, which includes interviewers, computer and laboratory technicians, clerical workers, research scientists, volunteers, managers, receptionists and nurses. This publication is the work of the authors, and JNK and LDH will serve as guarantors for the contents of this paper.

Funding

This work was supported by grant from the UK Economic and Social Research Council [ES/N000382/1, ES/N000498/1]. LDH is supported by a Career Development Award fellowship from the UK Medical Research Council [MR/M020894/1]. LMOK is supported by a UK Medical Research Council Population Health Scientist fellowship [MR/M014509/1]. JNK, AJA, LMOK, KHW, LCH, CLR, MS and LDH work in a unit that receives funding from the University of Bristol and the UK Medical Research Council [MC_UU_12013/2, MC_UU_12013/3, MC_UU_12013/4, MC_UU_12013/6, MC_UU_12013/9]. The UK Medical Research Council and the Wellcome Trust [grant ref.: 102215/2/13/2] and the University of Bristol provide core support for ALSPAC. JNK is a PhD student funded by the MRC Integrative Epidemiology Unit at Bristol University. ARIES was funded by the BBSRC (BBI025751/1 and BB/I025263/1). Supplementary funding to generate DNAm data which is (or will be) included in ARIES has been obtained from the MRC, ESRC, NIH and other sources. ARIES is maintained under the auspices of the MRC Integrative Epidemiology Unit at the University of Bristol (MC_UU_12013/2 and MC_UU_12013/8).

Authors' contributions

The study was conceived and designed by AJS and LDH. Statistical analyses were conducted by JNK and AJS. JNK was responsible for writing the first draft of the manuscript. All authors contributed to the interpretation of results and critical revisions of the manuscript and approved the final manuscript.

Competing interests

The authors declare that they have no competing interests.

Author details

[1]MRC Integrative Epidemiology Unit at the University of Bristol, Bristol, England. [2]Population Health Sciences, Bristol Medical School, University of Bristol, Bristol, England. [3]School of Experimental Psychology at the University of Bristol, Bristol, England.

References

1. Field D, Draper ES, Fenton A, Papiernik E, Zeitlin J, Blondel B, Cuttini M, Maier RF, Weber T, Carrapato M, et al. Rates of very preterm birth in Europe and neonatal mortality rates. Arch Dis Child-Fetal. 2009;94:F253–6.
2. de Jong F, Monuteaux MC, van Elburg RM, Gillman MW, Belfort MB. Systematic review and meta-analysis of preterm birth and later systolic blood pressure. Hypertension. 2012;59:226–34.
3. Evensen KA, Steinshamn S, Tjonna AE, Stolen T, Hoydal MA, Wisloff U, Brubakk AM, Vik T. Effects of preterm birth and fetal growth retardation on cardiovascular risk factors in young adulthood. Early Hum Dev. 2009;85:239–45.
4. Tinnion R, Gillone J, Cheetham T, Embleton N. Preterm birth and subsequent insulin sensitivity: a systematic review. Arch Dis Child. 2014;99:362–8.
5. Pike KC, Lucas JS. Respiratory consequences of late preterm birth. Paediatr Respir Rev. 2015;16:182–8.
6. Kotecha SJ, Edwards MO, Watkins WJ, Henderson AJ, Paranjothy S, Dunstan FD, Kotecha S. Effect of preterm birth on later FEV1: a systematic review and meta-analysis. Thorax. 2013;68:760–6.
7. Baron IS, Litman FR, Ahronovich MD, Baker R. Late preterm birth: a review of medical and neuropsychological childhood outcomes. Neuropsychol Rev. 2012;22:438–50.
8. Hoffman CS, Messer LC, Mendola P, Savitz DA, Herring AH, Hartmann KE. Comparison of gestational age at birth based on last menstrual period and ultrasound during the first trimester. Paediatr Perinat Ep. 2008;22:587–96.
9. Knight AK, Craig JM, Theda C, Baekvad-Hansen M, Bybjerg-Grauholm J, Hansen CS, Hollegaard MV, Hougaard DM, Mortensen PB, Weinsheimer SM, et al. An epigenetic clock for gestational age at birth based on blood methylation data. Genome Biol. 2016;17:206.
10. Bohlin J, Haberg SE, Magnus P, Reese SE, Gjessing HK, Magnus MC, Parr CL, Page CM, London SJ, Nystad W. Prediction of gestational age based on genome-wide differentially methylated regions. Genome Biol. 2016;17:207.
11. Horvath S. DNA methylation age of human tissues and cell types. Genome Biol. 2013;14:R115.
12. Zheng Y, Joyce BT, Colicino E, Liu L, Zhang W, Dai Q, Shrubsole MJ, Kibbe WA, Gao T, Zhang Z, et al. Blood epigenetic age may predict cancer incidence and mortality. Cancer Res. 2016;76:68–73.
13. Lin Q, Wagner W. Epigenetic aging signatures are coherently modified in cancer. PLoS Genet. 2015;11:e1005334.
14. Levine ME, Hosgood HD, Chen B, Absher D, Assimes T, Horvath S. DNA methylation age of blood predicts future onset of lung cancer in the women's health initiative. Aging-Us. 2015;7:690–700.
15. Levine ME, Lu AT, Bennett DA, Horvath S. Epigenetic age of the pre-frontal cortex is associated with neuritic plaques, amyloid load, and Alzheimer's disease related cognitive functioning. Aging-Us. 2015;7:1198–211.
16. Marioni RE, Shah S, McRae AF, Chen BH, Colicino E, Harris SE, Gibson J, Henders AK, Redmond P, Cox SR, et al. DNA methylation age of blood predicts all-cause mortality in later life. Genome Biol. 2015;16:25.
17. Christiansen L, Lenart A, Tan QH, Vaupel JW, Aviv A, McGue M, Christensen K. DNA methylation age is associated with mortality in a longitudinal Danish twin study. Aging Cell. 2016;15:149–54.
18. Horvath S, Pirazzini C, Bacalini MG, Gentilini D, Di Blasio AM, Delledonne M, Mari D, Arosio B, Monti D, Passarino G, et al. Decreased epigenetic age of PBMCs from Italian semi-supercentenarians and their offspring. Aging-Us. 2015;7:1159–70.
19. Marioni RE, Shah S, Mcrae AF, Ritchie SJ, Muniz-Terrera G, Harris SE, Gibson J, Redmond P, Cox SR, Pattie A, et al. The epigenetic clock is correlated with physical and cognitive fitness in the Lothian Birth Cohort 1936. Int J Epidemiol. 2015;44:1388–96.
20. Breitling LP, Saum K, Perna L, Schöttker B, Holleczek B, Brenner H. Frailty is associated with the epigenetic clock but not with telomere length in a German cohort. Clin Epigenetics. 2016;8:21.
21. Simpkin AJ, Suderman M, Howe LD. Epigenetic clocks for gestational age: statistical and study design considerations. Clin Epigenetics. 2017;9:100.
22. Simpkin AJ, Hemani G, Suderman M, Gaunt TR, Lyttleton O, McArdle WL, Ring SM, Sharp GC, Tilling K, Horvath S, et al. Prenatal and early life influences on epigenetic age in children: a study of mother-offspring pairs from two cohort studies. Hum Mol Genet. 2016;25:191–201.
23. Girchenko P, Lahti J, Czamara D, Knight AK, Jones MJ, Suarez A, Hamalainen E, Kajantie E, Laivuori H, Villa PM, et al. Associations between maternal risk

factors of adverse pregnancy and birth outcomes and the offspring epigenetic clock of gestational age at birth. Clin Epigenetics. 2017;9:49.
24. Osler M, Kriegbaum M, Christensen U, Holstein B, Nybo Andersen AM. Rapid report on methodology: does loss to follow-up in a cohort study bias associations between early life factors and lifestyle-related health outcomes? Ann Epidemiol. 2008;18:422–4.
25. Greene N, Greenland S, Olsen J, Nohr EA. Estimating bias from loss to follow-up in the Danish National Birth Cohort. Epidemiology. 2011;22:815–22.
26. Howe LD, Tilling K, Galobardes B, Lawlor DA. Loss to follow-up in cohort studies bias in estimates of socioeconomic inequalities. Epidemiology. 2013;24:1–9.
27. Winding TN, Andersen JH, Labriola M, Nohr EA. Initial non-participation and loss to follow-up in a Danish youth cohort: implications for relative risk estimates. J Epidemiol Community Health. 2014;68:137–44.
28. Gervin K, Page CM, Aass HCD, Jansen MA, Fjeldstad HE, Andreassen BK, Duijts L, van Meurs JB, van Zelm MC, Jaddoe VW, et al. Cell type specific DNA methylation in cord blood: a 450K-reference data set and cell count-based validation of estimated cell type composition. Epigenetics. 2016;11:690–8.
29. Boyd A, Golding J, Macleod J, Lawlor DA, Fraser A, Henderson J, Molloy L, Ness A, Ring S, Smith GD. Cohort profile: the 'children of the 90s'—the index offspring of the Avon Longitudinal Study of Parents and Children. Int J Epidemiol. 2013;42:111–27.
30. Fraser A, Macdonald-Wallis C, Tilling K, Boyd A, Golding J, Smith GD, Henderson J, Macleod J, Molloy L, Ness A, et al. Cohort profile: the Avon Longitudinal Study of Parents and Children: ALSPAC mothers cohort. Int J Epidemiol. 2013;42:97–110.
31. Relton CL, Gaunt T, McArdle W, Ho K, Duggirala A, Shihab H, Woodward G, Lyttleton O, Evans DM, Reik W. Data resource profile: accessible resource for integrated epigenomic studies (ARIES). Int J Epidemiol. 2015;44:1181–90.
32. Dedeurwaerder S, Defrance M, Calonne E, Denis H, Sotiriou C, Fuks F. Evaluation of the Infinium Methylation 450K technology. Epigenomics. 2011;3:771–84.
33. Simpkin AJ, Suderman M, Gaunt TR, Lyttleton O, McArdle WL, Ring SM, Tilling K, Smith GD, Relton CL. Longitudinal analysis of DNA methylation associated with birth weight and gestational age. Hum Mol Genet. 2015;24:3752–63.

Trajectories of inflammatory biomarkers over the eighth decade and their associations with immune cell profiles and epigenetic ageing

Anna J. Stevenson[1,6,7*], Daniel L. McCartney[1], Sarah E. Harris[1,2], Adele M. Taylor[3], Paul Redmond[3], John M. Starr[2,4], Qian Zhang[5], Allan F. McRae[5], Naomi R. Wray[5], Tara L. Spires-Jones[6,7], Barry W. McColl[6,7], Andrew M. McIntosh[2,8], Ian J. Deary[2,3] and Riccardo E. Marioni[1,2]

Abstract

Background: Epigenetic age acceleration (an older methylation age compared to chronological age) correlates strongly with various age-related morbidities and mortality. Chronic systemic inflammation is thought to be a hallmark of ageing, but the relationship between an increased epigenetic age and this likely key phenotype of ageing has not yet been extensively investigated.

Methods: We modelled the trajectories of the inflammatory biomarkers C-reactive protein (CRP; measured using both a high- and low-sensitivity assay) and interleukin-6 (IL-6) over the eighth decade in the Lothian Birth Cohort 1936. Using linear mixed models, we investigated the association between CRP and immune cell profiles imputed from the methylation data and examined the cross-sectional and longitudinal association between the inflammatory biomarkers and two measures of epigenetic age acceleration, derived from the Horvath and Hannum epigenetic clocks.

Results: We found that low-sensitivity CRP declined, high-sensitivity CRP did not change, and IL-6 increased over time within the cohort. CRP levels inversely associated with CD8+T cells and CD4+T cells and positively associated with senescent CD8+T cells, plasmablasts and granulocytes. Cross-sectionally, the Hannum, but not the Horvath, measure of age acceleration was positively associated with each of the inflammatory biomarkers, including a restricted measure of CRP (≤ 10 mg/L) likely reflecting levels relevant to chronic inflammation.

Conclusions: We found a divergent relationship between inflammation and immune system parameters in older age. We additionally report the Hannum measure of epigenetic age acceleration associated with an elevated inflammatory profile cross-sectionally, but not longitudinally.

Keywords: Inflammation, DNA methylation, Epigenetics, Epigenetic age acceleration, Immune cells

Background

Epidemiological studies have long associated ageing with a progressive move to a chronic inflammatory state, a phenomenon often referred to as 'inflammaging' [1, 2]. This low-grade, and typically sub-acute, elevation of peripheral pro-inflammatory mediators in the absence of overt infection is strongly associated with the susceptibility to, and progression of, many age-associated diseases such as cancer, type 2 diabetes and Alzheimer's disease, and is a key risk factor for mortality [3].

Many studies of inflammation in older adults have focused on the acute-phase protein C-reactive protein (CRP) and the pro-inflammatory cytokine interleukin 6 (IL-6), both of which are sensitive biomarkers of low-grade inflammation. Akin to other biomarkers, inflammatory mediators can be highly variable, yet much of the research

* Correspondence: anna.stevenson@ed.ac.uk
[1]Centre for Genomic and Experimental Medicine, Institute of Genetics and Molecular Medicine, University of Edinburgh, Edinburgh, UK
[6]UK Dementia Research Institute, Edinburgh Medical School, University of Edinburgh, Edinburgh, UK
Full list of author information is available at the end of the article

into their alterations in ageing has been cross-sectional [4, 5]. Multiple-time point measurements are critical to establish the chronicity of inflammatory biomarkers and their trajectories with age, which in itself is key to unravelling the mechanisms behind the process. Several putative pathways have been identified as playing a role in chronic systemic inflammation including increased visceral adiposity, oxidative stress and telomeric and mitochondrial dysfunction [6, 7], and genetic studies have produced candidate polymorphisms associated with the process [8–10]. There remains, however, a lack of understanding of the aetiology of chronic inflammation and its relationship with molecular ageing rates [3, 6].

DNA methylation is an epigenetic mechanism by which methyl groups are added to the DNA molecule, typically at cytosine-guanine (CpG) dinucleotides. Chronological age has been shown to have a significant effect on methylation levels, and as such, several highly accurate DNA methylation-based biological markers of ageing, or 'epigenetic clocks', have been proposed [11, 12]. Accelerated epigenetic ageing, as evinced by a greater methylation age compared to chronological age, has been linked to various age-associated health outcomes such as frailty [13], lung cancer [14] and Parkinson's disease [15], as well as all-cause mortality [16, 17]. There have been many diverse applications of the epigenetic clock to studies of ageing and disease, but relatively little is known about the relationship between accelerated epigenetic ageing and a likely key intermediary process of ageing and age-related morbidity: inflammation. Investigating such relationships may give further insight into the molecular aetiology of inflammation and the pathways that regulate it in the ageing process.

In the current study, we investigate the dynamics of inflammation across the eighth decade and its relationship with epigenetic age. We established the trajectories of the inflammatory biomarkers CRP and IL-6 and their association with imputed immune cells in the Lothian Birth Cohort 1936 (LBC1936). We then assessed their cross-sectional and longitudinal associations with epigenetic age acceleration, using two widely used measures: intrinsic epigenetic age acceleration (IEAA) and extrinsic epigenetic age acceleration (EEAA) (described in the 'Methods' section). Chronic inflammation is considered to be a pervasive feature of ageing and, as epigenetic age robustly correlates with chronological age, we hypothesise that a faster running epigenetic clock will associate with greater levels of systemic inflammatory biomarkers.

Results

Baseline cohort demographics

Of the 1091 (543 female; 49.8%) participants recruited at wave 1, CRP measures (mg/L) were available for 1054 participants (mean = 5.26 mg/L, SD = 6.68) and epigenetic age acceleration measures for 906 (IEAA: mean = – 0.465 years, SD = 5.99; EEAA: mean = – 0.319 years, SD = 7.09). Ninety-five participants were taking anti-inflammatory medication at baseline (8.7%).

Trajectories of inflammatory biomarkers

Spaghetti plots of the trajectories of both raw and log-transformed CRP and IL-6 over time are shown in Fig. 1. Low-sensitivity log(CRP) was found to decline over the 9 years of follow-up by an average of 0.01 SD per year ($p = 0.004$). The slight increase in high-sensitivity log(CRP) levels over the two waves seen in the plot was not found to be significant ($p = 0.718$). log(IL-6) increased with age, by an average of 0.15 SD per year ($p = 2 \times 10^{-16}$).

Due to the discrepancy between the trajectories of the high- and low-sensitivity CRP measures, we repeated the analysis of the low-sensitivity measure, restricted to the same time points as were available for the high-sensitivity measure (waves 2 and 3). Akin to the high-sensitivity measure, no change was seen over these two waves (beta = – 0.005, $p = 0.836$) indicating that the 3-year time period between waves is perhaps too brief to capture significant variations in CRP.

Correlations

Correlations between the inflammatory biomarkers both within and between waves are presented in Fig. 2. The high- and low-sensitivity CRP measures correlated strongly within waves ($r \geq 0.93$), and both measures had moderate intra-wave correlations with IL-6 ($r = 0.41$–0.45). The low-sensitivity CRP correlations across the four waves were low ($r = 0.14$–0.26). Similar coefficients were seen over the two waves for the high-sensitivity CRP measure ($r = 0.14$) and IL-6 ($r = 0.33$).

Associations with imputed immune cells

Due to the association between inflammation and immunosenescence, we examined the dynamics of the immune cells imputed from the methylation data, and their association with CRP levels.

We initially established the correlations between both the high- and low-sensitivity CRP measures and the imputed cell profiles across the four waves of data (Table 1). There was no significant difference between the correlation coefficients of the two measures across the two waves of overlap (Wilcoxon signed-rank test: wave 2: $p = 0.76$; wave 3: $p = 0.44$), and the directions of the coefficients were consistent. This indicated the lower-sensitivity measure of CRP was representative, and its use in our analyses was unlikely to skew results.

All lymphocyte cells declined over time: CD8+T total (beta = – 0.01 SD/year, $p = 4.46 \times 10^{-7}$); naïve CD8+T (beta = – 0.01 SD/year, $p = 4.22 \times 10^{-5}$); total CD4+T (beta = – 0.06 SD/year, $p = 2 \times 10^{-16}$); naïve CD4+T

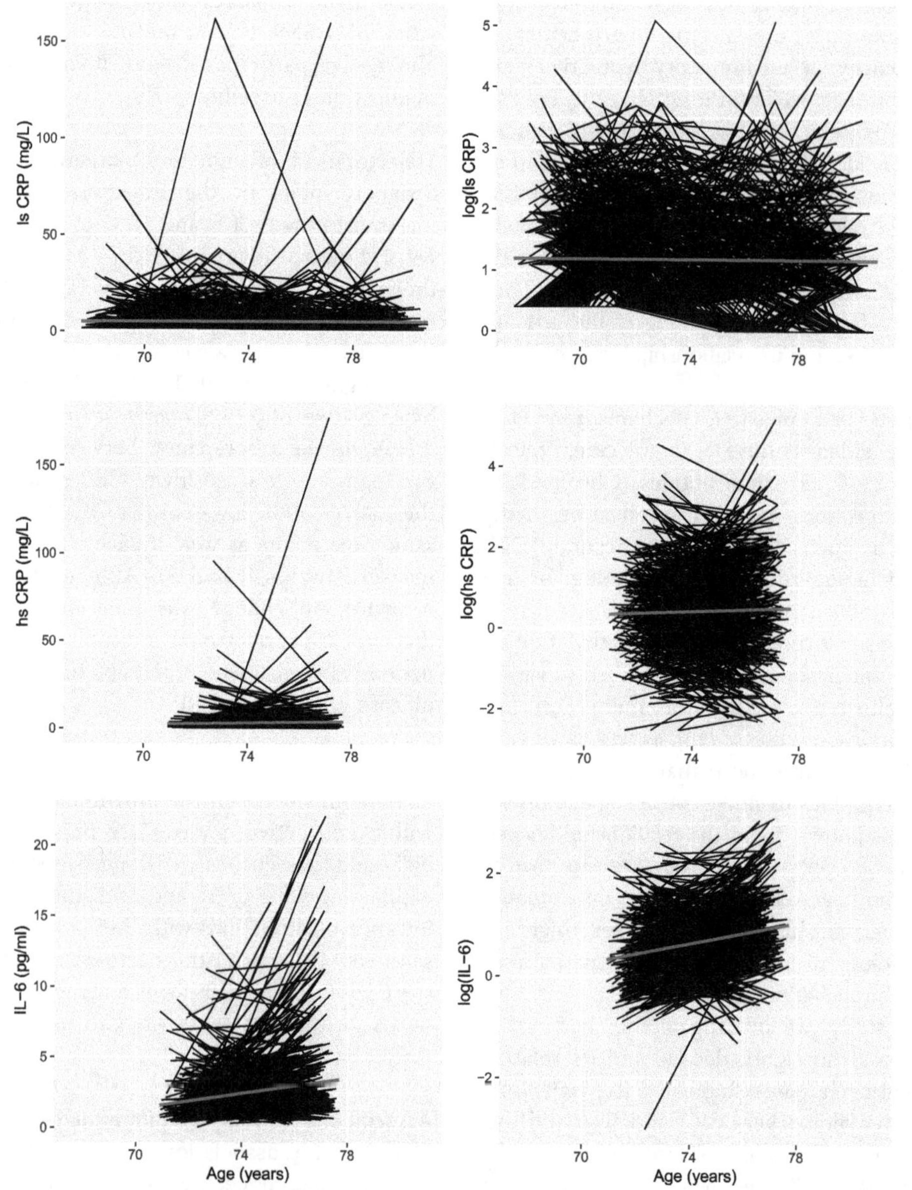

Fig. 1 Spaghetti plots of change in CRP and IL-6 over time. CRP: C-reactive protein; IL-6: interleukin-6; hs: high-sensitivity; ls: low-sensitivity; log(): log-transformed

(beta = – 0.05 SD/year, $p = 2 \times 10^{-16}$); NK (beta = – 0.04 SD/year, $p = 2 \times 10^{-16}$); B (beta = – 0.04 SD/year, $p = 2 \times 10^{-16}$). Exhausted/senescent CD8+T cells increased with age (beta = 0.03 SD/year, $p = 1.18 \times 10^{-14}$) as did monocytes (beta = 0.06 SD/year, $p = 2 \times 10^{-16}$), granulocytes (beta = 0.04 SD/year, $p = 2 \times 10^{-16}$) and plasmablasts (beta = 0.08 SD/year, $p = 2 \times 10^{-16}$) (Fig. 3.)

The baseline associations between the blood cellular composition and low-sensitivity log(CRP) within the cohort are presented in Table 2. An inverse association was observed between CRP and CD8+T cells (total: beta = – 0.073, $p = 0.026$; naïve: beta = – 0.142, $p = 2.54 \times 10^{-5}$) and CD4+T cells (total: beta = – 0.132, $p = 6.74 \times 10^{-5}$, naïve: beta = – 0.072, $p = 0.032$). A positive association was found between CRP and senescent CD8+T cells (beta = 0.134, $p = 3.79 \times 10^{-5}$), plasmablasts (beta = 0.148, $p = 1.38 \times 10^{-5}$) and granulocyte counts (beta = 0.133, $p = 4.17 \times 10^{-5}$). No associations were found between log(CRP) and B cells, NK cells or monocytes. A CRP level of ≤ 10 mg/L is often cited as reflecting the non-acute, chronic inflammation, relevant to what has been reported in ageing [18]. Because of this, we ran a sensitivity analysis excluding those with CRP > 10 mg/L to test if the associations were altered with more chronic levels of inflammation. Here, the associations with CD4+T cells, total CD8+T cells and granulocytes were attenuated, though the coefficients were in

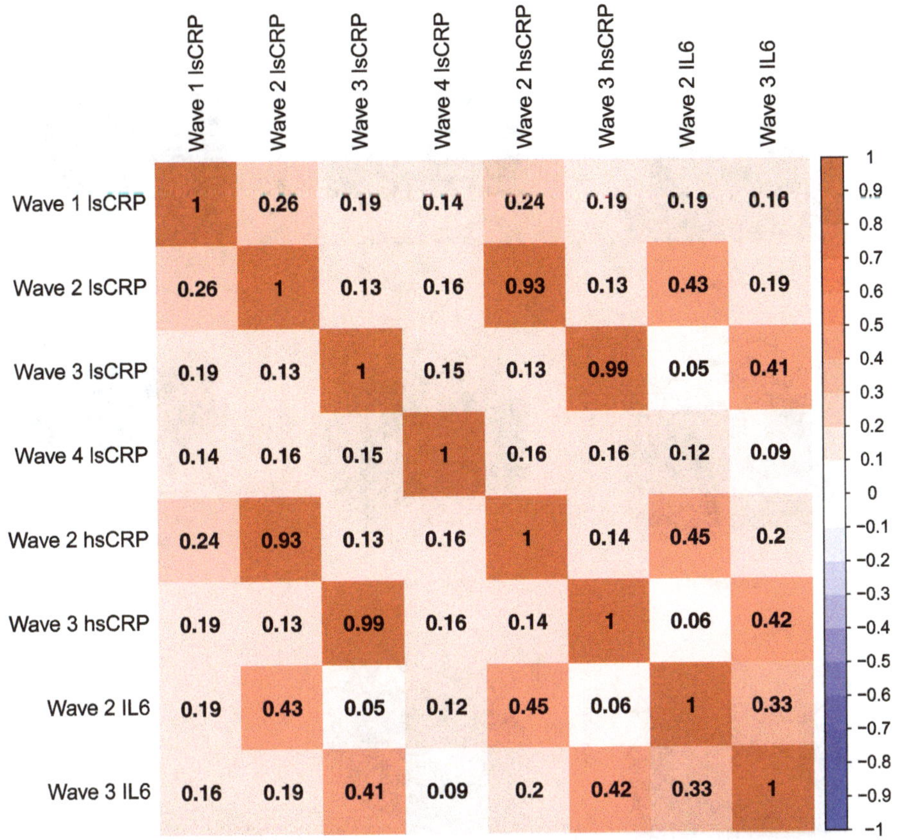

Fig. 2 Heatmap of correlations between inflammatory biomarkers within and across the four waves of data collection. lsCRP was available at all four waves of data collection; hsCRP and IL-6 were available at waves 2 and 3 only. CRP: C-reactive protein; IL-6: interleukin-6; ls: low-sensitivity; hs: high-sensitivity

the same direction as previously. All other results remained the same though with larger p values (Additional file 1).

Associations with age acceleration

We assessed the cross-sectional and longitudinal relationship between each inflammatory biomarker and methylation-based age acceleration using IEAA and EEAA (Table 3). Positive baseline associations were found between both the low- and high-sensitivity CRP measures and EEAA (low-sensitivity log(CRP): beta = 0.154, $p = 2.48 \times 10^{-5}$, high-sensitivity log(CRP): beta = 0.111, $p = 0.004$). No baseline correlations were seen between either CRP measure or

Table 1 Pearson correlations between high- and low-sensitivity CRP measures and imputed immune cell profiles

	Wave 1		Wave 2		Wave 3		Wave 4	
	ls	hs	ls	hs	ls	hs	ls	hs
Total CD8+T	−0.077	NA	− 0.057	−0.041	− 0.053	−0.053	− 0.098	NA
Total CD4+T	−0.167	NA	−0.104	−0.107	− 0.12	−0.112	− 0.079	NA
Natural killer	−0.108	NA	−0.067	−0.086	− 0.094	−0.083	− 0.15	NA
B cells	−0.093	NA	−0.053	−0.029	− 0.084	−0.071	0.006	NA
Senescent CD8+T	0.119	NA	0.077	0.072	0.039	0.044	0.003	NA
Naïve CD8+T	−0.068	NA	−0.055	−0.054	0.089	0.071	−0.102	NA
Naïve CD4+T	−0.066	NA	−0.024	−0.022	0.01	0.015	−0.033	NA
Monocytes	0.037	NA	0.099	0.101	0.079	0.087	0.134	NA
Granulocytes	0.192	NA	0.106	0.097	0.146	0.119	0.112	NA
Plasmablasts	0.186	NA	0.133	0.127	0.132	0.119	0.103	NA

ls low-sensitivity CRP, *hs* high-sensitivity CRP, *NA* not available

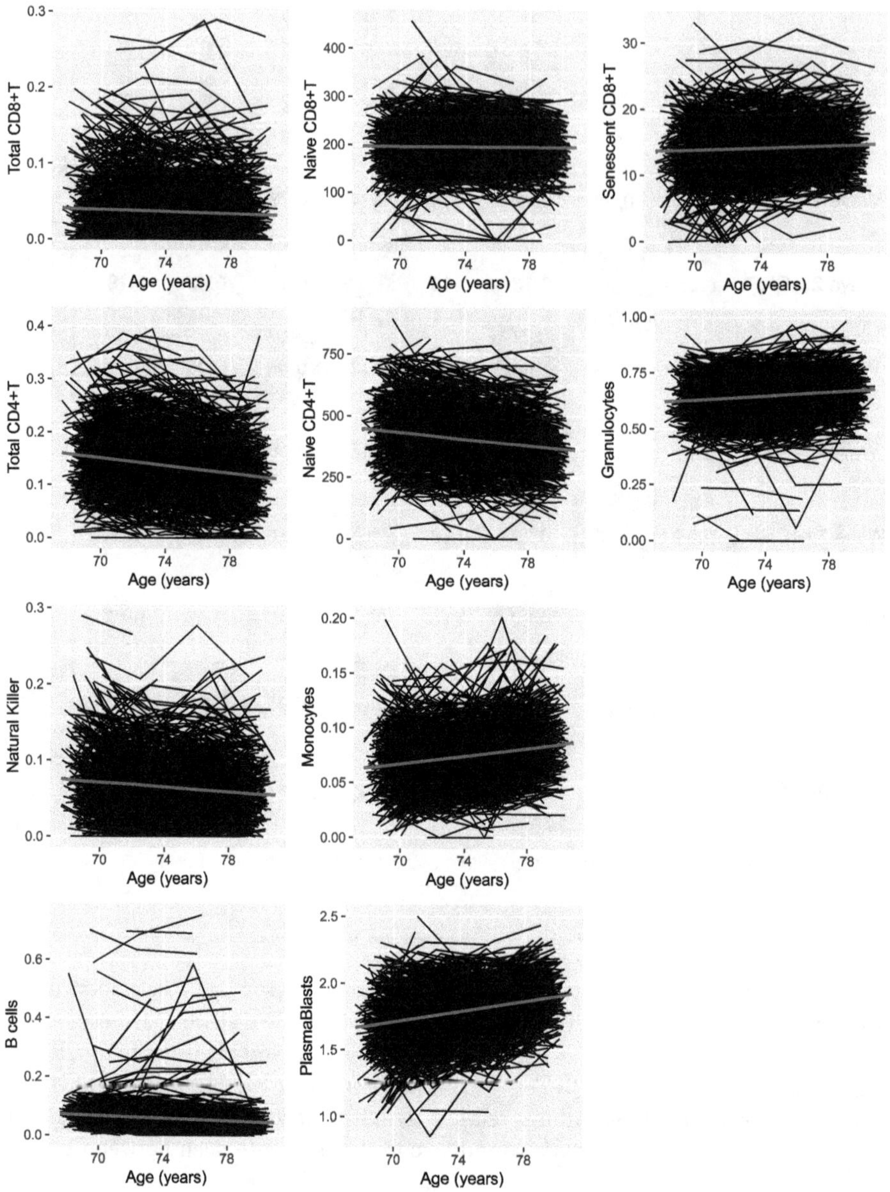

Fig. 3 Spaghetti plots of change in imputed immune cell profiles over time

IEAA ($p \geq 0.087$). Neither baseline IEAA nor EEAA was associated with longitudinal change in log(CRP) ($p \geq 0.360$).

log(IL-6) also showed a positive baseline association with EEAA (beta = 0.114, $p = 0.003$) but not with IEAA ($p = 0.563$). There was no longitudinal association between the log(IL-6) measure and either measure of epigenetic age acceleration ($p \geq 0.392$).

We additionally investigated the relationship between epigenetic age acceleration and log(CRP) in the subset of the cohort with CRP levels of ≤ 10 mg/L, as measured by the low-sensitivity assay (Table 3). A positive cross-sectional association was present between EEAA and CRP levels (beta = 0.129, $p = 0.0009$). No equivalent association was observed with IEAA ($p = 0.081$). There were no longitudinal associations with either measure of epigenetic age acceleration ($p \geq 0.303$).

Discussion

In the current study, we found a decline over time in the serum levels of the inflammatory mediator CRP, measured using a low-sensitivity assay in LBC1936. The CRP levels measured from the high-sensitivity assay did not exhibit similarly significant changes with

Table 2 Baseline associations between low-sensitivity C-reactive protein and imputed immune cell profiles

	Standardised beta	SE	*p*
Total CD8+T	−0.073	0.033	0.026
Total CD4+T	−0.132	0.033	6.74×10^{-5}
Naïve CD8+T	− 0.142	0.033	2.54×10^{-5}
Naïve CD4+T	−0.072	0.034	0.032
B cell	−0.063	0.033	0.052
Natural killer	−0.055	0.033	0.094
Senescent CD8+T	0.134	0.033	3.79×10^{-5}
Monocytes	0.052	0.034	0.123
Plasmablasts	0.148	0.034	1.38×10^{-5}
Granulocytes	0.133	0.033	4.17×10^{-5}

age, whereas the pro-inflammatory cytokine IL-6 was found to increase in the cohort across the two waves of follow-up from age 73 to 76. We found a decline over time in naïve and total CD8+T cells, naïve and total CD4+T cells, NK cells and B cells. Congruent with flow cytometric data, senescent CD8+T cells were found to increase with age, as did monocytes, granulocytes and plasmablasts [16]. Negative baseline associations were found between CRP and both naïve and total CD8+T cells and CD4+T cells, and positive associations between CRP and senescent CD8+T cells, plasmablasts and granulocytes. We report associations between both high- and low-sensitivity measures of CRP, IL-6 and a restricted CRP measure (≤ 10 mg/L) with extrinsic estimates of epigenetic age acceleration. These findings suggest a higher epigenetic age is associated with an increased inflammatory profile, in relation to both general inflammation, and to levels likely reflecting chronic, low-grade inflammation.

The dynamics of the low-sensitivity CRP in the cohort were paradoxical to what we might have predicted in a longitudinal study of ageing as previous studies have shown a progressive increase in CRP levels as a function of age [7, 19]. Furthermore, IL-6 is a major driving factor in CRP production, yet, despite observing a rise in the cytokine over waves 2 and 3, no corresponding increase is seen in the low-sensitivity CRP levels; in fact, the opposite is seen. These findings may be due to the poor sensitivity of the assay used to quantify the CRP levels, particularly at the lower range of values, though levels were found to correlate strongly with those from the more sensitive measure. It is possible that a disruption in the pathway of CRP production impacted our results. CRP is of hepatic origin and it is feasible that impaired liver function, which is common in older adults, influenced its production within individuals in the cohort. Similarly, CRP production is influenced by other cytokines alongside IL-6, such as IL-1 and IL-17, and as these were not measured in the current study, their potential influence is unknown [20]. Another explanation may lie in the fact the LBC1936 is a largely healthy older ageing cohort. Multiple chronic conditions are common in elderly populations, and our results may reflect a more successful ageing process revealed through more static or declining CRP levels. Though part of the innate immune system, inflammation may be a somewhat adaptive response in older age and research has indicated it might confer protection when under tight control [18, 21]. Indeed, centenarians often have signs of systemic inflammation but are not afflicted by age-associated diseases [22]. It is often argued that inflammation is beneficial in neutralising harmful stimuli in early life but becomes detrimental in older age; however, it may be that optimum levels of inflammation change, but continue to exist, in old age and excessive, insufficient, or

Table 3 Baseline and longitudinal associations between log-transformed inflammatory biomarkers and epigenetic age acceleration

	IEAA*			EEAA†		
	Standardised beta	SE	*p*	Standardised beta	SE	*p*
Baseline						
Low-sensitivity CRP	0.057	0.033	0.087	0.154	0.034	2.48×10^{-5}
High-sensitivity CRP	0.047	0.036	0.189	0.111	0.037	0.004
IL-6	0.021	0.036	0.563	0.114	0.037	0.003
Low-sensitivity CRP ≤ 10 mg/L	0.062	0.035	0.081	0.129	0.039	0.0009
Longitudinal						
Low-sensitivity CRP	−0.017	0.019	0.360	−0.008	0.019	0.672
High-sensitivity CRP	0.005	0.039	0.888	−0.006	0.039	0.888
IL-6	0.034	0.041	0.392	0.009	0.042	0.829
Low-sensitivity CRP ≤ 10 mg/L	−0.020	0.020	0.303	−0.006	0.020	0.759

CRP C-reactive protein, *IL-6* interleukin 6
*Intrinsic epigenetic age acceleration
†Extrinsic epigenetic age acceleration

highly fluctuating, levels could exacerbate the risk of disease. Finally, the mean age of the cohort at wave 1 was 70 years, and it is possible participants had already undergone a transition to an increased inflammatory profile and this is why we did not capture a rise in CRP over time. This is in line with findings from a previous study which reported an increased serum level of CRP between a 20–30-year-old age group and 60–70-year-olds, but no significant difference in levels between 60–70-year-olds and the 70–90-year-olds [23].

Because of the complexity in the inflammatory trajectories, and given that adaptive immune dysregulation is thought to be an important reciprocal mechanism to age-related inflammation, we additionally examined the dynamics of the immune cells imputed from the methylation data, and their association with CRP. It is important to highlight, however, that whilst we modelled the cell trajectories, the Houseman algorithm does not quantify actual cell counts, but instead yields cellular proportions, and the Horvath method estimates abundances (interpreted on an ordinal scale). We therefore cannot definitively establish whether the alterations in their profiles were due to a true change in the dimensions of the cell population or were instead a consequential shift due to alterations in other cell numbers. The baseline associations between CRP and the cells were not congruent, indicating the relationship between inflammatory mediators and individual immune cells is not uniform, with different compartments of the system displaying different relative characteristics. The interrelationship between inflammation and the immune system is clearly complex and the dyad is probably influenced further by other additional pathophysiological pathways activated in older age. Our results fit with the remodelling theory of ageing which postulates that immunosenescence or 'immuno remodelling' is a dynamic process involving both loss and gains of immune function [21, 24]. This theory hypothesises that those with a superior capacity to adapt their inflammatory and immune responses, rather than necessarily generating the most robust response, age most successfully. Exactly which of these alterations may be beneficial, and which detrimental, remains to be determined.

Despite no evidence of an increase in CRP with chronological age within the cohort, we found positive associations between all inflammatory biomarkers and extrinsic epigenetic age acceleration, suggesting a faster running epigenetic clock is associated with an increased inflammatory profile. No parallel association was seen between any of the inflammatory mediators and the intrinsic (cell-adjusted) measure of age acceleration. This discordance may be due to the difference in the two estimates. IEAA is calculated independently of the blood cellular composition, measures cell-intrinsic methylation changes, and likely captures an ageing process that is mostly conserved across cell types. Contrastingly, EEAA does capture age-related alterations in leukocyte composition and correlates with health-related characteristics [25]. Evidently, systemic inflammation is closely tied to the blood tissue and so is perhaps more likely to be discerned by a blood-based measure than one that focuses on multiple tissue types. Our results are similar to a recent cross-sectional study on a cohort of middle-aged adults where EEAA was found to correlate strongly with CRP and IL-6 but no similar association was found with IEAA [26].

The main strength of this study is its basis in a relatively large sample of older people with long-term follow-up. The repeated measures of the serum biomarkers have permitted both a description of their trajectories across the eighth decade, and the investigation of longitudinal associations with biological age. The study may have been limited by the cohort effect; as discussed above, the sample is representative of healthier older ageing and findings may not be relevant to typical ageing in which multi-morbidity is common. Further investigation in independent cohorts is necessary to validate these findings. Additionally, we only examined a restricted number of inflammatory variables and the observed associations with epigenetic age acceleration do not provide evidence of causation. As the trajectories of the inflammatory biomarkers were complex, it is difficult to determine which is most representative. IL-6, which showed a significant increase, may be a more indicative or reliable measure of inflammation, but as it was only available for two time--points we focused our analyses on CRP. Recent results have questioned the utility of DNA methylation patterns as biomarkers of ageing, as a reduced prediction error of chronological age was found in studies using larger sample sizes to train the age predictor [27]. These findings indicate a limitation in the variation in biological age that is captured by DNA methylation and so caution is needed in the interpretation of results from epigenetic age predictors. Finally, we did not apply a correction for multiple testing. Applying a strict Bonferonni-corrected threshold of significance would result in the attenuation of the less highly significant finding of the association between total CD8+T cells and CRP.

Conclusion

The dynamics of the assessed inflammatory markers did not conclusively confirm an increased inflammatory state with older chronological age. We found, however, that a faster running epigenetic clock, as measured by extrinsic epigenetic age acceleration, associated with a raised inflammatory profile cross-sectionally. This association should be investigated further in other independent populations and with respect to causal inference. The relationship between CRP and imputed immune cell counts suggest a divergent association between inflammatory mediators and immune parameters. Whether these are adaptive responses or detrimental changes is unclear and should be addressed by future studies.

Methods

The Lothian Birth Cohort 1936 (LBC1936)

Details of the LBC1936 study have been described previously [28]. Briefly, the cohort comprises individuals born in 1936, most of whom who took part in the Scottish Mental Survey 1947, aged about 11 years. One thousand and ninety-one participants were recruited to the study at a mean age of 70 years and, to date, have completed up to four waves of testing at mean ages of 70, 73, 76 and 79. Data collection for wave 5 is ongoing [29]. At each wave, participants have been extensively phenotyped with data obtained on a wide range of health outcomes, lifestyle factors, psycho-social variables, genetics and epigenetics, and cognition.

CRP and IL-6

Serum CRP (mg/L) and IL-6 (pg/ml) were measured from venesected whole-blood samples. CRP levels were quantified using both a regular-sensitivity assay (low-sensitivity CRP) at all four waves of data collection, and a high-sensitivity assay (high-sensitivity CRP) at waves 2 and 3. The low-sensitivity assay was performed using a dry-slide immuno-rate method on an OrthoFusion 5.1 F.S analysers (Ortho Clinical Diagnostics). This assay cannot distinguish values less than 3 mg/L, and all readings less than 3 mg/L were assigned a value of 1.5 mg/L. The high-sensitivity assay was performed at the University of Glasgow using an enzyme-linked immunosorbent assay (ELISA; R&D Systems, Oxford, UK) [30]. Though the high-sensitivity assay is more accurate and would have been preferred in analysis, more longitudinal data was available from the lower-sensitivity assay, so both measures were included to establish the equivalence in their trajectories and associations with epigenetic age. IL-6 levels were determined using high-sensitivity ELISA kits (R&D Systems, Oxford, UK) at waves 2 and 3 [31].

To account for skewed distributions, both CRP and IL-6 levels were log-transformed (natural log) prior to analyses.

Cell counts

Blood cell proportions were estimated based on DNA methylation signatures as described by Chen et al. [16]. Briefly, two approaches were used: Houseman's estimation method and the Horvath method. Houseman's method uses methylation signatures from purified leukocytes to estimate the proportion of CD8+T cells, CD4+T cells, natural killer cells, B cells, monocytes and granulocytes [32]. The Horvath method, calculated via the advanced analysis option of the epigenetic age calculator software, was used to estimate the ordinal abundance of exhausted/senescent CD8+T cells, naïve CD4+T and CD8+T cells and plasmablasts [11, 33]. Imputed cell counts have been shown to have a moderate correlation with reciprocal flow cytometric data [34].

Epigenetic age acceleration

Methodological details of the methylation profiling for LBC1936 are provided in (Additional file 2).

Age acceleration was calculated for each subject at each wave using the online calculator developed by Horvath (https://dnamage.genetics.ucla.edu/) [11].

Two established measures of methylation-based age acceleration were used in this study: intrinsic epigenetic age acceleration (IEAA) and extrinsic epigenetic age acceleration (EEAA). IEAA, based on methylation at 353 CpG sites across multiple tissues as described by Horvath, captures 'pure', cell-intrinsic epigenetic ageing, independent of age-related changes in blood cell composition [11]. It is defined as the residual resulting from a multivariate regression model of Horvath methylation age on chronological age and estimates of various blood immune cell counts imputed from methylation data.

Conversely, EEAA, an enhanced version of the Hannum clock based on 71 CpGs, up-weights the contribution of immune blood cell counts, in addition to tracking intrinsic methylation changes [12]. EEAA is calculated through use of a weighted average of Hannum's methylation age with three cell types that are known to change with age—naïve cytotoxic T cells, exhausted cytotoxic T cells and plasmablasts—using the Klerma-Doubal approach [35]. EEAA is defined as the residual variation resulting from regressing the weighted estimated age on chronological age [16].

Statistical analysis

Linear mixed models were used to investigate the baseline relationship between the inflammatory biomarker levels and the imputed cell counts and epigenetic age acceleration measures independently. In each model, age, sex and anti-inflammatory drug status (collected at baseline and coded as a dichotomous variable: on medication = 1; not on medication = 0) were included as covariates. Batch effects (set, position, array, plate and date) were included as random effects to control for technical artefacts.

Mixed effect models were used to examine the longitudinal change in cell counts and inflammatory biomarkers over the four waves for the low-sensitivity CRP, and two waves for the high-sensitivity CRP and IL-6. Here, sex and baseline use of anti-inflammatory medication were included as covariates, and age (years) as the timescale. Participant ID and batch effects were fitted as random effects on the intercept. Interaction terms (between chronological age and baseline epigenetic age acceleration, both centred to have mean 0 and SD 1) were included to investigate the changes in inflammatory biomarker levels with age predicted by baseline epigenetic age acceleration. Thus, the model formula was the following: inflammatory_biomarker ~ age*baseline_DNAm_age + sex + anti_inflammatory_status + (1|ID) + (1|set) + (1|date) + (1|array) + (1|position) + (1|plate).

Pearson correlations were calculated between IL-6 and the high- and low-sensitivity CRP measures, and between low-sensitivity CRP and the imputed cell counts at each wave separately.

Analyses were performed in R Version 3.5.0 using the 'lmerTest' library (Version 3.0–1) [36, 37].

Abbreviations

CRP: C-reactive protein; EEAA: Extrinsic epigenetic age acceleration; IEAA: Intrinsic epigenetic age acceleration; IL-6: Interleukin-6; LBC1936: Lothian Birth Cohort 1936; SD: Standard deviation; SE: Standard error

Acknowledgements

The authors thank all LBC1936 study participants and research team members who have contributed, and continue to contribute, to ongoing LBC1936 study.

Funding

The Lothian Birth Cohort 1936 is supported by Age UK (Disconnected Mind programme) and the Medical Research Council (MR/M01311/1). Methylation typing was supported by the Centre for Cognitive Ageing and Cognitive Epidemiology (Pilot Fund award), Age UK, The Wellcome Trust Institutional Strategic Support Fund, The University of Edinburgh, and The University of Queensland. This work was conducted in the Centre for Cognitive Ageing and Cognitive Epidemiology, which is supported by the Medical Research Council and Biotechnology and Biological Sciences Research Council (MR/K026992/1). This current study was partly supported by funding from the Wellcome Trust 4-year PhD in Translational Neuroscience – training the next generation of basic neuroscientists to embrace clinical research [108890/Z/15/Z to AJS]. The funders played no role in the design of the study, collection, analysis or interpretation of the data or in writing of the manuscript.

Authors' contributions

REM, DLM and AJS designed the research. AJS analysed the data and wrote the manuscript. PR, QZ, AFM, JMS and SEH prepared the data. AMT and IJD collected the data. All authors read, revised and approved the final manuscript.

Competing interests

The authors declare that they have no competing interests.

Author details

[1]Centre for Genomic and Experimental Medicine, Institute of Genetics and Molecular Medicine, University of Edinburgh, Edinburgh, UK. [2]Centre for Cognitive Ageing and Cognitive Epidemiology, University of Edinburgh, Edinburgh, UK. [3]Department for Psychology, University of Edinburgh, Edinburgh, UK. [4]Alzheimer Scotland Dementia Research Centre, University of Edinburgh, Edinburgh, UK. [5]Institute for Molecular Bioscience, University of Queensland, Brisbane, Queensland, Australia. [6]UK Dementia Research Institute, Edinburgh Medical School, University of Edinburgh, Edinburgh, UK. [7]Centre for Discovery Brain Sciences, University of Edinburgh, Edinburgh, UK. [8]Division of Psychiatry, Centre for Clinical Brain Sciences, University of Edinburgh, Edinburgh, UK.

References

1. Franceschi C, Bonafe M, Valensin S, Olivieri F, De Luca M, Ottaviani E, et al. Inflamm-aging. An evolutionary perspective on immunosenescence. Ann N Y Acad Sci. 2000;908:244–54.
2. Baylis D, Bartlett DB, Patel HP, Roberts HC. Understanding how we age: insights into inflammaging. Longevity & Healthspan. 2013;2:8.
3. Xia S, Zhang X, Zheng S, Khanabdali R, Kalionis B, Wu J, et al. An update on Inflamm-aging: mechanisms, prevention, and treatment. J Immunol Res. 2016;2016:8426874.
4. Kaptoge S, Di Angelantonio E, Lowe G, Pepys MB, Thompson SG, Collins R, et al. C-reactive protein concentration and risk of coronary heart disease, stroke, and mortality: an individual participant meta-analysis. Lancet (London, England). 2010;375(9709):132–40.
5. Puzianowska-Kuźnicka M, Owczarz M, Wieczorowska-Tobis K, Nadrowski P, Chudek J, Slusarczyk P, et al. Interleukin-6 and C-reactive protein, successful aging, and mortality: the PolSenior study. Immunity & Ageing : I & A. 2016;13:21.
6. Fougere B, Boulanger E, Nourhashemi F, Guyonnet S, Cesari M. Chronic inflammation: accelerator of biological aging. J Gerontol A Biol Sci Med Sci. 2017;72(9):1218–25.
7. Singh T, Newman AB. Inflammatory markers in population studies of aging. Ageing Res Rev. 2011;10(3):319–29.
8. Bonafe M, Olivieri F, Cavallone L, Giovagnetti S, Mayegiani F, Cardelli M, et al. A gender--dependent genetic predisposition to produce high levels of IL-6 is detrimental for longevity. Eur J Immunol. 2001;31(8):2357–61.
9. Suk HJ, Ridker PM, Cook NR, Zee RY. Relation of polymorphism within the C-reactive protein gene and plasma CRP levels. Atherosclerosis. 2005;178(1):139–45.
10. Vickers MA, Green FR, Terry C, Mayosi BM, Julier C, Lathrop M, et al. Genotype at a promoter polymorphism of the interleukin-6 gene is associated with baseline levels of plasma C-reactive protein. Cardiovasc Res. 2002;53(4):1029–34.
11. Horvath S. DNA methylation age of human tissues and cell types. Genome Biol. 2013;14(10):R115.
12. Hannum G, Guinney J, Zhao L, Zhang L, Hughes G, Sadda S, et al. Genome-wide methylation profiles reveal quantitative views of human aging rates. Mol Cell. 2013;49(2):359–67.
13. Breitling LP, Saum KU, Perna L, Schottker B, Holleczek B, Brenner H. Frailty is associated with the epigenetic clock but not with telomere length in a German cohort. Clin Epigenetics. 2016;8:21.
14. Levine ME, Hosgood HD, Chen B, Absher D, Assimes T, Horvath S. DNA methylation age of blood predicts future onset of lung cancer in the women's health initiative. Aging (Albany NY). 2015;7(9):690–700.
15. Horvath S, Ritz BR. Increased epigenetic age and granulocyte counts in the blood of Parkinson's disease patients. Aging (Albany NY). 2015;7(12):1130–42.
16. Chen BH, Marioni RE, Colicino E, Peters MJ, Ward-Caviness CK, Tsai P-C, et al. DNA methylation-based measures of biological age: meta-analysis predicting time to death. Aging (Albany NY). 2016;8(9):1844–59.
17. Marioni RE, Shah S, McRae AF, Ritchie SJ, Muniz-Terrera G, Harris SE, et al. The epigenetic clock is correlated with physical and cognitive fitness in the Lothian Birth Cohort 1936. Int J Epidemiol. 2015;44(4):1388–96.
18. Lassale C, Batty GD, Steptoe A, Cadar D, Akbaraly TN, Kivimaki M, et al. Association of 10-year C-reactive protein trajectories with markers of healthy aging: findings from the English Longitudinal Study of Ageing. The journals of gerontology Series A, Biological sciences and medical sciences. 2018.
19. Ferrucci L, Corsi A, Lauretani F, Bandinelli S, Bartali B, Taub DD, et al. The origins of age-related proinflammatory state. Blood. 2005;105(6):2294–9.
20. Eklund CM. Proinflammatory cytokines in CRP baseline regulation. Adv Clin Chem. 2009;48:111–36.
21. Fulop T, Larbi A, Dupuis G, Le Page A, Frost EH, Cohen AA, et al. Immunosenescence and inflamm-aging as two sides of the same coin: friends or foes? Front Immunol. 2017;8:1960.
22. Franceschi C, Campisi J. Chronic inflammation (inflammaging) and its potential contribution to age-associated diseases. J Gerontol A Biol Sci Med Sci. 2014;69(Suppl 1):S4–9.
23. Wyczalkowska-Tomasik A, Czarkowska-Paczek B, Zielenkiewicz M, Paczek L. Inflammatory markers change with age, but do not fall beyond reported normal ranges. Arch Immunol Ther Exp. 2016;64:249–54.
24. Franceschi C, Valensin S, Bonafe M, Paolisso G, Yashin AI, Monti D, et al. The network and the remodeling theories of aging: historical background and new perspectives. Exp Gerontol. 2000;35(6–7):879–96.

25. Lu AT, Xue L, Salfati EL, Chen BH, Ferrucci L, Levy D, et al. GWAS of epigenetic aging rates in blood reveals a critical role for TERT. Nat Commun. 2018;9(1):387.
26. Irvin MR, Aslibekyan S, Do A, Zhi D, Hidalgo B, Claas SA, et al. Metabolic and inflammatory biomarkers are associated with epigenetic aging acceleration estimates in the GOLDN study. Clin Epigenetics. 2018;10:56.
27. Zhang Q, Vallerga C, Walker R, Lin T, Henders A, Montgomery G, et al. Improved prediction of chronological age from DNA methylation limits it as a biomarker of ageing. In: bioRxiv; 2018.
28. Deary IJ, Gow AJ, Pattie A, Starr JM. Cohort profile: the Lothian Birth Cohorts of 1921 and 1936. Int J Epidemiol. 2012;41(6):1576–84.
29. Taylor AM, Pattie A, Deary IJ. Cohort profile update: the Lothian Birth Cohorts of 1921 and 1936. Int J Epidemiol. 2018;41(6):1576–84.
30. Aribisala BS, Wiseman S, Morris Z, Valdes-Hernandez MC, Royle NA, Maniega SM, et al. Circulating inflammatory markers are associated with magnetic resonance imaging-visible perivascular spaces but not directly with white matter hyperintensities. Stroke. 2014;45(2):605–7.
31. Mõttus R, Luciano M, Starr JM, Pollard MC, Deary IJ. Personality traits and inflammation in men and women in their early 70s. Psychosom Med. 2013; 75(1):11–9.
32. Houseman EA, Accomando WP, Koestler DC, Christensen BC, Marsit CJ, Nelson HH, et al. DNA methylation arrays as surrogate measures of cell mixture distribution. BMC bioinformatics. 2012;13:86.
33. Horvath S, Levine AJ. HIV-1 infection accelerates age according to the epigenetic clock. J Infect Dis. 2015;212(10):1563–73.
34. Horvath S, Gurven M, Levine ME, Trumble BC, Kaplan H, Allayee H, et al. An epigenetic clock analysis of race/ethnicity, sex, and coronary heart disease. Genome Biol. 2016;17(1):171.
35. Klemera P, Doubal S. A new approach to the concept and computation of biological age. Mech Ageing Dev. 2006;127(3):240–8.
36. Kuznetsova A, Brockhoff PB, Christensen RHB. lmerTest: Tests in Linear Mixed Effects Models. R package version 2.0-33. 2016.
37. R Core Team. R: a language and environment for statistical computing. Vienna, R Foundation for Statistical Computing; 2018.

19

Differential open chromatin profile and transcriptomic signature define depot-specific human subcutaneous preadipocytes

Adeline Divoux[1,2*†], Katalin Sandor[2,6†], Dora Bojcsuk[3], Amlan Talukder[4], Xiaoman Li[5], Balint L. Balint[3], Timothy F. Osborne[2,6] and Steven R. Smith[1,2]

Abstract

Background: Increased lower body fat is associated with reduced cardiometabolic risk. The molecular basis for depot-specific differences in gluteofemoral (GF) compared with abdominal (A) subcutaneous adipocyte function is poorly understood. In the current report, we used a combination of Assay for Transposase-Accessible Chromatin followed by sequencing (ATAC-seq), RNA-seq, and chromatin immunoprecipitation (ChIP)-qPCR analyses that provide evidence that depot-specific gene expression patterns are associated with differential epigenetic chromatin signatures.

Methods: Preadipocytes cultured from A and GF adipose tissue obtained from premenopausal apple-shaped women were used to perform transcriptome analysis by RNA-seq and assess accessible chromatin regions by ATAC-seq. We measured mRNA expression and performed ChIP-qPCR experiments for histone modifications of active (H3K4me3) and repressed chromatin (H3K27me3) regions respectively on the promoter regions of differentially expressed genes.

Results: RNA-seq experiments revealed an A-fat and GF-fat selective gene expression signature, with 126 genes upregulated in abdominal preadipocytes and 90 genes upregulated in GF cells. ATAC-seq identified almost 10-times more A-specific chromatin-accessible regions. Using a combined analysis of ATAC-seq and global gene expression data, we identified 74 of the 126 abdominal-specific genes (59%) with A-specific accessible chromatin sites within 200 kb of the transcription start site (TSS), including HOXA3, HOXA5, IL8, IL1b, and IL6. Interestingly, only 14 of the 90 GF-specific genes (15%) had GF-specific accessible chromatin sites within 200 kb of the corresponding TSS, including HOXC13 and HOTAIR, whereas 25 of them (28%) had abdominal-specific accessible chromatin sites. ChIP-qPCR experiments confirmed that the active H3K4me3 chromatin mark was significantly enriched at the promoter regions of HOXA5 and HOXA3 genes in abdominal preadipocytes, while H3K27me3 was less abundant relative to chromatin from GF. This is consistent with their A-fat specific gene expression pattern. Conversely, analysis of the promoter regions of the GF specific HOTAIR and HOXC13 genes exhibited high H3K4me3 and low H3K27me3 levels in GF chromatin compared to A chromatin.

(Continued on next page)

* Correspondence: adeline.divoux@flhosp.org
†Adeline Divoux and Katalin Sandor contributed equally to this work.
[1]Translational Research Institute for Metabolism and Diabetes, Florida Hospital, 301 E. Princeton Street, Orlando, FL 32804, USA
[2]Diabetes and Obesity Research Center, Sanford Burnham Prebys Medical Discovery Institute at Lake Nona, Orlando, FL, USA
Full list of author information is available at the end of the article

(Continued from previous page)

Conclusions: Global transcriptome and open chromatin analyses of depot-specific preadipocytes identified their gene expression signature and differential open chromatin profile. Interestingly, A-fat-specific open chromatin regions can be observed in the proximity of GF-fat genes, but not vice versa.

Keywords: Chromatin openness, Gene expression, Histone marks, Preadipocytes, Fat distribution, Abdominal fat, Gluteofemoral fat

Introduction

As body weight increases, the distribution of body fat becomes an important factor that determines metabolic health [1]. Excess intra-abdominal fat storage is well-known to be associated with increased cardiovascular and metabolic risks [2, 3]. As compared to other fat depots, visceral adipose tissue has increased metabolic activity, specifically both lipid uptake and lipolysis. Free fatty acids, the product of lipolysis, induce peripheral insulin resistance thereby inhibiting skeletal muscle uptake. However, over the past 15 years, growing evidence supports a primary role of subcutaneous adipose tissue in the metabolic complications of obesity and in the development of insulin resistance [4–7]. Importantly, Jensen demonstrated that the upper body non-visceral fat was the major source of free fatty acids in humans, with intra-abdominal (visceral) adipose tissue contributing to only 15% of the total systemic free fatty acids [6]. A very recent study where the authors collected the data from the National Health and Nutrition Examination Survey for the years 1999–2006 established in the same manner a strong association between upper body fat and metabolic risk factors independent of visceral fat [8]. In contrast, preferential fat accumulation in the lower body, or gluteal-femoral (GF) depot, is now recognized to be protective against the deleterious cardiometabolic effects of obesity [9, 10]. A common hypothesis is that lower body fat serves as a "sink" for excess energy sequestering lipid away from visceral adipose tissue and also preventing fat accumulation in other unhealthy areas such as the liver, pancreas, and muscle [11]. Regional gene expression differences that influence preadipocyte proliferation, differentiation, and subtype abundance likely contribute to regional variations in fat tissue function (for reviews, see [12–14]). However, the exact physiological, metabolic, or endocrine mechanisms underlying the beneficial effects of lower body fat deposition remain unknown.

Multiple studies, including our own work, reported that the homeobox (HOX) family and HOX domain-encoding genes (SHOX2 and IRBX2) are differentially expressed between the two major subcutaneous tissue depots, abdominal and GF [15–17]. Interestingly, preadipocytes isolated from these depots, cultured and differentiated under the same conditions, retain the unique gene expression profile characteristic of depot origin, and the differences are maintained during conversion into lipid-laden adipocytes [18, 19]. Importantly, we discovered that the lncRNA HOTAIR known to be involved in the epigenetic regulation of cancer progression [20, 21] is only expressed at appreciable levels in GF-fat and isolated preadipocytes from GF [22]. Altogether, these observations strongly indicate there is a depot-specific epigenetic program that is involved in adipose tissue patterning which may be also influence pathologic downstream effects in obesity.

Current knowledge is limited concerning the chromatin status of adipose tissue from different anatomical locations. To date, only one study investigated the DNA methylome of the human A- and GF-fat by using DNA methylation array in a heterogenous group of subjects [15]. Chromatin accessibility represents another essential level of genome regulation. In the present study, we investigated depot-specific chromatin structure and gene expression using preadipocytes isolated from human subcutaneous adipose tissue. We report on the differences in chromatin openness and transcriptomic signatures of the A and GF preadipocytes in order to better understand the basis for the differential programming of anatomically distinct scWAT depots.

Methods

Participants

Six healthy premenopausal, weight-stable females aged 20–40 years with a body mass index (BMI) (calculated as weight in kilograms divided by height in meters squared) between 27 and 40 kg/m^2 were recruited in Orlando using advertisements approved by an institutional review board. Subjects were excluded if they reported a history of chronic disease (diabetes, heart or liver disease, high blood pressure, gastrointestinal disorder), recent weight loss or gain (> 3 kg over the past 8 weeks), had abnormal blood or urine values, or use of oral contraceptives or hormone replacement therapy. Adipose tissue biopsies were collected with a three-hole 2.5-mm liposuction cannula from the mid-abdomen approximately 5–8 cm lateral to the umbilicus. Gluteofemoral adipose tissue was collected 10–20 cm below the greater trochanter on the most lateral side of the upper thigh. Samples were cleaned at the bedside; a fraction of it was snap frozen in liquid nitrogen, and the rest was immediately used for preadipocyte isolation.

The characteristics of the study group are presented in Table 1. Two subjects of this group were randomly selected to perform genome-wide analysis.

Isolation of preadipocytes and culture conditions

Stromal vascular fractions were isolated from scWAT abdominal and GF depot, plated, and grown as previously described [23] with the addition of hEGF and hFGF (Life Technologies, 10 μg/ml and 4 μg/ml, respectively) during the expansion phase [24]. The preadipocyte population was initially purified by depletion of the stromal vascular fraction from macrophages (CD14- and CD206-positive cells) and endothelial cells (CD31-positive cells) using fluorescence-activated cell sorting. At confluence, cells were harvested and used for Assay for Transposase-Accessible Chromatin followed by sequencing (ATAC-seq) or chromatin isolation as described above. A fraction of the cells were frozen for RNA extraction.

RNA-seq

RNA was isolated using RNeasy Mini Kit (Qiagen) from abdominal and GF preadipocytes. Approximately 2 μg was used for library preparation with TruSeq RNA Sample Preparation Kit (Illumina). Following purification, RNA was fragmented with divalent cations at 85 °C, and then cDNA was generated by random primers and SuperScript II enzyme (Life Technologies). Second-strand synthesis was performed followed by end repair, single "A" base addition, and ligation of barcode indexed adaptors to the DNA fragments. Adapter-specific PCRs were performed to generate sequencing libraries. Libraries were size selected with E-Gel EX 2% agarose gels (Life Technologies) and purified by QIAquick Gel Extraction Kit (Qiagen). The result is libraries with inserts ranging in size from 120 to 210 bp with a median size of 155 bp. Libraries were sequenced on HiSeq 2500 instrument.

Table 1 Clinical parameters of women subjects (mean ± standard deviation)

Clinical parameters	Obese subjects (*n* = 6)
Age (years)	34 ± 4.7
Adiposity markers	
BMI (kg/m^2)	34.0 ± 2.81
Body weight (kg)	95.4 ± 6.80
Waist to hip ratio	0.94 ± 0.04
Total fat mass (kg)	40.6 ± 4.73
Total lean mass (kg)	53.2 ± 3.92
% fat mass	43.0 ± 2.92
Metabolic markers	
Systolic blood pressure (mm Hg)	113 ± 4.85
Diastolic blood pressure (mm Hg)	68.0 ± 6.02
Glucose (mg/dL)	94.5 ± 12.9
Insulin (mU/L)	6.24 ± 2.85
FFA (mmol/L)	0.43 ± 0.06
TSH (mUI/L)	1.59 ± 0.36

ATAC-seq

ATAC-seq was carried out as described earlier [25]. After trypsinization, abdominal and GF preadipocytes nuclei were isolated. Nuclei were used for tagmentation using Nextera DNA Library Preparation Kit (Illumina). After tagmentation, DNA was purified with MinElute PCR Purification Kit (Qiagen). Tagmented DNA was amplified with Kapa HiFi Hot Start Kit (Kapa Biosystems) using 16 PCR cycles. Amplified libraries were purified with Agencourt AMPure XP (Beckman Coulter). Fragment distribution of libraries was assessed with Agilent Bioanalyzer, and libraries were sequenced on a HiSeq 2500 platform.

Real-time quantitative RT-PCR

Total RNA from adipose tissue and preadipocytes were extracted using the lipid RNeasy kit and the RNeasy mini kit (Qiagen), respectively. Gene expression was assessed by real-time PCR using a ViiA7 sequence detection system (Life Technologies) and Taqman technology suitable for relative gene expression quantification using the following parameters: 1 cycle of 95 °C for 10 min, followed by 40 cycles at 95 °C for 10 s and 60 °C for 1 min. All samples were normalized to PPIA showing low variability between A and GF samples (Additional file 1: Figure S1).

Chromatin Immunoprecipitation-PCR assay

Chromatin immunoprecipitations (ChIPs) were performed and analyzed as described [26]. Briefly, cells were crosslinked for 10 min with 1% formaldehyde and quenched 8 min with glycine (125 mM). Cells were incubated in buffer A (10 mM Tris, 1 mM KCl, 1.5 mM MgCl2) for 10 min on ice then dounce homogenized with 10 strokes. The mixture was centrifuged, and the pellet was resuspended in buffer B (50 mM Tris-HCl, 10 mM EDTA, 1% SDS) and kept for 10 min on ice. DNA was sonicated to obtain 300–1000 bp fragments with the Diagenode Bioruptor sonicator (high setting with 30 s on/off cycle during 15 min). The rabbit polyclonal H3K4me3 and H3K27me3 antibodies (Diagenode) were used to study the histone marks; a Rabbit IgG was used as a negative control. Dynabeads (Life Technologies) blocked with PBS 1% BSA were used to immunoprecipitate the complexes.

ChIP-PCR primers (Table 2) were designed to amplify the promoter regions from the specific HOX genes as detailed in Figs. 5 and 6. Primers were also designed for a region of the GAPDH locus for a positive control and G6Pase for a negative control.

RNA-seq analysis

Raw sequence data were aligned to the hg19 reference genome assembly (GRCh37) by using TopHat (v2.0.7). The fragments per kilobase of transcript per million mapped reads (FPKM) values were calculated by Cufflinks (v2.0.2) with default parameters [27]. Differentially expressed genes per subjects were determined by the Cuffdiff algorithm of Cufflinks, and only genes with $p \leq 0.05$ in both subjects were used to further analyses (Additional file 2: Table S1). Gene expression heat map was visualized by using the *pheatmap* function of the pheatmap package in R. The values were normalized per rows.

ATAC-seq analysis

Raw sequence reads were aligned to the hg19 reference genome assembly (GRCh37) by using the Burrows-Wheeler Alignment (BWA) tool (v07.10) [28], and then BAM files were generated with SAMtools (v0.1.19) [29]. "Peaks" were predicted using the Model-based Analysis of ChIP-Seq (MACS2) tool (v2.0.10) [30]. To remove the artifacts from the predicted peaks, we used the blacklisted genomic regions of the Encyclopedia of DNA Elements (ENCODE) [31]. Fragment length was set to 150 nucleotides by the *makeTagDirectory* program of the Hypergeometric Optimization of Motif EnRichment (HOMER) package (v4.2) [32].

Coverage (bedgraph) files were created by the *makeUCSCfile.pl* program of HOMER. A consensus set was generated from those peaks which could be predicted from at least two samples, and "summit coverage" values (on the middle 50-bp bins) were calculated based on this set by *annotatePeaks.pl* (HOMER) with *-hist 50* and *-ghist* parameters. Each value within the coverage files was divided with the median value of "summit coverage." Upon this normalization, bedgraph files were converted to tiled data formats (.tdf) by using the *toTDF* command of the IGVtools program (v2.3.9) [33]. Median normalized read distribution plots of overlapping and depot-specific peaks were also generated. Peak annotation was determined by *annotatePeaks.pl.* Histograms, created also with *annotatePeaks.pl*, show the average tag densities of the peaks relative to the transcription start site (TSS) ± 250 bp in 1-bp resolution. Overlapping and depot- or subject-specific peaks were determined using the *intersectBed* program of BedTools (v2.23.0) [34].

DiffBind analysis

Correlation heat maps of ATAC-seq peak densities were created by differential binding analysis (DBA) using the DiffBind package (v1.2.4) in R. Regions that were predicted from at least two samples (minOverlap parameter was set to 2) and were found differently opened between the depots according to a $P \leq 0.005$ threshold were used for visualization and further analyses. For volcano plots, significance and log fold change values were calculated by DiffBind. ATAC-seq peaks within ± 100 kb to the TSS of depot-specific genes but not farther than the neighboring gene (BedTools) were used for further DiffBind analyses.

Motif analysis

Motif enrichment analysis was carried out by *findMotifsGenome.pl* (HOMER). It was performed on the ± 100 bp flanking regions of the peak summits or in the ± 250 bp regions of genes TSSs. The search lengths of the motifs were 8, 10, 12, and 14 bp. *p* values were calculated by comparing the enrichments within the target regions and those of a random set of regions (background) generated by HOMER.

Visualization of the ATAC-seq data

Volcano plots, box plots, and histograms were created with GraphPad Prism 6. Coverage files were visualized by Integrative Genomics Viewer (IGV).

RT-qPCR and ChIP-qPCR analysis

To compare A-fat vs. GF-fat gene expression and histone marks in obese subjects, individual data are presented and paired *t* tests were used. ChIP-PCR data are presented as a percent of 5% input. All statistical analyses on clinical data were performed in SAS (V11.2.1).

Table 2 List of primer sequences used for real-time PCR to quantify the ChIP-assays

Gene	Forward	Reverse
HOTAIR (−329)	GTGAGCTCGCGGCATTTTTA	GCATTTTCGACCCAGGCATC
HOXA3 (− 313)	GGGGGTAGGGAGGAATTTGC	CCTGACCCCCAAGAACTCAC
HOXA5 (− 398)	TGGCTAAATGGCTTTCCCCC	CCGTTTTGCAGCCCCTCTTA
HOXC13 (+ 42)	CCAATCCAGAGACTTCAGGA	GAGGAGAGCGCTGTAACTG

Results

Characterization of the accessible chromatin profile of human subcutaneous preadipocytes

We set out to study the open chromatin profile of human subcutaneous white adipose tissue (WAT), using abdominal (A) and gluteofemoral (GF) depot-derived preadipocytes isolated from two obese apple-shaped women (age = 33 ± 2.3 years, BMI = 34 ± 1.4 kg/m^2, waist to hip ratio = 0.93 ± 0.02). In order to gain a genome-wide view of accessible chromatin regions from the isolated preadipocytes, we utilized Assay for Transposase-Accessible Chromatin followed by sequencing (ATAC-seq). We sequenced two technical replicates from each individual's A- and GF-derived preadipocytes yielding four samples from each depot. We identified 112,362 and 104,957 peaks in A and GF samples respectively, 91,022 peaks being common to both depots (81% of the A peaks and 87% of the GF peaks). Differential binding analysis of the ATAC-seq data and hierarchical clustering revealed that A and GF samples are clustered together as expected based on their distinct anatomical origin (Additional file 3: Figure S1). Further analysis of the ATAC-seq data identified the significantly different open chromatin regions between A and GF preadipocytes. We observed 7160 A-specific and 780 GF-specific open chromatin regions (Fig. 1a and Additional file 3: Figure S1). Genome browser visualizations of the top 5 A- and GF-specific regions in each sample were summarized in supplemental data (Additional file 3: Figure S2).

Genome-wide distribution of depot-specific accessible chromatin regions revealed that around half of these were localized in intergenic regions (43% of A-specific regions and 63% of GF-specific regions) as shown in Fig. 1b. In addition, a higher percentage of abdominal-specific regions were found in gene promoter regions (7%) compared to the GF-specific peaks (only 3%) (Fig. 1b). De novo motif analysis at these specific open chromatin regions identified some of the well-known transcription factors involved in adipogenesis, such as GATA and C/EBP (Fig. 1c). As expected, a clear majority of the depot-specific peaks showed enrichment for the transcription factor binding motif AP-1, which is known to promote WAT formation (Fig. 1c).

Gene expression profiling of human subcutaneous preadipocytes

After we determined the accessible chromatin regions of depot-specific preadipocytes, we investigated the associated gene expression profiles. In the first subject, 2117 genes were differentially expressed between abdominal and GF preadipocytes. The difference was much smaller for the second subject with only 536 differentially expressed genes (Fig. 2a). In this study, we have focused on the 216 genes that were differentially regulated in both subjects. Of these, 126 genes exhibited significantly higher expression in abdominal preadipocytes, and 90 genes showed significantly higher expression in GF preadipocytes (Fig. 2b, Additional file 2: Table S1). Consistent with our previously described results from adipose tissue [16], some of the HOX gene family members showed the greatest fold change difference in our datasets between the two depots (HOXA5 and HOXA3 in the abdominal depot—fold change 86 and 26, respectively; HOXC11 in GF depot—fold change 24). Interestingly, inflammatory cytokines (IL1α, IL1β) and chemokines (IL8, GCP2, GRO1/2/3, CXCL5, MCP1) were upregulated in abdominal preadipocytes whereas expression of extracellular matrix components (SFRP2, ADD2, MMP9, SPON1, HTRA3, CDON) were found preferentially increased in GF cells. We performed Ingenuity Pathway Analysis (IPA) to gain further insight into the possible functional implications of these gene expression signatures. Potential upstream regulators of the depot-specific gene sets show that abdominal-specific genes are highly likely to be regulated by inflammatory cytokines (TNF, IL1B, IL1A, IL17F, and C5) than GF-specific genes; however, chemokines were observed as the upstream regulators of both gene groups (Fig. 2c). GF-specific genes were enriched for the activators of the WNT-signaling pathway consistent with decreased adipose expansion for the GF depot in apple-shaped women (Fig. 2c).

Integration of transcriptional and chromatin openness data

To examine the correlation between depot-specific open chromatin regions from the ATAC-seq analysis with depot-specific gene expression signatures, we integrated our ATAC-seq and RNA-seq datasets. We first focused on the ATAC-seq signals at the proximal promoter that we defined as a region covering 250 bp upstream and downstream from the transcriptional start site (TSS) of the differentially expressed genes (Fig. 3a). Normalized read enrichments at the promoter regions of the 126 abdominal-specific genes reported significantly higher chromatin accessibility in the abdominal depot compared to the GF depot, for both subjects (Fig. 3b). Importantly, the same analysis on the gene promoters of the 90 GF signature genes did not show major differences, although we observed significantly less reads from the GF preadipocytes of subject 2 (Fig. 3b).

To provide a much more detailed view on chromatin openness on the abdominal- and GF-specific gene promoters, we calculated the ratio of the RPKM values of the ATAC-seq data from the two depots on each promoter for genes that showed depot-specific expression. This analysis allowed us to define more accessible promoter regions using a 1.5-fold change cutoff. Interestingly, more than 39% of abdominal- and close to 65% of

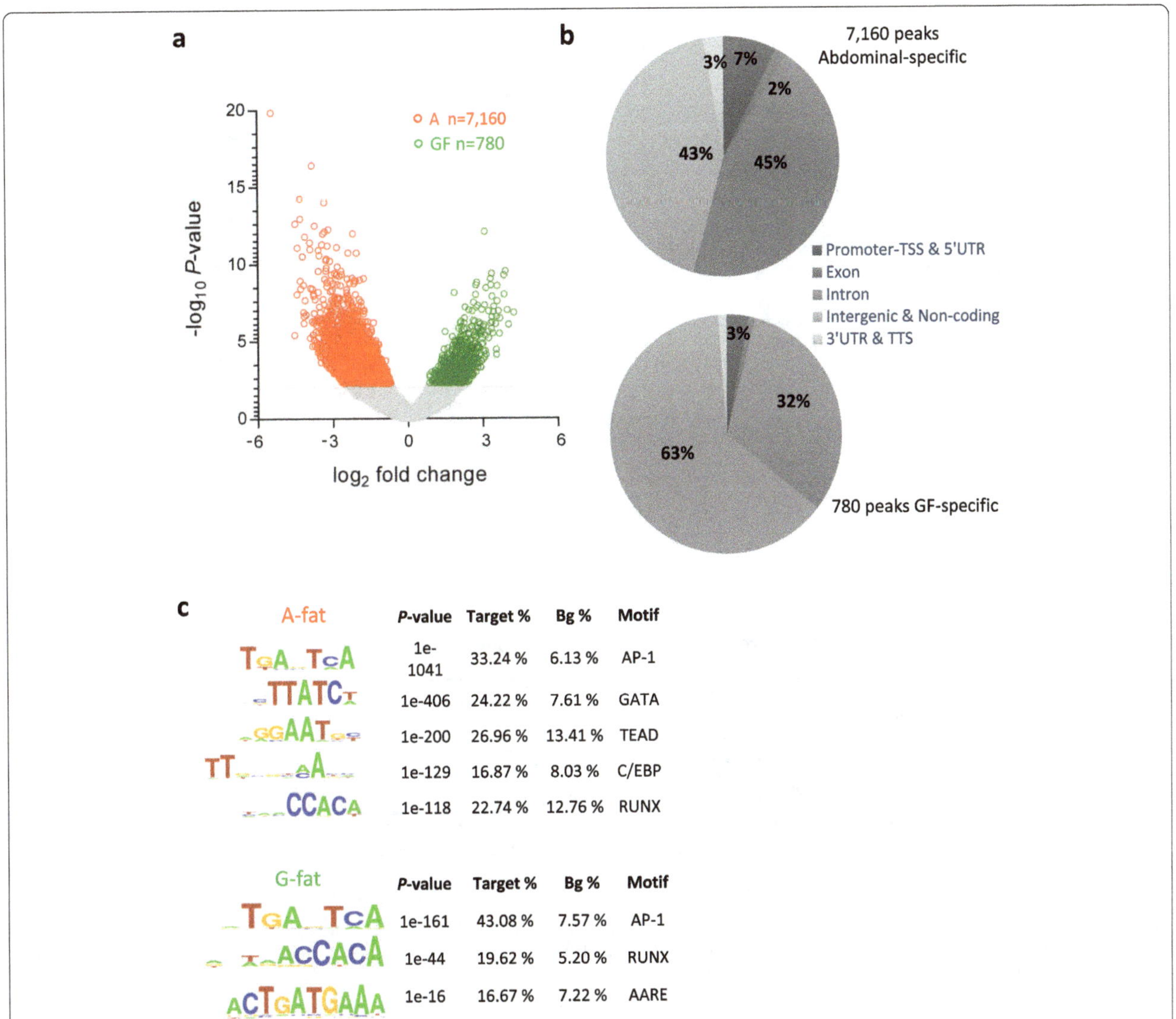

Fig. 1 Depot-specific open chromatin regions identify specific transcription factor motifs. **a** Volcano plot representation of depot-specific open chromatin regions in preadipocytes. Abdominal- (highlighted in red) and GF-specific (highlighted in green) open chromatin regions are presented ($p < 0.005$). **b** Genomic distribution of the depot-specific open chromatin regions. **c** Motif analysis of the depot-specific open chromatin regions. Enriched motif matrices are presented along with the p values; the percentages of each motif are found in the target (Target %) and background (Bg %) genomic regions

GF-specific genes promoters did not follow the expression of the corresponding gene with regard to their chromatin openness (Fig. 3c). As expected, 61% of the abdominal specific-genes promoters exhibited more accessibility in abdominal, and none of the abdominal-specific genes showed more open chromatin in GF cells (Fig. 3c). Surprisingly, the GF-specific gene promoters showed a mixed open chromatin profile between the depots, 19% being more open in GF cells and 17% being more open in abdominal cells (Fig. 3c).

To further investigate the relationship between chromatin openness and gene expression, we decided to extend our analysis to a broader genomic region around the TSSs of the depot-specific genes. Therefore, we annotated depot-specific open chromatin regions that are located in a genomic region of 100 kbs up- and downstream of the TSSs of the depot-specific genes (Fig. 4a). Our analysis identified 157 abdominal dominant open chromatin regions in the proximity of the abdominal-specific genes that are linked to 74 differentially expressed genes based on our annotation criteria (Fig. 4b left panel and Additional file 2: Table S2). The two well-established markers of abdominal depot HOXA5 and HOXA3 exhibited abdominal-specific expression and could be linked to seven and five abdominal-specific open chromatin regions, respectively. As expected, only two GF-specific regions could be annotated to abdominal genes (Fig. 4b left panel and

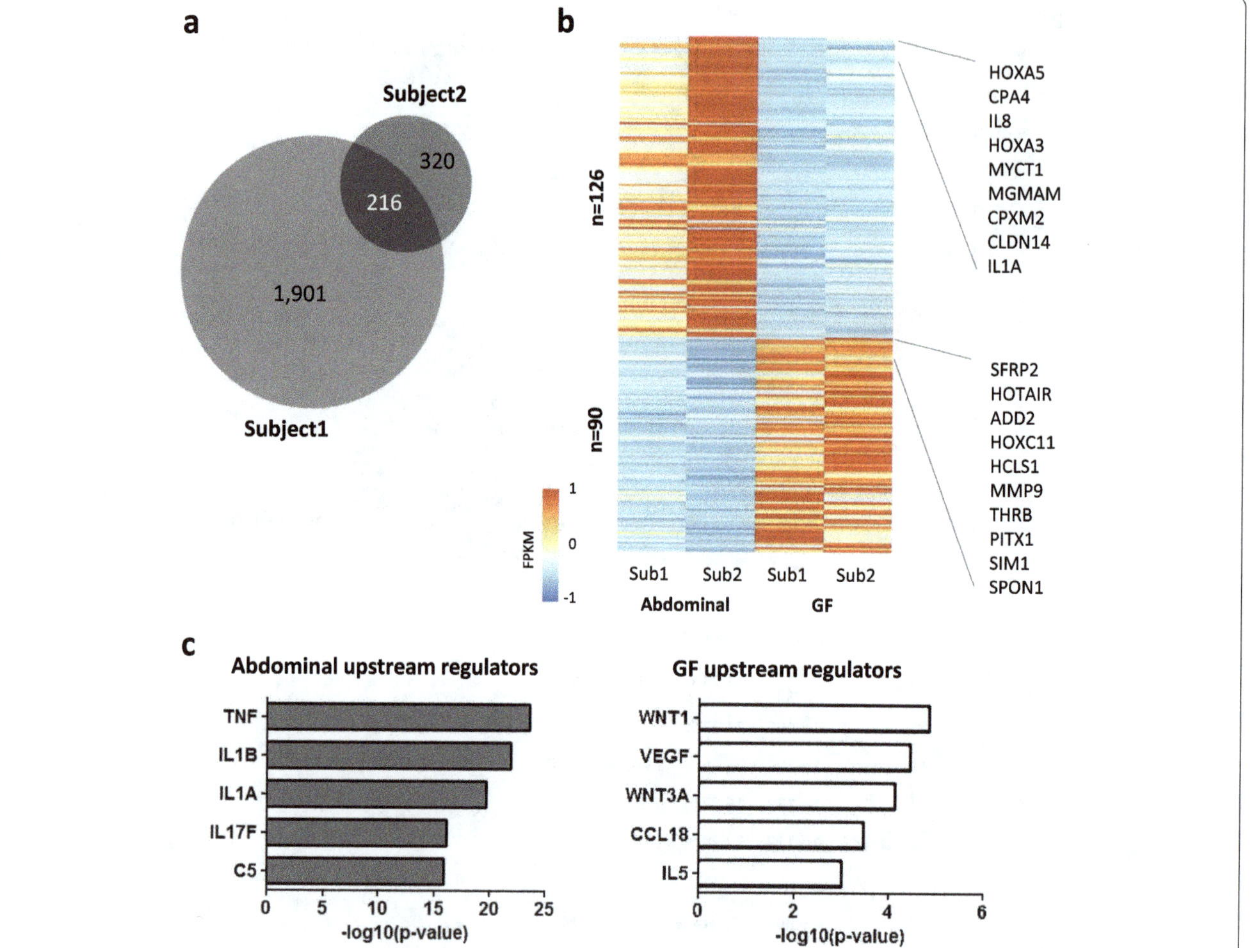

Fig. 2 Depot-specific gene expression in preadipocytes. **a** Venn diagram depicts the number of genes that were differentially expressed between abdominal and GF preadipocytes in each subject or in both ($p < 0.05$). **b** Heat map representation of depot-specific gene expression determined by RNA-seq from the abdominal and GF depots of two subjects (Sub). The top 10 signature genes of each depot are listed. **c** Ingenuity Pathway Analysis of the potential upstream regulators of abdominal- and GF-specific gene sets. Upstream regulators that fall into the category of cytokines and growth factors are presented

Additional file 2: Table S2). We observed a total of 66 GF-dominant open chromatin regions in the proximity of the GF-dominant genes, linked to 39 unique genes (Fig. 4b right panel and Additional file 2: Table S2). Surprisingly, 25 of these genes had significantly more open chromatin regions in the abdominal depot (corresponding to 40 ATAC-seq peaks), and only 14 genes had more open chromatin regions in the GF depot (corresponding to 26 ATAC-seq peaks) (Fig. 4b right panel). The already reported GF-specific HOXC13 gene possessed one of the most reliably detected GF-specific open chromatin regions.

After annotating the depot-dominant/specific open chromatin regions to the depot-specific genes, we next carried out de novo motif analysis on the 157 abdominal-specific open chromatin regions. Our results revealed transcription factor motifs involved in the regulation of inflammation (AP-1, NFκB-like motif) (Fig. 4c). Motif analysis on the abdominal-dominant open chromatin regions near GF-specific genes did not reveal significantly enriched motifs compared to the background, which can be explained by the low number [35] of target regions included in this analysis; however, the motifs found may function as response elements of transcriptional repressors (Additional file 3: Figure S3).

Active and repressive histone modifications positively correlate with promoter openness and gene expression of depot-specific genes

To confirm the validity of the data obtained by genome-wide sequencing technologies on these two subjects, we selected four depot-specific genes (abdominal-specific: HOXA5, HOXA3; GF-specific: HOXC13, HOTAIR) (Figs. 5a and 6a), isolated preadipocytes on a larger cohort of subjects ($n = 6$ obese, apple-shaped women, including the two subjects previously studied), and carried

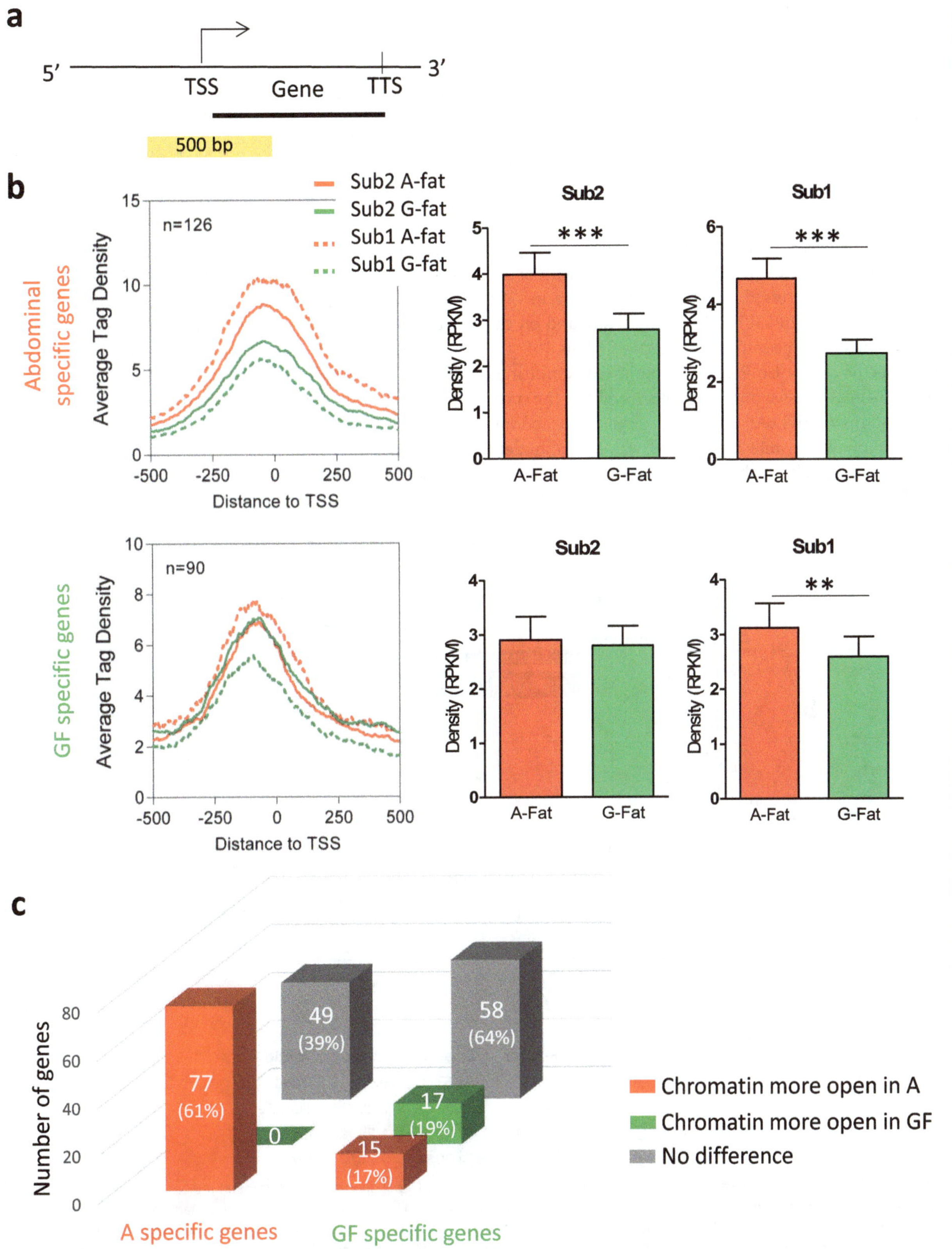

Fig. 3 (See legend on next page.)

(See figure on previous page.)
Fig. 3 Promoter accessibility of depot-specific genes. **a** Schematic representation of the investigation of promoter accessibility using ATAC-seq. ATAC-seq signals were calculated around the transcription start sites (TSSs) of the depot-specific genes in a 500-bp-wide window (250 bp up- (5′) and downstream (3′) relative to the TSSs). **b** Histogram-based depiction of the average tag density at the promoter regions of abdominal- ($n = 126$) and GF-specific ($n = 90$) genes in a 1-kb window centered on the TSSs. ATAC-seq density around the TSS of abdominal and GF depot-specific genes in each depot and for each subject (DiffBind). Sub1 = Subject 1, Sub2 = Subject 2 paired *t* test; $^{**}p < 0.01$, $^{***}p < 0.005$. **c** The number of genes with open promoter in abdominal (red) or GF (green) depot, according to their expression specificity (on the left side are the genes upregulated in abdominal preadipocytes, on the right side are the genes upregulated in GF preadipocytes). The gray bars represent the genes with no differential opened chromatin between A and GF depot

out promoter-based ChIP-qPCR for a select group of histone modifications known to be associated with active (H3K4me3) or repressed (H3K27me3) chromatin. We also performed RT-qPCR on the whole tissue and on the preadipocytes to measure the mRNA levels of the depot-specific genes. ChIP-qPCR experiments confirmed that H3K4me3 was significantly enriched at the promoter regions of HOXA5 and HOXA3 genes in abdominal preadipocytes, while H3K27me3 was less abundant (Fig. 5b). Conversely, analysis of the promoter regions of the GF-specific HOTAIR and HOXC13 genes exhibited high H3K4me3 and low H3K27me3 levels compared to abdominal preadipocytes (Fig. 6b). mRNAs of the HOXA5 and HOXA3 genes were consistent with the RNA-seq datasets and showed significantly higher expression in the abdominal depot and cells (Fig. 5b), whereas HOXC13 and HOTAIR mRNA were expressed significantly higher in the GF depot and cells (Fig. 6b).

Discussion

A substantial number of studies have focused on identifying extrinsic regulators of preadipocytes and adipocytes,

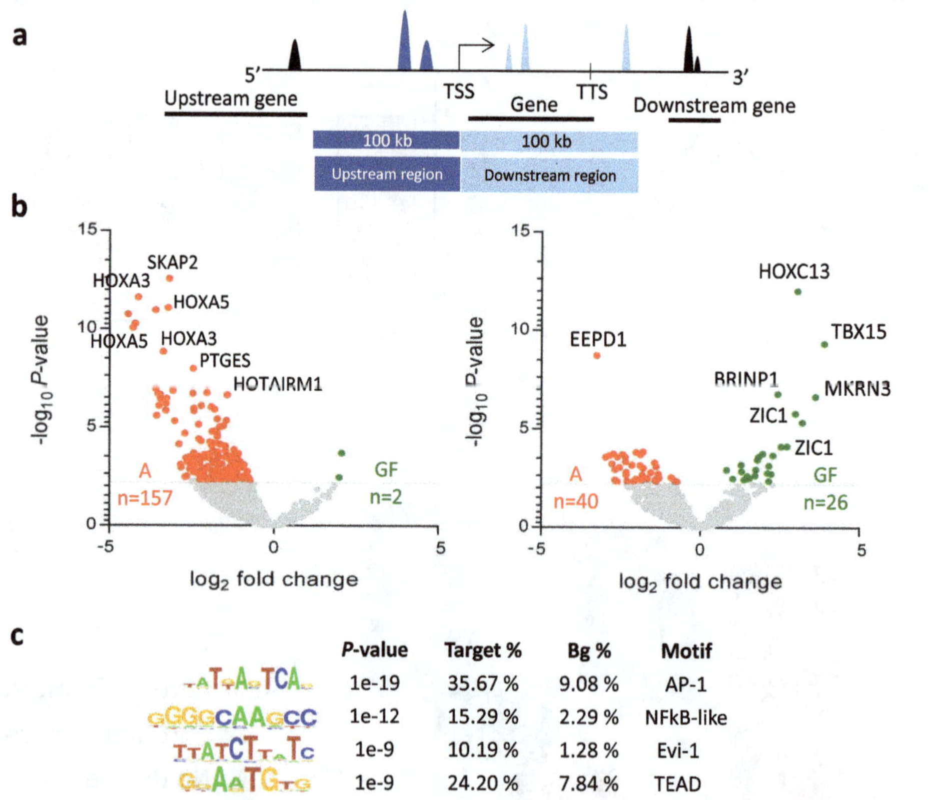

Fig. 4 Identification of the putative regulatory regions of depot-specific genes. **a** Depot-specific open chromatin regions determined by ATAC-seq were annotated to the nearest depot-specific genes in a ± 100-kb genomic region relative to the transcription start sites (TSSs) and (transcription termination site (TTS)). **b** Volcano plots portray the depot-specific open chromatin regions annotated to the abdominal- (left graph) and GF-specific genes (right graph). Abdominal-specific open chromatin regions are highlighted in red, while GF-specific open chromatin regions are highlighted in green. **c** Motif analysis of the 159 abdominal-specific open chromatin regions annotated to abdominal specific genes. Enriched motif matrices are presented along with the *p* values; the percentages of each motif are found in the target (Target%) and background (Bg%) genomic regions

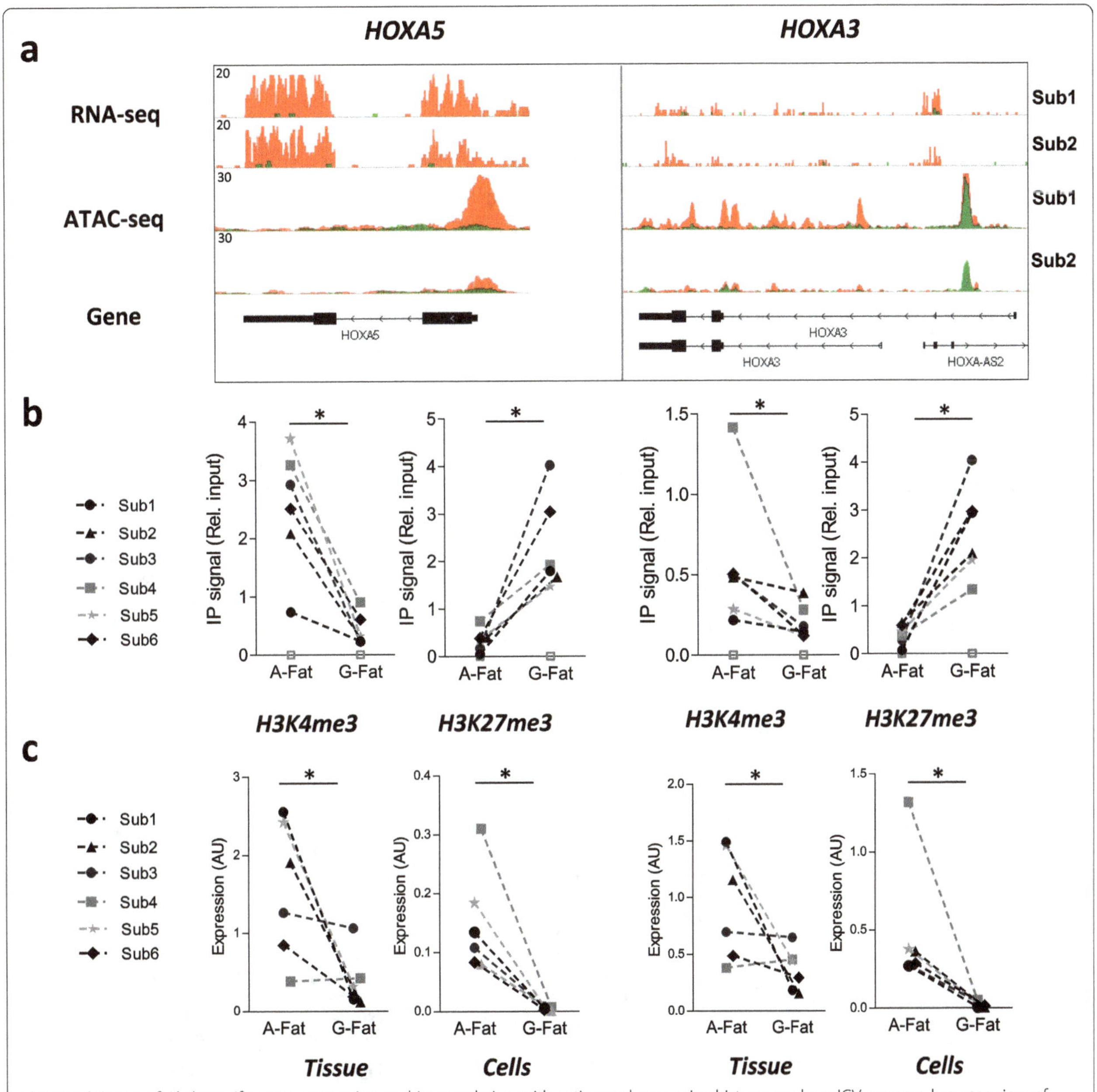

Fig. 5 Validation of Abd-specific gene expression and its correlation with active and repressive histone marks. **a** IGV genome browser view of RNA-seq and ATAC-seq signals on the indicated loci from abdominal (red) and GF (green) preadipocytes. Overlay tracks are presented for each gene loci. **b** ChIP-qPCR assay in abdominal and GF preadipocytes with H3K4me3 antibody and H3K27me3 antibody at the promoter region of the selected genes. **c** RT-qPCR assay for HOXA5 and HOXA3 in abdominal and GF preadipocytes. Wilcoxon test $^{*}p < 0.05$. White squares represent the IgG negative control

whereas comparatively very little is known about the chromatin structure differences that might control their identity and/or functions. A recent study showed the importance of chromatin modifications in the maintenance of the preadipocyte state by keeping the levels of the adipogenic master regulatory genes (PPARγ and C/EBPα) low. Similarly, high expression levels of these transcription factors upon adipocyte differentiation were also dependent on the presence of certain chromatin modifications [36], suggesting the importance of unique epigenetic signatures in the control of fat-specific gene expression. Global DNA methylomes of human scWAT have been related to BMI and body fat distribution [37], but only a small fraction of DNA methylation changes have been correlated to unique patterns of gene expression. However, this study did not take into consideration the cell composition of adipose tissue that can shift according to the degree of adiposity and inflammation. In our study, we investigated and compared the chromatin

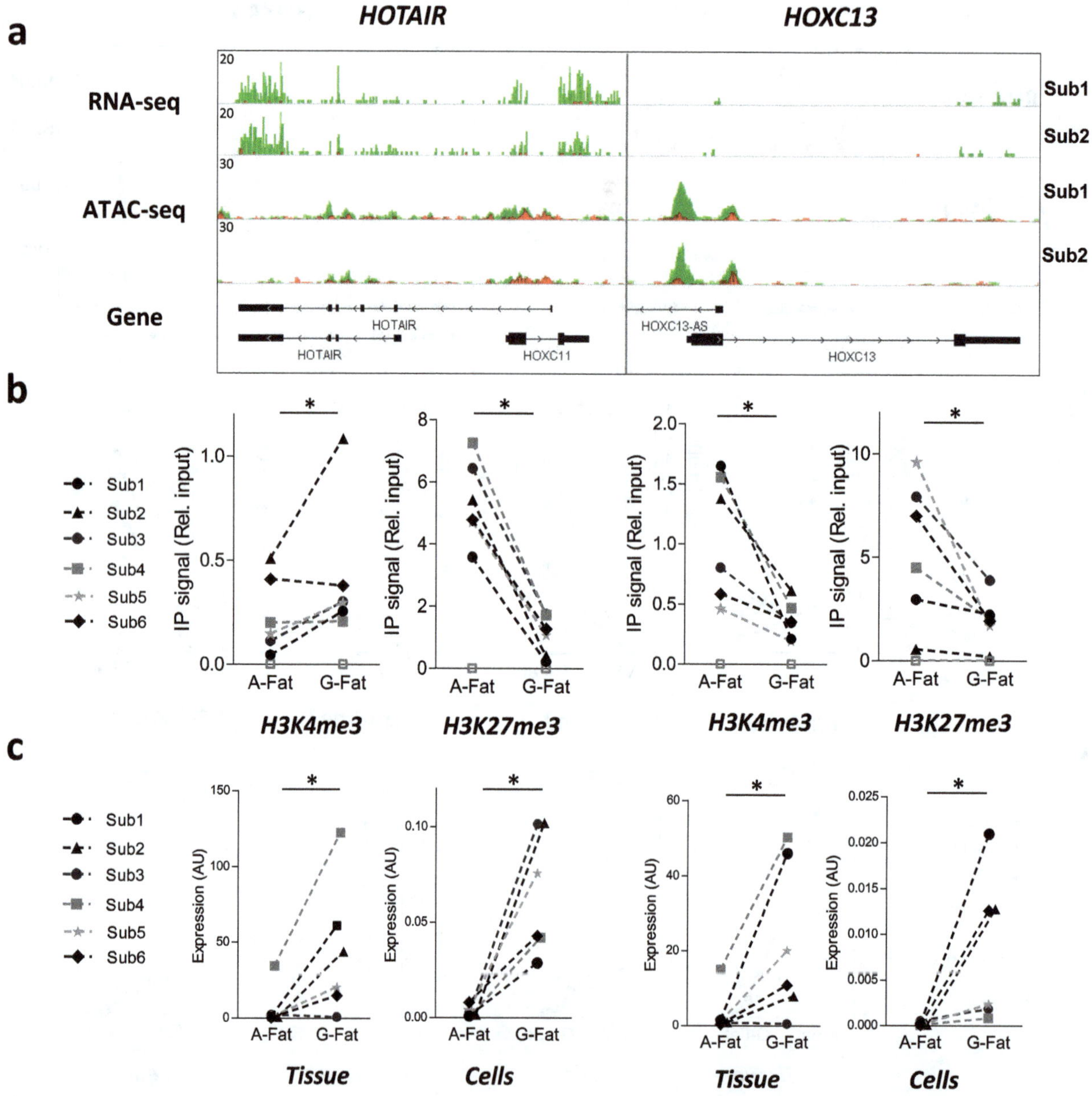

Fig. 6 Validation of GF-specific gene expression and its correlation with active and repressive histone marks. **a** IGV genome browser view of RNA-seq and ATAC-seq signals on the indicated loci from abdominal (red) and GF (green) preadipocytes. Overlay tracks are presented for each gene loci. **b** ChIP-qPCR assay in abdominal and GF preadipocytes with H3K4me3 antibody and H3K27me3 antibody at the promoter region of the selected genes. **c** RT-qPCR assay for HOXC13 and HOTAIR in abdominal and GF preadipocytes. Wilcoxon test $*p < 0.05$. White squares represent the IgG negative control

state of preadipocytes isolated from human abdominal and GF-fat and its correlation with cell gene expression signatures. Chromatin accessibility profiles of each depot were highly similar at a qualitative level, yet thousands of regions exhibiting quantitative differences in chromatin accessibility were also identified. Almost 8000 differentially accessible regions were observed between the depots. Using DNase hypersensitive site (DHS)-seq (technology comparable to ATAC-seq) during 3 T3-L1 adipogenesis, Mandrup's group identified 22,383 novel DHS sites at the early phase of differentiation, the majority of which being transiently open [38]. At the end of the differentiation, only 11,936 new DHS sites were observed in mature adipocytes. In another study performed on human α- and β-cells previously sorted, Ackermann et al. revealed 27,000 β-cell-specific ATAC-seq peaks whereas only 1850 ATAC-seq peaks were identified as α-cell-specific [39]. In our study, we compared two kinds of subcutaneous preadipocytes, defined by their differential anatomical localization, culture in the exact same condition. "8000 hits" is in the range of the data previously described and seems a reasonable number. Additional experiments on human adipose tissue are however necessary to discuss more in detail the number of differentially open regions we found. Interestingly, chromatin isolated from abdominal preadipocytes showed ten times more ATAC-seq signals compared to the GF cells, suggesting a global increase of open chromatin in this depot. Given the fact that the two participants included in our analysis have a predominant accumulation of fat in their abdominal region, the specific chromatin signature observed in this depot may reflect changes in preadipocytes activity such as proliferation and differentiation into mature adipocytes, both occurring during adipose development. Arner et al. reported a similar pattern with higher global mean DNA methylation observed in obese women compared to never obese women [40]. In our study, motif analysis performed on the abdominal-specific open chromatin regions also highlighted transcription factors known to be involved in proliferation (TEAD), adipocyte differentiation (GATA) [35], and adipocyte commitment (AP-1) [41] (Fig. 1c), consistent with the previous literature. GF-specific ATAC-seq signals showed a surprising enrichment for amino acid response elements (AARE) binding sites, implying for the first time a role for amino acid signaling in scWAT distribution. Amino acid deficiency has been shown to induce endoplasmic reticulum (ER) stress, itself known to couple obesity to other metabolic dysfunctions [42, 43]. By extrapolation, we speculate an increase of ER stress in GF-fat that may lead to potential preadipocyte dysfunction, making preadipocytes unable to properly differentiate into mature adipocytes to sequester excess calories. These events could lead to abnormal fat accumulation in the upper body and the emergence of metabolic disorder. However, our actual study did not show any evidence of differential ER stress level between the two scWAT depots. It is important to note that the two subjects we analyzed here were obese but did not show further signs of metabolic dysfunction. To validate our hypothesis, it would be necessary to investigate in more detail the GF depot in subjects presenting comorbidities.

Using RNA-seq, we identified 126 genes upregulated in abdominal cells and 90 genes upregulated in GF cells. In accordance with our previous studies [16, 22], the fat depot specificity of some HOX genes and the lncRNA HOTAIR is maintained in isolated preadipocytes. Pathway analysis with ingenuity suggested an upregulation of inflammatory signaling in the abdominal depot, whereas the GF depot seems to be more affected by extracellular matrix remodeling-related signaling pathways, suggesting a depot-specific pattern. Future studies need to confirm these preliminary observations in a larger number of apple-shaped subjects and to also explore the transcriptional patterns of cells isolated from pear-shaped women.

The strong association observed between open chromatin and active gene expression in A-fat supports the role of differential chromatin signatures in the transcriptional regulation of abdominal-specific genes. Inversely, GF-specific genes displayed a loss in GF chromatin accessibility within 200 kb of the TSS, reflecting a more complex situation in lower body fat depots. Surprisingly, we observed abdominal-specific ATAC-seq signals around the TSS of 25 GF-specific genes, which may suggest the presence of active transcriptional repressors at these open chromatin regions. Transcription factor motif analysis confirmed the presence of the DNA-binding motif for the transcriptional repressors, NF1, and/or ZNF263 at these abdominal-dominant open chromatin regions. ATAC-seq regions identified in abdominal depot near the TSS of GF-specific genes were also enriched for H3K27me3, which is the marker of repressed chromatin territories (data not shown). Altogether, these observations suggest the presence of abdominal-specific repressive mechanisms that affect the chromatin landscape of GF-specific gene loci and gene expression signature, but further functional studies are required to provide evidence about the existence of such phenomenon.

As described in our previous study [22], we observed a dramatic upregulation of the linc HOTAIR in the obese GF depot compared to the abdominal depot (fold change 28 in tissue and cells—Fig. 6c). The role of HOTAIR is well described in cancer where HOTAIR acts as a modular scaffold and interacts directly with PRC2 and LSD1 complexes, recruiting them to target gene loci, and represses their transcription via H3K27-trimethylation (PRC2 complex and EZH2 activity) and H3K4-demethylation (LSD1 activity) (for review [44]). Interestingly, there is a strong support that these two methyltransferases EZH2 and LSD1 promote adipogenesis [45, 46]. Overall, our limited ChIP-qPCR analysis for H3K27 and H3K4me3 is consistent with the changes in PRC2 and LSD1 activity and suggests that HOTAIR may play a deterministic role in the association observed between gene expression and chromatin structure in scWAT that merits further investigation.

Several studies revealed adipose tissue depot-specific expression of multiple HOX genes [47] and their implication in metabolic diseases [48]. HOXA1, A4, and HOXC4 have been previously found directly involved in the differentiation and further generation of human white and brown adipose tissue, showing the importance of HOX genes at the early stages of adipocyte differentiation and commitment. In the present study, chromatin structure and histone marks of some of the HOX genes were associated with their gene expression in both scWAT depots (HOXA5, HOXA3, and HOXC13). Their expression pattern is also preserved between adipose tissue and cells (Figs. 5 and 6), suggesting an epigenetic mechanism for control of their transcription. This correlation may be a simple consequence of their differential anatomical origin; however, the robust HOX gene signature observed in tissue and cells remains intriguing, and the question of their involvement in fat development and distribution remains unresolved.

Regarding the limitations of our study, our genome-wide analysis was performed only on two apple-shaped women. Future studies must involve more subjects not only for validation purposes but also to extend our analysis and provide a more comprehensive view on the potential epigenomic programming of depot-specific adipocytes, especially on women presenting with a gynoid fat pattern. A previous analysis of adipogenesis regulator genes performed in human mesenchymal stem cells revealed dynamic changes in histone marks during the differentiation [49]. However, other studies have found that histone modifications were globally stable throughout differentiation and showed distinct and highly dynamic distribution patterns at specific genes, indicating that histone modifications in mesenchymal stem cells appear to be gene-specific [50]. Here, we investigated the chromatin and histone modifications only in preadipocytes isolated from scWAT depots, and thus, we did not address their stability through the process of differentiation. It would be important to carry out follow-up experiments in fully differentiated adipocytes as well as in adipocytes freshly isolated from abdominal and GF-fat tissue to more fully investigate epigenomic control of transcriptional regulation of scWAT depot-specific genes.

In conclusion, our analysis revealed that the open chromatin landscapes for abdominal vs. GF preadipocytes exhibit significant differences, suggesting depot specific mechanisms that shape the cellular epigenome, according to their anatomical origin. In addition, the different open chromatin profile positively associates with a depot-specific gene expression signature, supporting a role for chromatin status in the regulation of the depot-selective patterns of scWAT gene expression. Finally, our gene-specific analyses show that our findings are reproducible with available technologies and highlight a strong positive correlation between chromatin openness and the presence of active and repressive chromatin marks in preadipocytes.

Additional files

Additional file 1: Additional figure with data on PPIA gene expression. Representation of the individual PPIA gene Ct value obtained by RT-qPCR in cells (white squares) and tissue (black squares). A = abdominal depot, G = GF depot.

Additional file 2: Additional tables with data on RNA-seq and ATAC-seq list of genes. **Table S1.** Differentially expressed genes between abdominal and GF depot in subject 1, subject 2, and in both. **Table S2.** List of open chromatin regions in the proximity of the depot-specific genes

Additional file 3: Additional figures with data on ATAC-seq. **Figure S1.** Differential binding analysis identifies depot-specific chromatin accessibility in preadipocytes. a) Correlation plot of accessible chromatin regions defined by ATAC-seq from different subjects (Sub1 and Sub2), fat depots (gluteofemoral-GF, abdominal-A), and technical replicates (rep#1 and rep#2). b) Identification of differentially open chromatin regions from GF and abdominal preadipocytes using differential binding analysis (DiffBind). Heat map representation of the abdominal- ($n = 7160$) and the GF-specific ($n = 780$) open chromatin regions. Sub = subject, Rep = technical replicate. The pairwise correlation scores were used for hierarchical clustering ($p < 0.005$, DiffBind). **Figure S2.** Depot-specific open chromatin regions of preadipocytes. IGV genome browser view of depot-specific ATAC-seq signals from abdominal (red) and GF (green) preadipocytes. Abdominal- (left) and GF-specific open chromatin regions are shown. Results are shown from two subjects and from 2-2 technical replicates. Chromosomal locations are indicated at the bottom for each genomic loci. Figure S3. Motif analysis on the 40 abdominal-specific open chromatin regions annotated to GF specific genes. Enriched motif matrices are presented along with the p values, the percentages of each motif found in the target (Target%) and background (Bg%) genomic regions.

Abbreviations

A-fat: Abdominal fat; ATAC: Assay for transposase-accessible chromatin; BMI: Body mass index; ChIP: Chromatin immunoprecipitation; FFA: Free fatty acid; FPKM: Fragments per kilobase of transcript per million mapped reads; GF-fat: Gluteofemoral fat; hEGF: Human epidermal growth factor; hFGF: Human fibroblast growth factor; HOX: Homeobox; IPA: Ingenuity Pathway Analysis; lncRNA: Long non-coding RNA; RPKM: Reads per kilobase of transcript per million mapped reads; scWAT: Subcutaneous white adipose tissue; TSS: Transcription start site; WHR: Waist to hip ratio

Acknowledgements

The authors thank the study volunteers for their participation and the TRI-MD clinical research staff for their contributions. The authors thank the personnel of the genomic core at Sanford-Burnham Prebys Medical Discovery Institute, Orlando, FL, who performed the sequencing and more particularly Subramaniam Shyamala Govindarajan and John Marchica.

Funding

This work was supported by the National Institutes of Health Grant R01DK107009-02; for BLB and DB, the work was supported by the MOLMEDEX FUN-OMICS (GINOP-2.3.3-15-2016-00007), Debrecen Venture Catapult Program (EFOP-3.6.1-16-2016-00022), by the University of Debrecen Medical Faculty through the Bridging Fund system, and by the internal research funding provided by the Department of Biochemistry and Molecular Biology; BLB was a Szodoray Fellow of the University of Debrecen, Faculty of Medicine, and an alumni of the Magyary Zoltan Fellowship supported by the TAMOP 4.2.4.A/2-11-1-2012-0001 grant. These funds were implemented through the New Hungary Development Plan co-financed by the European Social Fund and the European Regional Development Fund. DB is a recipient of the ÚNKP-18-3-III-DE-253New National Excellence Program grant of the Ministry of Human Capacities.

Disclosure

The authors have no conflicts of interest and nothing to disclose.

Authors' contributions

AD designed the experiments; collected the human samples; isolated the preadipocytes; performed the RNA extraction, ChIP-qPCR, and RT-qPCR experiments; participated in all data analysis; and wrote the draft manuscript.

KS designed and performed the ATAC-seq experiments, participated in all data analyses, and wrote the draft manuscript. DB performed the RNA-seq and ATAC-seq analysis. AT participated in the RNA-seq and ATAC-seq analysis. SRS designed and was the principal investigator of the clinical study. TFO and SRS planned the project. All authors commented on the manuscript. All authors read and approved the final manuscript.

Competing interests
The authors declare that they have no competing interests.

Author details
[1]Translational Research Institute for Metabolism and Diabetes, Florida Hospital, 301 E. Princeton Street, Orlando, FL 32804, USA. [2]Diabetes and Obesity Research Center, Sanford Burnham Prebys Medical Discovery Institute at Lake Nona, Orlando, FL, USA. [3]Genomic Medicine and Bioinformatic Core Facility, Department of Biochemistry and Molecular Biology, Faculty of Medicine, University of Debrecen, Nagyerdei krt 98, Debrecen 4032, Hungary. [4]Department of Computer Science, University of Central Florida, 4000 Central Florida Blvd, Orlando 32816, USA. [5]Burnett School of Biomedical Sciences, College of Medicine, University of Central Florida, 6900 Lake Nona Boulevard, Orlando, FL, USA. [6]Present address: Department of Medicine, Johns Hopkins All Children's Hospital, Johns Hopkins University School of Medicine, St. Petersburg, FL 33701, USA.

References

1. Vague J. The degree of masculine differentiation of obesities: a factor determining predisposition to diabetes, atherosclerosis, gout, and uric calculous disease. 1956. Obes Res. 1996;4(2):204–12.
2. Fontbonne A, Thibult N, Eschwege E, Ducimetiere P. Body fat distribution and coronary heart disease mortality in subjects with impaired glucose tolerance or diabetes mellitus: the Paris Prospective Study, 15-year follow-up. Diabetologia. 1992;35(5):464–8.
3. Pouliot MC, Despres JP, Nadeau A, Moorjani S, Prud'Homme D, Lupien PJ, Tremblay A, Bouchard C. Visceral obesity in men. Associations with glucose tolerance, plasma insulin, and lipoprotein levels. Diabetes. 1992;41(7):826–34.
4. Patel P, Abate N. Role of subcutaneous adipose tissue in the pathogenesis of insulin resistance. J Obes. 2013;2013:489187.
5. Fried SK, Lee MJ, Karastergiou K. Shaping fat distribution: new insights into the molecular determinants of depot- and sex-dependent adipose biology. Obesity (Silver Spring). 2015;23(7):1345–52.
6. Jensen MD. Is visceral fat involved in the pathogenesis of the metabolic syndrome? Human model. Obesity (Silver Spring). 2006;14 Suppl 1:20s–4s.
7. Jialal I, Devaraj S. Subcutaneous adipose tissue biology in metabolic syndrome. Horm Mol Biol Clin Invest. 2018;33(1):1868-91.
8. Grundy SM, Williams C, Vega GL. Upper body fat predicts metabolic syndrome similarly in men and women. Eur J Clin Investig. 2018;48(7):e12941.
9. Pinnick KE, Nicholson G, Manolopoulos KN, McQuaid SE, Valet P, Frayn KN, Denton N, Min JL, Zondervan KT, Fleckner J, et al. Distinct developmental profile of lower-body adipose tissue defines resistance against obesity-associated metabolic complications. Diabetes. 2014;63(11):3785–97.
10. Yusuf S, Hawken S, Ounpuu S, Bautista L, Franzosi MG, Commerford P, Lang CC, Rumboldt Z, Onen CL, Lisheng L, et al. Obesity and the risk of myocardial infarction in 27,000 participants from 52 countries: a case-control study. Lancet. 2005;366(9497):1640–9.
11. Tchkonia T, Thomou T, Zhu Y, Karagiannides I, Pothoulakis C, Jensen MD, Kirkland JL. Mechanisms and metabolic implications of regional differences among fat depots. Cell Metab. 2013;17(5):644–56.
12. Karpe F, Pinnick KE. Biology of upper-body and lower-body adipose tissue--link to whole-body phenotypes. Nat Rev Endocrinol. 2015;11(2):90–100.
13. Tchkonia T, Giorgadze N, Pirtskhalava T, Thomou T, DePonte M, Koo A, Forse RA, Chinnappan D, Martin-Ruiz C, von Zglinicki T, et al. Fat depot-specific characteristics are retained in strains derived from single human preadipocytes. Diabetes. 2006;55(9):2571–8.
14. Van Harmelen V, Rohrig K, Hauner H. Comparison of proliferation and differentiation capacity of human adipocyte precursor cells from the omental and subcutaneous adipose tissue depot of obese subjects. Metab Clin Exp. 2004;53(5):632–7.
15. Gehrke S, Brueckner B, Schepky A, Klein J, Iwen A, Bosch TC, Wenck H, Winnefeld M, Hagemann S. Epigenetic regulation of depot-specific gene expression in adipose tissue. PLoS One. 2013;8(12):e82516.
16. Karastergiou K, Fried SK, Xie H, Lee MJ, Divoux A, Rosencrantz MA, Chang RJ, Smith SR. Distinct developmental signatures of human abdominal and gluteal subcutaneous adipose tissue depots. J Clin Endocrinol Metab. 2013; 98(1):362–71.
17. Passaro A, Miselli MA, Sanz JM, Dalla Nora E, Morieri ML, Colonna R, Pisot R, Zuliani G. Gene expression regional differences in human subcutaneous adipose tissue. BMC Genomics. 2017;18(1):202.
18. Hauner H, Entenmann G. Regional variation of adipose differentiation in cultured stromal-vascular cells from the abdominal and femoral adipose tissue of obese women. Int J Obes. 1991;15(2):121–6.
19. Tchoukalova YD, Koutsari C, Votruba SB, Tchkonia T, Giorgadze N, Thomou T, Kirkland JL, Jensen MD. Sex- and depot-dependent differences in adipogenesis in normal-weight humans. Obesity (Silver Spring). 2010;18(10): 1875–80.
20. Gupta RA, Shah N, Wang KC, Kim J, Horlings HM, Wong DJ, Tsai MC, Hung T, Argani P, Rinn JL, et al. Long non-coding RNA HOTAIR reprograms chromatin state to promote cancer metastasis. Nature. 2010;464(7291):1071–6.
21. Tsai MC, Manor O, Wan Y, Mosammaparast N, Wang JK, Lan F, Shi Y, Segal E, Chang HY. Long noncoding RNA as modular scaffold of histone modification complexes. Science (New York, NY). 2010;329(5992):689–93.
22. Divoux A, Karastergiou K, Xie H, Guo W, Perera RJ, Fried SK, Smith SR. Identification of a novel lncRNA in gluteal adipose tissue and evidence for its positive effect on preadipocyte differentiation. Obesity (Silver Spring). 2014;22(8):1781–5.
23. Lee MJ, Wu Y, Fried SK. A modified protocol to maximize differentiation of human preadipocytes and improve metabolic phenotypes. Obesity (Silver Spring). 2012;20(12):2334–40.
24. Hebert TL, Wu X, Yu G, Goh BC, Halvorsen YD, Wang Z, Moro C, Gimble JM. Culture effects of epidermal growth factor (EGF) and basic fibroblast growth factor (bFGF) on cryopreserved human adipose-derived stromal/stem cell proliferation and adipogenesis. J Tissue Eng Regen Med. 2009;3(7):553–61.
25. Buenrostro JD, Giresi PG, Zaba LC, Chang HY, Greenleaf WJ. Transposition of native chromatin for fast and sensitive epigenomic profiling of open chromatin, DNA-binding proteins and nucleosome position. Nat Methods. 2013;10(12):1213–8.
26. Barish GD, Yu RT, Karunasiri MS, Becerra D, Kim J, Tseng TW, Tai LJ, Leblanc M, Diehl C, Cerchietti L, et al. The Bcl6-SMRT/NCoR cistrome represses inflammation to attenuate atherosclerosis. Cell Metab. 2012; 15(4):554–62.
27. Trapnell C, Williams BA, Pertea G, Mortazavi A, Kwan G, van Baren MJ, Salzberg SL, Wold BJ, Pachter L. Transcript assembly and quantification by RNA-Seq reveals unannotated transcripts and isoform switching during cell differentiation. Nat Biotechnol. 2010;28(5):511–5.
28. Li H, Durbin R. Fast and accurate short read alignment with Burrows-Wheeler transform. Bioinformatics. 2009;25(14):1754–60.
29. Li H, Handsaker B, Wysoker A, Fennell T, Ruan J, Homer N, Marth G, Abecasis G, Durbin R. The sequence alignment/map format and SAMtools. Bioinformatics. 2009;25(16):2078–9.
30. Zhang Y, Liu T, Meyer CA, Eeckhoute J, Johnson DS, Bernstein BE, Nusbaum C, Myers RM, Brown M, Li W, et al. Model-based analysis of ChIP-Seq (MACS). Genome Biol. 2008;9(9):R137.
31. Dunham I, et al. An integrated encyclopedia of DNA elements in the human genome. Nature. 2012;489(7414):57–74.
32. Heinz S, Benner C, Spann N, Bertolino E, Lin YC, Laslo P, Cheng JX, Murre C, Singh H, Glass CK. Simple combinations of lineage-determining transcription factors prime cis-regulatory elements required for macrophage and B cell identities. Mol Cell. 2010;38(4):576–89.
33. Thorvaldsdottir H, Robinson JT, Mesirov JP. Integrative Genomics Viewer (IGV): high-performance genomics data visualization and exploration. Brief Bioinform. 2013;14(2):178–92.
34. Quinlan AR, Hall IM. BEDTools: a flexible suite of utilities for comparing genomic features. Bioinformatics. 2010;26(6):841–2.
35. Tong Q, Dalgin G, Xu H, Ting CN, Leiden JM, Hotamisligil GS. Function of GATA transcription factors in preadipocyte-adipocyte transition. Science. 2000;290(5489):134–8.
36. Matsumura Y, Nakaki R, Inagaki T, Yoshida A, Kano Y, Kimura H, Tanaka T, Tsutsumi S, Nakao M, Doi T, et al. H3K4/H3K9me3 bivalent chromatin

domains targeted by lineage-specific DNA methylation pauses adipocyte differentiation. Molecular Cell. 2015;60(4):584–96.
37. Agha G, Houseman EA, Kelsey KT, Eaton CB, Buka SL, Loucks EB. Adiposity is associated with DNA methylation profile in adipose tissue. Int J Epidemiol. 2015;44(4):1277–87.
38. Siersbaek R, Nielsen R, John S, Sung MH, Baek S, Loft A, Hager GL, Mandrup S. Extensive chromatin remodelling and establishment of transcription factor 'hotspots' during early adipogenesis. EMBO J. 2011;30(8):1459–72.
39. Ackermann AM, Wang Z, Schug J, Naji A, Kaestner KH. Integration of ATAC-seq and RNA-seq identifies human alpha cell and beta cell signature genes. Mol Metab. 2016;5(3):233–44.
40. Arner P, Sinha I, Thorell A, Ryden M, Dahlman-Wright K, Dahlman I. The epigenetic signature of subcutaneous fat cells is linked to altered expression of genes implicated in lipid metabolism in obese women. Clin Epigenetics. 2015;7:93.
41. Luther J, Ubieta K, Hannemann N, Jimenez M, Garcia M, Zech C, Schett G, Wagner EF, Bozec A. Fra-2/AP-1 controls adipocyte differentiation and survival by regulating PPARgamma and hypoxia. Cell Death Differ. 2014; 21(4):655–64.
42. Lee J, Ozcan U. Unfolded protein response signaling and metabolic diseases. J Biol Chem. 2014;289(3):1203–11.
43. Scheuner D, Kaufman RJ. The unfolded protein response: a pathway that links insulin demand with beta-cell failure and diabetes. Endocr Rev. 2008; 29(3):317–33.
44. Bhan A, Mandal SS. LncRNA HOTAIR: a master regulator of chromatin dynamics and cancer. Biochim Biophys Acta. 2015;1:151–64.
45. Wei Y, Chen YH, Li LY, Lang J, Yeh SP, Shi B, Yang CC, Yang JY, Lin CY, Lai CC, et al. CDK1-dependent phosphorylation of EZH2 suppresses methylation of H3K27 and promotes osteogenic differentiation of human mesenchymal stem cells. Nat Cell Biol. 2011;13(1):87–94.
46. Musri MM, Carmona MC, Hanzu FA, Kaliman P, Gomis R, Parrizas M. Histone demethylase LSD1 regulates adipogenesis. J Biol Chem. 2010;285(39):30034–41.
47. Hilton C, Neville MJ, Karpe F. MicroRNAs in adipose tissue: their role in adipogenesis and obesity. Int J Obes (2005). 2013;37(3):325–32.
48. Procino A, Cillo C. The HOX genes network in metabolic diseases. Cell Biol Int. 2013;37(11):1145–8.
49. Mikkelsen TS, Xu Z, Zhang X, Wang L, Gimble JM, Lander ES, Rosen ED. Comparative epigenomic analysis of murine and human adipogenesis. Cell. 2010;143(1):156–69.
50. Zhang Q, Ramlee MK, Brunmeir R, Villanueva CJ, Halperin D, Xu F. Dynamic and distinct histone modifications modulate the expression of key adipogenesis regulatory genes. Cell Cycle. 2012;11(23):4310–22.

Permissions

All chapters in this book were first published in CE, by Springer; hereby published with permission under the Creative Commons Attribution License or equivalent. Every chapter published in this book has been scrutinized by our experts. Their significance has been extensively debated. The topics covered herein carry significant findings which will fuel the growth of the discipline. They may even be implemented as practical applications or may be referred to as a beginning point for another development.

The contributors of this book come from diverse backgrounds, making this book a truly international effort. This book will bring forth new frontiers with its revolutionizing research information and detailed analysis of the nascent developments around the world.

We would like to thank all the contributing authors for lending their expertise to make the book truly unique. They have played a crucial role in the development of this book. Without their invaluable contributions this book wouldn't have been possible. They have made vital efforts to compile up to date information on the varied aspects of this subject to make this book a valuable addition to the collection of many professionals and students.

This book was conceptualized with the vision of imparting up-to-date information and advanced data in this field. To ensure the same, a matchless editorial board was set up. Every individual on the board went through rigorous rounds of assessment to prove their worth. After which they invested a large part of their time researching and compiling the most relevant data for our readers.

The editorial board has been involved in producing this book since its inception. They have spent rigorous hours researching and exploring the diverse topics which have resulted in the successful publishing of this book. They have passed on their knowledge of decades through this book. To expedite this challenging task, the publisher supported the team at every step. A small team of assistant editors was also appointed to further simplify the editing procedure and attain best results for the readers.

Apart from the editorial board, the designing team has also invested a significant amount of their time in understanding the subject and creating the most relevant covers. They scrutinized every image to scout for the most suitable representation of the subject and create an appropriate cover for the book.

The publishing team has been an ardent support to the editorial, designing and production team. Their endless efforts to recruit the best for this project, has resulted in the accomplishment of this book. They are a veteran in the field of academics and their pool of knowledge is as vast as their experience in printing. Their expertise and guidance has proved useful at every step. Their uncompromising quality standards have made this book an exceptional effort. Their encouragement from time to time has been an inspiration for everyone.

The publisher and the editorial board hope that this book will prove to be a valuable piece of knowledge for researchers, students, practitioners and scholars across the globe.

List of Contributors

Matthew Devall, Rebecca G. Smith, Eilis Hannon, Michael Weedon and Katie Lunnon
University of Exeter Medical School, RILD, University of Exeter, Barrack Road, Devon, UK

Aaron Jeffries and Jonathan Mill
University of Exeter Medical School, RILD, University of Exeter, Barrack Road, Devon, UK
Institute of Psychiatry, Psychology and Neuroscience, King's College London, De Crespigny Park, London, UK

Matthew N. Davies
Department of Twin Research & Genetic Epidemiology, King's College London, Lambeth Palace Road, London, UK

Leonard Schalkwyk
School of Biological Sciences, University of Essex, Essex, UK

Junya Liang
Department of Biostatistics, School of Public Health, Nanjing Medical University, Nanjing 211166, China
China International Cooperation Center (CICC) for Environment and Human Health, Nanjing Medical University, Nanjing 211166, China

Yongyue Wei, Ruyang Zhang, Sipeng Shen, Yang Zhao and Feng Chen
Department of Biostatistics, School of Public Health, Nanjing Medical University, Nanjing 211166, China
China International Cooperation Center (CICC) for Environment and Human Health, Nanjing Medical University, Nanjing 211166, China
Department of Environmental Health, Harvard T.H. Chan School of Public Health, Harvard University, Boston, MA 02115, USA

Li Su
China International Cooperation Center (CICC) for Environment and Human Health, Nanjing Medical University, Nanjing 211166, China

David C. Christiani
China International Cooperation Center (CICC) for Environment and Human Health, Nanjing Medical University, Nanjing 211166, China
Department of Environmental Health, Harvard T.H. Chan School of Public Health, Harvard University, Boston, MA 02115, USA
Pulmonary and Critical Care Unit, Massachusetts General Hospital, Department of Medicine, Harvard Medical School, Boston, MA 02114, USA

Yichen Guo
Department of Environmental Health, Harvard T.H. Chan School of Public Health, Harvard University, Boston, MA 02115, USA

Xihong Lin
Department of Biostatistics, Harvard T.H. Chan School of Public Health, Harvard University, Boston, MA 02115, USA

Sebastian Moran and Manel Esteller
Cancer Epigenetics and Biology Program (PEBC), Bellvitge Biomedical Research Institute (IDIBELL), 08908 L'Hospitalet, Barcelona, Catalonia, Spain

Åslaug Helland, Maria M. Bjaanæs and Thomas Fleischer
Department of Genetics, Institute for Cancer Research, Oslo University Hospital, Oslo, Norway

Anna Karlsson, Maria Planck and Johan Staaf
Division of Oncology and Pathology, Department of Clinical Sciences Lund, Lund University, Medicon Village, SE 22381 Lund, Sweden

Yu-Qian Xiang, Jun-Yu Zhang, Ye Liu and Ya-Jing Tan
The International Peace Maternity and Child Health Hospital, School of Medicine, Shanghai Jiao Tong University, Shanghai 200030, China

He-Feng Huang
The International Peace Maternity and Child Health Hospital, School of Medicine, Shanghai Jiao Tong University, Shanghai 200030, China
The Key Laboratory of Reproductive Genetics, Ministry of Education (Zhejiang University), Hangzhou, Zhejiang 310006, China

Jie-Xue Pan
The International Peace Maternity and Child Health Hospital, School of Medicine, Shanghai Jiao Tong University, Shanghai 200030, China

The Key Laboratory of Reproductive Genetics, Ministry of Education (Zhejiang University), Hangzhou, Zhejiang 310006, China
Reproductive Medicine Center, The First Affiliated Hospital of Wenzhou Medical University, Wenzhou 325000, China

Fang-Fang Wang, Ning-Ning Hou, Fan Qu, Qing Meng and Jian Xu
The Key Laboratory of Reproductive Genetics, Ministry of Education (Zhejiang University), Hangzhou, Zhejiang 310006, China

Jian-Zhong Sheng
The Key Laboratory of Reproductive Genetics, Ministry of Education (Zhejiang University), Hangzhou, Zhejiang 310006, China
Department of Pathology and Pathophysiology, School of Medicine, Zhejiang University, Hangzhou 310058, China

Maxwell V. Meng and Sima P. Porten
Department of Urology, University of California, Mail code 1695, 550 16th Street, 6th Floor, San Francisco, CA 94143, USA

Thomas Sanford, Reema Railkar and Piyush K. Agarwal
Urologic Oncology Branch, Center for Cancer Research, National Cancer Institute, Building 10—Hatfield CRC, Room 2-5952, Bethesda, MD 20892-1210, USA

Alexander Beck, Franziska Trippel, Alexandra Wagner, Saskia Joppien, Dietrich von Schweinitz and Roland Kappler
Department of Pediatric Surgery, Dr. von Hauner Children's Hospital, Ludwig-Maximilians-University Munich, Lindwurmstr. 2a, 80337 Munich, Germany

Gernot Längst and Max Felle
Department of Biochemistry III, University Regensburg, Regensburg, Germany

Christian Vokuhl
Institute of Paidopathology, Pediatric Tumor Registry, Christian-Albrecht's-University Kiel, Kiel, Germany

Thomas Schwarzmayr and Tim M. Strom
Institute of Human Genetics, Helmholtz Zentrum München, Neuherberg, Germany
Institute of Human Genetics, Technische Universität München, Munich, Germany

Alexander S. Hölscher, Wolfgang A. Schulz, Maria Pinkerneil, Günter Niegisch and Michèle J. Hoffmann
Department of Urology, Medical Faculty, Heinrich-Heine-University, Duesseldorf, Moorenstr. 5, 40225 Duesseldorf, Germany

Inês Graça, David Bidarra, Eva Pereira-Silva and Sofia Salta
Cancer Biology & Epigenetics Group - Research Center (CI-IPOP), Portuguese Oncology Institute of Porto (IPO Porto), F Bdg, 1st floor, Rua Dr António Bernardino de Almeida, 4200-072 Porto, Portugal

João Ramalho-Carvalho
Cancer Biology & Epigenetics Group - Research Center (CI-IPOP), Portuguese Oncology Institute of Porto (IPO Porto), F Bdg, 1st floor, Rua Dr António Bernardino de Almeida, 4200-072 Porto, Portugal
Cancer Epigenetics and Biology Program, Bellvitge Biomedical Research Institute, Barcelona, Catalonia, Spain
Biomedical Sciences Graduate Program, Institute of Biomedical Sciences Abel Salazar- University of Porto (ICBAS-UP), Porto, Portugal
Division of Oncogenomics, Netherlands Cancer Institute, Plesmanlaan 121, 1066 CX Amsterdam, the Netherlands

Céline S. Gonçalves and Bruno M. Costa
Life and Health Sciences Research Institute (ICVS), School of Medicine, University of Minho, Campus de Gualtar, Braga, Portugal
ICVS/3B's- PT Government Associate Laboratory, Braga/Guimarães, University of Minho, Campus de Gualtar, Braga, Portugal

Maria Inês Godinho
Department of Immunology, Portuguese Oncology Institute of Porto, Porto, Portugal

Manel Esteller
Cancer Epigenetics and Biology Program, Bellvitge Biomedical Research Institute, Barcelona, Catalonia, Spain
Institucio Catalana de Recerca i Estudis Avançats (ICREA), Barcelona, Catalonia, Spain
Physiological Sciences Department, School of Medicine and Health Sciences, University of Barcelona (UB), Barcelona, Catalonia, Spain

Antonio Gomez
Cancer Epigenetics and Biology Program, Bellvitge Biomedical Research Institute, Barcelona, Catalonia, Spain
Gene Regulation, Stem Cells and Cancer Programme, Centre for Genomic Regulation (CRG), The Barcelona Institute of Science and Technology, Barcelona, Spain

Rui Henrique
Cancer Biology & Epigenetics Group - Research Center (CI-IPOP), Portuguese Oncology Institute of Porto (IPO Porto), F Bdg, 1st floor, Rua Dr António Bernardino de Almeida, 4200-072 Porto, Portugal
Department of Pathology, Portuguese Oncology Institute of Porto, Porto, Portugal
Department of Pathology and Molecular Immunology, Institute of Biomedical Sciences Abel Salazar- University of Porto (ICBAS-UP), Porto, Portugal

Carmen Jerónimo
Cancer Biology & Epigenetics Group - Research Center (CI-IPOP), Portuguese Oncology Institute of Porto (IPO Porto), F Bdg, 1st floor, Rua Dr António Bernardino de Almeida, 4200-072 Porto, Portugal
Department of Pathology and Molecular Immunology, Institute of Biomedical Sciences Abel Salazar- University of Porto (ICBAS-UP), Porto, Portugal

Yimin Zhu and Xiaohui Sun
Department of Epidemiology and Biostatistics, School of Public Health, Zhejiang University, Hangzhou 310058, China

Meiyan Li
BGI-Shenzhen, Shenzhen 518083, China

Hanlin Lu and Fei Gao
BGI-Shenzhen, Shenzhen 518083, China
Agricultural Genomics Institute at Shenzhen, Chinese Academy of Agricultural Sciences, Shenzhen 518120, China

Ledong Wan, Dan Yu, Yiping Tian and Dandan Zhang
Key Laboratory of Disease Proteomics of Zhejiang Province and Department of Pathology, School of Medicine, Zhejiang University, Hangzhou 310058, China

Maode Lai
Key Laboratory of Disease Proteomics of Zhejiang Province and Department of Pathology, School of Medicine, Zhejiang University, Hangzhou 310058, China
Department of Pathology, School of Medicine, Zhejiang University, 866 Yuhangtang Road, Zhejiang, Hangzhou 310058, China

Hongchuan Jin
Laboratory of Cancer Biology, Provincial Key Lab of Biotherapy in Zhejiang, Sir Runrun Shaw Hospital, Medical School of Zhejiang University, Hangzhou, China

Aifen Lin
Human Tissue Bank/Medical Research Center, Taizhou Hospital of Zhejiang Province, Wenzhou Medical University, Linhai, Zhejiang 317000, China

Marguerite R. Irvin, Stella Aslibekyan, Anh Do and Bertha Hidalgo
Department of Epidemiology, University of Alabama at Birmingham, 1665 University Blvd, RPHB 230J, Birmingham, AL 35294, USA

Degui Zhi
School of Biomedical Informatics, University of Texas Health Science Center at Houston, Houston, TX, USA

Steven A. Claas and Donna K. Arnett
College of Public Health, University of Kentucky, Lexington, KY, USA

Vinodh Srinivasasainagendra and Hemant K. Tiwari
Department of Biostatistics, University of Alabama at Birmingham, Birmingham, AL, USA

Steve Horvath
Human Genetics, David Geffen School of Medicine, University of California Los Angeles, Los Angeles, CA 90095, USA
Biostatistics, School of Public Health, University of California Los Angeles, Los Angeles, CA 90095, USA
Human Genetics, Gonda Research Center, David Geffen School of Medicine, University of California Los Angeles, Los Angeles, CA 90095-7088, USA

Devin M. Absher
HudsonAlpha Institute for Biotechnology, Huntsville, AL, USA

Jolein Mijnes, Nadine T. Gaisa, Eduard Burghardt, Sonja Gostek and Ruth Knüchel
Institute of Pathology, RWTH Aachen University, Pauwelsstr. 30, 52074 Aachen, Germany

Tim C. de Ruijter
Division of Medical Oncology, Maastricht University Medical Centre, Maastricht, The Netherlands
GROW—School for Oncology and Developmental Biology, Maastricht University Medical Centre, Maastricht, The Netherlands

Edgar Dahl and Michael Rose
Institute of Pathology, RWTH Aachen University, Pauwelsstr. 30, 52074 Aachen, Germany
RWTH Centralized Biomaterial Bank (RWTH cBMB), Medical Faculty, RWTH Aachen University, Aachen, Germany

David Pfister
Department of Urology, RWTH Aachen University, Aachen, Germany
Department of Urology, Uro-Oncology, Robot Assisted and Reconstructive Urologic Surgery, University Hospital Cologne, Cologne, Germany

Sebastian C. Schmid
Department of Urology, Klinikum rechts der Isar, Technical University Munich, Munich, Germany

Jürgen Veeck
Institute of Pathology, RWTH Aachen University, Pauwelsstr. 30, 52074 Aachen, Germany
Division of Medical Oncology, Maastricht University Medical Centre, Maastricht, The Netherlands
GROW—School for Oncology and Developmental Biology, Maastricht University Medical Centre, Maastricht, The Netherlands
RWTH Centralized Biomaterial Bank (RWTH cBMB), Medical Faculty, RWTH Aachen University, Aachen, Germany

Mary Prunicki, Xiaoying Zhou and Tara Paglino
Sean N. Parker Center for Allergy and Asthma Research at Stanford University, Stanford, CA 94305, USA
Department of Medicine, Stanford University, Stanford, CA 94305, USA

Deendayal Dinakarpandian
Department of Medicine, Stanford University, Stanford, CA 94305, USA
Center for Biomedical Informatics Research, Stanford University, Stanford, CA 94305, USA

Laurel Stell
Department of Biomedical Data Science, Stanford University, Stanford, CA 94305, USA

Mariangels de Planell-Saguer and Rachel L. Miller
Department of Medicine, Columbia University, New York, NY 10032, USA

Chiara Sabatti
Department of Biomedical Data Science, Stanford University, Stanford, CA 94305, USA
Department of Statistics, Stanford University, Stanford, CA 94305, USA

Richard W. Lucas
Southwest Environmental Institute, Phoenix, AZ 85087, USA

S. Katharine Hammond
School of Public Health, University of California, Berkeley, Berkeley, CA 94720, USA

John R. Balmes
School of Public Health, University of California, Berkeley, Berkeley, CA 94720, USA
Department of Medicine, University of California, San Francisco, San Francisco, CA 94143, USA

Kari C. Nadeau
Sean N. Parker Center for Allergy and Asthma Research at Stanford University, Stanford, CA 94305, USA
Department of Medicine, Stanford University, Stanford, CA 94305, USA
Division of Pulmonary and Critical Care Medicine, Department of Medicine, Stanford University, Stanford University School of Medicine, 269 Campus Drive, CCSR 3215, MC 5366, Stanford, CA 94305-5101, USA

Huijuan Zhang and Weiwei Cheng
International Peace Maternity and Child Health Hospital, Shanghai Jiao Tong University School of Medicine, No. 910. Hengshan Road, Xuhui District, Shanghai 200030, China

Xiaopeng Hu and Ji Wu
International Peace Maternity and Child Health Hospital, Shanghai Jiao Tong University School of Medicine, No. 910. Hengshan Road, Xuhui District, Shanghai 200030, China
Bio-X Institutes, Shanghai Jiao Tong University, No. 800. Dongchuan Road, Minhang District, Shanghai 200240, China
Key Laboratory of Fertility Preservation and Maintenance of Ministry of Education, Ningxia Medical University, Yinchuan 750004, China

Xinyue Li
Bio-X Institutes, Shanghai Jiao Tong University, No. 800. Dongchuan Road, Minhang District, Shanghai 200240, China

Junping Ao
State Key Laboratory of Oncogenes and Related Genes, Shanghai Cancer Institute, Renji Hospital, Shanghai Jiao Tong University School of Medicine, Shanghai 200032, China

Francesca Marta Elli
Endocrinology Unit, Department of Clinical Sciences and Community Health, University of Milan, Via Francesco Sforza, 35-20122 Milan, Italy

Paolo Bordogna
Endocrinology and Metabolic Diseases Unit, Fondazione IRCCS Ca' Granda Ospedale Maggiore Policlinico, Milan, Italy

Maura Arosio, Anna Spada and Giovanna Mantovani
Endocrinology Unit, Department of Clinical Sciences and Community
Health, University of Milan, Via Francesco Sforza, 35-20122 Milan, Italy
Endocrinology and Metabolic Diseases Unit, Fondazione IRCCS Ca' Granda Ospedale Maggiore Policlinico, Milan, Italy

Xiaoling Wang, Yue Pan, Haidong Zhu, Guang Hao, Yisong Huang, Vernon Barnes, Yanbin Dong and Shaoyong Su
Department of Pediatrics, Georgia Prevention Institute, Medical College of Georgia, Augusta University, HS-1640, Augusta, GA 30912, USA

Huidong Shi
Cancer Center, Augusta University, Augusta, GA, USA

Harold Snieder
Department of Epidemiology, University of Groningen, University Medical Center Groningen, Groningen, the Netherlands

James Pankow, Weihua Guan and Ellen Demerath
Division of Epidemiology and Community Health, School of Public Health, University of Minnesota, Minneapolis, MN 55454, USA

Kari North
Department of Epidemiology, University of North Carolina at Chapel Hill, Chapel Hill, NC 27514, USA

Megan Grove
Human Genetics Center, School of Public Health, University of Texas Health Sciences Center at Houston, Houston, TX 77030, USA

Lexie Prokopuk, Kirsten Hogg and Patrick S. Western
Centre for Reproductive Health, Hudson Institute of Medical Research, Clayton, Victoria 3168, Australia
Department of Molecular and Translational Science, Monash University, Clayton, Victoria 3168, Australia

Mercè Mateu-Jimenez, Víctor Curull, Albert Sánchez-Font, Joaquim Gea and Esther Barreiro
Pulmonology Department, Lung Cancer and Muscle Research Group, Hospital del Mar-IMIM, Parc de Salut Mar, Health and Experimental Sciences Department (CEXS), Universitat Pompeu Fabra (UPF), Parc de Recerca Biomèdica de Barcelona (PRBB), C/ Dr. Aiguader, 88, E-08003 Barcelona, Spain
Centro de Investigación en Red de Enfermedades Respiratorias (CIBERES), Instituto de Salud Carlos III (ISCIII), Barcelona, Spain

Alberto Rodríguez-Fuster and Rafael Aguiló
Thoracic Surgery Department, Hospital del Mar-IMIM, Parc de Salut Mar, Barcelona, Spain

Lara Pijuan
Pathology Department, Hospital del Mar-IMIM, Parc de Salut Mar, Barcelona, Spain

Andrew J. Simpkin, Linda M. O'Keeffe, Kaitlin H. Wade, Lotte C. Houtepen, Caroline L. Relton, Matthew Suderman and Laura D. Howe
MRC Integrative Epidemiology Unit at the University of Bristol, Bristol, England
Population Health Sciences, Bristol Medical School, University of Bristol, Bristol, England

Jasmine N. Khouja
MRC Integrative Epidemiology Unit at the University of Bristol, Bristol, England
Population Health Sciences, Bristol Medical School, University of Bristol, Bristol, England
School of Experimental Psychology at the University of Bristol, Bristol, England

Daniel L. McCartney
Centre for Genomic and Experimental Medicine, Institute of Genetics and Molecular Medicine, University of Edinburgh, Edinburgh, UK

Sarah E. Harris and Riccardo E. Marioni
Centre for Genomic and Experimental Medicine, Institute of Genetics and
Molecular Medicine, University of Edinburgh, Edinburgh, UK
Centre for Cognitive Ageing and Cognitive Epidemiology, University of Edinburgh, Edinburgh, UK

Adele M. Taylor and Paul Redmond
Department for Psychology, University of Edinburgh, Edinburgh, UK

Ian J. Deary
Centre for Cognitive Ageing and Cognitive Epidemiology, University of Edinburgh, Edinburgh, UK
Department for Psychology, University of Edinburgh, Edinburgh, UK

John M. Starr
Centre for Cognitive Ageing and Cognitive Epidemiology, University of Edinburgh, Edinburgh, UK
Alzheimer Scotland Dementia Research Centre, University of Edinburgh, Edinburgh, UK

Andrew M. McIntosh
Centre for Cognitive Ageing and Cognitive Epidemiology, University of Edinburgh, Edinburgh, UK
Division of Psychiatry, Centre for Clinical Brain Sciences, University of Edinburgh, Edinburgh, UK

Qian Zhang, Allan F. McRae and Naomi R. Wray
Institute for Molecular Bioscience, University of Queensland, Brisbane, Queensland, Australia

Tara L. Spires-Jones and Barry W. McColl
UK Dementia Research Institute, Edinburgh Medical School, University of Edinburgh, Edinburgh, UK
Centre for Discovery Brain Sciences, University of Edinburgh, Edinburgh, UK

Anna J. Stevenson
Centre for Genomic and Experimental Medicine, Institute of Genetics and Molecular Medicine, University of Edinburgh, Edinburgh, UK
UK Dementia Research Institute, Edinburgh Medical School, University of Edinburgh, Edinburgh, UK
Centre for Discovery Brain Sciences, University of Edinburgh, Edinburgh, UK

Adeline Divoux and Steven R. Smith
Translational Research Institute for Metabolism and Diabetes, Florida Hospital, 301 E. Princeton Street, Orlando, FL 32804, USA
Diabetes and Obesity Research Center, Sanford Burnham Prebys Medical Discovery Institute at Lake Nona, Orlando, FL, USA

Katalin Sandor and Timothy F. Osborne
Diabetes and Obesity Research Center, Sanford Burnham Prebys Medical Discovery Institute at Lake Nona, Orlando, FL, USA
Department of Medicine, Johns Hopkins All Children's Hospital, Johns Hopkins University School of Medicine, St. Petersburg, FL 33701, USA

Balint L. Balint and Dora Bojcsuk
Genomic Medicine and Bioinformatic Core Facility, Department of Biochemistry and Molecular Biology, Faculty of Medicine, University of Debrecen, Nagyerdei krt 98, Debrecen 4032, Hungary

Amlan Talukder
Department of Computer Science, University of Central Florida, 4000 Central Florida Blvd, Orlando 32816, USA

Xiaoman Li
Burnett School of Biomedical Sciences, College of Medicine, University of Central Florida, 6900 Lake Nona Boulevard, Orlando, FL, USA

Index

www.ingramcontent.com/pod-product-compliance
Lightning Source LLC
LaVergne TN
LVHW080914210926
848485LV00004B/652
* 9 7 8 1 6 3 9 2 7 2 5 5 6 *